EXTRACORPOREAL LIFE SUPPORT

EXTRACORPOREAL LIFE SUPPORT

Robert M. Arensman, M.D.
Professor of Surgery and Pediatrics
The University of Chicago
Surgeon-in-Chief
Wyler Children's Hospital
Chicago, Illinois

J. Devn Cornish, M.D.
Associate Professor of Pediatrics
Emory University School of Medicine
Director, Egleston Children's ECMO Center
Atlanta, Georgia

Boston
BLACKWELL SCIENTIFIC PUBLICATIONS

Oxford   London   Edinburgh   Melbourne   Paris   Berlin   Vienna

BLACKWELL SCIENTIFIC PUBLICATIONS
Editorial offices:
238 Main Street, Cambridge, Massachusetts 02142, USA
Osney Mead, Oxford OX2 0EL, England
25 John Street, London WC1N 2BL, England
23 Ainslie Place, Edinburgh EH3 6AJ, Scotland
54 University Street, Carlton, Victoria 3053, Australia
Arnette SA, 2 rue Casimir-Delavigne, 75006 Paris, France
Blackwell-Wissenschaft, Meinekestrasse 4, D-1000 Berlin 15, Germany
Blackwell MZV, Feldgasse 13, A-1238 Vienna, Austria

Distributors:
USA
  Blackwell Scientific Publications
  238 Main Street
  Cambridge, MA 02142
  (Telephone orders: 800-759-6102 or 617-876-7000)
Canada
  Times Mirror Professional Publishing
  130 Flaska Drive
  Markham, Ontario L6G 1B8
  (Telephone orders: 800-268-4178 or 416-470-6739)
Australia
  Blackwell Scientific Publications (Australia) Pty Ltd
  54 University Street
  Carlton, Victoria 3053
  (Telephone orders: 03-347-0300)
Outside North America and Australia:
  Blackwell Scientific Publications, Ltd.
  c/o Marston Book Services, Ltd.
  P.O. Box 87
  Oxford OX2 0DT
  England
  (Telephone orders: 44-865-791155)

Typeset by Huron Valley Graphics
Printed and bound by Hamilton Printing Company
© 1993 by Blackwell Scientific Publications
Printed in the United States of America
93 94 95 96 5 4 3 2 1

All rights reserved. No part of this book may be reproduced in any form or by any electronic or mechanical means, including information storage and retrieval systems, without permission in writing from the publisher, except by a reviewer who may quote brief passages in a review.

Library of Congress Cataloging in Publication Data

Extracorporeal life support / edited by Robert M. Arensman, J. Devn Cornish.
    p.   cm.
  Includes bibliographical references and index.
  ISBN 0-86542-197-8
  1. Extracorporeal membrane oxygenation. 2. Respiratory therapy for newborn infants. I. Arensman, Robert M. II. Cornish, J. Devn.
   [DNLM: 1. Extracorporeal Membrane Oxygenation. WG 188 E978]
  RJ312.E95   1993
  618.B2'01—dc20
  DNLM/DLC
  for Library of Congress   92-48685
                                                       CIP

Dedicated to

Robert E. Gross, whose vision made pediatric cardiac surgery and cardiopulmonary bypass a reality

Robert H. Bartlett, whose questioning mind has extended greatly the use of cardiopulmonary bypass and our understanding of pulmonary failure in children

Esperanza, whose name and life continue to inspire hope in all who are interested in the field of extracorporeal life support

Contents

❖

Contributors   xi

Foreword   xv

Preface   xvii

1. An Introduction to Extracorporeal Membrane Oxygenation   1
   J. Devn Cornish and Robert M. Arensman

2. History of the Development of Extracorporeal Circulation   9
   C. Walton Lillehei

3. The Development of Prolonged Extracorporeal Circulation   31
   Robert H. Bartlett

4. Clinical Studies of Neonatal ECMO   42
   P. Pearl O'Rourke

5. Optimizing Conventional Respiratory Support   51
   Jen-Tien Wung and L. Stanley James

6. Alternative Therapies for Respiratory Failure   68
   J. Devn Cornish and Reese H. Clark

7. Physiology of Extracorporeal Life Support   89
   Robert H. Bartlett and Robert E. Cilley

8.	Interactions of Blood and Artificial Surfaces: In Search of "Heparin-free" Cardiopulmonary Bypass *Robert C. Eberhart*	105
9.	Cardiac Changes During Prolonged Extracorporeal Membrane Oxygenation *Gerard R. Martin*	126
10.	ECMO and the Brain *Christine A. Gleason*	138
11.	Pre-ECMO Considerations for Neonatal Patients *Billie L. Short*	156
12.	Vascular Access for Extracorporeal Life Support *Steven L. Moulton, Ralph E. Delius, and Robert M. Arensman*	175
13.	Clinical Management of the Neonatal ECMO Patient *Billie L. Short*	195
14.	Emergencies During Extracorporeal Membrane Oxygenation and Their Management *Joseph B. Zwischenberger and Charles S. Cox, Jr.*	207
15.	Risks of Neonatal ECMO *R. E. Schumacher*	226
16.	Patient Neurodevelopmental Outcomes after Neonatal ECMO *Penny Glass*	241
17.	Management of Infants with Congenital Diaphragmatic Hernia Using ECMO *Charles J.H. Stolar, Mitchell R. Price, Marilyn W. Butler, and Eric L. Lazar*	252
18.	Venovenous ECMO *Martin Keszler and Theodor Kolobow*	262
19.	Extracorporeal Life Support in Children *Robert M. Arensman and Vincent R. Adolph*	274
20.	Extracorporeal Respiratory Support in Patients with Adult Respiratory Distress Syndrome *Eckhard Müller*	286
21.	Extracorporeal Membrane Oxygenation for Cardiac Disease *Michael D. Klein and Grant C. Whittlesey*	302

22.	ECMO as a Tool for Physiologic Research *Carlos E. Blanco*	320
23.	The Economics of ECMO *Billie L. Short and Gail D. Pearson*	331
24.	Prospects for the Future *Robert H. Bartlett*	337
	Appendix 1: Cannula Specifications *Steven L. Moulton*	345
	Appendix 2: Venovenous Extracorporeal Membrane Oxygenation in Neonates Using the Double-Lumen Catheter *Robert H. Bartlett*	351

Index   355

Contributors

Vincent R. Adolph, M.D.
Pediatric Surgery Fellow, Montreal Children's Hospital, Montreal, Canada

Robert M. Arensman, M.D.
Professor of Surgery and Pediatrics, The University of Chicago; Surgeon-in-Chief, Wyler Children's Hospital; Chicago, Illinois

Robert H. Bartlett, M.D.
Professor of Surgery, University of Michigan, Ann Arbor, Michigan

Carlos E. Blanco, M.D., PH.D.
Professor in Pediatrics/Director of Neonatology, Academic Hospital Maastricht, Maastricht, The Netherlands

Marilyn W. Butler, M.D.
General Surgery Resident, Presbyterian Hospital, New York, New York

Robert E. Cilley, M.D.
Assistant Professor of Surgery and Pediatrics, Pennsylvania State University, Milton S. Hershey Medical Center, Hershey, Pennsylvania

Reese H. Clark, M.D.
Assistant Professor of Pediatrics, Emory University School of Medicine, Atlanta, Georgia

J. Devn Cornish, M.D.
Associate Professor of Pediatrics, Emory University School of Medicine; Director, Egleston Children's ECMO Center; Atlanta, Georgia

Charles S. Cox, Jr., M.D.
Fellow in Cardiothoracic Surgery, John Sealey Hospital, Galveston, Texas

Ralph E. Delius, M.D.
ECMO Fellow, University of Michigan Medical Center, Ann Arbor, Michigan

Robert C. Eberhart, PH.D.
Professor and Chairman, Joint Program in Biomedical Engineering, University of Texas Southwestern Medical Center at Dallas, University of Texas at Arlington, Dallas, Texas

Penny Glass, PH.D.
Director, ECMO Follow-up; Associate Professor of Pediatrics, Center for Child Development, Children's National Medical Center, Washington, DC

Christine A. Gleason, M.D.
Associate Professor, Pediatrics; Director, Division of Neonatology; Johns Hopkins University School of Medicine, Baltimore, Maryland

L. Stanley James, M.D.
Professor of Pediatrics and Obstetrics and Gynecology; Director, Division of Perinatal Medicine; Department of Pediatrics, Columbia University, College of Physicians and Surgeons, New York, New York

Martin Keszler, M.D.
Associate Professor of Pediatrics, Director of ECMO Program, Georgetown University Medical Center, Washington, DC

Michael D. Klein, M.D.
Chief, Pediatric General Surgery, Children's Hospital of Michigan; Professor of Surgery, Wayne State University School of Medicine; Detroit, Michigan

Theodor Kolobow, M.D.
Chief, Section on Pulmonary and Cardiac Assist Devices, LCB, National Heart Lung and Blood Institute, National Institutes of Health, Bethesda, Maryland

Eric L. Lazar, M.D.
Research Fellow, Pediatric Surgery, The Babies' Hospital, College of Physicians and Surgeons, Columbia-Presbyterian Medical Center; Resident in Surgery, New York University Medical Center; New York, New York

C. Walton Lillehei, PH.D., M.D.
Professor of Surgery, University of Minnesota Medical Center, Minneapolis, Minnesota

Gerard R. Martin, M.D.
Associate Professor of Pediatrics, The George Washington University Medical Center; Director of Echocardiography, Children's National Medical Center; Washington, DC

Steven L. Moulton, M.D.
Chief Surgical Resident, University of California, San Diego, California

Eckhard Müller, M.D.
Department of Anesthesiology and Intensive Care Therapy, Philipps-University Hospital, Marburg, Germany

P. Pearl O'Rourke, M.D.
Associate Professor of Pediatric Anesthesia, University of Washington School of Medicine; Director, Pediatric ICU; Co-Director, ECMO Program; Children's Hospital, Seattle, Washington

Gail D. Pearson, M.D., SC.D.
Resident in Pediatrics, Children's National Medical Center, Washington, DC

Mitchell R. Price, M.D.
Department of Surgery, New York University Medical Center, New York, New York

Robert E. Schumacher, M.D.
Associate Professor of Pediatrics, Section of Newborn Services, University of Michigan Medical Center, Ann Arbor, Michigan

Billie Lou Short, M.D.
Professor of Pediatrics, The George Washington University School of Medicine; Director, ECMO Program, The Children's National Medical Center; Washington, DC

Charles J.H. Stolar, M.D.
Associate Professor, Department of Surgery, Division of Pediatric Surgery, Columbia University College of Physicians and Surgeons, New York, New York

Grant C. Whittlesey, C.C.P.
Children's Hospital of Michigan, Detroit, Michigan

Jen-Tien Wung, M.D.
Professor of Clinical Anesthesiology/Pediatrics, Columbia University College of Physicians and Surgeons; Attending Anesthesiologist, Columbia-Presbyterian Medical Center; New York, New York

Joseph B. Zwischenberger, M.D.
Associate Professor of Cardiothoracic Surgery; Director, ECMO Program; The University of Texas Medical Branch at Galveston, Galveston, Texas

Foreword

ECMO, the acronym for long-term extracorporeal membrane oxygenation, carries a crisp, definitive ring that mirrors the exciting new technology it labels. Complete, effective rest for temporarily deranged lungs has been dreamed about since surgeons first laid a scalpel on a patient's chest. The advent of extracorporeal oxygenation in 1953 followed two decades of investigation spearheaded by and first brought to success on a human patient by John H. Gibbon, Jr. The subsequent step-by-step development of this technical revolution in cardiac surgery is recorded here in the chapter by C. Walton Lillehei, a major player in the events. It remained for Robert H. Bartlett to synthesize all the foregoing work and bring to fruition an extension of extracorporeal oxygenation using a functioning heart to offer immature lungs the luxury of two or three weeks to gain or regain their ability to oxygenate a patient's blood.

As a surgical houseofficer in Boston, Bob Bartlett was strongly influenced by the surgical research accomplishments of Francis D. Moore and Robert E. Gross. His wife, Wanda, supplemented the then meager salary of a surgical resident by signing on to handwash, dry, and reassemble Dr. Gross's pump oxygenator at the Boston Children's Hospital. This association led to several dinner visits for the young couple at Four Winds, Dr. Gross's home in Framingham. There, junior resident Bartlett learned about the success and limitation of the disc-oxygenator then in use for the repair of children's heart deformities. At that time, in the early 1960s, extended pump use of more than several hours ended in failure due to the destruction of red cells and other elements of the blood. Even the far-thinking Dr. Gross discouraged his young guest's questions about possible long-term pump runs for lung recovery.

As Dr. Bartlett describes in the chapter entitled "The Development of Prolonged Extracorporeal Circulation", Kolff (the father of renal dialysis), Kolobow, Bramson, Clowes, and others each independently began to experiment with the new substance silicone for building membrane oxygenators. This new methodology permitted a gentler, less destructive, more physiologic oxygenation of blood. Yet it took daily painstaking work for more than a decade to bring forward for clinical use a system of extracorporeal oxygenation that could be successfully sustained for one, then two, then three weeks. As Gibbon was the unflagging leader for the two decades it took to consummate the development of the pump oxygenator for open heart surgery, so has Bartlett been the indefatigable champion of long-term extracorporeal circulation for recoverable lungs.

This timely volume embraces all features of this signal advance in pulmonary therapeutics. Heretofore restricted to special newborn centers, prolonged lung rest provided by ECMO must become available to every neonate who can be saved. As Bartlett and other investigators extend the methodology to older subjects and to a wider range of clinical indications, the existing state of this art, so well described in the following pages, must be made available in all total-care facilities. Cornish and Arensman bring their extensive experience in all phases of ECMO to fashion a masterful compendium of all current information on prolonged extracorporeal membrane oxygenation. This volume stands as a gift to those currently toiling in this vineyard and to those who should and must guarantee that this technology reaches all needy patients everywhere.

Judson G. Randolph, M.D.
Nashville, Tennessee

Preface

The technological revolution has transformed American hospitals. Critical care units now rival the command module of a spaceship for complexity of technological devices. Even general medical/surgical units have become extensions of the intensive care units and employ a wide variety of advanced monitoring devices. Nowhere has this explosion of technology been more dramatic than in extracorporeal life support (ECLS). The cardiopulmonary bypass pump, once considered extraordinarily complex and difficult to run and monitor, has passed beyond the operating room doors and become an integral part of the therapeutic interventions for patients with pulmonary failure.

In this book, Centers throughout the world report their experience with ECLS over the past two decades. This text traces some of the major developments in extracorporeal life support, reviews basic physiology, reports on the establishment or organization of an ECMO team, reviews general principles of ECLS initiation, discusses patient management during and after ECLS, and then reviews the major current indications for ECLS in neonates, older children, and adults.

In a field of therapeutic intervention that is changing so often and so dramatically, this text should be considered a primer to create familiarity with basic concepts and techniques in the extracorporeal life support process. On behalf of the Communications Committee of the Extracorporeal Life Support Organization (ELSO), we thank all the authors who have worked so diligently on the preparation of this book.

Robert Arensman
University of Chicago
Chicago, Illinois

Devn Cornish
Emory University
Atlanta, Georgia

Notice

The indications and dosages of all drugs in this book have been recommended in the medical literature and conform to the practices of the general medical community. The medications described do not necessarily have specific approval by the Food and Drug Administration for use in the diseases and dosages for which they are recommended. The package insert for each drug should be consulted for use and dosage as approved by the FDA. Because standards of usage change, it is advisable to keep abreast of revised recommendations, particularly those concerning new drugs.

EXTRACORPOREAL LIFE SUPPORT

1

An Introduction to Extracorporeal Membrane Oxygenation

❖

J. Devn Cornish, M.D.
Robert M. Arensman, M.D.

WHAT IS ECMO?

ECMO is an acronym for extracorporeal membrane oxygenation. From early on, this term, as opposed to the more conventional "extracorporeal circulation," connoted not only perfusion support (i.e., "heart-lung bypass"), but the application of such support to neonates with life-threatening lung disease for periods of days to weeks. Long-term perfusion support of patients with acute cardiac and/or respiratory failure was attempted in the late 1960s and early 1970s by a number of surgical teams (1–5). The first successful outcome was reported in an adult patient by Hill and colleagues (6) in 1972. Bartlett and co-workers (7) reported the first neonatal survivor in 1975.

Subsequent favorable outcomes paved the way for a multicenter prospective controlled trial sponsored by the National Institutes of Health (NIH) which was summarized by Zapol and others (8) in 1979. Ninety patients in nine hospitals were admitted to the study, of whom 48 were treated with mechanical ventilation alone and 42 were treated with mechanical ventilation plus partial venovenous, venoarterial, or mixed bypass support. Ultimately, only three of the control patients and four of the ECMO patients survived. The implication of the study was obvious: ECMO did not work!

While that was the almost universal conclusion drawn from this study, that is not what the study showed. The entry criteria used were expected to identify patients with a 50% mortality risk related to their acute respiratory failure. As may be seen, the actual mortality approached 90% in both groups, independent of therapy. Subsequent data have reinforced the high mortality rate predicted by these criteria. In truth, all that may appropriately be concluded from the NIH controlled trial of ECMO is that neither therapy improved patient outcome. This is not equivalent to documenting that neither is capable of improving outcomes in patients with acute respiratory failure. Testing of that hypothesis would have to await the identification of a less severely affected patient population.

Much has happened since 1979. Bartlett's ability to demonstrate consistently favorable results in neonatal patients treated with ECMO (9–12) inspired others to adopt his technique. Soon series of survivors were reported by Hardesty and others (13), Krummel et al. (14), Kirkpatrick and colleagues (15), Loe et al. (16), and Short and co-workers (17). The largest published experience to date was drawn from the National Neonatal ECMO Registry (18). Survival in this group of 715 patients was 81%, a figure that has been matched or bettered in every semiannual Registry report to the present, with the number of included patients now in excess of 3,000. Improved ECMO technology has begun to be employed again to treat adults with life-threatening pulmonary failure. The encouraging reports of Gattinoni and colleagues (19–21) have been accompanied by similar results in other adult ECMO centers. As a consequence, ECMO is now offered for neonatal patients at 62 centers worldwide, with adult ECMO available in a few more.

ECMO, as it is currently practiced, differs from the heart-lung bypass used in the operating room in several important ways. It requires only cervical rather than intrathoracic cannulation which can be performed under local rather than general anesthesia. It is continued not for one to four hours, as during cardiac surgery, but for periods generally ranging from three to ten days. Also, the purpose of the procedure is not to provide support during the surgical repair of a cardiac lesion but rather to "buy time" during which the healing process may occur. In all patients at present, ECMO requires systemic heparinization, and in neonates it involves the cannulation and permanent ligation of both the right common carotid artery and the right internal jugular vein. Consequently, recourse to ECMO in any particular case is reserved as a last resort.

The substantial success that has been experienced in applying ECMO to the support of neonates with cardiac and/or respiratory failure is attributable in large measure to the ability of Bartlett and other pioneers to define a population for whom the benefits of the technique were likely to be greater than its risks. Thus, neonates of less than 34 weeks' gestation are generally excluded since their immature cerebral vascular structure is felt to render the risk of dying from an intracranial hemorrhage after systemic heparinization approximately the same as the risk of dying from the underlying heart or lung disease. Neonates with long-established fibrotic and scarring lung disease are also excluded since it is unlikely that a period of 5–14 days on ECMO would produce sufficient healing to change the patient's ultimate prognosis. Using this kind of reasoning, a set of broadly accepted entry criteria has been developed for neonatal ECMO patients (Table 1.1).

A problem that plagues such last-resort therapies for any disease is that even extreme measures are unlikely to succeed if implemented only very late in the course of the illness. Thus, a means is needed to identify those patients who are likely to die without ECMO well before they are in critical condi-

TABLE 1.1 Representative patient selection criteria for neonatal ECMO

1. Gestational age ≥34 weeks, birthweight at least 2.0 kg.
2. Pulmonary disease likely to be reversible within 1–2 weeks of support.
3. Absence of severe nonpulmonary disorders that might dictate ultimate prognosis (e.g., significant intracranial hemorrhage or intractable bleeding at any site, major malformation syndromes, major chromosomal anomalies, untreatable renal dysfunction, evidence of severe neurologic impairment).
4. Evidence of severe, refractory respiratory failure as indicated by
   a. "Oxygenation index" over 40 on three out of five postductal blood gases at least 30 minutes apart but not more than 60 minutes apart (oxygenation index defined as mean airway pressure × fractional inspired oxygen concentration × 100/postductal Pao_2). This is reported to correlate with an 80% mortality rate *or*
   b. $AaDo_2 = P_{atm} - 47 - Pao_2 - Pco_2 \cdot 610$ for 8 hours (80% mortality) >600 for 12 hours (100% mortality) *or*
   c. Severe, refractory respiratory failure with sudden decompensation (defined loosely as Pao_2 less than 40 mm Hg for 2 hours) unresponsive to maximal medical management.

tion. To this end, a number of statistical predictors of mortality risk have been developed for use in neonatal patients who meet the first three criteria listed. These are summarized under item 4 in Table 1.1. Initially, each of these indicators was proposed because it had been shown through retrospective chart review of patients at a given center (12,22,23) to predict a mortality rate of 80% or more. Various authors (24–29) have shown that one or several of these failed to identify a high mortality population under their management (i.e., that patients meeting a given indicator of severity did not experience the high mortality rate reported in one of the previous studies). They have utilized this lack of local validity in the predictors to support the contention that ECMO may not have been needed in the reported patient groups and that therefore ECMO may not be superior to conventional ventilator support for this population.

One may quite credibly argue that these criteria do not allow the assignment of a specific mortality risk to any given patient, since they were derived from retrospectively collected data and are influenced to a large extent by specific characteristics of the patient population and of management techniques at any given institution. Moreover, the validity of such predictors would be expected to erode with time as conventional medical therapy improves (27). However, one cannot argue that because a given predictor is not currently valid at one center it was never valid at the original reporting center. Moreover, one can not imply that the failure of a given criterion to predict a high mortality indicates that ECMO was not beneficial in the original report. Unfortunately, no set of mortality predictors is likely to apply over an extended period of time, since, even if they were derived from carefully controlled prospective studies, the nature of the intensive care environment in which they are applied continues to advance.

Selection criteria such as those summarized in Table 1.1 are at best only examples of the kind of predictors that may be used to identify candidate patients. To be meaningful, criteria must be derived and tested at each institution and must be reviewed frequently (30–32). What can be said for these criteria is that they have been successful at a number of centers, on an empirical basis, at identifying the population of neonates for whom ECMO should be considered.

HOW IS IT DONE?

The mechanics of ECMO are quite straightforward. The ECMO system consists essentially of a blood pump, a membrane oxygenator, a countercurrent heat exchanger to warm the blood, and a servo-control module. The blood pump is usually a simple roller pump, though some centers employ either a "constrained vortex" centrifugal pump or a pulsatile pump. The membrane lung used may be the traditional SciMed-Kolobow Silastic spiral coil design or one of the newer hollow fiber devices. The membrane accomplishes both carbon dioxide removal from and oxygen delivery to the blood. The heat exchanger rewarms the blood by exposing it through metal tubing to the heat of warmed water which is circulating in the opposite direction from the blood. A broad variety of control modules are currently in use, but all function by regulating pump speed so that the rate of gravity drainage of blood from the patient equals that of blood return to the patient.

Other devices may be added to the basic ECMO system. Some ECMO centers, such as ours, insert an arterial line filter in the circuit between the heat exhcanger and the arterial cannula to trap any air, thrombi, or particulate material. Pressure monitors are often placed before and after the membrane to monitor the pressure of the circulating blood and to identify increasing resistance in the artificial lung. Several different types of sensors have been applied to the blood path of ECMO circuits to measure the P_{O_2}, hemoglobin saturation, and other blood gas parameters in the circulating blood. A variety of other technologies are being introduced to make the system safer, simpler, and easier to use.

Conceptually, the procedure is also quite elementary. First, the ECMO system is primed with fresh banked blood, and the acid-base balance and blood gases in the prime are adjusted appropriately. Next, the tissues of the neck are anesthetized, or the infant is given a general anesthetic, and a catheter is inserted into the right internal jugular vein through a small incision in the neck. This catheter (usually 14 French in size) is advanced centrally to the level of the mid-right atrium. Through the same skin incision, the right common carotid artery is isolated and cannulated (commonly with an 8–12 French catheter) to the level of the aortic arch. The drainage and return lines of the ECMO system are then connected to the venous and arterial catheters, respectively, and pump flow is started. Blood flows by gravity from the patient to the control module which regulates pump speed, then onto the pump, then to the heat exchanger, and finally back to the patient. In simplistic terms, ECMO follows the old adage, "out goes the bad blood, in goes the good blood."

Although the plumbing of ECMO is quite simple, its clinical application is rather more complicated. A detailed description of the management of neonatal ECMO patients is contained in Chapter 11. In addition, several excellent summaries of technical methods and clinical management protocols have been prepared previously to which the interested reader may also refer (33–36).

WHAT ARE THE RESULTS?

Although it is conceivable that there are hospitals quietly offering ECMO support to neonates without either reporting their results or participating in national and international meetings on the subject, it is felt that the overwhelming majority of infants treated with this modality have been reported to the National Neonatal ECMO Registry which has been maintained at the University of Michigan under the direction of Dr. Robert H. Bartlett since 1980. At present, 62 ECMO centers have been identified to the Registry worldwide.

The Registry is now managed under the auspices of the Extracorporeal Life Support Organization, an international association of clinicians, researchers, inventors, and industry representatives formed to foster the development and application of long-term perfusion support technology. It is instructive to note the variations in survival by disease category as recorded by the Registry (37). These are summarized in Table 1.2. Also tabulated by the Registry are the patient and mechanical complications reported by participating centers. The more significant of these are summarized in Tables 1.3 and 1.4.

Obviously, the question as to whether and for whom ECMO improves survival can only be definitively addressed by a prospective, controlled clinical trial. Two such trials have been conducted in neonatal patients (38,39). These are reviewed in detail in Chapter 4 of this volume. Also, a new controlled trial among adult patients is in progress (40). The impact of ECMO on patient morbidity must be assessed through carefully conducted follow-up studies. Such studies are summarized in Chapter 14.

Much concern and considerable controversy

TABLE 1.2 Survival of neonatal ECMO patients by diagnosis

Diagnosis	Number	Survived	Percent
Meconium aspiration syndrome	1215	1121	92.3
Respiratory distress syndrome	474	390	82.3
Congenital diaphragmatic hernia	493	310	62.9
Sepsis	351	267	76.1
Persistent pulmonary hypertension	432	373	86.3
Pneumothorax	10	6	60.0
Cardiac	40	23	57.5
Other	68	57	83.8
Total	3083	2547	82.6

TABLE 1.3 Patient and mechanical complications associated with neonatal ECMO

Complication	Number affected	Survived	Percent survival
Intracranial hemorrhage (US)	403	207	51.4
Intracranial hemorrhage (CT)	87	73	83.9
Gastrointestinal hemorrhage	112	72	64.3
Bleeding at surgical site	319	214	67.1
Hemolysis	232	168	72.4
Other hemorrhagic complications	227	150	66.1
Brain death	57	3	5.3
Seizures	499	338	67.7
Jitteriness	113	97	85.8
Other neurological problems	101	67	66.3
Serum creatinine >3.0	51	23	45.1
Arrhythmia	92	60	65.2
Miscellaneous cardiovascular	330	232	70.3
Pneumothorax	150	102	68.0
Other pulmonary complications	134	84	62.7
Positive culture	147	100	68.0
White blood cell count <1500	41	24	58.5
Other infectious complications	31	22	71.0
Systemic hypertension	355	289	81.4

have centered on the question of ECMO-related complications, and properly so. The risks of neurological injury, including those associated with ligation of the right common carotid artery and the right internal jugular vein, have been discussed at length in the literature (41–51). The risk of bleeding during systemic heparinization is obviously increased (52,53). And the potential for a sudden and catastrophic mishap is not trivial (54). However, considering all of the available data in combination, ECMO would appear to add little to the risks associated with the underlying diseases when managed with conventional therapy. It is difficult to know the true risks of the procedure itself, since only the very sickest of term and near-term neonates are offered ECMO. Many of these have suffered substantial morbidity before ECMO is ever instituted. Hopefully, follow-up studies of patients from the few controlled trials will assist in answering this question. Nonetheless, it must be stated that, given the risks currently associated with neonatal ECMO, this procedure should not be offered to a patient unless there is no significant likelihood of survival using other less invasive and less risky therapies. This approach should prevail until the apparent risks can be clearly shown to have been reduced.

TABLE 1.4 Mechanical complications associated with neonatal ECMO

Complication	Number affected	Survived	Percent survival
Oxygenator failure	159	106	66.7
Tubing rupture	74	59	79.7
Pump failure	42	35	83.3
Heat exchanger malfunction	38	28	73.7
Cannula problems	219	165	75.3
Other mechanical complications	340	275	80.9

CONCLUSION

The development of perfusion support technology and its clinical applications is progressing rapidly. Much has been written about ideal selection criteria for candidate patients, the methodologies of the procedure, and its effects on patient outcomes. The increasing acceptance of this technology must be accompanied by improvements in its safety and ease of use.

REFERENCES

(1) Rashkind WJ, Freeman A, Klein D, Toft RW. Evaluation of a disposable plastic low volume, pumpless oxygenator as a lung substitute. J Ped 1965;66:94–102.

(2) Dorson WJ, Baker E, Cohen ML, et al. A perfusion system for infants. Trans Am Soc Artif Intern Organs 1969;15:155.

(3) White JJ, Andrews HG, Risemberg H, Mazur D, Haller JA Jr. Prolonged respiratory support in newborn infants with a membrane oxygenator. Surgery 1971;70:288–96.

(4) Pyle RB, Helton WC, Johnson FW, et al. Clinical use of the membrane oxygenator. Am Surg 1975;110:966–70.

(5) Bartlett RH, Gazzaniga AB, Fong SW, Burns NE. Prolonged extracorporeal cardiopulmonary support in man. J Thorac Cardiovasc Surg 1974;68:918.

(6) Hill JD, O'Brien TG, Murray JJ, et al. Prolonged extracorporeal oxygenation for acute post-traumatic respiratory failure (shock-lung syndrome). Use of the Bramson Membrane Lung. N Engl J Med 1972;286:629–34.

(7) Bartlett RH, Gazzaniga AB, Jefferies MR, et al. Extracorporeal membrane oxygenation (ECMO) cardiopulmonary support in infancy. Trans Am Soc Artif Intern Organs 1976;22:80–93.

(8) Zapol WM, Snider MT, Hill DJ, et al. Extracorporeal membrane oxygenation in severe acute respiratory failure: a randomized prospective study. JAMA 1979;242:2193–6.

(9) Bartlett RH, Gazzaniga AB, Huxtable RF, Schippers HC, O'Connor JJ, Jeffries MR. Extracorporeal circulation (ECMO) in neonatal respiratory failure. J Thorac Cardiovasc Surg 1977;74:826–33.

(10) Bartlett RH, Andrews AF, Toomasian JM, Haiduc NJ, Gazzaniga AB. Extracorporeal membrane oxygenation for newborn respiratory failure: forty-five cases. Surgery 1982;92:425–33.

(11) Andrews AF, Roloff DN, Bartlett RH. Use of extracorporeal membrane oxygenation in persistent pulmonary hypertension of the newborn. Clin Perinatol 1984;11:729–35.

(12) Bartlett RH, Gazzaniga AB, Toomasian J, Corwin AG, Roloff D, Rucker R. Extracorporeal membrane oxygenation (ECMO) in neonatal respiratory failure. 100 cases. Ann Surg 1986;204:236–45.

(13) Hardesty RL, Griffith BP, Debski RF, Jeffries MR, Borovetz HS. Extracorporeal membrane oxygenation. Successful treatment of persistent fetal circulation following repair of congenital diaphragmatic hernia. J Thorac Cardiovasc Surg 1981;81:556–63.

(14) Krummel TM, Greenfield LJ, Kirkpatrick BV, Mueller DG, Ormazabal M, Salzberg AM. Clinical use of an extracorporeal membrane oxygenator in neonatal pulmonary failure. J Pediatr Surg 1982;17:525–31.

(15) Kirkpatrick BV, Krummel TM, Mueller DG, Ormazabal MA, Greenfield LJ, Salzberg AM. Use of extracorporeal membrane oxygenation for respiratory failure in term infants. Pediatrics 1983;72:872–6.

(16) Loe WA Jr, Graves ED III, Ochsner JL, Falterman KW, Arensman RM. Extracorporeal membrane oxygenation for newborn respiratory failure. J Pediatr Surg 1985;20:684–8.

(17) Short BL, Pearson GD. Neonatal extracorporeal membrane oxygenation: a review. J Intens Care Med 1986;1:47–54.

(18) Toomasian JM, Snedecor SM, Cornell RG, Cilley RE, Bartlett RH. National experience with extracorporeal membrane oxygenation for newborn respiratory failure: data from 715 cases. Trans Am Soc Artif Intern Organs 1988;34:140–7.

(19) Gattinoni L, Pesenti A, Kolobow T, Damia G. A new look at therapy of the adult respiratory distress syndrome: motionless lungs. Int Anaesth Clin 1983;21:97–117.

(20) Gattinoni L, Pesenti A, Mascheroni D, et al. Low-frequency positive-pressure ventilation with extracorporeal CO_2 removal in severe acute respiratory failure. JAMA 1986;256:881–910.

(21) Pesenti A, Gattinoni L, Kolobow T, Damia G. Extracorporeal circulation in adult respiratory failure. Trans Am Soc Artif Intern Organs 1988;34:43–7.

(22) Beck R, Anderson KD, Pearson GD, Cronin J, Miller MK, Short BL. Criteria for extracorporeal membrane oxygenation in a population of infants with persistent pulmonary hypertension of the newborn. J Pediatr Surg 1986;21:297–302.

(23) Krummel TM, Greenfield LJ, et al. Alveolar-arterial oxygen gradients versus the Neonatal Pulmonary Insufficiency Index for prediction of mortality in ECMO candidates. J Pediatr Surg 1984;19:380–4.

(24) Wung J-T, James LS, Kilchevsky E, James E. Management of infants with severe respiratory failure and persistence of the fetal circulation, without hyperventilation. Pediatrics 1985;76:488–94.

(25) Hageman JR, Dusik J, Keuler H, Bergman J, Gardner TH. Outcome of persistent pulmonary hypertension in relation to severity of presentation. AJDC 1988;142:293–6.

(26) Cole CH, Jillson E, Kessler D. ECMO: Regional evaluation of need and applicability of selection criteria. AJDC 1988;142:1320–4.

(27) Dworetz AR, Moya FR, Sabo B, Gladstone I, Gross I. Survival in infants with persistent pulmonary hypertension without extracorporeal membrane oxygenation. Pediatrics 1989;84:1–6.

(28) Ortega M, Ramos AD, Platzker ACG, Atkinson JB, Bowman CM. Early prediction of ultimate outcome in newborn infants with severe respiratory failure. J Pediatr 1988;113:744–747.

(29) Nading JH. Historical controls for extracorporeal membrane oxygenation in neonates. Crit Care Med 1989;17:423–5.

(30) Short BL. The extracorporeal membrane oxygenation debate (letter). Pediatrics 1990;85:380–1.

(31) Rhine WD, Fischer AF, Stevenson DK. The extracorporeal membrane oxygenation debate (letter). Pediatrics 1990;85:381–2.

(32) Clark RH, Kinsella JP, McCurnin DC, Null DM, deLemos RA. The extracorporeal membrane oxygenation debate (letter). Pediatrics 1990;85:382–3.

(33) Bartlett RH, Gazzaniga AB. Extracorporeal circulation for cardiopulmonary failure. Curr Probl Surgery 1978;15:1–96.

(34) Bartlett RH, Gazzaniga AB. Physiology and pathophysiology of extracorporeal circulation. In: Ionescu MI, Wooler GH, eds. Current techniques in extracorporeal circulation. Boston: Butterworths, 1981: 1–44.

(35) Hirschl RB, Bartlett RH. Extracorporeal membrane oxygenation support in cardiorespiratory failure. Adv Surg 1987;21:189–212.

(36) Zwischenberger JB, Barlett RH. Extracorporeal circulation for respiratory or cardiac failure. In: Civetta, Taylor, Kirby, eds. Critical care. Philadelphia: Lippincott, 1988:1629–37.

(37) The National Neonatal ECMO Registry. Neonatal ECMO Registry report October 1989. Ann Arbor: University of Michigan Hospitals, 27 October 1989.

(38) Bartlett RH, Roloff DW, Cornell RG, Andrews AF, Dillon PW, Zwischenberger JB. Extracorporeal circulation in neonatal respiratory failure: a prospective randomized study. Pediatrics 1985;76:479–87.

(39) O'Rourke PP, Crone RK, Vacanti JP, et al. Extracorporeal membrane oxygenation and conventional medical therapy in neonates with persistent pulmonary hypertension of the newborn: a prospective randomized study. Pediatrics 1989;84:957–63.

(40) Morris AH, Menlove RL, Rollins RJ, Wallace CJ, Beck E. A controlled clinical trial of a new 3-step therapy that includes extracorporeal CO_2 removal for ARDS. Trans Am Soc Artif Intern Organs 1989;34:48–53.

(41) Bowerman RA, Zwischenberger JB, Andrews AF, Bartlett RH. Cranial sonography of the infant treated with extracorporeal membrane oxygenation. AJNR 1985;6:377–382.

(42) Cilley RE, Zwischenberger JB, Andrews AF, Bowerman RA, Roloff DW, Bartlett RH. Intracranial hemorrhage during extracorporeal membrane oxygenation in neonates. Pediatrics 1986;78:699–704.

(43) Taylor GA, Glass P, Fitz CR, Miller MK. Neurologic status in infants treated with extracorporeal membrane oxygenation: correlation of imaging findings with developmental outcome. Radiology 1987;165:679–82.

(44) Schumacher RE, Barks JDE, Johnston MV, Donn SM, Scher MS, Roloff DW, Bartlett RH. Right-sided brain lesions in infants following extracorporeal membrane oxygenation. Pediatrics 1988;82:155–161.

(45) Campbell LR, Chantrapa B, Holmes GL, Howell CG Jr, Kanto WP. Right common carotid artery ligation in extracorporeal membrane oxygenation. J Pediatr 1988;113:110–113.

(46) Mitchell DG, Merton D, Desai H, et al. Neonatal brain: color Doppler imaging. Part II. Altered flow patterns from extracorporeal membrane oxygenation. Radiology 1988;167:307–10.

(47) Luisiri A, Graviss ER, Weber T, Silberstein MJ, Tantana S, Connors R, Brodeur AE. Neurosonographic changes in newborns treated with extracorporeal membrane oxygenation. J Ultrasound Med 1988;7:429–38.

(48) Raju TNK, Kim SY, Meller JL, Srinivasan G, Ghai V, Reyes H. Circle of Willis blood flow velocity and flow direction after common carotid artery ligation for neonatal extracorporeal membrane oxygenation. Pediatrics 1989;83:343–7.

(49) Taylor GA, Fitz CR, Kapur S, Short BL. Cerebrovascular accidents in neonates treated with extracorporeal membrane oxygenation: sonographic-pathologic correlation. AJR 1989; 153:355–61.

(50) Lewin JS, Masaryk TJ, Modic MT, Ross JS, Stork EK, Wiznitzer M. Extracorporeal membrane oxygenation in infants: angiographic and parenchymal evaluation of the brain with MR imaging. Radiology 1989;173:361–5.

(51) Pearlman JM, Altman DI, Powers WS, Volpe JJ. Cerebral injury and regional cerebral blood flow in newborn infants undergoing extracorporeal membrane oxygenation. Ann Neurol 1987; 22:421.

(52) Sell LL, Cullen ML, Whittlesey GC, Yedlin ST, Philippart AI, Bedard MP, Klein MD. Hemorrhagic complications during extracorporeal membrane oxygenation: prevention and treatment. J Pediatr Surg 1986;21:1087–91.

(53) Anderson HL III, Cilley RE, Zwischenberger JB, Bartlett RH. Thrombocytopenia in neonates after extracorporeal membrane oxygenation. Trans Am Soc Artif Intern Organs 1986; 32:534–7.

(54) Zwischenberger JB, Cilley RE, Hirschl RB, Heiss KF, Conti VR, Bartlett RH. Life-threatening intrathoracic complications during treatment with extracorporeal membrane oxygenation. J Pediatr Surg 1988;23:599–604.

2

History of the Development of Extracorporeal Circulation

C. Walton Lillehei, PH.D., M.D.

What mankind can dream—research and technology can achieve!

As recently as 1952, a physician at the bedside of a child dying of an intracardiac malformation could only pray for a recovery. Today, with the heart-lung machine, correction is routine.

Open heart surgery has been widely regarded as one of the most important medical advances of the twentieth century. Today, its application is so widespread (2,000 such surgeries performed every 24 hours worldwide) and it is performed so effortlessly and with such low risk at all ages from neonates to octogenarians that it may be very difficult for the current generation of cardiologists and cardiac surgeons, much less the lay public, to appreciate that just 38 years ago, the outer wall of the living human heart represented an impenetrable anatomical barrier to the surgeon's knife. These past 38 years have seen the evolution of methods for the diagnosis and correction of all types of congenital and acquired cardiac conditions. For those few that are not correctable, heart replacement has become a reality.

The keystone to this astonishing progress has been extracorporeal circulation (ECC). This procedure has allowed surgeons to empty the heart of blood, stop its beat as necessary, open any desired chamber, and safely carry out reparative procedures or even total replacement in an unhurried manner. A number of the developments that made the transition from research laboratory to clinical open heart surgery possible and successful occurred in the Department of Surgery at the University of Minnesota beginning in 1952 (Table 2.1).

This institution boasted two unique assets. One was the world's first heart hospital devoted entirely to the medical and surgical treatment of heart diseases. This 80-bed facility was donated to the University of Minnesota by the Variety Club of the Northwest and opened its doors July 1, 1951. The second and perhaps even more important asset was the presence of Owen H. Wangensteen, a truly visionary surgeon, as chairman of the Department of Surgery. He was not a cardiac surgeon, but he had made immense contributions in the field of general surgery. He had the ability to spot talent and capabilities in younger col-

TABLE 2.1 Original open heart operations and techniques developed at the University of Minnesota, 1952–1957

Operation/Technique	Date*	Technique
Atrial septal defect	September 2, 1952	General hypothermia
Ventricular septal defect closure	March 26, 1954	Extracorporeal circulation (by cross-circulation)
Atrioventricularis communis correction	August 6, 1954	Same as above
Tetralogy of Fallot correction	August 31, 1954	Same as above
Disposable bubble oxygenator	May 13, 1955	
First use of direct cardiac stimulation by myocardial electrodes with a pacemaker for complete heart block	January 30, 1957	

*Dates indicate first successful use in patients.

leagues, whose aptitudes were not at all obvious to others—often not even to themselves. Dr. Wangensteen was an enemy of tradition and frequently said, "Tradition is great for the French Foreign Legion or the Notre Dame football team, but it is frequently a disaster in science because tradition so often represents errors that the student inherits, without question, from his teachers."

THE OPEN HEART ERA IS BORN

In this stimulating milieu, major accomplishments were soon forthcoming. The first of these occurred on September 2, 1952 when, after a period of laboratory research on dogs, Dr. F. John Lewis, a medical school classmate and close personal friend of the author, successfully closed an atrial secundum defect (1) in a five-year-old girl under direct vision utilizing inflow stasis and moderate total body hypothermia. (The patient remains entirely well 38 years after her operation.) The date has considerable historical significance because that operation was the world's first successful operation on the open human heart under direct vision. Dr. Lewis had been inspired by Bigelow's experimental studies (2) upon hypothermia as a technique for open heart repairs. Such operations soon became routine at the University of Minnesota Hospital, and news of these successes spread rapidly throughout the medical world. Swan was the next surgeon to report successful direct vision intracardiac operations in humans utilizing general hypothermia and inflow stasis (3).

Hypothermia with inflow stasis proved to be an excellent method for simple atrial secundum defects. Lewis reported that eight out of his first nine patients had their atrial septal defects successfully closed, with only one death (4). Also, hypothermia proved excellent for isolated congenital pulmonic or aortic stenoses (3). However, failure was uniform when this technique was applied to more complex lesions such as ostium primum, atrioventricularis communis, or ventricular septal defect (VSD). These experiences reconfirmed the oft-predicted need for a perfusion method for the more complex intracardiac lesions.

The first attempt to use a heart-lung machine for total cardiopulmonary bypass (CPB) to permit intracardiac surgery in humans was also carried out at the University of Minnesota Hospital by Dennis and colleagues on April 5, 1951 (5). Two patients were operated upon within a month's time, but both died in the operating room. The first patient had an erroneous preoperative diagnosis despite two heart catheterizations and finger exploration of the heart's interior five months earlier. Instead of the anticipated atrial secundum defect, she had an unexpected partial atrioventricularis communis lesion. This pathology was baffling at the time. The second patient, operated upon two weeks later, had an atrial secundum defect repaired, but died intraoperatively from massive air embolism (6).

In both of these operations, the failures were related to the high perfusion rates that were considered necessary. In the first patient, in addition to the unfamiliar pathology, Drs. Dennis and Varco stated that they were visually handicapped by "an amazing amount of blood" from the coronary sinus/thebesian loss, and that "adjacent tissue anteriorly was employed to attempt closure in spite of the recognition of a good deal of encroachment upon the tricuspid orifice" (5). The cardiac specimen was studied by Dr. Jesse Edwards who found that the tricuspid orifice had been severely stenosed in the attempt to close the primum (personal communication, 1992). In the second patient, the arterial reservoir was emptied suddenly (by the high flow), resulting in air being pumped into the patient's systemic circuit (6). Later in 1951, Dr. Dennis and many of his team moved to New York City to continue their work.

The next milestone was reached in May of 1953 by Dr. John H. Gibbon, Jr., who had started working on a pump oxygenator in 1937 (7). He had developed his apparatus and techniques to the point where 12 of 20 dogs survived the closure of a surgically created VSD for one week to six months (8). By 1953, he thought that he was ready to venture into the clinical arena. His first patient died, but the second case, operated upon May 6, 1953 with an atrial secundum defect, was a complete success (9). Similar to the experience of Dennis, Gibbon's first patient selected for intracardiac surgery to close an atrial septal defect was a 15-month-old infant with an erroneous preoperative diagnosis. At operation, no septal defect was found. Autopsy disclosed a large unrecognized patent ductus arteriosus. Case 2 was the 18-year-old girl with the successful atrial defect closure. Cases 3 and 4 were both five-and-a-half-year-old girls operated upon in July 1953, and both died intraoperatively. Case 3 had an atrial secundum defect, and repair was attempted. Case 4 had been diagnosed preoperatively as an atrial septal defect, but also had a VSD and small patent ductus. None of the defects could be repaired "because of the flooding of the intracardiac field by blood" in the bypassed heart (9). Kirklin has written (10) (and also confirmed in a letter to this author) that Gibbon operated upon four patients after his May 1953 success, and none survived. These last two patients were never reported by Gibbon nor associates, and details are not available.

This success was well received in a report in the lay press 12 days later (11) but aroused surprisingly little enthusiasm or interest among cardiologists and cardiac surgeons at the time. There were several reasons for this. First, Dr. Gibbon had been able only to duplicate Dr. Lewis's successes beginning eight months earlier, but had not been able to repeat nor extend his one success. Second, Dr. Lewis was regularly closing atrial secundum defects (ASD) under direct vision using inflow stasis and moderate hypothermia with excellent results. In his first 11 patients (Table 2.2), he reported eight successful atrial septal repairs, one patient explored but not repaired (survived), and only two operative deaths (12). Swan (3,13) and others were also duplicating these excellent results with ASD. Third, and perhaps most importantly, Dr. Gibbon was never able to repeat his one success with the ASD or to achieve success with the more complex VSD. He became discouraged after five failures (Table 2.3) and abandoned open heart surgery as a means for repair of human heart lesions.

From 1951 to early 1954, there were many reported (Table 2.4) as well as many more unreported attempts to utilize CPB for intracardiac operations. In all of the reported clinical attempts at open heart operations, there was a common scenario: namely, good-to-acceptable survival in the experimental animals, but universal failure when the same apparatus and techniques were applied to humans. Thus, virtually all of the most experienced investigators of that era concluded with seemingly impeccable logic that the problems were not with the perfusion techniques nor the

TABLE 2.2 Direct vision closure, atrial (secundum) defects, systemic hypothermia, and caval occlusion 1952–1953, F.J. Lewis, M.D. (4,12), University of Minnesota

Patients	Defect closed	Deaths
11*	8	2 (18%)

*One patient developed ventricular fibrillation and was not repaired, but recovered.

TABLE 2.3 Total cardiopulmonary bypass by J.H. Gibbon, using the screen oxygenator (10,11)

Patient	Age	Date of operation	Diagnosis Preoperative	Diagnosis Postoperative	Results
1	15 months	1953	ASD	PDA (only)*	Died (in OR)
2	18 years	May 6, 1953	ASD	Same	Lived (long-term)
3	5.5 years	July 1953	ASD	Same	Died (in OR)
4	5.5 years	July 1953	ASD	ASD, VSD, PDA	Died (in OR)
5	Data NA	—	—	—	Died
6	Data NA	—	—	—	Died
Total 6 patients					1 lived (ASD) 5 died

*PDA = patent ductus arteriosus, OR = operating room.

heart-lung machines, but that the sick human heart ravaged by failure could not possibly be expected to tolerate the magnitude of the operations required and then recover immediately with adequate output as occurred when the same machines and techniques were applied to dogs with healthy hearts. Thus, discouragement was rampant, and pessimism about the future of open heart surgery became widespread.

The prevalent belief was that the concept of open heart repair, however attractive, was doomed for patients with more complex pathological conditions who urgently required and would benefit the most from corrective procedures. What was necessary, many thought, was a means of mechanical support for the heart during its recovery period. Even today, more than three decades later, prolonged mechanical support of the failing heart presents many unsolved problems.

TABLE 2.4 Open heart surgery with total cardiopulmonary bypass, all reported cases 1951–1954 (prior to cross-circulation March 26, 1954)

Physician	Patients	Age range	Defects*	Method	Date	Result Died	Result Lived
Dennis (5,6)	2	6–8 years	ASD, AV canal	Film oxygenator	1951	2	0
Gibbon (10,11)	6	15 months–18 years	PDA, ASD(2), ASD & VSD(1), NA(2)	Film oxygenator	1953	5	1 (ASD)
Helmsworth (15)	1	4 years	ASD	Bubble oxygenator	1952	1	0
Dodrill (16)	1	NA	Pulmonary stenosis	Autogenous	1953	1	0
Mustard (17)	5	10 months–11 years	Tetralogy	Monkey lungs	1951–1953	5	0
Clowes (18)	3	Neonate–55 years	Lung disease, AO stenosis, LA Myxoma	Bubble oxygenator	1953	3	0
Total	18 patients					17 (11 OR)	1 (5.5%)

*ASD = atrial secundum, PDA = patent ductus arteriosus, AV canal = atrioventricular communis, VSD = ventricular septal defect.

As happens from time to time in research, some simple and apparently unrelated experiments were performed that suggested an entirely fresh outlook on these seemingly insurmountable problems. This new information, which we have termed the "azygos flow concept," made possible a perfusion breakthrough totally unprecedented in scope. It is my opinion that the single most important discovery that made clinical open heart surgery successful was the realization of the vast discrepancy between the total body flow rate that was *thought* necessary and what was *actually* necessary.

THE AZYGOS FLOW CONCEPT

During some canine experiments in which the cavae were temporarily occluded to test tolerance limits of the brain and heart to ischemia (18), we discovered that if the azygos vein alone were not clamped, the resulting very small cardiac output (19) (measured at 8 to 14 mL/kg body wt/min) was sufficient to sustain the vital organs safely in every animal for a minimum of 30 minutes at normothermia. To even mention, at that time, that such a low flow might be adequate for perfusion was heresy. We were pleased to learn of a similar observation in 1952 in England by Andreason and Watson (20). Both of these studies agreed that only about 10% of the so-called basal cardiac output was needed to sustain animals unimpaired physiologically for a reasonable period of time at normothermia. From the earliest days, the universally accepted minimum for cardiopulmonary bypass (at normothermia) was considered by the authorities (5,10,14,17,21) of that time to be 100 to 165 mL/kg body wt/min in animals and humans. Our findings of this remarkable tolerance to drastically lower flows of only 8 to 14 cc/kg/min was very surprising, but the animal (dog) results were unmistakably clear. In analyzing these findings, we described at that time at least three identifiable important physiologic adjustments that were occurring in response to lowered blood flow (19). These compensating readjustments were additive and in their entirety at normal body temperatures accounted very well for the fact that these animals

survived for 30 minutes with their vital organs (brain, liver, heart, and kidneys) well protected.

At that time in our studies, we quickly found that "low flow" was a pejorative term, and that advocacy of systemic flows much lower than the so-called basal cardiac output of 100 to 120 kg/min was considered totally wrong. What most clinicians and even physiologists did not appreciate was the simple fact that, at basal cardiac output, venous blood was returning with 65% to 75% of its oxygen content unused. There was no physiologic harm whatsoever in utilizing fully the oxygen contained in the blood. Thus, the azygos flow was really not low flow but *physiologic flow*.

Reducing the volume of blood necessary to be pumped had immediate and immense benefits. It has been observed that one of the problems responsible in part for the failures with extracorporeal circulation by Dennis (5), Gibbon (9), Helmsworth (14), and others was the enormous and unexpected blood return into the open hearts, which made accurate vision almost impossible. Also, these unanticipated blood losses often made the perfusions physiologically precarious.

We immediately appreciated at that time that the discovery of the "azygos flow concept" represented the sword that would eventually sever the Gordian knot of complexity that had garroted perfusion technology. I was convinced that some simple way could be found to successfully perfuse only 20 to 25 mL/kg/min which we set as a desirable flow rate with a comfortable safety margin. This "low flow" or "physiologic flow" quantity was only 10% to 20% of what others deemed necessary. Consequently, armed with this information in 1952, I believed that successful open heart surgery was not only possible, but inevitable in the near future.

THE AUTOGENOUS LUNG

The low-flow principle made autogenous lung oxygenation much simpler and more attractive (22). However, the extra cannulae and tubing in the operative field were sensitive to even slight displacements with the subsequent rapid onset of pulmonary edema. This rather frequent complication in our animal studies dampened our enthusiasm for potential clinical use. However, these venous drainage kinking problems led directly to the idea of moving the extra pulmonary cannulas completely out of the operative field by utilizing a separate donor animal for oxygenation (cross-circulation).

Initially, our extracorporeal perfusions using cross-circulation in dogs had been intended only as an interim method to permit some open heart experience in animals without the need for a complex conventional pump-oxygenator, which was unavailable to us at the time. However, as the experiments progressed, it became apparent that the dogs undergoing a 30-minute open heart interval utilizing low-flow cross-circulation not only survived at a far higher percent, but recovered far more rapidly when compared with dogs we had observed undergoing a similar period of high-flow pump-oxygenator perfusions. (In 1950–1951, Dr. Dennis and the author had adjoining experimental laboratories at the University of Minnesota Medical School.) The differences were truly astonishing, and, for the first time, we realized that this might be the simple and effective clinical method for intracardiac operations for which we were searching. The experimental and clinical data on cross-circulation perfusions and the reduced or physiological perfusion flow rates based on the "azygos flow" studies have been documented elsewhere (23–26).

CLINICAL APPLICATION OF CROSS-CIRCULATION

Cross-circulation for clinical intracardiac operations was an immense departure from established surgical practice at the time. The thought of taking a normal human being to the operating room to provide a donor circulation (with potential risks, however small), even temporarily, was considered unacceptable and even immoral by some critics. However, we had begun to suspect that there were massive

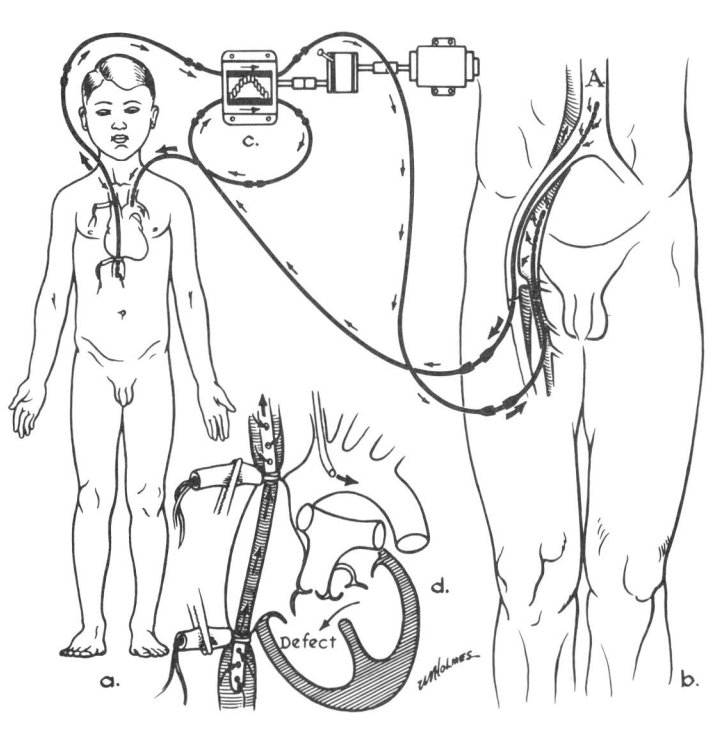

FIGURE 2.1 Method for direct vision intracardiac surgery utilizing extracorporeal circulation by means of controlled cross-circulation. (a) Patient, showing sites of arterial and venous cannulations. (b) Donor, showing sites of arterial and venous (superficial femoral and great saphenous) cannulations. (c) The single pump controlling the reciprocal exchange of blood between patient and donor. (d) Close-up of the patient's heart showing the vena caval catheter positioned so as to draw venous blood from both the superior and inferior venae cavae during the cardiac bypass interval. The arterial blood from the donor was circulated to the patient's body through the catheter inserted into the left subclavian artery.

physiological disturbances evoked by total body perfusion and open cardiotomy about which we knew very little and that, by temporarily instituting a "placental" circulation, we might minimize or even correct those to permit otherwise impossible operations (Figure 2.1).

The continued lack of any success in the other centers around the world that were working actively on heart-lung bypass (Table 2.4) and the widespread doubt about the feasibility of open heart surgery in humans contributed to our decision to go ahead clinically on March 26, 1954 (Figure 2.2).

The cross-circulation technique was a dramatic success in humans (24–32). In the months that followed its first use to close a VSD, a rapid succession of surgical firsts occurred for correction of congenital heart defects that previously had been inoperable (Table 2.1). Cross-circulation as the means for extracorporeal circulation to permit work inside the human heart was utilized for 45 operations (Table 2.5). There was no donor mortality and no long-lasting donor sequelae (32).

Almost overnight, the "sick human heart theory" was refuted because the patients operated upon with cross-circulation, mostly infants in terminal congestive failure, could not

FIGURE 2.2 The scene on March 26, 1954 in Operating Room B, University of Minnesota Medical Center, during the first controlled cross-circulation operation, at which time a ventricular septal defect in a 12-month-old infant was successfully visualized by ventricular cardiotomy and closed by direct suture during a bypass interval of 19 minutes. The average flow rate was 40 cc/kg body wt/min at normothermia. The Sigmamotor pump that served as the mechanical heart is not visible in this photo. The lightly anesthetized donor with groin cannulations (patient's father), serving as the extracorporeal oxygenator, may be seen to the far right. C. W. Lillehei is immediately to the right of the scrub nurse, and opposite him is Dr. R. L. Varco. Behind Dr. Lillehei is Dr. H. E. Warden, and next to him looking over the scrub nurse is Dr. M. Cohen. Drs. Cohen and Warden are the two residents who had perfected this technique in the experimental dog laboratory.

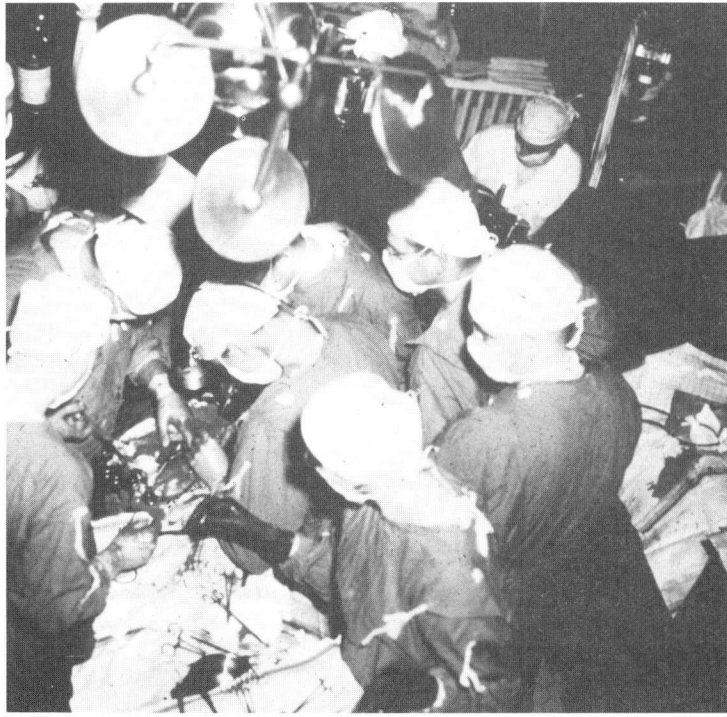

TABLE 2.5 Results of direct vision intracardiac operations with cross-circulation on 45 patients from March 26, 1954 to July 9, 1955* (25–31, 33–35)

			Mortality	
Abnormality	Corrective operations†	Patients	Hospital	Late (30 years)
VSD	Suture closure	27	8	2
PDA (with severe pulmonary hypertension)	Exploratory ventriculotomy, division of ductus	1	0	0
Tetralogy of Fallot	Suture closure of VSD, repair of infundibular/valvular pulmonary stenosis	10	5	3
Atrioventricular communis	Closure of ostium primum, VSD; repair of valvular deformities	5	3	1
Isolated infundibular pulmonary stenosis	Resection of infundibulum	1	0	0
Pulmonary stenosis, ASD, anomalous pulmonary venous return	Pulmonary valvotomy, ventricular and atrial cardiotomies, transposition of anomalous pulmonary veins, closure of septal defects	1	1	0
Totals		45	17	6

*Cross-circulation was used exclusively from its inception through February 1955. Beginning March 1, 1955, other bypass methods (bubble oxygenator, dog-lung oxygenator, arterial reservoir) were employed for lower-risk patients. Cross-circulation was reserved for high-risk patients. By July 1955, the bubble oxygenator had become the sole method.
†VSD = ventricular septal defect, PDA = patent ductus arteriosus, ASD = atrial (secundum) septal defect.

have been worse operative risks. Thus, after 15 years in the experimental laboratory, open heart surgery moved permanently into the clinical arena.

A THREE-DECADE FOLLOW-UP

The follow-up of a minimum of 30 years on these first patients with VSD, AV canal, infundibular pulmonic stenosis, and tetralogy of Fallot who had successful intracardiac corrections has been particularly informative and impressively sanguine (32). Twenty-eight of the 45 (62%) patients undergoing extracorporeal circulation survived the operation and were discharged from the hospital. Even more impressive was the finding that only six of these patients had died in 30 years, and thus twenty-two of the 45 patients (49%) initially operated upon were alive 30 years later, and all were in good health.

The 27 patients with VSDs constituted the largest category to have repair, and 17 (63%) were living and well 30 or more years later. The only two late VSD patient deaths in all of the years following hospital discharge occurred in two patients with closed defects but inexorable progression of their pulmonary vascular disease. The late follow-up on the more complex tetralogy patients has been equally rewarding (30,33,34).

Cross-circulation was so successful because

the donor automatically corrected all of the various hematologic and metabolic derangements. At that time, we had no idea what these physiological aberrations were, and thus no knowledge about measuring them, much less treating them. In 1954–1955, pH and blood gases were not obtainable clinically. Even emergency plasma electrolytes took four to six hours. There was no respiratory assistance equipment for infants and children, and there were no intensive care units, much less any monitors, pacemakers, or external defibrillators. In effectively reconstituting the placental circulation with cross-circulation, we rediscovered the world's greatest ICU: "the intrauterine environment." It was some years before we could duplicate these remarkable results in equally sick patients using the pump oxygenator.

PROBLEMS REQUIRING SOLUTION FOR SUCCESSFUL OPEN HEART SURGERY

For open intracardiac operations in humans to be regularly successful, workable solutions had to be identified for the three major obstacles that had stalled progress for so long. First, an effective method for safely emptying the heart of blood for a reasonable length of time was needed. Extracorporeal circulation by cross-circulation fulfilled that need. Next, having gained access to the interior of the living human heart, it became evident that these malformations existed in a very broad spectrum, and in many forms not yet described or even recognized by clinicians or pathologists. Surgical methods for dealing with these unfamiliar lesions required rapid technical development, often improvised on the spot, and sometimes with poignant failures. Moreover, given the existing state of technology, the preoperative diagnoses were often wrong or incomplete. Finally, these patients, often critically ill preoperatively, required postoperative care on a much higher level of sophistication than was known or available at the time.

Knowing now what we did not know in 1951–1954, it seems very probable that the only method for extracorporeal circulation that could possibly have succeeded so rapidly in the face of such formidable problems, and with such limited knowledge in the many high-risk infants and children with complex anatomical lesions, was cross-circulation. The homeostatic mechanisms of the donor automatically corrected the untold number of mostly unknown physiological aberrations evoked by total body perfusion.

Thirty years ago, we wrote that "clinical experience with cross-circulation has made it apparent that it is unlikely that a technique for total cardiopulmonary bypass will be developed which excels this one for the patients' safety" (28). The spectacular success of clinical cross-circulation operations stimulated intensive laboratory work upon alternative methods of clinical oxygenation without the need for a living human donor.

HETEROLOGOUS BIOLOGIC OXYGENATORS

Beginning on March 1, 1955, a series of clinical open heart operations was started at the University of Minnesota utilizing a pair of canine lungs as oxygenators. Twelve patients were operated upon, with four long-term survivors (35,36). Subsequent to those two reports, two more patients were operated upon for a total of 14, with five long-term survivors. In none of these patients was the death attributable to oxygenator dysfunction. The only other attempt to use heterogeneous lungs at that time was the report of Mustard and associates (16,37) using monkey lungs. In their series of seven patients, there were no survivors. Mustard and Thomson (16) subsequently reported 21 infants and children having ECC utilizing monkey lungs between 1952–1956, with three survivors.

EXTRACORPOREAL CIRCULATION FROM A RESERVOIR OF OXYGENATED BLOOD

Beginning March 3, 1955, the first of a series of five patients was operated on at the University of Minnesota for intracardiac repair of

VSD or transposition of the great vessels by continuous perfusion from a reservoir of oxygenated blood (25,38,39). This very simple technique was particularly applicable to infants requiring relatively simple intracardiac repairs and lesser blood volumes. (Patient L.O. (male) was operated on March 29, 1955, at age 6 months, weighing 4.7 kg, for closure of a ventricular septal defect, utilizing reservoir perfusion. This patient has now been followed for 35 years. He was recatheterized in 1964, with findings of normal pulmonary pressures and a completely closed defect.) The arterialized venous blood for perfusion was drawn in the blood bank a few hours before surgery, utilizing an ordinary venipuncture in donors whose arms had been immersed in water heated to 45°C for 15 minutes, which effectively oxygenated the venous blood.

THE MECHANICAL PUMP OXYGENATOR FOR CARDIOPULMONARY BYPASS: BEGINNING OF AN ERA

In two publications in 1955 from the Mayo Clinic, Kirklin, Wood, and associates (40,41)

TABLE 2.6 Mayo Clinic open heart experience (43), first series (March–May 1955) with Gibbon-Mayo screen oxygenator

Lesion	Number of patients	Lived	Hospital deaths
Atrial (secundum)	1	1	0
Ventricular defect	4	2	2
AV canal	2	1	1
Tetralogy of Fallot	1	0	1
Totals	8	4	4

described their experimental results utilizing a Gibbon-type pump oxygenator as originally built by International Business Machines Corporation (IBM) and modified by them. Their first clinical application was March 22, 1955, and a report followed on their first eight patients undergoing open heart surgery (42) (Figure 2.3). Their four survivors had atrial septal defect (1 patient), ventricular septal defect (2), and an AV canal (1). Their four deaths were: VSD (2), AV canal (1), and tetralogy of Fallot (1) (Table 2.6). Their flow rates varied from 100–200 cc/kg body wt/min at normothermia. By September 1958, 245 patients had been operated upon at the Mayo Clinic by Kirklin et al. (43).

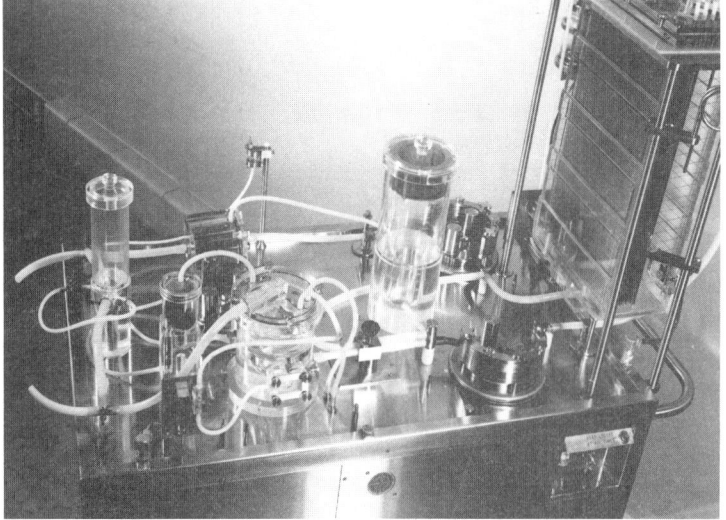

FIGURE 2.3 The Mayo-Gibbon screen oxygenator. This model was used in 1955 during the first series of open heart operations performed by Dr. John Kirklin and associates at the Mayo Clinic, Rochester, Minnesota. (Photo courtesy of J. W. Kirklin.)

ADVENT OF THE DeWALL-LILLEHEI DISPOSABLE BUBBLE OXYGENATOR

Prior to 1955, there was universal agreement among the world's authorities that the one way that blood could not be arterialized was by a bubble oxygenator. On May 13, 1955, DeWall and Lillehei, based upon their dog laboratory research, began routine clinical use of a very simple disposable bubble oxygenator (Figure 2.4A). In their first report, Lillehei, DeWall, et al. (44) described seven patients having VSDs closed, with five long-term survivors. The operations took place at normothermia, with perfusion rates (utilizing a Sigmamotor pump) of 25 to 30 cc/kg body weight. All of the seven patients awoke postoperatively, and there was no evidence of neurologic, hepatic, or renal impairment.

In an addendum to their paper (44), DeWall and Lillehei reported that a total of 36 patients ranging in age from 16 weeks to 21 years had their hearts and lungs totally bypassed for intracardiac correction utilizing this bubble oxygenator with similar excellent results. The congenital defects successfully corrected were VSD, tetralogy of Fallot, AV canal, complete transposition, and atrial secundum defects. As the number of patients having open heart surgery with ECC increased rapidly, the bubble oxygenator was refined to increase capacity for adult patients (45) (Figures 2.4–2.7).

In the early clinical open heart operations, considerable physiologic and biochemical data (46) were collected, analyzed, and compared to the earlier animal studies (47). This information confirmed the excellence of the patients' physiologic status while undergoing perfusion at the lower (more physiologic) flow rates (the azygos flow concept) with support from the bubble oxygenator. Tests done by psychologists and neurologists upon our patients before and after perfusion detected no significant abnormalities in cerebral function attributable to the perfusions (48). In a 26–31-year follow-up of 106 patients operated on for correction of tetralogy (33), 32% had college or graduate degrees, including two M.D.'s, two Ph.D.'s and one lawyer (LLB). Obviously, putting people on the bubble oxygenator would not be expected to increase intelligence, but these figures were far beyond the average for a random group from the general population

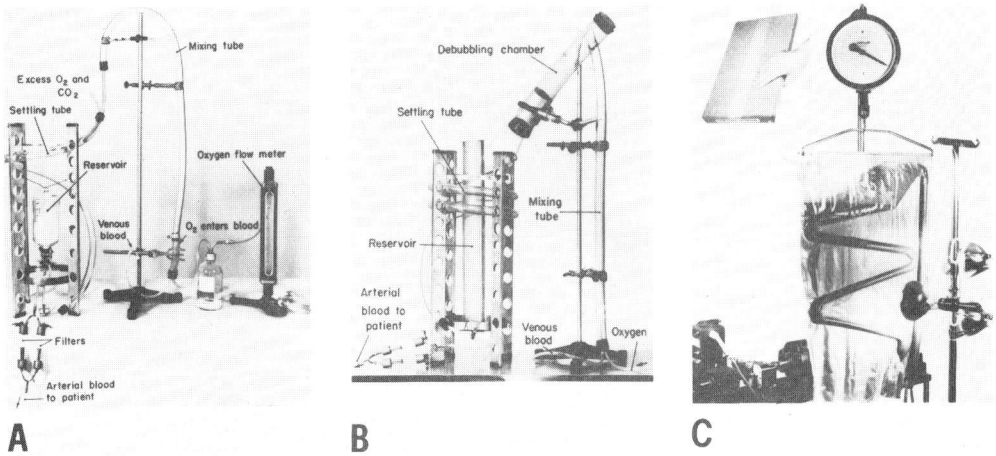

FIGURE 2.4 Evolution of the simple disposable DeWall-Lillehei bubble oxygenator for open heart surgery. (A) First 1955 model, successful in infants and small children. (B) Later 1955 helix reservoir model suitable for adults. (C) 1956 commercially manufactured model shipped sterile in a package (inset) ready to hand up and use.

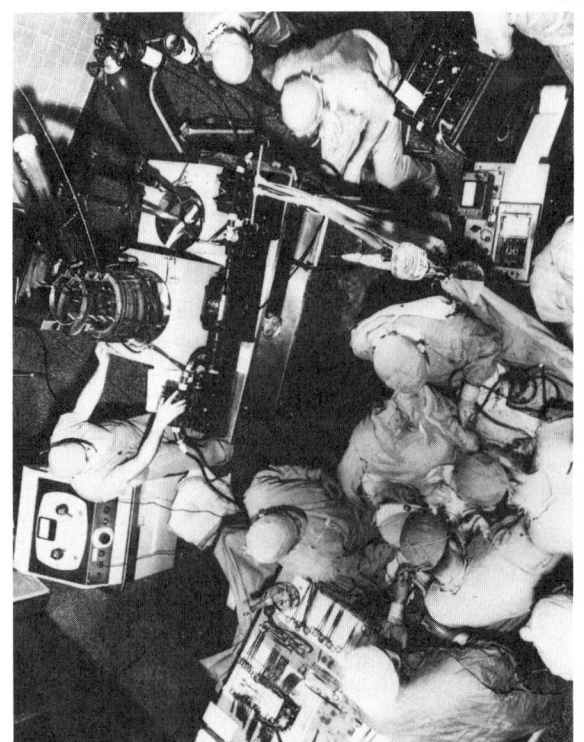
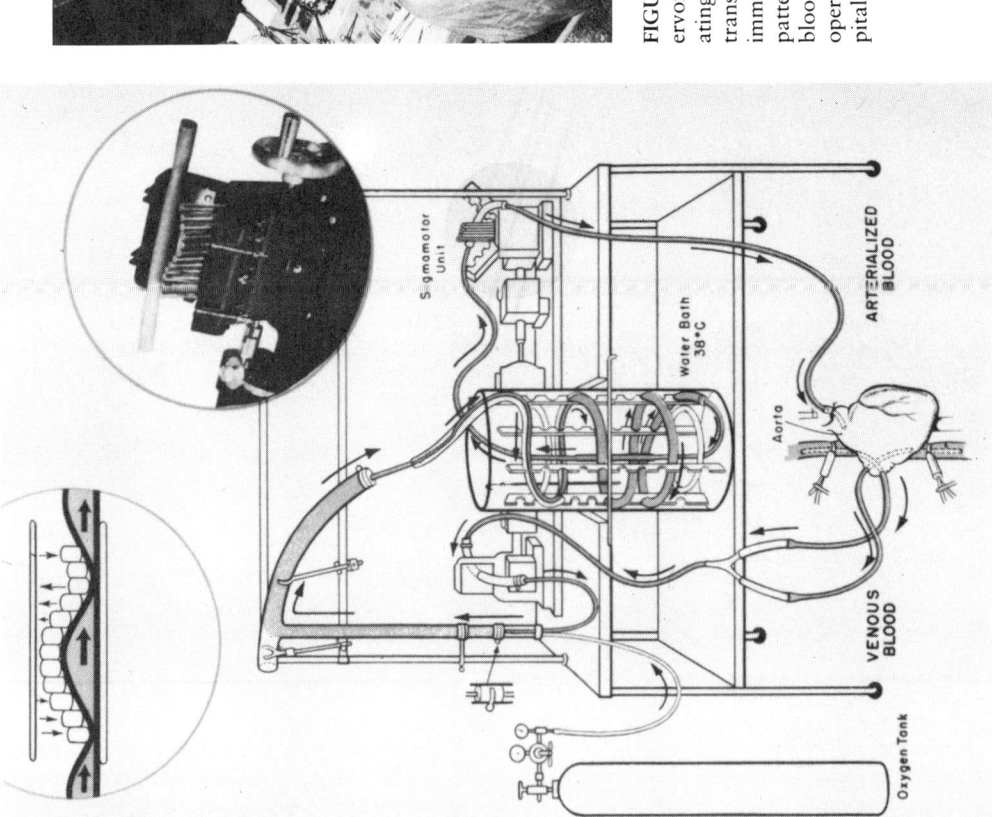

FIGURE 2.5 (A) Diagrammatic portrayal of 1955 DeWall-Lillehei helix reservoir disposable pump oxygenator with adult capacity. The upright oxygenating column with the venous blood mixing with oxygen bubbles at base, transverse debubbling chamber, and the spiral (helix) debubbling/reservoir immersed in a water bath are evident. The two insets show the wavelike pattern of the Sigmamotor pump's 12 metallic "fingers" as they stroke the blood through the plastic tubing without direct contact. (B) An open heart operation in an adult patient in progress at the University of Minnesota Hospital (1956).

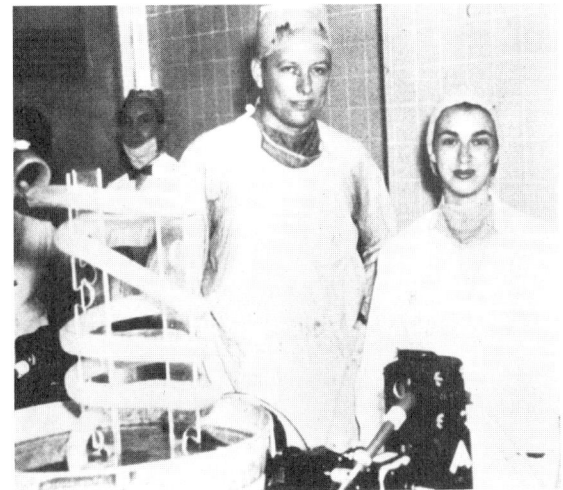
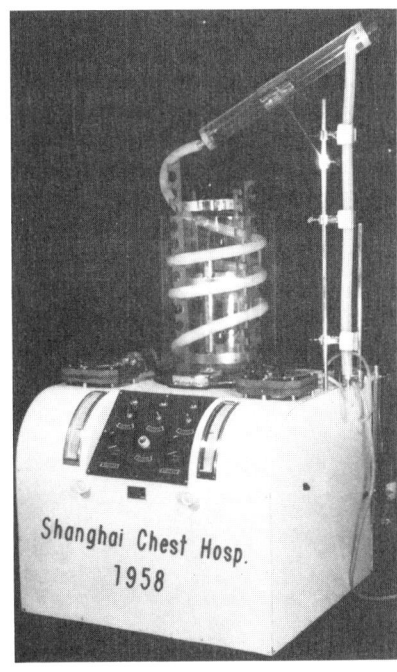

FIGURE 2.6 The availability of the simple, effective, disposable helix reservoir bubble oxygenator had an explosive effect upon worldwide growth of open heart surgery. (A) Dr. Denton Cooley with perfusionist after an atrial septal defect closure, September 12, 1957, in Caracas, Venezuela. (B) Equipment utilized by Professor Pan Chih and associates for many successful open heart operations at the Shanghai Chest Hospital, China, 1957–1958.

and at the very least supported the absence of any significant cerebral dysfunction.

The DeWall-Lillehei bubble oxygenator was an instant success because it had so many practical advantages. It was efficient, inexpensive, heat sterilizable, easy to assemble and check, had no moving parts, and was disposable (Figures 2.4, 2.5). The development of the self-contained unitized plastic sheet oxygenator (Figure 2.4C, 2.7) in 1956 by Gott, DeWall, Lillehei, and others (49,50) further improved this system and played an important role in the tremendous expansion of open heart surgery that occurred after 1956. The revelation that safe perfusion of the body could be achieved with several lengths of plastic tubing, a few clamps, and some oxygen had an explosive effect upon the worldwide development of cardiac surgery (Figure 2.6). The surgeon's dream of routinely performing intracardiac corrections on the open heart had become a reality (51) (Table 2.7).

It is interesting to note that, in the year 1954, the only place in the world doing regu-

TABLE 2.7 Open cardiotomy: summary of the early clinical experience at the University of Minnesota Hospitals (52)

Method	Period	Number of patients
Hypothermia only	1952–1956	70
Cross-circulation	1954–1955	45
Arterial reservoir (26,39,40)	1955	5
Dog-lung oxygenator (36,37)	1955	14
Bubble oxygenator	1955–1966	2,581
Total		2,715

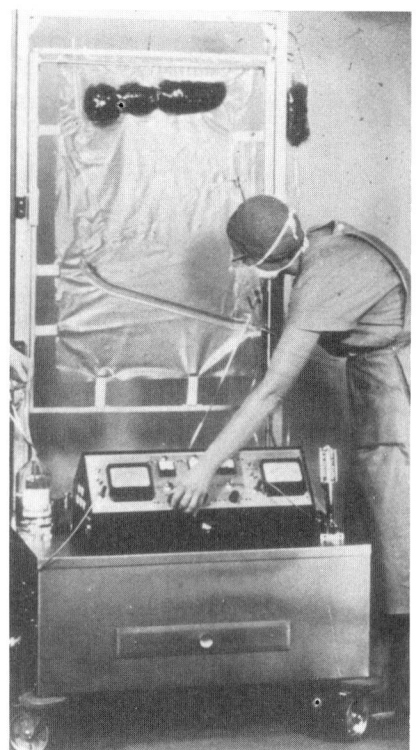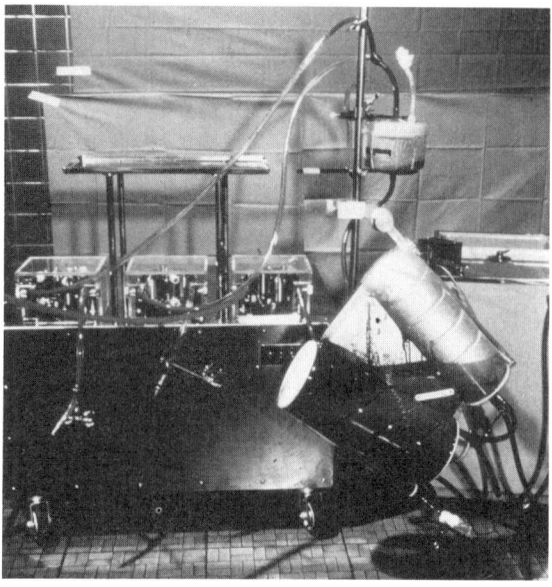

FIGURE 2.7 (A) DeWall-Lillehei unitized plastic sheet oxygenator was commercially manufactured, and shipped sterile—ready to hang up, prime, and use, as shown here. (Photo courtesy of D. A. Cooley.) (B) The Temptrol disposable bubble oxygenator with self-contained heat exchanger during a perfusion. In this unit, Dr. DeWall introduced the rigid, presterilized plastic outer shell that has been the basis of all subsequent oxygenator designs for both bubble and membrane units.

larly scheduled open heart surgery by extracorporeal circulation was the University of Minnesota Hospital in Minneapolis (utilizing cross-circulation). Throughout the year 1955 and well into 1956, there were only two places in the world performing these operations, the University of Minnesota in Minneapolis and the Mayo Clinic in Rochester, only 90 miles apart. Visitors from all parts of the world traveled to these two places to observe open heart surgery. On the one hand was the Mayo-Gibbon apparatus which was very expensive, handcrafted, and unobtainable at any price. On the other hand was the unbelievably simple, disposable, heat-sterilized bubble oxygenator of DeWall-Lillehei, costing only a few dollars to assemble. It is no wonder that many visiting surgeons left these two clinics totally confused as to which method to pursue.

Dr. Denton Cooley, an early observer in June of 1955, was to write later (52) that "the contrast between the two institutions and the two surgeons was striking. We observed Lillehei and a team composed mostly of house staff correct a ventricular septal defect using cross-circulation. During the visit, we also saw an oxygenator developed by Richard DeWall at the University of Minnesota. The next day we observed John Kirklin and his impressive team in Rochester that was made up of physiologists, biochemists, cardiologists, and others as they performed operations using the Mayo-Gibbon apparatus. Such a device was beyond my organizational capacity and financial reach. Thus I was deeply disappointed on our return to Houston when Dr. McNamara stated that he would not permit me to operate on his patients unless I had a Mayo-Gibbon apparatus." However, Cooley succeeded in convincing some of his cardiologists that "the era of open heart surgery had arrived," and in 1956 began to perform open heart surgery utilizing the DeWall-Lillehei bubble oxygenator with considerable success (52).

Professor Naef also later wrote, "The homemade helix bubble of DeWall and Lillehei, first used clinically on May 13, 1955, went on to conquer the world and helped many teams to embark on the correction of malformations inside the heart in a precise and unhurried manner. The road to open-heart surgery had been opened" (53).

THE ROTATING DISC FILM OXYGENATOR (KAY-CROSS)

After finishing his surgical training at the University of Minnesota in 1953, Dr. Frederick Cross moved to Cleveland where he developed with Earl Kay in 1956 a rotating disc oxygenator which had wide use in the 1950s, particularly in the United States. This oxygenator, called the Kay-Cross apparatus (54, 55), was based on the earlier experimental work of Björk (56). It had multiple vertical discs placed on a horizontal axis which rotated with the discs dipping into a pool of venous blood, creating a film on the discs in an atmosphere of oxygen. This filming unit, like the Mayo-Gibbon film oxygenator was capable of good oxygenation, but both, being nondisposable, shared similar problems. They were cumbersome to use, required large priming volumes, and were difficult to clean and sterilize. However, the Kay-Cross unit became commercially available, in contrast to the Mayo-Gibbon machine which was extremely expensive to handcraft, and therefore largely unobtainable in those early years.

The Kay-Cross filming unit appealed to the cardiac surgeons who could not believe that bubble oxygenation was far more efficient, probably safer, and very effective, yet vastly simpler to use and less expensive. Even the Mayo Clinic had by 1971 converted almost entirely to the use of the bubble oxygenator (57). By 1976, it was estimated that 90% of all open heart operations worldwide involved the use of a bubble oxygenator (58).

Other oxygenators that were publicly known and worthy of mention, but had limited or in some cases ephemeral clinical applications, were those of Rygg (59), Dennis et al. (5) (film), Clark et al. (60) (bubble), Craaford and Senning (61) (film and bubble), Clowes et al. (17) (bubble) and (62) (membrane), Melrose (63) (film), and Bramson et al. (64) (membrane). The Rygg bubble oxygenator was a replica of the DeWall-Lillehei technology that was manufactured in Denmark and had usage in countries where U.S. patents did not apply. For more information on these devices, the reader is referred to the fine review articles of DeWall and colleagues (65,66).

MEMBRANE OXYGENATORS

Kolff and associates (67) described a disposable membrane oxygenator for experimental use in 1956. Clowes and Neville (62) described their experimental studies with membrane oxygenation and an apparatus suitable for clinical perfusions in 1958.

The belief that membrane oxygenation gives a better perfusion than the bubble or film has been clear only with perfusions of 12 to 24 hours in duration. Confusion has arisen over the innumerable comparative studies of membrane versus bubble oxygenators in shorter perfusions. With perfusions lasting six to eight hours, the membrane oxygenator is associated with less reduction of platelets, complement activation, postoperative bleeding, and microemboli. Since ECC times for most cardiac procedures are two to three hours or less, it has been difficult to prove that these changes, which are for the most part readily reversible, have any permanent ill effects. Some studies have failed to show the theoretical benefits of membrane over bubble oxygenation (68–70), while other published data demonstrate improved hematologic tolerance of CPB with membrane oxygenators (71–73). The author, with Lande and others (74), described the first compact disposable membrane oxygenator for clinical use.

FURTHER DEVELOPMENTS IN BUBBLE OXYGENATION

In 1966, DeWall et al. (75) made a significant advance in oxygenator design with the introduction of a hard shell bubble oxygenator with an integrated oxygenator and omnithermic heat exchanger in a disposable, presterilized polycarbonate unit (Figure 2.7). The adequacy of oxygenation and acid-base balance was well documented (76,77). The integrated hard shell concept has been the basis of all subsequent refinements both in bubble and membrane oxygenators (Figure 2.8).

FIGURE 2.8 Maxima (Medtronic) hollow fiber membrane oxygenator is a widely used state-of-the-art device. This disposable unit and similar competitive devices, such as those of Cobe, Terumo, Sarns, Shiley, Bard, etc., have rigid outer shells with integrated heat exchangers, easily attached venous and cardiotomy reservoirs, suction chambers, low priming volumes, and efficient gas transfer. Their ease of use and more competitive price differentials versus the bubblers have resulted in increasing use for routine open heart procedures.

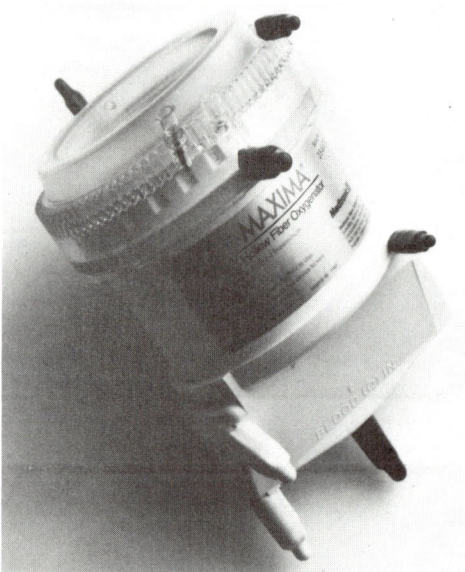

CURRENT STATUS OF EXTRACORPOREAL CIRCULATION

In the early days of open heart surgery, postoperative cerebral dysfunction was a subject of intensive interest. As the major causes were identified and resolved (48), concern over this matter decreased. However, there has been a resurgence of interest in the detection and prevention of more subtle changes in personality and intellect that may be associated with otherwise successful CPB (78–81). The reality and frequency of these changes, as well as the use of continuous EEG monitoring to allow immediate correction of problems, are under study (82).

HEMODILUTION

One of the technologic advances that has had a tremendous effect upon the growth of ECC has been the appreciation that pump oxygenators could be primed with nonblood solutions, reducing the need for blood and at the same time improving the quality of perfusions. The hemodilution innovators were Zuhdi and colleagues in 1961 (83–85). DeWall and colleagues (86,87) confirmed the benefits of hypothermic hemodilution in ECC. Other hemodilution studies were reported from the Minnesota group confirming the value of low molecular weight dextran (88–90). Comparative studies demonstrated the value of hemodilution with differing perfusates for improving renal blood flow and lessening hemolysis (91,92). Further, the beneficial effects of hemodilution and antiadrenergic drugs on prevention of renal ischemia during ECC were confirmed (93,94).

PROGRESS IN PUMP DESIGN

In the earliest days of ECC, the multicam-activated Sigmamotor pump was used. Then the roller pumps, because of their ease of use and reliability, gained popularity. In more recent years, the centrifugal pump described by Rafferty, Kletschka, and co-workers in 1968

(95) has become commercially available as the Biopump (marketed by BioMedicus, Inc., a division of Medtronic, Inc., 7000 Central Ave., N.E., Minneapolis, Minnesota 55432). Some of the advantages of this pump are reliability, ease of use over a wide range of flows, inability to pump air, absence of spallation, and low hemolysis. This pump was originally developed and applied for perfusions lasting hours or days. However, surgeons in growing numbers have been impressed by the centrifugal pump's performance and advantages and have begun to use it for routine ECC.

OTHER DEVELOPMENTS

As extracorporeal circulation became routine for a wide variety of congenital malformations, open cardiotomy was successfully applied in 1956 to revolutionize the treatment of acquired valvular heart disease (96,97) and subsequently, to the even larger group afflicted with coronary arteriosclerosis (98,99). By 1967, the ultimate landmark was reached with the successful transplantation of a human heart by Drs. Barnard and Shumway, who had trained together in the late 1950s in the author's cardiac program at the University of Minnesota.

The current challenge is to make the benefits of heart replacement more broadly available both by increasing the number of donors and by developing an effective, permanent intracorporeal mechanical heart. This latter seems a likelihood in the foreseeable future. Because of the shortage of donors, only about 10% to 12% of potential recipients are being served. Short of a breakthrough with xenotransplantation (which is quite possible), the gap inevitably will have to be filled by a reliable, practical, fully implantable total artificial heart (TAH).

AN IMPLANTABLE TOTAL ARTIFICIAL HEART: THE PRESENT CHALLENGE

There is no conflict between transplantation and the total artificial organ. Both methods are urgently needed. During the past two decades, the goal of implantation of an effective TAH has been one of the most exciting in medicine, but the failures have been among the most agonizing. This cycle of recurrent enthusiasm alternating with pessimism and failures is very reminiscent of the earlier history of open heart surgery as noted herein. The development of a successful TAH is obviously a complex problem involving many disciplines. However, this author believes that the greater the complexity of a problem, the greater is the need for decisive simplification in solving it.

Table 2.8 outlines some theories on the essentials for a successful implantable heart to function long term without the need for anticoagulants. The TAH has to be fully implantable; that means no tubes or even wires penetrating the skin. There are at least two options here. In 1975, Westinghouse developed and tested a fully implantable TAH powered by plutonium 238 (Figure 2.9). This

TABLE 2.8 Total artificial heart: some essential elements for success

Totally implanted power source (atomic, skeletal muscle/pacemaker)
Continuous flow pump
Eliminate all four valves
Eliminate all need for anticoagulation drugs

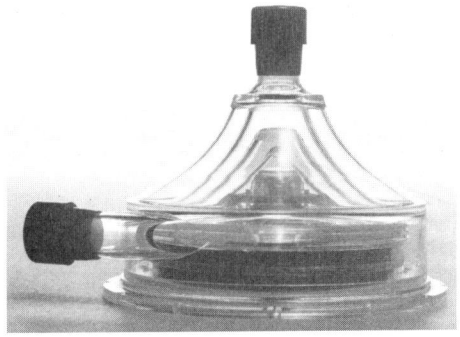

FIGURE 2.9 Westinghouse/University of Utah prototype pump (1975) powered by plutonium 238 for totally implanted nuclear-powered artificial hearts. This unit eliminates all transcutaneous wires/tubes and was designed to produce 12 watts of power.

unit put out 12 watts of power, which was sufficient for an adult circulation. Unfortunately, largely due to unwarranted fears about plutonium by highly vocal, misguided critics, this project has been tabled. Another option that may be feasible is to form a flap of autologous skeletal muscle trained to pump and driven by an appropriately implanted pacemaker (100).

A cherished belief of many is a "need for pulsatile flow." However, this investigator can find no convincing evidence in the extensive literature on this subject that pulsatile flow is a physiologic necessity or even advantageous. By going to continuous flow, an intracorporeal pump can be much simpler and less traumatic to the blood. Further, all cardiac valves can be eliminated completely with the coincidental elimination of many other significant problems such as durability, blood trauma, and thromboembolism with the need for chronic anticoagulation.

Another potential simplification is a concentric TAH utilizing all of the patient's own valves (101). This variation recognizes the fact that the great majority of hearts removed at transplant operations have undamaged valves. These ideas may or may not help solve the remaining problems, but they are illustrative of the fresh approach to the TAH that this writer believes is needed and long overdue.

SUMMARY

Extracorporeal circulation for open heart surgery and even replacement of the heart itself, which all were just dreams 38 years ago, have, after millions of total body perfusions, become standard, widely used, low-risk procedures with immense benefits to humankind.

REFERENCES

(1) Lewis FJ, Taufic M. Closure of atrial septal defects with the aid of hypothermia: experimental accomplishments and the report of one successful case. Surgery 1953;33:52–9.

(2) Bigelow, WG, Callaghan JC, Hopps JA. General hypothermia for experimental intracardiac surgery. Ann Surg 1950;132:531–9.

(3) Swan H, Zeavin I, Blount SG Jr, Virtue RW. Surgery by direct vision in the open heart during hypothermia. JAMA 1953;1081–5.

(4) Lewis JF. Discussion of Bigelow WG, Mustard WT, Evans JG. Some physiologic concepts of hypothermia and their applications to cardiac surgery. J Thorac Surg 1954;28:463–80.

(5) Spreng DS Jr, Nelson DS, et al. Development of a pump-oxygenator to replace the heart and lungs: an apparatus applicable to human patients and application to one case. Ann Surg 1951;134:709–21.

(6) Dennis C. Perspective in review: one group's struggle with development of a pump-oxygenator. Trans Am Soc Artif Intern Organs 1985;31:1–11.

(7) Gibbon JH Jr. Artificial maintenance of circulation during experimental occlusion of pulmonary artery. Arch Surg 1937;34:1105.

(8) Gibbon JH Jr, Miller BJ, Dobell AR, Engell HC, Voight GB. The closure of intraventricular septal defects in dogs during open cardiotomy with the maintenance of the cardiorespiratory functions by a pump oxygenator. J Thorac Surg 1954;28:235–40.

(9) Gibbon JR Jr. Application of a mechanical heart and lung apparatus to cardiac surgery. Minn Med 1954;37:171–85.

(10) Kirklin JW. Open heart surgery at the Mayo Clinic—the 25th anniversary. Mayo Clinic Proc 1980;50:339.

(11) Historic operation. Time 1953 May:70.

(12) Lewis JF, Varco RL, Taufic M. Repair of atrial septal defects in man under direct vision with the aid of hypothermia. Surgery 1954;36:538–56.

(13) Swan H. Discussion of Lewis JF, Varco RL, Taufic M. Repair of atrial septal defects in man under direct vision with the aid of hypothermia. Surgery 1954;36:538–56.

(14) Helmsworth JA, Clark LC Jr, Kaplan S, Sherman RT. An oxygenator pump for use in total bypass of heart and lungs. J Thorac Surg 1953;26:617–31.

(15) Dodrill FD. Discussion of Gibbon JR Jr. Application of a mechanical heart and lung apparatus to cardiac surgery. Minn Med 1954;37:171–85.

(16) Mustard WT, Thomson JA. Clinical experience with the artificial heart lung preparation. J Can Med Assoc 1957;76:265–9.

(17) Clowes GHA Jr, Neville WE, Hopkins A, Anzola J, Simeone A. Factors contributing to the success or failure in the use of a pump oxygenator for complete bypass of the heart and lung, experimental and clinical. Surgery 1954; 36:557–79.

(18) Cohen M, Hammerstrom RW, Spellman MW, Varco RL, Lillehei CW. The tolerance of the canine heart to temporary complete vena caval occlusion. Surg Form 1952;3:172.

(19) Cohen M, Lillehei CW. A quantitative study of the "azygos factor" during vena caval occlusion in the dog. Surg Gynecol Obstet 1954; 98:225.

(20) Andreason AT, Watson F. Experimental cardiovascular surgery. Br J Surg 1952;39:548.

(21) Gibbon JH Jr. The maintenance of life during experimental occlusion of the pulmonary artery followed by survival. Surg Gynecol Obstet 1939;69:602.

(22) Cohen M, Lillehei CW. Autogenous lung oxygenator with total cardiac bypass for intracardiac surgery. Surgical Forum, Clinical Congress of the American College of Surgeons. Philadelphia: WB Saunders & Co., 1953;4:34.

(23) Warden HE, Cohen M, DeWall RA, Schultz EA, Buckley JJ, Read RC, Lillehei CW. Experimental closure of intraventricular septal defects and further physiologic studies on controlled cross circulation. Surg Forum 1954;5:22.

(24) Warden HE, Cohen M, Read RC, Lillehei CW. Controlled cross circulation of open intracardiac surgery. J Thorac Surg 1954;28:331.

(25) Lillehei CW, Cohen M, Warden HE, et al. Direct vision intrafusion for correction of ventricular septal defects, atrioventricularis communis, isolated infundibular pulmonic stenosis, and tetralogy of Fallot. Proceeding of Henry Ford Hospital Symposium. Philadelphia: WB Saunders & Co., 1955:371–392.

(26) Lillehei CW. Controlled cross circulation for direct vision intracardiac surgery correction of ventricular septal defects, atrioventricularis communis, and tetralogy of Fallot. Postgrad Med 1955;17:388.

(27) Lillehei CW, Cohen M, Warden HEE, Varco RL. The direct vision intracardiac correction of congenital anomalies by controlled cross circulation: results in 32 patients with ventricular septal defects, tetralogy of Fallot, and atrioventricular communis defects. Surgery 1955;38:11.

(28) Lillehei CW, Cohen M, Warden HE, et al. Direct vision intracardiac surgical correction of the tetralogy of Fallot, pentalogy of Fallot, and pulmonary atresia defects: report of the first ten cases. Ann Surg 1955;142:418.

(29) Lillehei CW, Cohen M, Warden HE, et al. The results of direct vision closure of ventricular septal defects in eight patients by means of controlled cross circulation. Surg Gynecol Obstet 1955;101:446.

(30) Lillehei CW, Cohen M, Warden HE, Varco RL. Complete anatomical correction of the tetralogy of Fallot defects: report of a successful surgical case. Arch Surg 1956;73:526.

(31) Lillehei CW. A personalized history of extracorporeal circulation. ASAIO 1982;28:5–16.

(32) Lillehei CW, Varco RL, Cohen M, et al. The first open heart repairs of ventricular septal defect, atrioventricular communis, and tetralogy of Fallot using extracorporeal circulation by cross circulation: a 30-year follow-up. Ann Thorac Surg 1986;41:4–21.

(33) Lillehei CW, Varco RL, Cohen M, et al. The first open heart corrections of tetralogy of Fallot. A 26–31 year follow-up of 106 patients. Ann Surg 1986;204:490–502.

(34) Gott VL. C. Walton Lillehei and total correction of tetralogy of Fallot. Ann Thor Surg 1990;49:328–32.

(35) Campbell GS, Crisp NW, Brown EB. Total cardiac bypass in humans utilizing a pump and heterologous lung oxygenator (dog lungs). Surgery 1956;40:364.

(36) Campbell GS, Vernier R, Varco RL, Lillehei CW. Traumatic ventricular septal defect. Report of two cases. J Thorac Surg 1959;37:496.

(37) Mustard WT, Chute AL, Keith JD, Sirek A, Rowe RD, Valad P. A surgical approach to transposition of the great vessels with extracorporeal circuit. Surgery 1954;36:39.

(38) Warden HE, DeWall RA, Read RC, et al. Total cardiac bypass utilizing continuous perfusion from a reservoir of oxygenated blood. Proc Soc Exp Biol Med 1955;90:246–50.

(39) Warden HE, Read RC, DeWall RA, et al. Direct vision intracardiac surgery by means of a reservoir of "arterialized venous" blood. J Thorac Surg 1955;30:649–57.

(40) Jones RE, Donald DE, Swan HJC, Harshbarger HG, Kirklin JW, Wood EH. Apparatus of the Gibbon type for mechanical bypass of the heart and lungs. Proceedings of the staff meetings of the Mayo Clinic 1955 March 23; 30:105.

(41) Donald DE, Harshbarger HG, Hetzel PS, Patrick RT, Wood EH, Kirklin JW. Experiences

with a heart lung bypass (Gibbon type) in the experimental laboratory. Proceedings of the staff meetings of the Mayo Clinic 1955 March 23; 30:113.

(42) Kirklin JW, DuShane JW, Patrick RT, et al. Intracardiac surgery with the aid of a mechanical pump oxygenator system (Gibbon type): report of eight cases. Proceedings of the staff meetings of the Mayo Clinic 1955 May 18; 30:201.

(43) Kirklin JW, McGoon DC, Patrick RT, Theye RT. What is adequate perfusion. In: Moore FD, Morrow AG, Swan H, eds. Extracorporeal circulation. Springfield, IL: Charles C. Thomas, 1958.

(44) Lillehei CW, DeWall RA, Read RC, Warden HE, Varco RL. Direct vision intracardiac surgery in man using a simple, disposable artificial oxygenator. Dis Chest 1956;29:1–8.

(45) DeWall RA, Warden HE, Read RC, et al. A simple, expendable, artificial oxygenator for open heart surgery. Surg Clin North Am 1956;36:1025.

(46) DeWall RA, Warden HE, Gott VL, Read RC, Varco RL, Lillehei CW. Total body perfusion for open cardiotomy utilizing the bubble oxygenator. J Thorac Surg 1956;32:591–603.

(47) DeWall RA, Warden HE, Varco RL, Lillehei CW. The helix reservoir pump-oxygenator. Surg Gynecol Obstet 1957;104:699–710.

(48) Hodges PC, Sellers RD, Story JL, Stanley PH, Torres F, Lillehei CW. The effects of total cardiopulmonary bypass procedures upon cerebral function evaluated by the electroencephalogram and a blood brain barrier test. In: Moore FD, Morrow AG, Swan H, eds. Extracorporeal circulation. Springield, IL: Charles C. Thomas, 1958:279–94.

(49) Gott VL, DeWall RA, Matthias P, Zuhdi MN, Weirich W, Varco RL, Lillehei CW. A self-contained, disposable oxygenator of plastic sheet for intracardiac surgery. Thorax 1957;12:1–9.

(50) Gott VL, Sellers RD, DeWall RA, Varco RL, Lillehei CW. A disposable unitized plastic sheet oxygenator for open heart surgery. Dis Chest 1957;32:615–25.

(51) Lillehei CW, Varco RL, Ferlic RM, Sellers RD. Results in the first 2,500 patients undergoing open heart surgery at the University of Minnesota Medical Center. Surgery 1967;62:819–32.

(52) Cooley DA. Recollections of early development and later trends in cardiac surgery. J Thorac Cardiovasc Surg 1989;98:817–22.

(53) Naef AP. The story of thoracic surgery. Milestones and pioneers. Toronto: Hografe and Huber, 1990:113–9.

(54) Cross FS, Berne RM, Hirsoe Y, Kay EB. Description and evaluation of a rotating disc type reservoir oxygenator. Surg Forum 1956;7:274.

(55) Key EB, Zimmerman HA, Berne RM, Hirose Y, Jones RD, Cross FS. Certain clinical aspects in the use of the pump oxygenator. JAMA 1956; 162:639.

(56) Björk VO. Brain perfusions in dogs with artificially oxygenated blood. Acta Chir Scand 1948;96 (Suppl):137.

(57) Barnhorst DE, Moffitt EA, McGoon DC. Clinical use of the Bentley-Temptrol oxygenator system. In: Ionescu MI, Wooler GH, eds. Current techniques in extracorporeal circulation. London: Butterworths, 1976.

(58) Bartlett RH, Harken DE. Instrumentation for cardiopulmonary bypass—past, present and future. Med Instru 1976;10:119–124.

(59) Rygg IH, Kvvsgaard E. A disposable polyethylene oxygenator system applied in a heart-lung machine. Acta Chir Scand 1956;112:433.

(60) Clark LC Jr, Gollan F, Gupta VB. The oxygenation of blood by gas dispersion. Science 1950;111:85–7.

(61) Craaford CA, Senning A. Utvecklingen av extracorporeal cirkulation med hjart-lungmaskin. Nordisk Med 1956;56:1263.

(62) Clowes GHA Jr, Neville WE. The membrane oxygenator. In: Allen JG, ed. Extracorporeal circulation. Springfield, IL: Charles C. Thomas, 1958:81–100.

(63) Melrose DM. A mechanical heart-lung for use in man. Br Med J 1953;(4827):57–66.

(64) Gerbode F, Osborn JJ, Bramson ML. Experiences in the development of a membrane heart-lung machine. Am J Surg 1967;114:16.

(65) DeWall RA, Grage TB, McFee AS, Chiechi MA. Theme and variations on blood oxygenators. Surgery 1961;50:931–40.

(66) DeWall RA, Grage TB, McFee AS, Chiechi MA. Theme and variation on blood oxygenators. II. Film oxygenators. Surgery 1962;51:251–7.

(67) Kolff WJ, Effler DB, Groves LJ, Peereboom G, Moraca PP. Disposable membrane oxygenator (heart-lung machine) and its use in experimental surgery. Cleveland Clin Q 1956;23:69.

(68) Edmunds LH Jr, Ellison N, Colman RW, et al. Platelet function during cardiac operations. Comparison of membrane and bubble oxygenators. J Thorac Cardiovasc Surg 1982;83:805–12.

(69) Sade RM, Bartles DM, Dearing JP, Campbell LJ, Loadholt CB. A prospective randomized study

of membrane and bubble oxygenators in children. Ann Thorac Surg 1980;29:502–11.

(70) Trumbell HR, Howe J, Mottl K, Nicoloff DM. A comparison of the effects of membrane and bubble oxygenators on platelet counts and platelet size in elective cardiac operations. Ann Thorac Surg 1980;30:52–7.

(71) van den Dungen JJAM, Karlicek GF, Brenken U, Homan van der Heide JN, Wildevuur CRH. Clinical study of blood trauma during perfusion with membrane and bubble oxygenators. J Thorac Cardiovasc Surg 1982;83:108–16.

(72) Van Deveren W, Kazatchkine VDW, Descamps-Latscha B, et al. Deleterious effects of cardiopulmonary bypass. A prospective study of bubble versus membrane oxygenation. J Thorac Cardiovasc Surg 1985;89:888–9.

(73) Boers M, van den Dungen JJAM, Karlicek GF, Brenken U, Homan van der Heide JN, Wildevuur CRH. Two membrane oxygenators and a bubbler. A clinical comparison. Ann Thorac Surg 1983;35:455–62.

(74) Lande AJ, Dos SJ, Carlson RG, et al. A new membrane oxygenator-dialyzer. Surg Clin North Am 1967;47:1461–1470.

(75) DeWall RA, Bentley DJ, Hirose M, Battung V, Najafi H, Roden T. A temperature controlling (omnithermic) disposable bubble oxygenator for total body perfusion. Dis Chest 1966;49:207.

(76) DeWall RA, Najafi H, Roden T. A hard shell temperature controlling disposable blood oxygenator. JAMA 1966;197:1065.

(77) Kalke BR, Castaneda A, Lillehei CW. A clinical evaluation of the new Temptrol (Bentley) disposable blood oxygenator. J Thorac Cardiovasc Surg 1969;57:679.

(78) Aberg T, Kihlgren M, Jonsson L, et al. Improved cerebral protection during open-heart surgery. A psychometric investigation on 339 patients. In: Becker R, et al., eds. Psychopathological and neurological dysfunctions following open-heart surgery. Berlin: Springer-Verlag 1982: 343–51.

(79) Aberg T. Intellectual function late after open-heart operation. Ann Thorac Surg 1983;36: 680–3.

(80) Henriksen L. Evidence suggestive of diffuse brain damage following cardiac operations. Lancet 1984;1:816–20.

(81) Shaw PJ, Bates D, Carlidge NEF, et al. Early neurological complications of coronary artery bypass surgery. Br Med J 1985;291:1384–7.

(82) Arom KV, Cohen DE, Strobl FT. Effect of intraoperative intervention on neurological outcome based on electroencephalographic monitoring during cardiopulmonary bypass. Ann Thorac Surg 1989;48:476–83.

(83) Zuhdi N, McCollough B, Carey J, Krieger K, Greer A. Hypothermic perfusion for open heart surgical procedures—report of the use of a heart lung machine primed with five percent dextrose in water inducing hemodilution. J Int Coll Surg 1961;35:319.

(84) Zuhdi N, McCollough B, Carey J, Krieger K, Greer A. Double helical reservoir heart lung machine designed for hypothermic perfusion primed with five percent glucose in water inducing hemodilution. Arch Surg 1961;82:320.

(85) Zuhdi N. Discussion. J Thorac Cardiovasc Surg 1961;42:827.

(86) DeWall R, Lillehei CW. Simplified total body perfusion reduced flows, moderate hypothermia, and hemodilution. JAMA 1962;179:430.

(87) DeWall R, Lillehei R, Sellers R. Hemodilution perfusions for open heart surgery. N Engl J Med 1962;266:1078.

(88) Lillehei CW. Hemodilution perfusions for open heart surgery. Use of low molecular dextran and 5 percent dextrose. Surgery 1962;52:30–1.

(89) Cuello-Mainardi L, Bhanganada K, Mack JD, Lillehei CW. Hemodilution in extracorporeal circulation: comparative study of low molecular weight dextran and 5 percent dextrose. Surgery 1964;56:349–54.

(90) Long DM Jr, Todd DB, Indeglia RA, Varco RL, Lillehei CW. Clinical use of dextran-40 in extracorporeal circulation—a summary of 5 years experience. Transfusion 1966;6:401–3.

(91) Todd DB, Indeglia RA, Simmons RL, Levy MJ, Lillehei CW. Comparative clinical study of hemolysis and renal function accompanying extracorporeal circulation utilizing hemodilution with different perfusates. Am J Cardiol 1965;15:149.

(92) Nakib A, Lillehei CW. Assessment of different priming solutions for oxygenators by renal blood flow and metabolism. Ann Thorac Surg 1966;2:814–22.

(93) Lillehei CW, Simmons RL, Miller ID, Bonnabeau RC Jr. Role of hemodilution and phenoxybenzamine (dibenzyline) in prevention of renal ischemia during cardiopulmonary bypass. Circulation 1965(Suppl 2);31,32:138.

(94) Todd DB Jr, Indeglia RA, Lillehei RC, Lillehei CW. An analysis of some factors influencing renal function following open heart surgery

utilizing hemodilution and antiadrenergic drugs. Am J Cardiol 1967;19:154.

(95) Rafferty EH, Kletschka HD, Wynyard M, Larkin JT, Smith LV. Cheathem B: Artificial heart: application of nonpulsatile force-vortex principle. Minn Med 1968;51:11.

(96) Lillehei CW, Gott VL, DeWall RA, et al. Surgical correction of pure mitral insufficiency by annuloplasty under direct vision. J Lancet 1957; 77:446–9.

(97) Lillehei CW, Gott VL, DeWall RA, et al. The surgical treatment of stenotic or regurgitant lesions of the mitral and aortic valves by direct vision utilizing a pump oxygenator. J Thorac Surg 1958;35:154–91.

(98) Favaloro RG. Saphenous vein graft in the surgical treatment of coronary artery disease, operative technique. J Thorac Cardiovasc Surg 1969;58:178–85.

(99) Johnson WD, Flemma RS, Lepley D Jr. Direct coronary surgery utilizing multiple-vein bypass grafts. Ann Thorac Surg 1970;9:436–44.

(100) Chiu R, ed. Biomechanical cardiac assist, cardiomyoplasty, and muscle powered devices. Mt. Kisco, NY: Futura Publishers, 1986.

(101) Lande AJ, Frazier OH, Lillehei CW. Concentric heart-TAH utilizing all the patient's own valves. ASAIO (abstracts) 1988;17:16.

3

The Development of Prolonged Extracorporeal Circulation

Robert H. Bartlett, M.D.

The problem that drove John Gibbon to the laboratory in 1932 was massive pulmonary embolism, and his quest was to develop a device for extracorporeal circulation to treat that problem. Sustaining cardiopulmonary function mechanically proved a difficult problem, however, and his goal turned from days to hours, from life support to cardiac surgery. The heart-lung machine described in Chapter 2 that was so successful for short cardiac operations became a lethal device when used for more than a few hours. The toxic manifestations included diffuse capillary leakage, poor perfusion, acidosis, hemolysis, thrombocytopenia, coagulopathy, and progressive organ failure. The toxicity was traced to the artificial lung, and specifically to the direct interface between blood and gas. Gross foaming, macro- and microbubbles, and hemolysis inevitably occurred if the procedure was continued long enough. Protein denaturation was identified by Lee et al. (1) and verified by Dobell et al. (2). The first serious attempts to construct a membrane lung to eliminate this gas interface were reported by Clowes et al. (3), perhaps stimulated by reports from Kolff and Berk (4) that venous blood became oxygenated during its sojourn through a membrane dialyzer. Although Clowes et al. constructed and successfully used a membrane lung for cardiopulmonary bypass (3), the various plastic and cellophane membranes available were almost impervious to respiratory gases so that very large and impractical surface areas were required, and the project was tabled.

In 1957, Kammermeyer synthesized a polymer of dimethypolysiloxane, a plastic that has come to be called "silicone rubber" (5). This remarkable material has the unique characteristic of permeability to gases, including oxygen, carbon dioxide, water vapor, and nitrogen. When prepared as a thin sheet or thin-walled tube and appropriately reinforced with silicates or supporting fabric, the material is strong enough to withstand considerable hydrostatic pressure, yet permit the transfer of ample amounts of respiratory gas, simulating the normal alveolus. Artificial lungs made from silicone rubber membrane were devised and tested by Kolff and Effler (6), Pierce (7), Kolobow and Bowman (8), Lande et al. (9), Day et al. (10), Bramson et al. (11), and others. The oxygen transfer capability of silicone rubber membrane 1 mL thick (0.025 mm) is

12,100 cc $O_2/m^2/min$, and the CO_2 transfer capability is even higher. So it seemed that a device made of 4-mL membrane, for example, would transfer 300 cc $O_2/m^2/min$. However, when the remarkable membrane was fabricated into sheets or channels, the actual oxygen transfer was approximately 30 $cc/m^2/min$, far short of what might have been predicted. It soon became obvious that the reason for this was the limitation imposed by oxygen diffusing through the venous blood and binding to hemoglobin. Several methods designed to narrow the blood path (12) and induce secondary flows by internal spacers (13) or external agitation (14) were tried. Oxygen transfer in an oscillating torus of silicone rubber membrane exceeded 200 $cc/O_2/m^2/min$ (15), but simpler, more practical designs with gas transfer rates in the range of 50 $cc/m^2/min$ proved adequate. The early membrane lungs often leaked and clotted, but these were solvable problems, and attention turned to the feasibility of prolonged extracorporeal circulation itself.

Now, in an era when perfusion runs of two or three weeks are common, it is hard to imagine the excitement that attended a perfusion of 12 or 24 hours in those years. We spoke of maintaining perfusion for one week in terms reserved for as-yet unaccomplished feats such as flying to the moon or transplanting the heart. Looking back, it is surprising how quickly these barriers fell during five years in the late 1960s. After development of membrane artificial lungs, the problems that limited the study of prolonged perfusion were vascular access, bleeding from the animal, clotting in the system, mechanical breakdowns, air embolism, deterioration of the chronically anesthetized animal, and the fatigue of the investigators. As each of these problems was solved, the apparatus and techniques of prolonged extracorporeal circulation evolved. Kolobow et al. demonstrated that the procedure could and should be studied in awake animals (16) (Figure 3.1). They designed vascular access catheters and demonstrated that adequate flow could be obtained through extrathoracic cannulation. Bartlett et al. developed a concept of titrating heparin to a defined clotting time (17). In their experiments, they eliminated reservoirs and stagnant zones and developed a simple method of servoregulating a roller pump, resulting in a tenfold decrease in the usual heparin dose and a system that did not require continuous attendance.

With these modifications in the equipment and technology of cardiopulmonary bypass, it was possible to characterize physiologic (18) and hematologic (19) responses of the normal animal during prolonged extracorporeal circulation. Several investigators (17–19,21) demonstrated that extracorporeal circulation for days was possible without causing significant

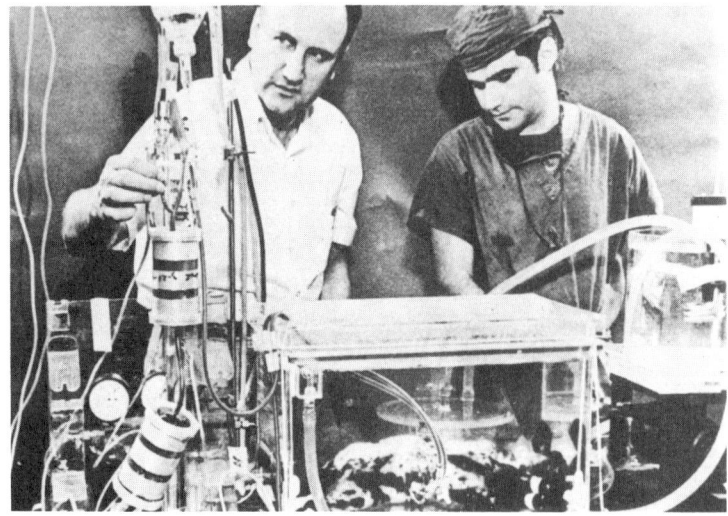

FIGURE 3.1 Theodor Kolobow (left) and Warren Zapol (right) conducting laboratory studies at NIH, 1968.

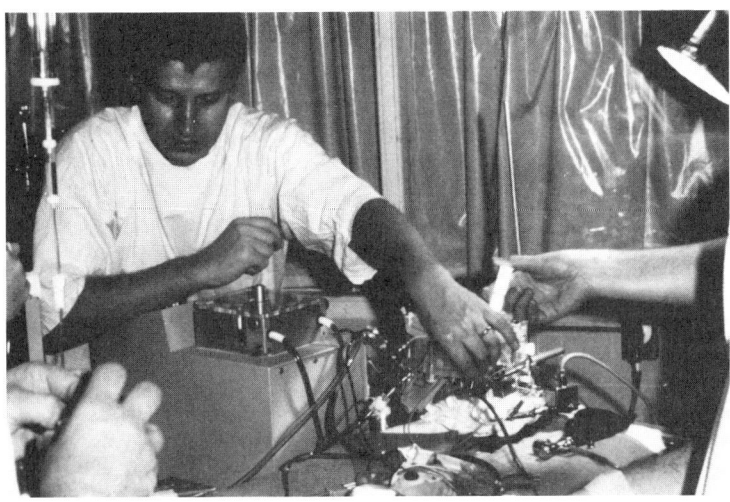

FIGURE 3.2 William Dorson using his umbilical access newborn support system, Phoenix 1969.

injury to normal animals. Hemodynamics were easy to regulate. Acidosis, capillary permeability, and organ deterioration, which often plagued prolonged cardiopulmonary bypass in the operating room, did not occur. Bleeding was minimal with adequate control of heparin. Hemolysis was negligible. Thrombocytopenia inevitably occurred but was manageable (19). All of these studies in the animal laboratory showed that the technique was feasible and provided the background for early clinical trials.

The first attempts at prolonged extracorporeal circulation in humans were by Callaghan et al. (21), Dennis (22), and others (23). The first attempts at respiratory support in infants were reported by Rashkind et al. (24), Dorson et al. (25), and White et al. (26) (Figures 3.2, 3.3). The first successful human

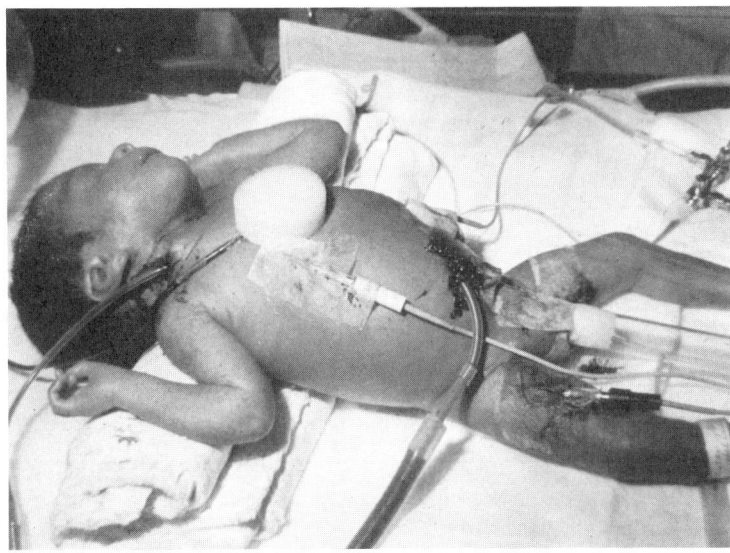

FIGURE 3.3 One of the infants treated by Jack White at Johns Hopkins, 1969. Venovenous access from jugular to umbilical vein was used.

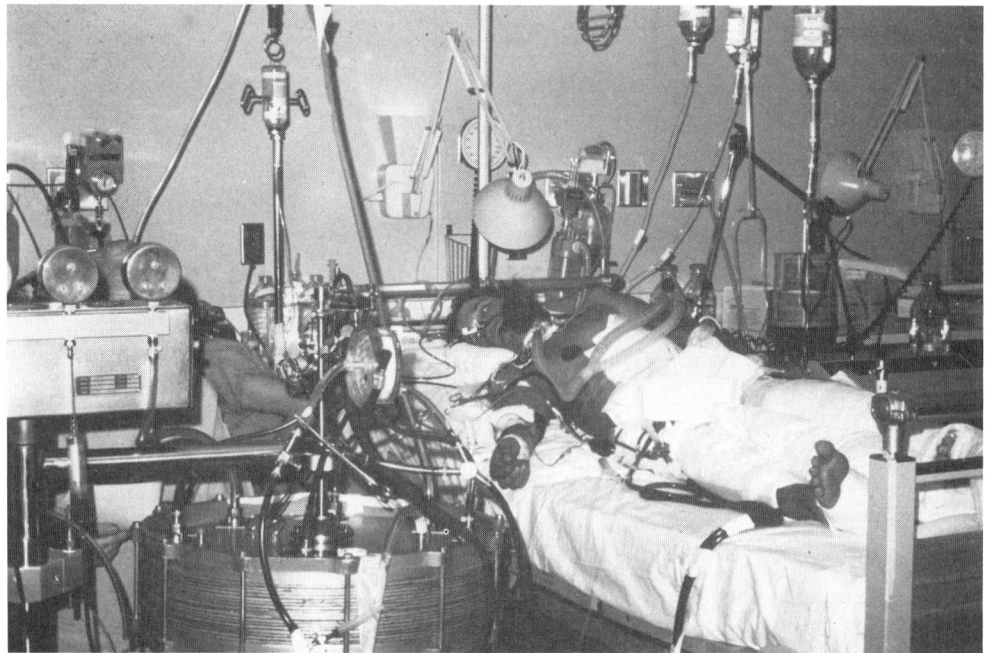

FIGURE 3.4 The first successful extracorporeal life support patient, treated by J. Donald Hill using the Bramson oxygenator (foreground), Santa Barbara, 1971.

case was reported by Hill, O'Brien, and others in 1972 (27). The patient was a young man who sustained a ruptured aorta and other injuries in a motorcycle accident in Santa Barbara, California (Figure 3.4). Don Hill and his team from San Francisco brought the equipment to Santa Barbara and managed the patient on venoarterial extracorporeal life support (ECLS) for three days. Reports of several other successful cases soon followed (28–30). In 1974, the Lung Division of the National Heart and Lung Institute proposed a multicenter prospective randomized study of extracorporeal membrane oxygenation (ECMO) in adult respiratory failure (Figure 3.5). This study began in 1975, a pivotal year for extracorporeal support.

In 1975, a meeting was held outside of Copenhagen that included most of the researchers on prolonged extracorporeal support. This meeting was hosted by Zapol and Qvist, and the proceedings were reported in a benchmark publication (31). The plans for the National Institutes of Health (NIH) ECMO study were reported and reviewed at that meeting (32). Four different membrane oxygenators were manufactured and used in 1975, the Kolobow Sci-Med, the Lande-Edwards, the Pierce-GE, and the Bramson. (The Food and Drug Administration did not become involved with devices until 1976.) The first successful ECMO treatment of a newborn infant was done in May 1975 and reported at the Copenhagen meeting.

NEONATAL RESPIRATORY FAILURE

Bartlett, Gazzaniga, and their colleagues at the University of California, Irvine, treated the first successful neonatal ECMO patient (33) (named "Esperanza" (Hope) by the nurses) (34) (Figure 3.6). This was soon followed by other successful neonatal cases (35). By mid-1980, they had treated 45 newborn cases, with 25 survivors (36). The technique for newborn

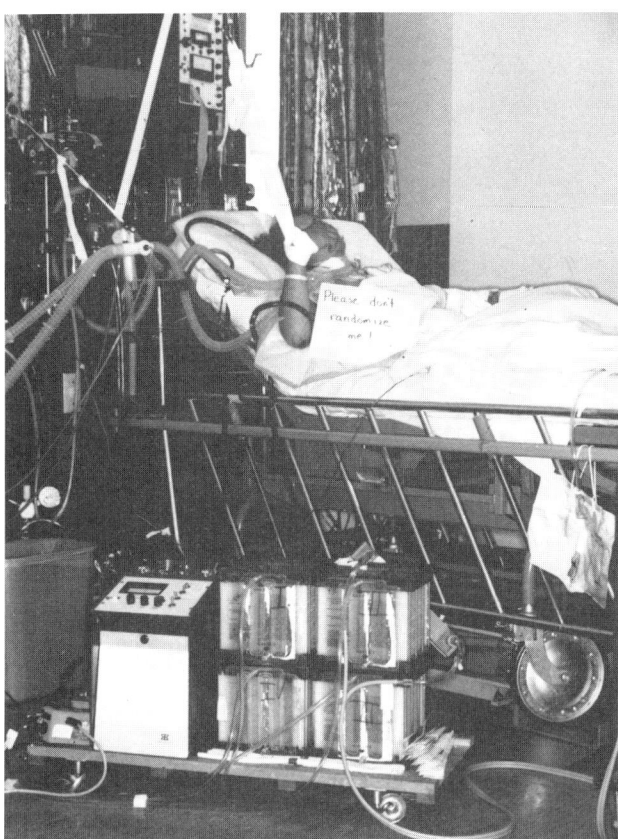

FIGURE 3.5 Adult patient on extracorporeal life support with Lande-Edwards oxygenator. This photograph was prepared for the planning session of the NIH ECMO study with the note "Please don't randomize me." Orange, California, 1974.

infants was fairly standardized, involving venoarterial access via the right internal jugular vein and right carotid artery, heparin titration based on whole blood activated clotting times, "lung rest" at low ventilator settings, and recognition of persistent pulmonary hypertension as the primary underlying pathophysiology. In 1979, the first neonatal ECMO seminar was held at the University of California, Irvine, demonstrating the circuit, the technology, the concept of the ECMO team, and specialists. This led to the development of ECMO research teams at Richmond, Pittsburgh, and Detroit. In 1980, the neonatal ECMO project moved from the University of California, Irvine, to the University of Michigan, and experience gradually increased from a few cases each year to a few cases each month (Figure 3.7). Representatives of other centers attended the annual seminar, and some established ECMO teams, all with a standardized system and protocol. By the end of 1986, 715 newborns had been treated in 18 centers (37), with excellent survival results reported from each center (38–42) (Figure 3.8).

With a standardized technique and an experienced, trained team, the Michigan group carried out a prospective randomized study in newborn infants between 1982 and 1984 (43). They used a statistical technique called randomized play-the-winner, in which assignment to any given treatment is randomized but influenced by all previous patients enrolled in the study (44). Statistical significance is reached when there is a significantly larger group of patients in one arm of the study than in the

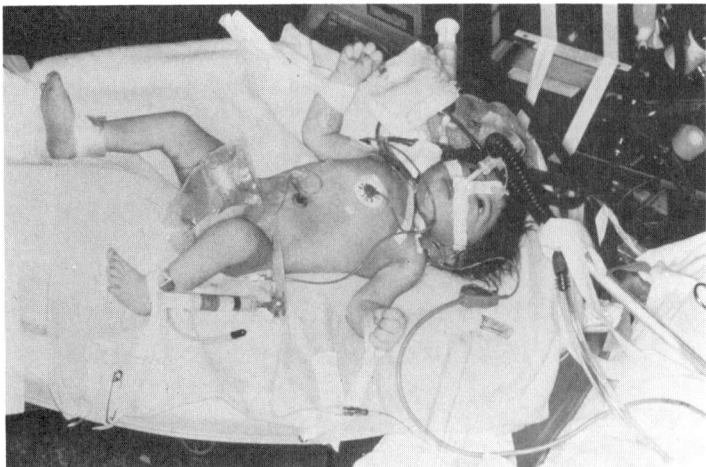

FIGURE 3.6 The first successful neonatal ECMO patient (Esperanza), treated by Bartlett and Gazzaniga at Orange County Medical Center. (A) The patient on ECMO (May 1975) and (B) at age one.

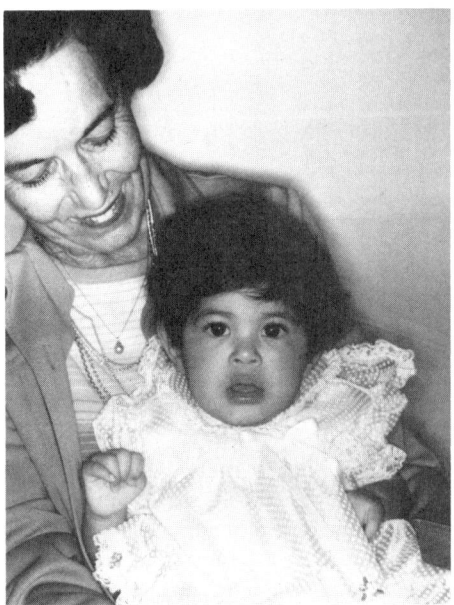

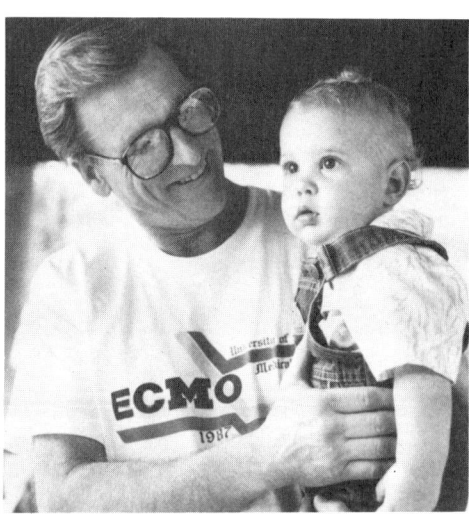

FIGURE 3.7 Robert Bartlett and the University of Michigan team conducted seminars in neonatal ECMO that standardized the technique and established the Registry.

other. This resulted in the unusual groupings of one control patient (who died) and 11 ECMO patients (all of whom survived). This proved that the results with ECMO were better than with conventional therapy, but the study was treated with skepticism (45). The most articulate of the critics—Ware and Epstein (46)—undertook to design a prospective, randomized study of ECMO in neonatal respiratory failure but soon encountered the same problems of ethics and logistics. They solved these problems by using a similar adaptive statistical design and reported their prospective randomized study (with similar results) in 1989 (47).

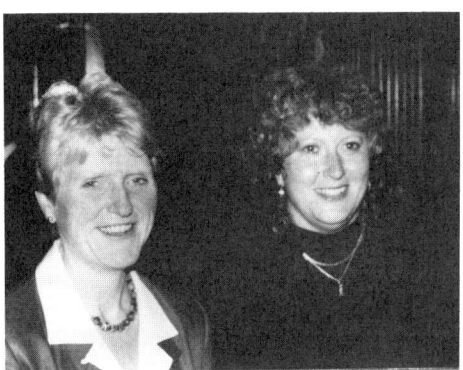

FIGURE 3.8 Pearl O'Rourke (left) and Billie Lou Short (right) were instrumental in introducing ECMO into pediatric intensive care and neonatology.

ADULT RESPIRATORY FAILURE

The NIH-sponsored study of ECMO in adult patients was completed in 1979 and reported in 1980 (48). Other related studies of pathology findings (49) and epidemiology of respiratory failure (50) in the study centers were reported. This was the first attempt at prospective, randomized study of a life support technique in which the end point was death. There were many problems with the study:

1. Nine centers were involved, some of which had no prior experience with ECMO before their first study patient.

2. The logistics of consent to the study tended to exclude the best-risk and worst-risk patients.

3. A nationwide epidemic of influenza pneumonia occurred in 1976, and these patients dominated the trial.

4. Bleeding complications were major, with average blood loss exceeding 2 L/day (51).

5. Although the purpose of ECMO is lung rest, many of the patients were maintained on high ventilator settings (51).

The study was planned for 300 patients, but it was terminated after entry of 92 patients because survival in both the control and ECMO groups was less than 10, and it seemed unlikely that the results would be any different after study of 300 patients. The cause of death was related to technical complications in a significant number of patients, but extensive and apparently irreversible fibrosis was uniformly found at autopsy, indicating that the major problem was not the technology but the underlying parenchymal lung disease (48). As a result of this study, clinical research on ECMO in adult patients essentially stopped in 1979. Since that time, only occasional cases have been reported in the United States, and the study of extracorporeal support in adults proceeded primarily in Europe.

EVOLUTION OF THE CONCEPT OF EXTRACORPOREAL CO_2 REMOVAL

Luciano Gattinoni worked with Kolobow at the NIH, learning the techniques of extracorporeal support in sheep (Figure 3.9). He returned to Milan with these hypotheses:

FIGURE 3.9 Luciano Gattinoni from Milan, Italy, persisted with clinical ECLS research for adult respiratory failure when others gave up. Emphasizing venovenous access, CO_2 removal, and low airway pressure, he reported 50% survival in 1986.

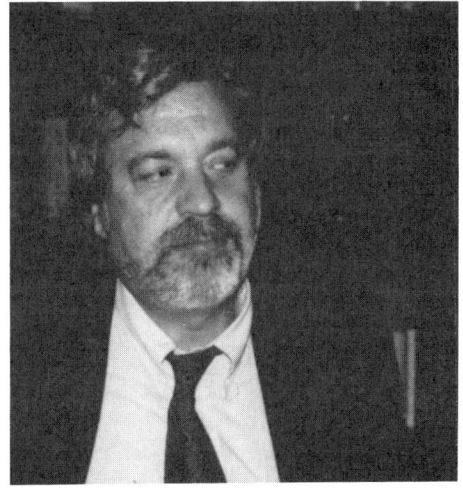

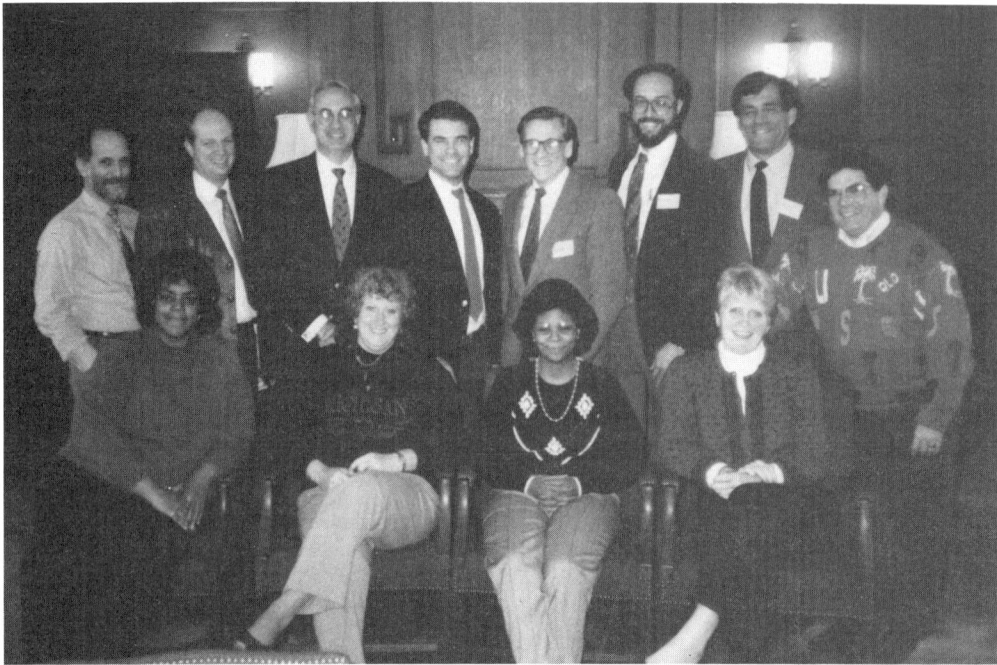

FIGURE 3.10 The Extracorporeal Life Support Organization (ELSO) Steering Committee includes many of the early neonatal ECMO Program Directors. Back row, left to right: Charles Stolar, Devn Cornish, Michael Klein, Fred Ryckman, Robert Bartlett, Martin Keszler, William Kanto, and Robert Arensman. Front row, left to right: Sandy Snedecor (ELSO Registry), Billie L. Short, Phoebe Hankins (ELSO Secretary), and P. Pearl O'Rourke. Larry Cook is absent from the photograph. Ann Arbor, Michigan, 1990.

1. The purpose of ventilation is to excrete CO_2; oxygenation can be achieved by inflation and airway oxygenation alone. Progressive lung injury in adult respiratory distress syndrome is caused in part by ventilator-induced, high-pressure injury of the most normal alveoli. When functional residual capacity is severely decreased, the remaining alveoli can be overinflated if high tidal volumes are used, leading quickly to alveolar injury and fibrosis. An extracorporeal support system should eliminate the need for high airway pressure and high Fio_2, although this was not always done in the NIH-sponsored ECMO study.

2. If the emphasis is on CO_2 removal to eliminate the need for high-pressure ventilation, this could be accomplished with venovenous access using reelatively low flow and large membrane oxygenator surface area. This system would allow for normal pulmonary blood flow, even if the lung were severely injured with large amounts of transpulmonary shunting. The venoarterial bypass used in the NIH ECMO study caused decreased pulmonary blood flow, which might have contributed to microthrombosis or inhibition of lung healing.

Gattinoni and his colleagues used these principles in venovenous extracorporeal gas exchange in a variety of adult patients selected by the same criteria used for the NIH ECMO study. In 1986, they reported 21 survivors in 43 patients (49%) (52). These results were corroborated by Lennartz and colleagues in Marburg (53), Falke and Schulte in Dusseldorf (54), Bindslev in Stockholm (55), and Todd in Toronto (Todd, personal communication, 1988). Similar results were reported by Morioka and Terasaki of Kumamoto (56). All of these investigators reported their results at a European communities conference held at Marburg, Germany, in 1988 (57).

CURRENT STATUS

In 1990, 65 centers used extracorporeal support as routine treatment for severe respiratory failure in newborn infants, and an additional dozen centers used extracorporeal support for adult respiratory failure. With more than 3,000 newborn cases reported, the overall survival rate is 83% (58). The most experienced centers reported survival of greater than 95% (59). Survival in centers treating adult respiratory failure is remarkably constant at 50%. Similar results are reported for support of older children (60,61) and support of patients with primary cardiac disease (62,63). In 1989, the active ECMO centers joined together to form a study group called the Extracorporeal Life Support Organization (Figure 3.10). The purpose of this group is to maintain the data registry, conduct clinical studies on extracorporeal support, and serve as the communication center for research and clinical practice on extracorporeal life support.

The subsequent chapters of this book describe the physiology, techniques, and devices currently used for extracorporeal life support, and applications of this technique to the management of respiratory and cardiac failure.

REFERENCES

(1) Lee WH Jr, Krumhar D, Fonkalsrud EW, et al. Denaturation of plasma proteins as a cause of morbidity and death after intracardiac operations. Surgery 1961;50:29.

(2) Dobel ARC, Mitri M, Galva R, et al. Biological evaluation of blood after prolonged recirculation through film and membrane oxygenators. Ann Surg 1965;161:617–22.

(3) Clowes GHA Jr, Hopkins AL, Neville WE. An artificial lung dependent upon diffusion of oxygen and carbon dioxide through plastic membranes. J Thorac Surg 1956;32:630–7.

(4) Kolff WJ, Berk HT Jr. Artificial kidney: a dialyzer with a great area. Acta Med Scand 1944;117:121.

(5) Kammermeyer K. Silicone rubber as a selective barrier. Ind Eng Chem 1957;49:1685.

(6) Kolff WJ, Effler DB. Disposable membrane oxygenator (heart lung machine) and its use in experimental and clinical surgery while the heart is arrested with potassium citrate according to the Melrose technique. Trans ASAIO 1956;2:13–21.

(7) Pierce EC II. Modification of the Clowes membrane lung. J Thorac Cardiovasc Surg 1960;39:438.

(8) Kolobow T, Bowman RL. Construction and evaluation of an alveolar membrane artificial heart lung. Trans ASAIO 1963;9:238.

(9) Lande AJ, Dos SJ, Carlson RG, et al. A new membrane oxygenator-dialyzer. Surg Clin North Am 1967;47:1461–70.

(10) Day SW, Crystal DK, Wagner CL, et al. Properties of synthetic membranes in extracorporeal circuits. Am J Surg 1967;114:314–9.

(11) Bramsom ML, Osborn JJ, Main FB, et al. A new disposable membrane oxygenator with integral heat exchanger. J Thorac Cardiovasc Surg 1965;50:391.

(12) Drinker PA. Progress in membrane oxygenator design. Anesthesiology 1972;37:242.

(13) Bellhouse BJ, Bellhouse FH, Curl CM, et al. A high efficiency membrane oxygenator and pulsatile pumping system, and its application to animal trials. Trans ASAIO 1973;19:72.

(14) Bartlett RH, Drinker PA, Burns NE, Fong SW, Hyans T. The toroidal membrane oxygenator: design, performance and bypass testing of a clinical model. Trans ASAIO 1972;18:369–73.

(15) Drinker PA, Bartlett RH, Bialer R, et al. Augmentation of membrane gas transfer by oscillation of a coiled tube. Surgery 1969;66:774.

(16) Kolobow T, Zapol W, Pierce JE, et al. Partial extracorporeal gas exchange in alert new born lambs with a membrane artificial lung perfused via an AV shunt for periods up to 96 hours. Trans ASAIO 1968;14:328.

(17) Bartlett RH, Isherwood J, Moss RA, Olszewski WL, Polet H, Drinker PA. A toroidal flow membrane oxygenator: four day partial bypass in dogs. Surg Forum 1969;20:152–3.

(18) Bartlett RH, Burns NE, Fong SW, Gazzaniga AB, Achauer BM, Fraille J. Prolonged partial venoarterial bypass: physiologic, biochemical, and hematologic responses. Surg Forum 1972;23: 178–80.

(19) Fong SW, Burns NE, Williams G, Woldanski C, Gazzaniga AB, Bartlett RH. Changes in coagulation and platelet function during prolonged extracorporeal circulation (ECC) in sheep and man. Trans ASAIO 1974;20:239–46.

(20) Lande AJ, Fillmore SJ, Subramanian V, et al. 24 hour venoarterial perfusions of awake dogs with a simple membrane oxygenator. Trans ASAIO 1969;15:181.

(21) Callaghan JC, Maynes EA, Hug HR. Studies in lambs of the development of an artificial placenta. Review of nine long-term survivors of extracorporeal circulation maintained in a fluid medium. Can J Surg 1965;8:208–13.

(22) Dennis C. Certain methods for artificial support of the circulation during intracardiac surgery. Surg Clin North Am 1956;36:423.

(23) Hill JD, Bramson ML, Rapaport E, et al. Experimental and clinical experiences with prolonged oxygenation and assisted circulation. Ann Surg 1969;170:448.

(24) Rashkind WJ, Freeman A, Klein D, et al. Evaluation of a disposable plastic, low volume, pumpless oxygenator as a lung substitute. J Pediatr 1965;66:94–102.

(25) Dorson W Jr, Meyer B, Baker E, et al. Response of distressed infants to partial bypass lung assist. Trans ASAIO 1970;16:345.

(26) White JJ, Andrews HG, Risemberg H, et al. Prolonged respiratory support in newborn infants with a membrane oxygenator. Surgery 1971;70: 288–96.

(27) Hill D, O'Brien TG, Murray JJ, et al. Extracorporeal oxygenation for acute post-traumatic respiratory failure (shock-lung syndrome): use of the Bramson Membrane Lung. N Engl J Med 1972;286:629–34.

(28) Schulte HD. Membrane oxygenators in prolonged assisted extracorporeal circulation. Dtsch Med Wochenschr 1973;98:508.

(29) Geelhoed GW, Adkins PC, Corso PJ, Joseph WL. Clinical effects of membrane lung support for acute respiratory failure. Ann Thorac Surg 1975;20:177–86.

(30) Gille JP, Bagniewski AM. Ten years of use of extracorporeal membrane oxygenation (ECMO) in the treatment of acute respiratory insufficiency (ARI). Trans ASAIO 1976;22:102.

(31) Zapol WM, Qvist J, eds. Artificial lungs for acute respiratory failure. New York: Academic Press, 1976.

(32) Blake LH. Goals and progress of the NHLI collaborative ECMO study. In: Zapol W, Qvist J, eds. Artificial lungs for acute respiratory failure. New York: Academic Press, 1976.

(33) Bartlett RH, Gazzaniga AB, Jefferies R, Huxtable RF, Haiduc N, Fong SW. Extracorporeal membrane oxygenation (ECMO) cardiopulmonary support in infancy. Trans ASAIO 1976;22:80–8.

(34) Bartlett RH. Esperanza (ASAIO Presidential Address). Trans ASAIO 1985;30:723–5.

(35) Bartlett RH, Gazzaniga AB, Huxtable RF, Schippers HC, O'Connor MJ, Jefferies MR. Extracorporeal circulation (ECMO) in neonatal respiratory failure. J Thorac Cardiovasc Surg 1977;74:826–33.

(36) Bartlett RH, Andrews AF, Toomasian JM, Haiduc NJ, Gazzaniga AB. Extracorporeal membrane oxygenation (ECMO) in neonatal respiratory failure: 45 cases. Surgery 1982;92:425–53.

(37) Toomasian JM, Snedecor SM, Cornell R, Cilley RE, Bartlett RH. National experience with extracorporeal membrane oxygenation (ECMO) for newborn respiratory failure: data from 715 cases. Trans ASAIO 1988;34:140–7.

(38) Krummel TM, Greenfield LJ, Kirkpatrick BV, et al. Clinical use of an extracorporeal membrane oxygenator in neonatal pulmonary failure. J Pediatr Surg 1982;17:525–31.

(39) Hardesty RL, Griffith BP, Debski RF, et al. Extracorporeal membrane oxygenation: successful treatment of persistent fetal circulation following repair of congenital diaphragmatic hernia. J Thorac Cardiovasc Surg 1981;81:556–63.

(40) Short BL, Pearson GD. Neonatal extracorporeal membrane oxygenation: a review. J Intens Care Med 1986;1:47–54.

(41) Loe W, Grave E, Ochsner J et al. Extracorporeal membrane oxygenation for newborn respiratory failure. J Pediatr Surg 1985;20:684–8.

(42) Weber TR, Pennington DG, Connors R, et al. Extracorporeal membrane oxygenation for newborn respiratory failure. Ann Thorac Surg 1986;42;529–35.

(43) Bartlett RH, Roloff DW, Cornell RG, Andrews AF, Dillon PW, Zwischenberger AB. Extracorporeal circulation in neonatal respiratory failure: a prospective randomized study. Pediatrics 1985;4:479–87.

(44) Cornell RG, Landenberger BD, Bartlett RH. Randomized play-the-winner clinical trials. Communications in Statistics: Theory and Methods 1986;1:159–78.

(45) Meinert CL. Extracorporeal membrane oxygenation trials (commentaries). Pediatrics 1990; 85:365–6.

(46) Ware JH, Epstein MF. Extracorporeal circulation in respiratory failure (commentaries). Pediatrics 1985;76:849–51.

(47) O'Rourke PP, Krone R, Vacanti J, et al. Extracorporeal membrane oxygenation and conventional medical therapy in neonates with persistent pulmonary hypertension of the newborn: a prospective randomized study. Pediatrics 1989; 84:957–63.

(48) Zapol WM, Snider MT, Hill JD, et al. Extracorporeal membrane oxygenation in severe respiratory failure. JAMA 1979;242:2193–6.

(49) Pratt PC, Vollmer RT, Shelburn JD, Cramp JD. Pulmonary morphology in a multihospital collaborative extracorporeal membrane oxygenation project. Am J Pathol 1979;95:191–212.

(50) Bartlett RH, Morris AH, Fairley HB, et al. A prospective study of acute hypoxic respiratory failure. Chest 1986;5:684–9.

(51) NHLI-NIH. Extracorporeal support for respiratory insufficiency. Washington, D.C.: DHEW Publication, 1980.

(52) Gattinoni L, Presenti A, Mascheroni D, et al. Low frequency positive pressure ventilation with extracorporeal CO_2 removal in severe acute respiratory failure. JAMA 1986;256:881–5.

(53) Knoch M. Treatment of severe ARDS with extracorporeal CO_2 removal. In: Gille JP, ed. Neonatal and adult respiratory failure. Paris: Elsevier, 1989.

(54) Falke K, Schulte HD. Extracorporal CO_2 elimination mit niedrigfrequenter beatmung zur behandlung des schwern akuten wengenversagens. Dtsch Med Wochenschr 1985;110:663–4.

(55) Bindslev L. Extracorporeal circulation using surface heparinized equipment. In: Gille JP, ed. Neonatal and adult respiratory failure. Paris: Elsevier, 1989.

(56) Morioka T, Terasaki H. Present status of extracorporeal lung assist (ECLA as ECMO or extracorporeal CO_2 removal) in Japan. In: Gille JP, ed. Neonatal and adult respiratory failure. Paris: Elsevier, 1989.

(57) Bartlett RH. Extracorporeal life support in neonatal respiratory failure. In: Gille JP, ed. Neonatal and adult respiratory failure. Paris: Elsevier, 1989.

(58) ECMO Data Registry. Ann Arbor, Michigan: University of Michigan, 1990.

(59) Bartlett RH, Gazzaniga AB, Toomasian JM, Roloff DW, Rucker R, Coran AG. Extracorporeal membrane oxygenation (ECMO) in neonatal respiratory failure: 100 cases. Ann Surg 1986; 204:36–45.

(60) Anderson HL, Attorri RJ, Custer JR, Chapman RA, Bartlett RH. Extracorporeal membrane oxygenation (ECMO) for pediatric cardiopulmonary failure. J Thorac Cardiovasc Surg 1990; 99:1011–9.

(61) Redmond CR, Graves ED, Falterman KW, et al. Extracorporeal membrane oxygenation for respiratory and cardiac failure in infants and children. J Thorac Cardiovasc Surg 1987;93: 199–204.

(62) Kanter KR, Pennington DG, Weber TG, et al. Extracorporeal membrane oxygenation for postoperative cardiac failure in children. J Thorac Cardiovasc Surg 1987;93:27–35.

(63) Klein MD, Arensman RM, Weber TR, et al. Pediatric ECMO: directions for new developments. Trans ASAIO 1988;34:978–85.

4

Clinical Studies of Neonatal ECMO

P. Pearl O'Rourke, M.D.

HISTORY OF ECMO

The modern history of extracorporeal membrane oxygenation (ECMO) began with the development of the bubble or disk oxygenator for cardiopulmonary bypass in the 1950s. These oxygenators effected oxygenation by directly mixing blood and oxygen in a common chamber. While effective, the direct physical interface of blood and gas produced enough hemolysis to limit the feasibility of this technology for long-term clinical support (1).

In 1956, Clowes and associates (2) described the first membrane oxygenator with a semipermeable membrane separating the blood and gas phases. This development made long-term extracorporeal support a possibility. Approximately 20 years later, the first patients with acute respiratory failure (ARF) were clinically supported with ECMO (3). The initial focus was the adult population. By the mid-1970s, anecdotal patient series reported modest results, with approximately 15% survival; despite the high mortality, the individual successes were dramatic (4,5).

After these initial reports, the question of the efficacy of ECMO for adults with ARF was formally addressed in a multicenter trial supported by the National Institutes of Health (NIH) (6). This prospective randomized study failed to show any difference between ECMO and conventional mechanical ventilation (CMV), with survival rates of 9.5% and 8.3%, respectively. A number of possible explanations for this unexpected ECMO failure were cited: 1) the heterogeneity of the population, 2) the possibility that patients already had irreversible lung disease at the time of randomization, and 3) the fact that, in this study, the lungs continued to be exposed to high levels of oxygen and inflating pressures. This study immediately extinguished clinical interest in ECMO for many centers and many clinical investigators.

At the time that the NIH study was published, a number of neonatal ECMO trials had been reported. In 1969, Dorson et al. (7) described a system of partial venoarterial (VA) bypass for infants, using the umbilical vessels for access. In 1970, Dorson applied this technology to five infants who were judged to have terminal respiratory failure. These infants also had preexistent evidence of internal bleeding. ECMO was used for 5 to 21 hours. Although all the infants died, during bypass there was improved gas exchange as well as cardiovascular function. Cannula-related problems proved the greatest technical difficulty.

White et al. (8) reported in 1971 the use of venovenous ECMO in three premature infants (28, 30, and 32 weeks' gestation) with respiratory failure. Oxygenation and ventilation were successfully supported in each infant, but all died secondary to central nervous system (CNS) hemorrhage occurring at 2, 3, and 10 days. In 1975, Bartlett et al. (9) reported the first survivor of neonatal ECMO. This was immediately followed by further successful reports of neonatal ECMO support (10,11). Thus, the present era of neonatal ECMO began.

NEONATAL ECMO

There are a number of obvious differences between potential adult and neonatal ECMO patients. Adults supported with ECMO often have ARF from a destructive primary lung disease or from adult respiratory distress syndrome (ARDS), which, in severe cases, results in parenchymal obliteration (12). In contrast, neonatal ARF is usually secondary to an abnormality of the pulmonary vascular bed, immaturity of the surfactant system, or, as in meconium aspiration syndrome, a chemical pneumonitis with small airway obstruction (13). It is unusual for a neonate to have a primary destructive pulmonary process. This gives the neonate a higher likelihood of having reversible lung disease. But despite this advantage, neonates as well as adults can develop secondary lung damage associated with barotrauma and elevated levels of FiO_2. In fact, these iatrogenic complications may be exaggerated in the hypoplastic or immature lung. While this secondary lung injury begins immediately with ventilator exposure, the severity of damage appears to be related to the duration of exposure (14,15). In the multicenter adult study, it was suggested that patients already had severe, irreversible lung damage either from their primary disease or secondary to ventilator management at the time they met study entry criteria. It became obvious that it would be important to try to identify patients earlier in the course of disease and possible therapy before secondary damage occurs. Fortunately, the natural history of neonatal respiratory failure usually makes it possible to identify infants with increased mortality risk within the first days of life, before major ventilator toxicity is incurred. The final difference in the neonatal ECMO experience was the early and almost exclusive use of venoarterial ECMO, which achieved enough blood flow to support adequate gas exchange without necessitating exposure of the lungs to continued aggressive ventilator management.

PHASE I: SAFETY AND EFFICACY STUDIES

Each of these factors predisposed to the relative success of neonatal ECMO. After a number of scattered case reports, the first series of neonatal patients was published by Bartlett et al. in 1982 (16) as a Phase I study evaluating the safety and efficacy of ECMO support. An experience of ECMO support in 45 infants from 1974–1982 was reported. The patient population was broad, with gestational ages of 27–44 weeks and birthweights of 1–5.2 kg. The investigators tried to identify patients with a less than 10% chance of survival by using the Neonatal Pulmonary Insufficiency Index (NPII) in the first 24 hours or the attending neonatologist's clinical judgment that the patient was "about to die" with routine management. Patient diseases included respiratory distress syndrome (RDS), meconium aspiration syndrome (MAS), or persistent pulmonary hypertension of the neonate (PPHN), and sepsis. The overall survival was 56%. (Broken down by diagnosis, survival was as follows: RDS 43%, MAS 68%, PPHN 60%, sepsis 25%.) Survival was dramatically improved over the anticipated survival of 10%. The conclusion was made that ECMO was effective and had improved benefit over conventional management.

In Bartlett's Phase I Study, the infants were also evaluated for morbidity. Sixteen (35%) of the infants had intracranial bleeding; 15 of these children died. Twenty (80%) of the survivors were normal. This was compared to historical groups of infants treated conventionally: 4% to 38% developed chronic lung disease, and up to 60% had evidence of intracranial hemorrhage at autopsy. The authors expanded their conclusion by stating that ECMO resulted in reduced morbidity (16).

The premature infants who were supported with ECMO had much higher morbidity and mortality. Technical problems with the circuit and intracranial bleeding were common. Because of these initial observations, prematurity was considered an exclusion criteria for ECMO support. Subsequent ECMO experience has been limited to infants 34 weeks' gestational age or older.

Neonatal ECMO received further support with reports from the Medical College of Virginia and the University of Pittsburgh. In 1983, Kirkpatrick et al. (17,18) reported eight term infants who were supported with VA ECMO at the Medical College of Virginia. These infants were selected for ECMO when they fulfilled the institutional criteria for 100% predicted mortality with an $AaDo_2$ greater than 620 mm Hg for 6 to 12 hours. In this series, six infants survived, for a 75% survival rate. Trento et al. (19) described the Pittsburgh ECMO experience between 1981 and 1985. Thirty-three infants were supported; 18 (54%) survived. These reports encouraged the development of ECMO services at other institutions. By the end of 1984, nine centers in the United States offered ECMO to neonates. The cumulative experience of these centers was reported by Short and Pearson in 1985 (5): 221 neonates had been supported with ECMO; 143 (54.7%) survived. These early data functionally represented two patient populations. At most institutions, the first ECMO patients commonly were moribund and received ECMO as rescue therapy, often after sustaining cardiac arrests and requiring aggressive resuscitation. Once ECMO technology was better understood and each institution gained experience and confidence, the rescue approach was changed to identify patients before they were moribund. Clinicians then started to offer ECMO support when infants met criteria for 80% predicted mortality. Since 1984, there has been dramatic growth in the number of ECMO centers, with 62 active centers identified today.

NEONATAL ECMO REGISTRY DATA

A very important aspect of the growth of neonatal ECMO is the fact that the national experience has been collected continuously in the Neonatal ECMO Registry. This registry was created for the purpose of capturing the ECMO experience and hence being able to track growth, success, or failure. While the Registry has the strength of numbers, it also has significant limitations. Registry reporting is voluntary, and the only incentive for participation is the shared appreciation for an accurate date base. Fortunately, most, if not all, ECMO centers in the United States now participate. Another limitation lies in the fact that the Registry includes different institutions and hence reflects different ECMO learning curves, different modes of conventional support, and different criteria for predicted mortality. This results in a very heterogeneous population. In 1988, Toomasian et al. (20) reported the first formal review of the Registry. A total of 715 infants treated at 18 centers between 1980 and 1987 were included. These infants met their own institutional criteria for 80% predicted mortality. With ECMO support, 81% survived. Stratification of this population by disease is given in Table 4.1.

A number of conclusions could be made from this review. While ECMO resulted in an

TABLE 4.1   National ECMO Registry (1987) (20)

Primary diagnosis	Total	Survivors	% Survived
MAS	310	281	91
RDS	96	75	78
CDH	121	78	65
Sepsis	64	46	72
PPHN	100	84	84
Other	24	15	63
Total	715	579	81

excellent survival rate for the entire group, the survival rate was a function of the primary diagnosis. Infants with MAS or PPHN enjoyed the highest survival rate. By comparison, infants with congenital diaphragmatic hernia (CDH) had a much lower survival. Infants with CDH have always been problematic. Their associated lung hypoplasia and dysplasia automatically assign them to a higher mortality group. For this reason, many ECMO centers feel that infants with CDH should be considered separately from other neonates.

There were some interesting characteristics of the ECMO population. Only 7% were inborn infants treated primarily at the reporting hospital, whereas 93% were outborn patients referred specifically for ECMO. This number of outborn patients is probably artificially high, because many ECMO centers are children's hospitals with no inborn population; nonetheless, this suggests that conventional ventilator management of respiratory failure was good for inborn patients at the ECMO centers. These observations place in focus the need for improved perinatal and conventional respiratory care in referral hospitals.

This Registry review also emphasized the importance of the learning curve in ECMO. The patient data were analyzed to see if outcome improved with technologic experience. Survival of the first 10 patients at all centers was 73.5%, compared to an 83.7% survival if the first 10 patients were excluded. This difference could not be explained by any differences in pre-ECMO characteristics among these patients. Of note, the first 10 patients had a higher incidence of complications (2.26/patient) compared with patients studied later (1.6/patient). The Registry is not specifically designed to capture follow-up data, but it appears that 10% to 25% of patients suffer some neurologic injury, and 5% to 10% have some degree of chronic lung disease. Currently, there are 2,900 neonates in the Registry; disease stratification and survival results are similar to the 1988 report (Table 4.2) (21).

Proponents of ECMO use the Registry data to support the efficacy of ECMO support in the neonatal population. Opponents state that survival rates generated from the Registry data are difficult to interpret because true mortality with conventional support is unknown in this population. The criticism of historical control data for predicting mortality has been one of the major hurdles preventing ECMO from gaining acceptance as standard care. Without a concomitant control population, it is virtually impossible to corroborate any formulated predictors. Nonbelievers state that conventional care is changing so rapidly that predictors formulated from historical populations may be meaningless when applied prospectively.

TABLE 4.2 National Neonatal ECMO Registry (1989), University of Michigan, Ann Arbor, Michigan

Primary diagnosis	Total	Survivors	% Survived
MAS	1,161	1,069	92
RDS	444	364	82
CDH	465	293	63
Sepsis	337	260	77
PPHN	419	365	87
Other	120	85	71
Total	2,946	2,436	82.6

Mortality Prediction

It is important to understand the specific methods that have been used to predict mortality. The most simplistic approach, now used infrequently, is the purely clinical assessment that the patient is "about to die." This is obviously fraught with observer bias. The criteria used most commonly are the oxygenation index (OI) (22) and the Washington, D.C., criteria (23), which use the $AaDo_2$ in conjunction with time and peak airway pressure.

The OI is calculated by the following formula:

$$\frac{(Fio_2) \cdot (\text{Mean airway pressure}) \times 100}{Pao_2}$$

Various institutions have applied the OI to control populations in order to identify what value predicts mortality at 50%, 80%, or 100% levels. A commonly used OI value for 80% predicted mortality is 40, but the importance of tailoring the OI to one's own institution has been emphasized repeatedly.

The Washington, D.C., criteria (23) were compiled from a retrospective analysis of 30 infants with PPHN. The investigators found the following criteria to be retrospectively predictive:

$AaDo_2 \geq 610$ for 8 hours

or

Peak inspiratory pressure ≥ 38 cm H_2O plus $AaDo_2$ 605 for 4 hours

Again, the authors stated that these criteria were not universally applicable and that if other centers wanted to use them, a review should be completed at their own institution to test accuracy among their own patients. Despite these disclaimers and warnings, non-ECMO centers have prospectively applied these criteria to their own patients and have found that, rather than identifying an 80% mortality group, in fact, the true mortality may be as low as 10% (24,25).

Criticisms of patient selection are valid. The only way to absolutely prove or disprove ECMO efficacy would be to complete a prospective, randomized, controlled study comparing ECMO and CMV, accepting survival or death as the endpoints for each arm. To date, there have been two such studies. The difficulties associated with each were immense.

PHASE II: RANDOMIZED STUDIES

The Phase II study by Bartlett and associates (26), published in 1985, was the first randomized neonatal ECMO study. This study was proposed in an institution in which ECMO was already accepted as state-of-the-art therapy. Because of this bias, the investigators were unwilling to expose a large number of neonates to death on a conventional therapy limb for the purpose of completing a standard, randomized study. To accommodate this bias, an alternate statistical method, "play-the-winner," was used. The randomization regimen of play-the-winner affords the first patient a 50:50 randomization; every subsequent patient then has odds that favor assignment to the better therapy as determined by the previous patient experience. Patients in this study weighed more than 2 kg and had an 80% predicted mortality based on one of the following general categories: 1) acute deterioration, unresponsiveness to maximal therapy, barotrauma, CDH; and 2) unresponsiveness to maximal therapy, or a neonatal pulmonary insufficiency index (NPII) with a greater than 80% mortality. Twelve patients were randomized into the study. Eleven received ECMO and survived; one received conventional ventilation and died. Statistically, these results met significance, but ECMO critics were not convinced, stating that one patient in the CMV group was not reasonable comparison to a therapy group of 11.

An editorial (27) accompanying this study stated an appreciation for the ethical dilemma of clinical trials in critically ill patients with a potentially high mortality, but criticized the statistical design. The play-the-winner adaptive design was problematic in that it allowed extremely unbalanced patient allocation by altering the odds disproportionately in response to the first few patients treated. In addition, the use of a selective or ranking paradigm rather than the more usual hypothesis-testing paradigm was also criticized. The selection (ranking) paradigm preferentially ensures the selection of the superior therapy, resulting in a high false-positive rate. Finally, the need for data supporting the 90% predicted mortality rate was discussed. In summary, the editorial stated that this study raised interesting ethical and statistical design questions but failed to offer more than suggestive evidence that ECMO might be superior therapy.

A second prospective, randomized study was done at the Children's Hospital, Boston (CHB) (28). An adaptive design was chosen for this trial, again for the purposes of expeditious study completion and minimization of patient deaths. The selected design guaranteed a more even patient allocation than the previous study by Bartlett. The design had two phases. The first phase had 50:50 randomization, and ended when there were four deaths in either of the two arms. Phase II then started. In this phase, randomization ceased, and all patients were assigned to the "better" arm. Two potential endpoints were identified. If there were no differences between these two therapies, a fourth death would be expected in the second arm before a statistical difference in number of survivors could be demonstrated. In contrast, if one therapy were superior, the number of survivors would be statistically greater in the better arm before four deaths occurred. Patients in this study were 38 weeks' gestational age or older and had PPHN as documented by pre- and postductal differences, right-to-left shunt via echocardiogram, or both. All patients had an 80% predicted mortality by retrospective chart review. The accuracy of the predicted mortality would be tested by the outcome of the control group. The results are given in Table 4.3. The study supported ECMO as better therapy ($p = 0.05$). The study also presented the difficulty of predicting mortality using historical controls. While 80% predicted mortality was sought, the true mortality in a small number of patients was only 40%. Criticisms of this study include its atypical design and its definition of conventional management, which included aggressive hyperventilation and the use of muscle relaxants. While this was standard therapy at CHB, there is no universally accepted definition of CMV.

Despite the limitations of these two prospective studies, the future for further randomized trials is uncertain. Accepting death as a final outcome is ethically difficult in the face of an increasingly positive neonatal ECMO experience and its growing national acceptance; without concurrent control populations, the dilemmas of accurately predicting mortality and defining optimal CMV will remain.

The concerns regarding conventional treatment of infants with PPHN deserve further discussion. There are currently several approaches to ventilator management of these patients. Aggressive ventilation, with the goal of pulmonary vasodilation with induced respiratory alkalosis and relative hyperoxia, has been, and continues to be, considered the standard of care by many neonatologists. The downside of this approach is the fact that infants' lungs are exposed to elevated airway pressures and Fio_2. In addition, muscle relaxants are often required. A more conservative form of pulmonary support has been offered as an alternate approach. In this mode, hyperoxia and hypocarbia are not goals, hyperventilation is not used, and hence the patients' exposure to elevated airway pressures and Fio_2 is minimized (29). The success of this therapy in infants with PPHN has been reported. Wung et al. (29) treated 15 infants with PPHN having conservative support. All infants survived, and only one developed chronic lung disease. These results were presented as being superior to those achieved with aggressive management. The argument is thus made that if conservative management were better understood and applied, the death rate for PPHN would be lower and the need for ECMO miniscule.

CURRENT STATUS OF NEONATAL ECMO

The present status of neonatal ECMO can best be described as controversial and changing. The national experience has steadily grown over the past six years. The results of that experience suggest a very high survival rate. Short- and long-term follow-up studies suggest an acceptable morbidity. But like so many therapies for critically ill patients, despite a few prospective randomized trials, ECMO has not undergone the rigors of a large conventional, randomized study to prove or disprove its efficacy. In addition, the problems of defining the "best" CMV and identifying appropriate selection criteria continue to plague ECMO clinicians. While none of these problems has been forgotten, despite the lack of resolution, ECMO is expanding and this expansion raises new questions.

The growing clinical ECMO experience has had a number of effects. One has been the dramatic growth of ECMO centers. In 1984,

TABLE 4.3 Survival experience of patients randomized to ECMO and to conventional therapy (CMV) during Phase I, the randomized phase of the trial, and Phase II, the nonrandomized phase

	Phase I		Phase II	
	ECMO	CMV	ECMO	CMV
Lived	9	6	19	0
Died	0	4	1	0

there were nine centers. This increased to 17 in 1985, to 25 in 1986, to 45 in 1987, and to 52 in 1988 (21); currently, there are 62 reporting centers. The absolute number of ECMO centers and the rate of their proliferation raises a number of concerns. Given the present neonatal experience, is it possible to accurately predict the number of infants who may benefit from ECMO support? Is there a way to determine an optimum number of centers and a reasonable method of regionalization? Alternatively, should every tertiary care center have ECMO available on site? The problem of regionalization involves the risk of transporting desperately ill infants to another institution for therapy. To minimize the risk of transport, it makes sense to have an ECMO center in every tertiary-level neonatal intensive care unit. Yet this could result in too many centers managing too few cases. This could threaten the ability of existing programs to maintain an excellent standard of ECMO care. It seems obvious that a minimum frequency of ECMO runs is required to sustain an adequate level of expertise. These concerns are presently being addressed on a national level under the auspices of the Extracorporeal Life Support Organization (ELSO). ELSO is charged with creating guidelines and standards for ECMO centers, not only the issues of regionalization and how to maintain standards, but also guidelines for team composition, training and equipment, required consultant staff availability, etc.

While these guidelines and standards are important, it is necessary to realize that the potential ECMO population will be changing in both size and characteristics over the coming years. Current needs and anticipated future needs may well be quite different. Improvements in CMV may shrink the ECMO populations. Conversely, safety improvements in ECMO technology may expand application of ECMO.

Proponents of conservative ventilation argue that if this form of less aggressive ventilation could be mastered, the need for ECMO would decrease drastically. In addition, fewer infants would be eligible if surfactant were found to be beneficial in neonates with PPHN or if a selective pulmonary vasodilator were identified. Most practitioners would welcome decreased ECMO utilization resulting from improvements in any of these noninvasive therapies.

ECMO in 1990 appears to be safer than ECMO in 1980. To some extent, this reflects familiarity and experience gained from the large number of infants treated. There have also been a number of changes in ECMO over the past 10 years, such as an improved understanding of anticoagulation for long-term bypass and the availability of more standardized equipment (i.e., pumps, catheters, monitors). Anticipated developments include heparinized circuits and the use of single-catheter venovenous ECMO (30–32). As safety improves, target populations may increase. In the neonatal population, the two new categories of potential patients are premature infants and term infants with less than 80% predicted mortality. The main reason for using ECMO in these groups would be to avoid the pulmonary complications of barotrauma and oxygen toxicity. There have already been some preliminary investigations for both applications.

Regarding the use of ECMO earlier in the course of disease, at a time of lower predicted mortality, Bartlett et al. (33) recently completed a Phase III study comparing early ECMO versus late ECMO. Patients who met criteria for 50% predicted mortality using an OI greater than 25 were randomized to either ECMO or continued CMV. The CMV group either improved or, after meeting 80% predicted mortality, were offered late ECMO. The goal was not to assess differences in survival, since with the availability of ECMO survival was expected to be high in all groups. Instead, the goal was to evaluate differences in length of hospital stay, length of mechanical ventilation, cost, and patient morbidity among groups receiving early ECMO, late ECMO, and CMV. Preliminary results regarding patient morbidity suggest that the "best" group went on ECMO early (15/20 normal survivors versus 6/11 normal survivors in the group receiving late ECMO and 1/5 normal survivors in the group that never required ECMO; Table 4.4). There are no statistical differences in cost.

ECMO support for premature infants is attracting renewed interest. Recent expanded

TABLE 4.4 Patient morbidity with early, late, or no ECMO

	N	Normal	Handicaps Pulmonary	CNS
Early ECMO	20	15	5	0
Late ECMO	11	6	5	1
No ECMO	5	1	4	1

evaluation of the existing ECMO experience with premature infants was reported by Bui et al. (34). This group reviewed the initial Phase I study by Bartlett, with a specific look at the premature infants supported during that time. Sixteen preterm infants 27 to 35 weeks' gestational age received ECMO support between 1975 and 1984. The birthweight of these infants was 1.6 ± 0.36 kg, and the gestational age was 31.4 ± 2 weeks. Four (25%) infants survived. One survivor had a grade III intraventricular hemorrhage (IVH) and bronchopulmonary dysplasia. Comparing the survivor and nonsurvivor groups, the nonsurvivors had a lower gestational age (30.7 ± 1.8 weeks versus 33.5 ± 1.3 weeks) and lower Pao_2 before starting ECMO (39.8 ± 17.6 versus 53 ± 6). Fifty percent of the nonsurvivor group had technical problems related to the ECMO circuit which required interruption of ECMO and replacement of the circuit. While preterm infants have been excluded from ECMO because of potential IVH, this review suggests that much of the mortality may have been secondary to mechanical complications associated with early ECMO experience and a steep learning curve. ECMO for premature infants should be reexamined cautiously as ECMO technology becomes safer.

Neonatal ECMO has shown dramatic growth and change since the first successful patient outcome was reported in 1975. It remains an evolving technology, and its future holds a number of exciting advances. There will be a better understanding of the long-term morbidity and mortality as ECMO-supported patients are evaluated chronologically over several years. Some changes in the conventional management of neonates with respiratory failure may decrease morbidity and mortality without using ECMO. An improved understanding of the transitional pulmonary vascular bed may well provide us with new pharmacologic means by which to support the pulmonary circulation. ECMO technology will change, and with those changes, may become the safest way to support neonates with respiratory failure. The history of ECMO has not been static. The future promises to be both clinically and scientifically exciting.

REFERENCES

(1) Kenedi RM, Courey JM, Gaylor JDS, Gilchrist T. Artificial organs. Baltimore: University Park Press, 1976:11–9.

(2) Clowes GHA Jr, Hopkins AL, Neville WE. An artificial lung dependent upon diffusion of oxygen and carbon dioxide through plastic membranes. J Thorac Surg 1956;32:630–7.

(3) Hill DJ, O'Brien GO, Morray JJ, et al. Prolonged extracorporeal oxygenation for acute post-traumatic respiratory failure (shock lung syndrome). N Engl J Med 1972; 286:629–34.

(4) Pierce EC. Is extracorporeal membrane oxygenation a viable technique? Ann Thorac Surg 1981;31:102–4.

(5) Short BL, Pearson GD. Neonatal extracorporeal membrane oxygenation: a review. J Intens Care Med 1986;1:47–63.

(6) Zapol WM, Snider MT, Hill DJ, et al. Extracorporeal membrane oxygenation in severe acute respiratory failure: a randomized prospective study. JAMA 1979;242:2193–6.

(7) Dorson W Jr, Meyer B, Baker E, et al. Response of distressed infants to partial bypass lung assist. Trans Am Soc Artif Intern Organs 1970;16:345–51.

(8) White JJ, Andrews HG, Risenberg H, Mazur D, Haller JA Jr. Prolonged respiratory support in newborn infants with a membrane oxygenator. Surgery 1971;70:288–96.

(9) Bartlett RH, Gazzaniga AB, Jefferies MR, et al. Extracorporeal membrane oxygenation (ECMO) cardiopulmonary support in infancy. Trans Am Soc Artif Intern Organs 1976;22:80–93.

(10) Bartlett RH, Gazzaniga AB, Fong SW, et al. Extracorporeal membrane oxygenator support for cardiopulmonary failure. J Thorac Cardiovasc Surg 1977;73:375–86.

(11) Bartlett RH, Gazzaniga AG, Huxtable RF, et al. Extracorporeal circulation (ECMO) in neonatal respiratory failure. J Thorac Cardiovasc Surgery 1977;74:826–33.

(12) Maunder RJ, Hudson LD. The adult respiratory distress syndrome. In: Simons DH, ed. Current pulmonology. Vol 7. Chicago: Yearbook Medical Publishers Inc. 1986:97–116.

(13) Gersony WM. Neonatal pulmonary hypertension: pathophysiology, classification and etiology. Clin Perinatal 1984;11:517–24.

(14) Jackson RM. Pulmonary oxygen toxicity. Chest 1988;88:900–5.

(15) Haake R, Schlichtig R, Ulstad DR, Henschen RR. Bantrauma: pathophysiology, risk factors and prevention. Chest 1987;91:608–13.

(16) Bartlett RH, Andrews AF, Toomasian JM, et al. Extracorporeal membrane oxygenation for newborn respiratory failure: forty-five cases. Surgery 1982;92:425–33.

(17) Kirkpartrick BV, Krummel TM, Moeller DG, et al. Use of extracorporeal membrane oxygenation for respiratory failure in term infants. Pediatr 1983;72:872–6.

(18) Krummel TM, Greenfield LJ, Kirkpatrick BV, et al. Clinical use of an extracorporeal membrane oxygenator in neonatal pulmonary failure. J Pediatr Surg 1982;17:525–31.

(19) Trento A, Griffith BP, Hardesty RL. Extracorporeal membrane oxygenation experience at the University of Pittsburgh. Ann Thorac Surg 1986;1:47–53.

(20) Toomasian JM, Snedecor SM, Cornell RG, et al. National experience with extracorporeal membrane oxygenation for newborn respiratory failure. Trans Am Soc Artif Intern Organs 1988;34:140–7.

(21) National Neonatal ECMO Registry. Ann Arbor: University of Michigan.

(22) Ortiz RM, Cilley RE, Bartlett RH. Extracorporeal membrane oxygenation in pediatric respiratory failure. Pediatr Clin North Am 1987;34:39–46.

(23) Beck R, Anderson KD, Pearson GD, et al. Criteria for extracorporeal membrane oxygenation in a population of infants with persistent pulmonary hypertension of the newborn. J Pediatr Surg 1986;21:297–302.

(24) Cole CH, Jillson E, Kessler D. ECMO: regional evaluation of need and applicability of selection criteria. Am J Dis Child 1988;142:1320–5.

(25) Dworetz AR, Moya FR, Sabo B, Gladstone I, Gross I. Survival in infants with persistent pulmonary hypertension of the newborn without extracorporeal membrane oxygenation. Pediatrics 1989;84:1–6.

(26) Bartlett RH, Roloff DW, Cornell RG, et al. Extracorporeal circulation in neonatal respiratory failure: a prospective randomized study. Pediatrics 1985;76:479–87.

(27) War JH, Epstein MF. Extracorporeal circulation in neonatal respiratory failure: a prospective randomized study (Editorial). Pediatrics 1985;76:849–51.

(28) O'Rourke PP, Crone RK, Vacanti JP, et al. A prospective randomized study of extracorporeal membrane oxygenation (ECMO) and conventional medical therapy in neonates with persistent pulmonary hypertension of the newborn. Pediatrics 1989;84:957–63.

(29) Wung JT, James LJ, Kilchevsky E, James E. Management of severe respiratory failure with persistence of the fetal circulation without hyperventilation. Pediatrics 1985;76:488–94.

(30) Durandy Y, Chevalier JY, Petion AM. A new single lumen cannula allowing an original technique of cannulation for AREC. Ann Arbor, MI: ELSO Charter Meeting, October, 1989.

(31) Chevalier JY, Durandy Y. Use in AREC of a pediatric single cannula extracorporeal lung assist device. Ann Arbor, MI: ELSO Charter Meeting, October, 1989.

(32) Anderson H, Wortley R, Otsu T, et al. Double lumen catheter for neonatal VV ECMO. Ann Arbor, MI: ELSO Charter Meeting, October, 1989.

(33) Bartlett RH, Schumacher R, Rodolf DW, et al. Prospective randomized study of cost effectiveness of neonatal ECMO. Ann Arbor, MI: ELSO Charter Meeting, October, 1989.

(34) Bui KC, Bartlett RH, Van Dekerkove J, LaClair P. ECMO for premature infants with respiratory failure. Ann Arbor, MI: ELSO Charter Meeting, October, 1989.

5

Optimizing Conventional Respiratory Support

❖

Jen-Tien Wung, M.D.
L. Stanley James, M.D.

ECMO was first used successfully for the treatment of severe respiratory failure in the newborn in 1975 (1), and in the past decade the use of this technique has greatly accelerated. A high proportion of infants who are treated with ECMO have meconium aspiration syndrome (MAS) or persistent pulmonary hypertension (PPHN), or both. However, there is concern that the need for this procedure might result as much from ventilator-induced lung injury as from the primary disease (2,3), since a number of institutions report a high survival rate for infants suffering from MAS without the use of ECMO (2–4). Concern is also raised because of variations in the incidence of chronic lung disease across neonatal intensive care units (NICUs) (5,6). Barotrauma from overventilation appears to be a major factor in this variation (3–8).

The most widely practiced initial therapy for PPHN is hyperventilation with induced alkalosis. First proposed in 1978 (9), the treatment is based on the observed fall in pulmonary arterial pressure during hyperventilation and induced hypocapnia (10). We have adopted a more conservative approach that minimizes barotrauma and maintains adequate oxygenation while the disease process resolves. With that approach, we have been able to manage the majority of infants with severe PPHN without using ECMO, including those in profound respiratory failure who have received "maximal" therapy with hyperventilation.

The principles of our management are to provide graded assistance to ventilation depending upon the degree of respiratory distress or failure, with treatment initiated as soon as signs of respiratory difficulty are apparent. In order to minimize barotrauma and cardiovascular depression, respirator settings are kept at a low level compatible with adequate oxygenation, and no attempt is made to induce hypocarbia or to keep the $Paco_2$ in the normal range by increasing the level of ventilation. Infants are not paralyzed and are weaned aggressively so that the duration of intubation will be as short as possible. These principles apply to both the immature infant suffering from respiratory distress syndrome (RDS) and more mature infants suffering from MAS or PPHN. The methods of management are demonstrated in detail in a video tape that may be obtained from the authors.

IMMEDIATE CARE AT BIRTH

Because many infants treated with ECMO have aspirated meconium, early management of MAS is of prime importance in order to facilitate the establishment of the transitional circulation and to prevent the development of PPHN.

For infants born with meconium, it is mandatory to ensure that there is a good airway and that meconium, if present, is promptly removed. As soon as the infant's head is delivered, meconium is removed from the mouth manually with a gauze pad, followed by suctioning. Upon delivery, any meconium present in the trachea is removed by direct suctioning prior to ventilation. This procedure should be carried out in all infants in whom there is thick meconium, but it may be omitted when the amniotic fluid is merely meconium stained. If the infant does not breathe spontaneously after tracheal suctioning, the lungs are expanded mechanically with high concentrations of oxygen. For the next 30 min, close attention should be paid to the infant's oxygenation; chest physiotherapy and pharyngeal suctioning, if necessary, are used to ensure continued removal of meconium. An arterial Po_2 and pH should be obtained as soon as possible after birth since skin color in these infants is a very unreliable indication of oxygenation due to peripheral vasoconstriction. Hypoxia during this critical period will cause the pulmonary vasculature to remain constricted, maintaining a high pulmonary vascular resistance.

If breathing is established promptly, the endotracheal tube should be removed. If labored breathing or intercostal retractions are present, nasal continuous positive airway pressure (CPAP) is begun. Should the infant fail to respond to CPAP or be severely depressed, mechanical ventilation is used. All procedures should be carried out in a warmed crib under radiant heating because of the importance of maintaining body temperature; at the same time, care should be taken not to overheat the infant because this will increase the metabolic requirements and may also cause peripheral vasodilation, which may lead to systemic hypotension favoring the maintenance of the fetal pattern of circulation.

EARLY NASAL PRONG CPAP

For infants with respiratory distress, we initiate early treatment with nasal prong CPAP. This approach may avoid the subsequent need for more invasive mechanical ventilation. Indications for CPAP are tachypnea, inspiratory retractions, and nasal flaring with or without an audible grunt. CPAP is maintained at 5 cm of water pressure. Higher pressures usually result in air escaping through the mouth. The concentration of inspired oxygen is adjusted to keep the arterial oxygen tension between 50 and 70 mm Hg. As soon as the apparatus is properly applied, the baby will breathe more easily; respiratory rate and retractions will decrease. If 5 cm H_2O CPAP is insufficient to achieve a Pao_2 of 50–70 mm Hg while breathing 80% to 100% oxygen, the patient probably requires mechanical ventilation.

MECHANICAL VENTILATION

The major complications of mechanical ventilation are the result of barotrauma and adverse effects on the circulation. In order to minimize these complications, our approach has emphasized modest but adequate ventilator settings. The intermittent mandatory ventilation (IMV) mode allows spontaneous breathing to continue during the expiratory phase of the respirator cycle and permits gradation of ventilatory support depending upon the degree of respiratory failure. Hence, the ventilator cycling frequency can be set at a lower rate for the same level of minute ventilation. This reduces the danger of barotrauma and cardiovascular compromise and, at the same time, facilitates weaning.

Indications for mechanical ventilation (Table 5.1) are marked retractions, frequent apnea while on CPAP, a Pao_2 of less than 50 mm Hg with a fraction of inspired oxygen (Fio_2) of 80% to 100%, a $Paco_2$ greater than 65 mm Hg, or intractable metabolic acidosis with a

TABLE 5.1 Indications for mechanical ventilation

- Marked retractions on CPAP
- Frequent apnea on CPAP
- $Pao_2 < 50$ mm Hg with Fio_2 80%–100%
- $Paco_2 > 65$ mm Hg
- BD > 10 mEq/L after Rx with $NaHCO_3$
- Cardiovascular collapse
- Neuromuscular disorder

base deficit greater than 10 mEq/L despite bicarbonate therapy. Other conditions in which cardiovascular function is severely compromised or in which there is a neuromuscular disorder may also require ventilator support.

Prior to initiating mechanical ventilation, it is important to observe the patient's clinical condition. If the blood gas results are not compatible with the patient's clinical appearance, further investigation is needed. The blood gas machine may be malfunctioning, or the timing or technique of collecting the blood sample may be faulty. It is also important to make sure that the infant's deterioration is not due to improper application of CPAP or nasal obstruction from secretions.

Type of Ventilator

Most ventilators currently used for newborn infants are time-cycled, pressure-limited, and continuous flow devices, including the Baby Bird-2, the Bourns BP 200, the Bear Cub, the Healthdyne 105, and the Sechrist IV-100B. Many aspects of their design features are similar. For successful mechanical ventilation of infants in respiratory failure, it is essential that all personnel be knowledgeable about the function of each control parameter of the ventilator, i.e., flow rate, Fio_2, IMV rate, inspiration time (Ti), peak inspiratory pressure (PIP), and positive end-expiratory pressure (PEEP).

Ventilator Settings

There is no standard or uniformity in the selection of settings for mechanical ventilation among different institutions. This might account for the variability in the incidence of both successes and complications. Four methods of mechanical ventilation in the IMV mode have been practiced in our NICU over the past eight years using the Healthdyne 105 (Table 5.2).

Conventional method (Table 5.3) The settings for this method are based on standard principles of pulmonary mechanics.

1. *Flow rate.* The minimal flow rate should be two and a half times the infant's minute ventilation in order to wash out expired carbon dioxide; an additional flow rate should also be provided to compensate for leaks around the humidifier and tubing connections. The flow rate should also be high enough to generate a desired peak inspiratory pressure within the inspiratory time. We have arbitrarily set this flow rate at 7 L/min.

2. *Fractional inspired oxygen.* This is adjusted to maintain the arterial oxygen tension between 50 and 70 mm Hg. Although the minimal adequate Pao_2 is unknown, it might be 40 mm Hg or lower providing there is no circulatory insufficiency.

3. *Rate of IMV.* This will depend upon the infant's ability to breathe spontaneously. It is usually started at 20–30 breaths per minute and then adjusted to maintain the

TABLE 5.2. Four techniques of mechanical ventilation using conventional infant ventilators

1. Conventional technique.
2. High-frequency positive-pressure ventilation (HFPPV).
3. Prolonged inspiratory time with inspiratory pressure plateau.
4. IMV rate between 40 and 100/min.

TABLE 5.3 Settings for conventional technique

1. Flow rate 7 L/min.

2. FiO_2 to keep PaO_2 at 50–70 mm Hg.

3. IMV rate: usually started at 20–30/min. Avoid excessive labored breathing. Maintain $PaCO_2$ at 50–60 mm Hg.

4. Inspiration time (Ti) 0.6 s.

5. Peak inspiration pressure (PIP). Adequate chest excursion. Usually 20–30 cm H_2O.

6. PEEP 5 cm H_2O.

arterial tension of CO_2 in the range of 50–60 mm Hg; the rate should be sufficient to avoid the infant's need to make excessive respiratory efforts which will lead to exhaustion. The infant soon adapts to this rate and breathes spontaneously during the expiratory phase of the respirator cycle. A higher-than-normal level of CO_2 is accepted because it allows a lower level of minute ventilation while maintaining adequate oxygenation. To achieve a lower $PaCO_2$ requires a much higher level of ventilation (11), increasing the risk of barotrauma. An IMV rate greater than 40 is rarely used in the conventional method because it may create an "inadvertent" PEEP due to the short expiration time.

4. *Inspiratory time*. A Ti of 0.6 s is used for IMV rates of up to 40 per minute.

5. *Peak inspiratory pressure*. The inspiratory pressure depends upon the compliance of the lung but is usually started at 20 cm H_2O. It is then adjusted so that adequate, but not excessive, chest excursions are visible, indicating that the tidal volume is appropriate. Lower pressures are used for less severely ill infants with higher compliance. If the inspiratory pressure is too low, tidal volume will be inadequate, and the patient will develop atelectasis and intrapulmonary shunts, leading to hypoxemia. If, on the other hand, the inspiratory pressure is too high, the lung will be overinflated. This leads to three important consequences: 1) increased lung injury from barotrauma, 2) an increase in pulmonary vascular resistance, and 3) circulatory compromise with decreased venous return, pulmonary blood flow, cardiac output, systemic blood pressure, and oxygenation. If the infant remains hypoxic despite good chest excursions, it is important to exclude other causes such as cyanotic heart disease. To attempt to treat hypoxemia with continuous increases in PIP is a frequent error. In patients who are overventilated, blood gases will improve when ventilator settings are gradually decreased.

6. *PEEP*. This pressure is initially set at +5 cm H_2O and is used to prevent alveolar collapse and to increase functional residual capacity towards normal.

For infants ventilated by the conventional method, clinical improvement is indicated by decreasing tachypnea and retractions and an improvement in blood gas status. The IMV rate is reduced by two to five breaths per minute as the $PaCO_2$ falls into the range of 50 mm Hg or less, provided this is not accompanied by excessively labored spontaneous breathing. The inspiratory pressure is reduced by 2 to 5 cm H_2O for excessive chest excursions, and the FiO_2 is reduced by about one tenth of the inspired oxygen concentration when the arterial oxygen tension is greater than 60 mm Hg. PEEP, inspiratory time, and flow rate usually remain the same.

Worsening of the clinical condition is evidenced by hypoxemia, hypercarbia with a $PaCO_2$ rising above 60 mm Hg, or excessively labored breathing. For a low PaO_2, the FiO_2 is raised or PIP is gradually increased if chest excursions are inadequate. For a rising $PaCO_2$ or excessively labored breathing, the IMV rate is gradually increased to a limit of 40 per min. For severe retractions observed during spontaneous breathing, PEEP may be increased gradually by 2 cm H_2O to a limit of 10 cm H_2O, but this is rarely necessary. Inspiration time is maintained at 0.6 s.

High-Frequency Positive-Pressure Ventilation (HFPPV) This method of mechanical ventilation is tried in any of the following situations:

1. When the infant's Pao$_2$ is less than 50 mm Hg with an Fio$_2$ of 100% while on the conventional method.

2. When a PIP above 30 cm H$_2$O is necessary to achieve visible chest excursions.

3. If the Paco$_2$ is > 70 mm Hg with an IMV rate of up to 40 per min.

For such infants, the IMV rate is increased to 100/min, and the inspiratory time is reduced to 0.3 s. The inspiratory pressure should be lowered by 5 to 10 cm H$_2$O from the conventional setting, while the flow rate is increased to 10 to 20 L/min. The PEEP is set at 0 on the ventilator because a high rate of IMV creates an "inadvertent PEEP" at the tracheal level. If the patient's condition improves, as indicated by the blood gas status or a more stable oxygen tension recorded on the transcutaneous partial pressure of oxygen (TcPo$_2$) monitor, these settings are maintained. This technique is tried not for the purpose of hyperventilation but for the following reasons: the mechanism of gas exchange may be different on a high ventilator rate; a lower PIP will decrease barotrauma; and hypercarbia may decrease with increased minute ventilation.

Prolonged inspiratory time with an inspiratory plateau If the infant cannot maintain an adequate Po$_2$ using the conventional or HFPPV settings, we return to the conventional method and increase the inspiratory time from 0.6 to 0.8–1.0 seconds with an inspiratory pressure plateau. Infants who require these ventilator settings have very stiff lungs due to conditions such a congenital pneumonia or severe RDS. However, use of this method carries a greater risk of pulmonary air leak.

IMV rate of 40–100 breaths/minute When a vigorously breathing infant has not improved with the conventional or HFPPV method or with a prolonged inspiration time, an IMV rate of 40 to 100 breaths/min is tried. The IMV rate is set at the patient's spontaneous respiratory rate in an attempt to synchronize the rate with his spontaneous breathing. Ti is kept at 0.6 s or the I:E ratio at 1:1, whichever time is shorter. Most infants treated by this method have severe MAS.

WEANING

An attempt to wean the infant from mechanical ventilation is begun as soon as the patient is stable. The Fio$_2$ is lowered in decrements of 2% to 10% to maintain a Pao$_2$ between 50 and 70 mm Hg. The IMV rate is lowered in decrements of 2 to 5 per min, maintaining the Paco$_2$ between 50 and 60 mm Hg and allowing spontaneous but not excessively labored breathing. PIP is lowered as the patient's pulmonary compliance improves and chest excursions become excessive. If the patient was previously ventilated at a rate of 100 per min, weaning is accomplished by lowering the Fio$_2$ and PIP as indicated and leaving the IMV rate at 100 until a PIP of 20 mm Hg is reached. Then the management is changed back to the conventional method with an IMV of 40 breaths/min. Thereafter, the infant is weaned as in the conventional method. For the patient being ventilated with prolonged Ti, the inspiration time is gradually decreased to 0.6 s, at which point, weaning continues as with the conventional technique. For the infant on an IMV between 40 and 100 breaths, the IMV rate is reduced and Ti changed accordingly as the patient's condition improves.

EXTUBATION

Extubation is indicated when the rate of IMV is reduced to 6 breaths per minute. At this stage, the patient is usually stable, the Fio$_2$ is less than 40%, the Pao$_2$ is between 50 and 70 mm Hg, and the Paco$_2$ is between 50 and 60 mm Hg. Extubation is performed under direct laryngoscopy using an oxyscope or with supplemental oxygen flowing via a catheter attached to the laryngoscope blade. When the tube has been removed, pharyngeal secretions are suctioned, and the larynx is painted with Vaponephrine to decrease postextubation edema. After extubation, it is not unusual to see the Paco$_2$ fall to a lower level than noted previously with an IMV rate of 6 breaths per minute. This decrease is probably due to the lower airway resistance with spontaneous breathing after extubation. Following extubation, nasal CPAP at 5 cm H$_2$O is applied, and the Fio$_2$ is increased by 5%. Thereafter, the infant is weaned from CPAP as tolerated.

ADDITIONAL ASPECTS OF MANAGEMENT DURING MECHANICAL VENTILATION

Humidity

Maintenance of adequate humidity is essential in order to keep the infant's secretions thin and easily suctioned. This is achieved by using an efficient humidifier which provides a relative humidity of 100% at whatever water temperature is inside the humidifier. Water temperature is kept between 90–100°F, a lower temperature for patients with loose secretions and a higher temperature for those with thick secretions.

Nasotracheal Intubation

This route is preferred over the orotracheal route because it provides for better fixation of the endotracheal tube and minimizes accidental extubation or intubation of a main bronchus.

Endotracheal Tube Placement

The tube is inserted very carefully so that the tip lies 1–2 cm above the bifurcation of the trachea, depending on the size of the infant. The correct depth of insertion is derived from a reference chart (12) that relates the distance from the nares to the midtrachea. This length is marked on the tube prior to intubation.

Suctioning

The endotracheal tube is suctioned at a minimum of every two to three hours and more frequently if secretions are copious. Prior to suctioning, the concentration of inspired oxygen is increased by 20% and the IMV rate is raised to 20 or higher. Depending upon the size of the infant, the suction catheter is advanced only 3 to 5 cm beyond the tip of the endotracheal tube in order to avoid perforation of the lung while the mainstem bronchus is suctioned. The right and left side are suctioned by turning the infant's head in the opposing direction. We do not recommend the use of a ventilating bag before and after suctioning because of the difficulty in avoiding excessive inflating pressure. With careful attention to humidification of inspired gas in suctioning of the endotracheal tube, lung collapse or obstruction of the tube is very rare.

Muscle Relaxants

We discourage the use of muscle relaxants to paralyze the infant for a number of reasons. There is a better match between ventilation and perfusion with spontaneous breathing (13). For the paralyzed patient lying supine, the upper portion of the lung is ventilated more, while the lower dependent portion is better perfused. Adequate ventilation can be achieved at a lower rate in a nonparalyzed patient breathing spontaneously, thus reducing the risk of barotrauma to the lung. Long-term paralysis can also result in atrophy of the muscles of respiration, making weaning from mechanical ventilation more difficult. An additional important point is that the infant's clinical status can be assessed by his/her spontaneous activity. For infants referred from other centers whose Pao$_2$ may have been low for an unknown period, spontaneous activity and tone provide valuable guides in the assessment of hypoxic insults to the brain.

The patient who appears to be "fighting the respirator" may be doing so because of a problem. The endotracheal tube may be blocked by secretions and require suctioning, or the tube may be positioned incorrectly. A restless infant may also indicate that the respirator settings are incorrect or that the respirator is malfunctioning. Another possible reason for the patient's restlessness may be a pneumothorax. Whatever the cause of agitation, rather than paralyzing the patient, one should identify the problem. Once the cause is determined and corrected, the patient usually becomes quiet and breathes easily with the ventilator. If there is no obvious cause, the patient may merely need some "TLC" or a pacifier. For the rare patient who is agitated without a definable, correctable cause, mild sedation with phenobarbital or a narcotic is more appropriate than paralysis. Although a low incidence of pneumothorax has been reported when the infant is paralyzed (14), the incidence of pneumothorax at Babies' Hospital was less than 15% in infants with severe respiratory failure who were mechanically ventilated without paralysis.

Recording of Transcutaneous Po_2

During mechanical ventilation, continuous recording of the transcutaneous oxygen tension or saturation is essential. This enables one to more readily follow trends and to observe an infant's response to a ventilator setting immediately. The physician can determine promptly whether the new ventilator settings are in the right direction. This is particularly important for very unstable infants and may help in diagnosing the cause of deteriorating blood gases. Furthermore, considerable fluctuations in the Pao_2 are not unusual in patients with PPHN, and continuous recording of the Pao_2 will reveal whether or not the fluctuation is transient, thus avoiding unnecessary changes in the ventilator settings.

Persistently High $Paco_2$

Occasionally, a patient's $Paco_2$ remains elevated despite a high respirator rate and adequate chest excursions. This is probably due to a high physiological dead space or ventilation/perfusion ratio disturbances. Attempting to lower the $Paco_2$ by increasing the ventilator settings is not beneficial and will only serve to inflict lung damage. Should a pneumothorax occur as a result of the high ventilator settings, the infant's condition will promptly worsen. An elevated $Paco_2$ can be tolerated if hypoxia is not a problem. Infants with hypercarbia refractory to increases in IMV may often be weaned by decreasing the IMV without a further elevation in $Paco_2$. As the patient's pulmonary status improves with time, the $Paco_2$ will fall gradually.

Persistent Pulmonary Hypertension of the Neonate (PPHN)

The management of infants with PPHN and respiratory failure is extremely difficult and presents one of the major challenges to the neonatologist. These infants have pulmonary hypertension with right-to-left shunting at the foramen ovale and ductus arteriosus and a high alveolar-arterial oxygen gradient ($AaDo_2$). They are extremely labile and withstand any stress or handling poorly. The reasons for their extreme lability are not understood. It could be related to the abnormal vasoconstriction secondary to hypertrophy of the smooth muscle media of the pulmonary arterioles (15,16). Alternatively, it could be related to failure of the normal relaxation of pulmonary vascular tone due to an absence or decrease in the amount of the endothelial relaxing factor (17) secondary to damage to the lung parenchyma from hypoxia or barotrauma. Intrapulmonary shunting and abnormal distribution of ventilation leading to hypoxia probably also play a role.

For these patients, no attempt is made to induce alkalosis by hyperventilation or by the continuous infusion of alkali. Alkalosis will shift the oxygen hemoglobin dissociation curve to the left, which may impair tissue oxygenation. This situation is especially dangerous for a patient with a low Pao_2.

For an infant with PPHN who remains hypoxic despite proper mechanical ventilation and good chest excursions, tolazoline is given intravenously in a bolus injection of 1 mg/kg while the Pao_2 is recorded continuously with a transcutaneous electrode. If a beneficial effect is demonstrated after the initial bolus, a continuous infusion of tolazoline is given at 1 mg/kg/h. The drug is administered via a peripheral vein in an upper extremity or a scalp vein in order to favor circulation of the drug to the superior vena cava and then to the right side of the heart and the pulmonary vascular bed. Systemic blood pressure is monitored continuously with an indwelling arterial catheter. A decrease in systemic blood pressure of approximately 10 mm Hg usually occurs after the bolus injection of tolazoline and lasts no more than 15 minutes provided the infant is not hypovolemic or being hyperventilated. Rarely, the systolic blood pressure decreases to below 50 mm Hg. If hypotension persists, a bolus injection of 10 mL/kg normal saline is administered to expand the vascular volume. Occasionally, a patient who receives tolazoline becomes agitated because of cerebral vasodilation, which requires treatment with intravenous phenobarbital 5–10 mg/kg. Failure to respond to tolazoline could be due to overinflation which leads to pulmonary vasoconstriction, this effect overriding the vasodilating action of the drug. It could also be due to impairment of venous return, leading to a systemic arterial pressure which is lower than the pulmonary arterial pressure.

If tolazoline does not achieve the desired effect, we may use epinephrine or prostaglandin E_1, each in a dose of 0.1 μg/kg/min, in an effort to dilate the pulmonary vasculature. Both drugs have a short half-life; therefore, should there be no improvement in oxygenation, the drug administration can be stopped immediately.

Dopamine is not given routinely. It is used for the treatment of oliguria or for poor myocardial contractility demonstrated echocardiographically. For oliguria, a dose of 2.5 μg/kg/min is administered; for poor myocardial contractility, a dose of 5–10 μg/kg/min is indicated to augment myocardial function. More than 10 μg/kg/min is not used because of the danger of an alpha-adrenergic effect, which can lead to further pulmonary vascular constriction.

Four case histories of PPHN are presented to illustrate our management of PPHN with respiratory failure.

Case 1 (Table 5.4 and Figure 5.1) An infant weighing 3,350 g was delivered by emergency cesarean section in our obstetric unit at 42 weeks' gestation because of ruptured membranes for 24 hours, thick meconium, and a fetal scalp pH of 7.19. Apgar scores were 3, 5, and 7 at 1, 2, and 5 min, respectively. The infant cried and aspirated meconium prior to tracheal

TABLE 5.4   Case 1

Age (h)	IMV (min)	Ti (s)	PIP (cm H_2O)	PEEP (cm H_2O)	F_{IO_2} (%)	pH	$PaCO_2$ (mm Hg)	PaO_2 (mm Hg)	BE
0.5				CPAP +5	100	7.02	82	51	
2	30	0.6	25	5	100	7.28	44	71	−5
4	30	0.6	25	5	100	7.30	46	53	−3
7	100	0.3	25	3	100	7.43	35	39	0
8	40	0.6	30	5	100	7.27	47	38	−5
9	25	0.6	30	5	100	7.37	40	67	−2
19	20	0.6	28	5	100	7.33	49	51	0
19.5	Tolazoline 3.5 mg IV bolus ($TcPO_2$ 36–75) then 3.5 mg/h IV infusion								
20	20	0.6	28	5	100	7.33	44	58	0
29	20	0.6	28	5	100	7.41	37	62	0
	Tolazoline tapered and discontinued								
35	20	0.6	28	5	100	7.39	42	37	1
36	100	0.3	23	3	100	7.53	29	40	3.5
	Tolazoline 3 mg IV bolus, then 3.5 mg/h restarted								
41	100	0.3	25	3	100	7.46	32	45	1
84	100	0.3	25	3	100	7.45	29	51	−2
86	30	0.6	28	5	100	7.38	37	79	−2
93	30	0.6	28	5	90	7.37	35	88	−4
120	20	0.6	25	5	85	7.34	47	56	0
144	20	0.6	25	5	65	7.37	45	68	1
168	17	0.6	25	5	45	7.34	48	65	0
192	10	0.6	25	5	30	7.35	50	56	2
	Tolazoline tapered over 8 hours and discontinued								
200	6	0.6	25	5	30	7.35	49	61	2
206	Nasal CPAP +5				30	7.35	48	66	2

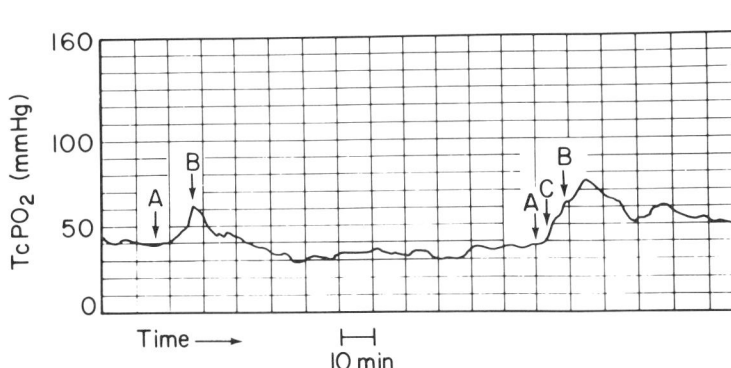

FIGURE 5.1 Tracing of transcutaneous Po_2 (Case 1). (A) Blood pressure cuffs were applied to both thighs at a pressure of 10–20 mm Hg above systemic systolic pressure. $TcPo_2$ rose. (B) Blood pressure cuffs were released and $TcPo_2$ fell. (C) Tolazoline was injected intravenously in a bolus dose of 1 mg/kg and $TcPo_2$ rose.

suctioning. Respiratory distress with tachypnea and inspiratory retraction developed immediately. Nasal CPAP at +5 cm H_2O was applied with an Fio_2 of 100%, with little improvement. Because of a pH of 7.02, $Paco_2$ of 82 mm Hg, and a Pao_2 of 51 mm Hg, mechanical ventilation was begun via a nasotracheal tube. Initial respirator settings of IMV 30, Ti of 0.6 s, PIP 25 cm H_2O, PEEP 5 cm H_2O, and Fio_2 100% resulted in a pH of 7.28, $Paco_2$ of 44 mm Hg, and a Pao_2 of 71 mm Hg. Because the $TcPo_2$ was labile and falling and the infant appeared to be deteriorating, IMV 100 was tried at age seven hours. Oxygenation deteriorated further despite a decrease in $Paco_2$ from 46 to 35 mm Hg, and the IMV was returned to 40. From 8 to 19 hours, IMV rates were decreased with some increase in oxygenation, but the infant remained very unstable. When the infant was 19.5 hours of age, a bolus of tolazoline 3.5 mg was given, and $TcPo_2$ increased from 40 to 75 (Figure 5.1). Thereafter, a continuous infusion of tolazoline was maintained in a dose of 3.5 mg/h. Between 29 and 36 hours, as the tolazoline was tapered, the Pao_2 gradually declined and became more unstable. A trial of IMV 100 produced no improvement. Tolazoline in a dose of 3 mg was again administered as a bolus, followed by a continuous intravenous infusion at the rate of 3.5 mg/h. This was followed by a more stable $TcPo_2$ and some improvement in Pao_2. Between 84 and 86 hours of age, the IMV rate was decreased from 100 to 30, and PIP increased from 25 to 28 cm H_2O; Pao_2 increased from 51 to 70 mm Hg (despite a rise

in $Paco_2$ from 29 to 37 mm Hg). The patient's respiratory status continued to improve on these settings. Tolazoline was tapered over eight hours and then stopped when the infant was 192 hours old. On the following day, the patient was extubated and placed on nasal CPAP +5 cm H_2O. By 14 days of age, the infant was off CPAP and breathing room air.

Comment This infant had severe MAS confirmed radiographically and PPHN evidenced by right-to-left shunts at the foramen ovale and ductus arteriosus and confirmed by echocardiogram. Initially, he was artificially ventilated by the conventional method and had a favorable response to an infusion of tolazoline. However, when the tolazoline was tapered between 29 and 36 hours, he deteriorated. The HFPPV technique was then tried, with little improvement. Tolazoline was restarted, and the infant stabilized on this regimen. When the infant was 86 hours of age, oxygenation markedly improved when the ventilation was changed to the conventional method. It is noteworthy that oxygenation improved despite an increase in the $Paco_2$ rather than the reverse. The infant made a complete recovery in nine days with no further respiratory complications.

In infants with severe PPHN, the magnitude of shunting at the foramen ovale and ductus arteriosus is determined by the relative resistance of the pulmonary and systemic vascular beds. In an attempt to raise the infant's systemic vascular resistance, we have applied blood pressure cuffs to both thighs with an inflation pressure 10–20 mm Hg above systolic blood pressure. Preliminary experience has shown an elevation of TcPo$_2$ (Figure 5.1), suggesting that the increase in the systemic vascular resistance has reduced the right-to-left shunt. We speculate that, if tolazoline is given during this maneuver, circulation of the drug to the pulmonary vascular bed may be favored and the adverse effect on the systemic circulation reduced.

Case 2 (Figure 5.2) A term male infant weighing 2,690 grams was delivered vaginally in our obstetrical unit; thick meconium was present at birth. The membranes had been ruptured for four days. Meconium was promptly removed by endotracheal suctioning under direct laryngoscopy; Apgar scores were 4 and 6 at 1 and 5 min, respectively. Breathing was labored with retractions, but air entry was good. Nasal prong CPAP +5 cm H$_2$O was applied, resulting in an improvement in breathing with only mild retractions. Echocardiography demonstrated right-to-left shunts at both the foramen ovale and ductus arteriosus without a congenital cardiac anomaly. When the infant was 7.5 hours of age with an Fio$_2$ of 100%, the preductal blood gases were pH 7.20, Paco$_2$ 59 mm Hg, and Pao$_2$ 32 mm Hg. At the age of eight hours, a bolus injection of tolazoline in a dose of 3 mg was given intravenously. This resulted in an increase in TcPo$_2$ from 19 to 50 in 10 min and to 75 in 20 min. Tolazoline was maintained as a continuous infusion at a dose of 3 mg/h. One hour later, at an Fio$_2$ of 100%, blood gas levels were pH 7.24, Paco$_2$ 57 mm Hg, and Pao$_2$ 211 mm Hg preductally, and pH 7.21, Paco$_2$ 61 mm Hg, and Pao$_2$ 54 mm Hg postductally. The infant continued to improve and, at 44.5 hours of age with an Fio$_2$ of 25% and CPAP of +5 cm H$_2$O, blood gas levels were pH 7.39, Paco$_2$ was 38 mm Hg, and Pao$_2$ was 87 mm Hg preductally, and pH was 7.4, Paco$_2$ was 40 and Pao$_2$ was 43 mm Hg postductally. When the infant was four days old, the CPAP was removed, and the infant began to breathe room air.

Comment This infant also has MAS and PPHN. Because air exchange with spontaneous respiration was adequate, the patient was treated with nasal prong CPAP only. Endotracheal intubation and mechanical ventilation were unnecessary and would only have stressed the patient without further ventilatory benefit. The infant had a remarkable improvement in oxygenation after a bolus injection of tolazoline and continued to improve over the next two days, although right-to-left shunt was still detected at the ductus level. He recovered by the fourth day.

Case 3 (Figure 5.3) An infant weighing 2,970 grams was delivered spontaneously vaginally at 41 weeks' gestation at a level I hospital. Apgar scores at 1 and 5 min were 8 and 9, respectively. Meconium was present at birth. Oral and nasal, but not endotracheal, suctioning were performed. The infant was admitted to a regular nursery, but at five hours of age

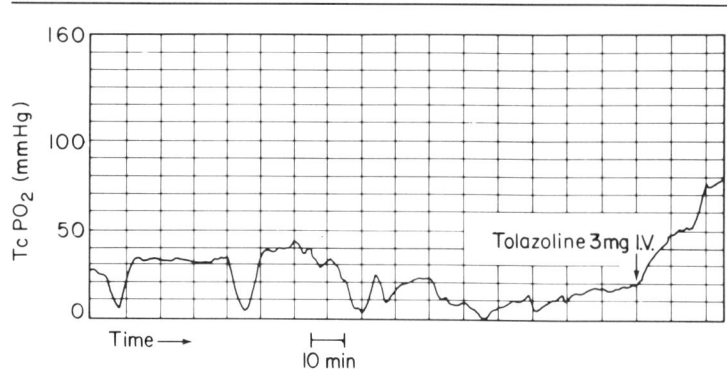

FIGURE 5.2 Tracing of transcutaneous Po$_2$ (Case 2). TcPo$_2$ rose after tolazoline was injected intravenously as a bolus in a dose of 1 mg/kg.

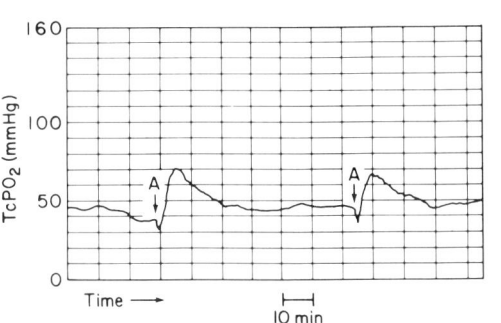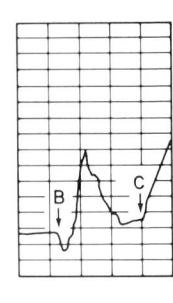

FIGURE 5.3 Tracing of transcutaneous Po_2 (Case 3). (A) Rise in $TcPo_2$ after stimulus of suction of endotracheal tube. (B) After insertion of intravenous catheter (note $TcPo_2$ started to decrease several minutes later). (C) Tolazoline 1 mg/kg injected intravenously as a bolus. $TcPo_2$ rose.

was found to be in respiratory distress. He was then transferred to a level III hospital where he was intubated and hyperventilated. On an IMV of 60, Ti of 0.5 s, PIP of 25 cm H_2O, and PEEP of +4 cm H_2O, his initial blood gases were pH 7.49, $Paco_2$ 25 mm Hg, and Pao_2 188 mm Hg. Later, the infant's blood gases gradually deteriorated despite continuous hyperventilation. Tolazoline was administered, resulting in a slight improvement, but the drug was subsequently discontinued because of hypotension. At 35 hours, the respirator settings were IMV 100, Ti 0.3 s, PIP 40 cm H_2O, PEEP +4 cm H_2O, Fio_2 100% with pH 7.56, $Paco_2$ 29 mm Hg, and Pao_2 44 mm Hg. The infant was also receiving dopamine 15 µg/kg/min, pavulon, and phenobarbital. The patient was then transferred to Babies' Hospital for ECMO. On arrival, excessive chest excursions were noted. The respirator settings were changed to IMV 100, Ti 0.3 s, PIP 30 cm H_2O, PEEP 0, and Fio_2 100%. Blood gases were pH 7.44, $Paco_2$ 37 mm Hg, Pao_2 52 mm Hg. IMV was gradually reduced to 40, with Ti of 0.6 s, PIP raised to 35 cm H_2O, and PEEP of +5 cm H_2O; thereafter, blood gases were pH 7.42, $Paco_2$ 42 mm Hg, and Pao_2 58 mm Hg. The patient was then ventilated using the conventional method. At 84 hours of age, on IMV of 25, Ti of 0.6 sec, PIP of 30 cm H_2O, PEEP of +5 cm H_2O, and Fio_2 100%, the patient's blood gases were pH 7.36, $Paco_2$ 50 mm Hg, and Pao_2 44 mm Hg. A bolus of tolazoline 3 mg was then administered intravenously, and the $TcPo_2$ increased from 40 to 85 over a 10-min period, while the blood pressure remained at 80/45 mm Hg. The infant continued to improve while respirator settings were lowered further. On the sixth day of life, the infant was extubated and placed on nasal prong CPAP at +5 cm H_2O, and by the eighth day of life he was breathing room air.

Comment This case suggests that tolazoline has little or no beneficial effect if the infant is being hyperventilated. Prior to transfer to our unit, while being hyperventilated, the patient was given tolazoline with some improvement; however, because of hypotension, the drug was discontinued. At Babies' Hospital, without hyperventilation, the patient was again given tolazoline, and a marked improvement in oxygenation was observed with no change in the blood pressure.

The $TcPo_2$ tracings (Figure 5.3) showed that Po_2 increased briefly over a 5-min period and then decreased following stimulation from suctioning the nasotracheal tube or inserting an intravenous line. We have observed this phenomenon in patients with PPHN but not in patients with hyaline membrane disease or pneumonia, in whom the Pao_2 usually falls with any form of stimulation. Patients demonstrating an increase in Pao_2 following brief stimulation usually have a favorable response to tolazoline provided hypovolemia is absent and the patient is not being hyperventilated.

Case 4 (Table 5.5) A male infant weighing 3,250 grams was delivered by repeat cesarean section at 38 weeks' gestation at a level I hospital. Delivery was complicated by maternal hypotension following epidural anesthesia and placental abruption. Apgar scores at 1 and

TABLE 5.5 Case 4

Age (h)	IMV (min)	Ti (s)	PIP (cm H$_2$O)	PEEP (cm H$_2$O)	FiO$_2$ (%)	pH	PaCO$_2$ (mm Hg)	PaO$_2$ (mm Hg)	MAP* (cm H$_2$O)	OI†	AaDO$_2$
1			Head hood		52	7.24	60	57			
2			Head hood		100	7.18	45	200			468
6	60	0.5	37	5	100	7.51	27	158	18.5	11.7	528
7.5	60	0.5	34	5	100	7.49	26	163	17.3	10.6	524
9.5	60	0.5	32	5	100	7.49	28	220	16	7.3	455
13.5	60	0.5	32	5	100	7.40	31	38	16	42.1	644
14.5	60	0.5	32	5	100	7.42	32	60	16	26.7	621
16	60	0.5	32	5	100	7.45	32	55	16	29.1	626
18	60	0.5	32	5	100	7.41	40	72	16	22.2	601
20.5	85	0.4	32	5	100	7.55	29	57	18.0	31.6	627
23	80	0.4	32	5	100	7.41	41	26	17.2	66.2	646
35	80	0.4	50	4	100	7.56	31	30	23.3	77.7	652
36.5	Transferred to Babies' Hospital										
37	40	0.6	46	5	100	7.50	33	40	17.6	44	640
37.5	40	0.6	40	5	100	7.54	35	49	16.4	33.5	629
46	30	0.8	35	5	100	7.36	52	50	14.6	29.2	611
55	30	0.8	28	5	100	7.31	47	54	12.6	23.3	612
62.5	25	0.8	28	5	95	7.30	49	73			
85	20	0.8	28	5	80	7.34	43	57			
114	18	0.7	25	5	65	7.36	46	56			
169	6	0.7	25	5	23	7.36	46	62			
171			Nasal CPAP + 5 cm H$_2$O		30	7.33	47	68			

*MAP = mean airway pressure.
†OI = Oxygen index: (MAP × FiO$_2$ [%]) ÷ PaO$_2$.

5 min were 5 and 7, respectively. The infant developed respiratory distress and, at one hour of age, had a pH of 7.24, PaCO$_2$ of 60 mm Hg, and a PaO$_2$ of 57 mm Hg on an FiO$_2$ of 52% (via head hood). A transport team from a level III hospital suspected PPHN, intubated the infant, and instituted hyperventilation. At 9.5 hours of age, the infant's blood gases were pH 7.49, PaCO$_2$ 28 mm Hg, and PaO$_2$ 220 mm Hg. Thereafter, the infant gradually deteriorated. By 35 hours of age, the infant was on IMV of 80, Ti of 0.4 s, PIP of 50 cm H$_2$O, PEEP of 4 cm H$_2$O, and FiO$_2$ of 100%; pH was 7.56, PaCO$_2$ was 31 mm Hg, and PaO$_2$ was 30 mm Hg. In addition, the infant had been given intravenous neosynephrine 0.2 µg/kg/min, dopamine 15 µg/kg/min, dobutamine 20 µg/kg/min, and THAM, digoxin, morphine, and pavulon.

At 36.5 hours of age, the infant was transferred for ECMO treatment to Babies' Hospital. On admission, all drugs were discontinued except for dopamine, which was decreased to 10 µg/kg/min. Because of excessive chest excursions, respirator settings were reduced to IMV 40, Ti 0.6 s, and PIP 46 cm H$_2$O. This resulted in pH 7.5, PaCO$_2$ 33 mm Hg, and PaO$_2$ 40 mm Hg. The blood gases continued to improve as the respirator settings were decreased. The infant was extubated at seven days of age and placed on nasal CPAP of 5 cm H$_2$O for four more days. By 11 days of age, the infant was doing well off CPAP and was breathing room air.

Comment It is likely that the major reason for this infant's deterioration before transfer for ECMO was overventilation, evidenced by the excessive chest excursions with high inspiratory pressures observed on the infant's arrival at Babies' Hospital. The infant's condition improved as the respirator settings were gradually decreased.

Discussion The case histories exemplify the adverse effects of hyperventilation and demonstrate how extremely ill infants may be managed successfully using conservative methods. The first two cases were inborn and more seriously ill than the two outborn infants, who initially had relatively normal blood gases. From the clinical descriptions, we would predict that the latter two infants would recover with CPAP alone. However, they were hyperventilated. This treatment was tolerated at first, but, within a few hours, they both began to deteriorate. This led to a further increase in the respirator settings, accompanied by a further compromise of their acid-base status. By 35 hours of age, these two infants were critically ill on very high respirator settings and met the current criteria for instituting ECMO (18,19). Case 4 sustained an oxygen index (OI) higher than 40 for more than 14 hours and an $AaDo_2$ greater than 620 for more than 17 hours. After transfer to Babies' Hospital, both patients improved when hyperventilation was discontinued, and the use of ECMO was avoided. The course of these two infants suggests that hyperventilation was a major contributor to the high OI index and $AaDo_2$, and demonstrates that the adverse effects of treatment can be reversed when respirator settings are lowered, even when the $AaDo_2$ gradient has met the usually accepted criteria for instituting ECMO.

Hyperventilation was introduced in the belief that hypocarbia and alkalosis could lower pulmonary vascular resistance (9,10). However, earlier experiments in humans and dogs (20) demonstrated that this effect is mediated through pH rather than $Paco_2$. Higher levels of hydrogen ion produced by either raising $Paco_2$ or infusing acid lead to an increase in pulmonary vascular resistance (PVR). The increase in PVR due to hypoxia was greater in the presence of acidosis. There was no evidence that alkalosis alone would lower PVR or that alkalosis and hypocarbia could prevent an increase in PVR in the presence of hypoxia. Later experiments in newborn calves (21) confirmed the additive effect of hypoxia and acidosis in raising PVR, an effect that was much greater than that observed in adult humans or in dogs. The effect of hypoxia was overriding, occurring in the presence of an elevated, normal, or low $Paco_2$. Thus, these experiments do not support the contention that hypocarbia or alkalosis has an independent effect that lowers pulmonary vascular resistance.

Pulmonary vascular resistance is also influenced by lung volume (27). At low lung volumes, PVR is high because the extraalveolar vessels become narrow; at high volumes, the capillaries are stretched and their caliber is reduced, increasing resistance. Thus, PVR is increased under conditions of either hypo- or hyperventilation.

The widely held belief that Pao_2 is directly proportional to mean airway pressure (MAP) (23) creates additional problems in the management of ventilation. When Pao_2 is falling, MAP is raised progressively in an effort to improve oxygenation. However, this concept is only partly true since MAP is altered by any change in flow rate, IMV, Ti, PIP, or PEEP, although each of these parameters has a different function. For example, in Case 4 (Table 5.5), when the patient was 35 hours of age, Pao_2 was 30 mm Hg with ventilation at an IMV of 80, Ti of 0.4 s, PIP of 50 cm H_2O, and PEEP of +4 cm H_2O with a MAP of 23.3. At 37 hours, after MAP had been lowered to 17.6 with IMV of 40, Ti of 0.6 s, PIP of 46 cm H_2O, and PEEP of +5 cm H_2O, Pao_2 had risen to 40 mm Hg. There was a further improvement in Pao_2 as lowering of ventilator settings was continued. By the same token, using oxygen index [OI = (MAP × Fio_2%)/Pao_2] to assess the severity of respiratory failure may also be misleading, since OI is also dependent upon MAP. The value of Pao_2 will depend not only on the respirator settings but also on the infant's cardiac and pulmonary status. A high MAP will adversely affect oxygenation in the presence of circulatory failure or overinflation of the lungs.

Finally, prolonged overventilation has been shown to cause severe impairment in lung function (24,25). Healthy paralyzed and anesthetized sheep ventilated with peak inspiratory pressure of 50 cm H_2O died within 2–35 hours of respiratory failure. The initial improvement that may be observed in an infant with PPHN when hyperventilation is first begun could be due to a rise in Pao_2 as a result of an increase in lung volume. This is followed by later deterioration due to an increase in PVR from overinflation, damage to lung parenchyma, and/or impairment of venous return and eventually respiratory failure.

Tolazoline has been reported to improve oxygenation (26–28) in 40% to 87% of cases, presumably through its vasodilating effect on the pulmonary vasculature. Our experience agrees with these earlier reports, in that a rise in Pao_2 is observed in approximately 90% of cases following administration of the drug. However, in infants who are hyperventilated, the response is variable, with a fall in Pao_2 occurring in some (9). This finding is confirmed in Case 3. It is notable that when hyperventilation was discontinued in this infant, he had a good response to tolazoline. These observations suggest that the beneficial effects of tolazoline on the pulmonary vasculature can be outweighed by adverse effects of hyperventilation on the circulation.

It has been suggested that the success of our management of PPHN is due to inclusion of infants with milder forms of the disease. This is unlikely since, over the past seven years, in a high-risk obstetric service, we have only made the diagnosis of PPHN and severe respiratory failure in 14 of 31,000 infants, an incidence of less than 1 in 2,000. All 14 survived with conservative management (Table 5.6). Infants with milder forms of PPHN, in which right-to-left shunting occurs only at the level of the ductus arteriosus, are not included in this group. During the same seven-year period, 47 outborn infants with severe PPHN *and who had received hyperventilation* have been referred to our unit for ECMO (excluding those with congenital diaphragmatic hernia) (Table 5.6). Most were in very poor condition upon admission. Nevertheless, 34 were treated successfully with ventilation alone. The remaining thirteen had deteriorated to such a degree that they met our criteria for ECMO (Table 5.7). Twelve were placed on ECMO. Of the 47 outborn infants, three died, two were declared brain dead while on ECMO, and in one instance the parents refused permission to place the infant on ECMO. Thus, over the past seven years, our overall survival among 60 infants with PPHN in severe respiratory failure is 95%, and the majority have been treated with ventilation alone *without the use of hyperventilation or by discontinuing this method of so-called "maximal" ventilatory support.*

Our criteria for ECMO (Table 5.7) require that 1) the infant have a Pao_2 of less than 40 mm Hg for at least four hours while receiving 100% oxygen *and optimal ventilatory settings;* or 2) the Pao_2 be in the low 40s and unstable with the infant on a PIP of 45 cm H_2O and an Fio_2 of 100%; or 3) sepsis and intractable metabolic acidosis are present. Additionally, the infant should have none of the generally accepted contraindications; whenever possible, the patient should receive an optimal trial of mechanical ventilation; and the patient must have failed to respond to tolazoline. The major difference between these criteria and those generally used (18,19) is our use of conservative ventilatory methods rather than hyperventilation.

The relatively low incidence of PPHN in our unit might be a direct reflection of the early management of infants with MAS or more severe degrees of asphyxia, together with graded assistance via ventilatory support that depends upon the patient's degree of respiratory distress. The majority of our patients, even those who aspirate thick meconium, are relatively asymptomatic after appropriate, immediate suctioning at delivery, followed by chest physiotherapy and further suctioning if

TABLE 5.7 Criteria for ECMO, Babies' Hospital

1. $Pao_2 < 40$ mm Hg $\times$ 4 h with Fio_2 100%.
2. Pao_2 low 40s, unstable. Required high PIP (>45 cm H_2O) with Fio_2 100%.
3. Intractable metabolic acidosis or sepsis.

Prerequisites
1. No contraindications, e.g., IVH or severe asphyxia, etc.
2. Optimal trial of mechanical ventilation.
3. Failure to respond to tolazoline.

TABLE 5.6 Severe PPHN, Babies' Hospital, 1983–1990

61 Patients

14 inborn; all survived.
47 outborn; 44 survived.
12 ECMO; 2 died of brain death.
35 no ECMO; 1 died (parents refused ECMO).

necessary in the transitional nursery; they can then be admitted to the regular nursery. This early treatment could be an important preventive procedure if the further complications of PPHN are to be avoided. The incidence of meconium observed at birth at our institution is approximately 10%. Only 4% of these infants have required admission to NICU or semiacute nursery for MAS, where the majority recover with nasal CPAP; only 12% of this group with MAS require treatment with IMV for severe depression or PPHN.

Infants with PPHN who have been treated with our methods of mechanical ventilation have not required prolonged hospitalization. Neurological follow-up has revealed a good outcome (29), and there have been no cases of sensorineural deafness, which have been reported by others as a significant sequela following hyperventilation (30,31). Adverse neurological outcome has also been reported following prolonged use of hyperventilation (32).

Two control trials have been conducted to determine the benefits of ECMO over "conventional" medical therapy (33,34). Unfortunately, hyperventilation, with all of the adverse effects enumerated above, was the standard used for "conventional" therapy. Therefore, although these trials demonstrate the superiority of ECMO, it is superior only to hyperventilation. The appropriate place for ECMO in the therapy of respiratory failure remains to be determined by comparison with optimal ventilatory therapy.

Information submitted to the ECMO Registry on the clinical diagnosis of infants receiving ECMO lists 39% with meconium aspiration, 13% with PPHN, 15% with hyaline membrane disease, 17% with congenital diaphragmatic hernia, and 12% with sepsis, excluding those with both congenital diaphragmatic hernia and sepsis. We believe that most of these infants could be managed with conservative techniques. The group listed as hyaline membrane disease is of particular concern, since this disease is very rare in larger, more mature infants. It is possible that they were suffering from transient tachypnea of the newborn or type II RDS, conditions rarely associated with mortality. If these infants had been treated early by hyperventilation, a mild self-limiting illness could have been changed to a severe one, ultimately necessitating ECMO.

SUMMARY

The adverse effects of hyperventilation include the risk of increasing pulmonary vascular resistance from overinflation of the lungs, damage to lung parenchyma, and impairment of venous return. Furthermore, prolonged overventilation alone can result in respiratory failure. There is no clear evidence that hypocarbia or alkalosis can lower PVR in the presence of hypoxemia. Additionally, the adverse effects of hypocarbia on the cerebral vasculature following hyperventilation must be considered (35,36). While some authors have concluded that hyperventilation appears not to cause significant deficits and that any mental or motor deficits may be attributable to perinatal asphyxia or other aspects of a complex course (37–39), a great deal of uncertainty remains (30–32). In our current state of knowledge, it would seem prudent to avoid hyperventilation with all its attendant risks, since infants with PPHN can usually be managed successfully by conservative methods.

REFERENCES

(1) Bartlett RH, Gazzaniga AB, Jefferies R, et al. Extracorporeal membrane oxygenation (ECMO) cardiopulmonary support in infancy. Trans ASAIO 1976;22:80–8.

(2) Dworetz AR, Moya FR, Sabo B, Gladstone I, Gross I. Survival of infants with persistent pulmonary hypertension without extracorporeal membrane oxygenation. Pediatrics 1989;84:1–6.

(3) Wung J-T, James LS, Kilchevsky E, James E. Management of infants with severe respiratory failure and persistence of the fetal circulation, without hyperventilation. Pediatrics 1985;76:488–94.

(4) Schapira D, Solimano A. Is extracorporeal membrane oxygenation necessary to reduce mortality and morbidity in patients with meconium aspiration syndrome? Pediatr Res 1988;23:424A.

(5) Avery ME, Tooley WH, Keller JB, et al. Is

chronic lung disease in low birth weight infants preventable? A survey of eight centers. Pediatrics 1987;79:26–30.

(6) Kraybill EN, Runyan DK, Bose CL, Khan JH. Risk factors for chronic lung disease in infants with birth weights of 751 to 1000 grams. J Pediatr 1989;115–20.

(7) Tooley WH. Epidemiology of bronchopulmonary dysplasia. J Pediatr 1979;95:851–5.

(8) Rhodes PG, Graves GR, Patel OM, Campbell SB, Blumenthal BL. Minimizing pneumothorax and bronchopulmonary dysplasia in ventilated infants with hyaline membrane disease. J Pediatr 1983;103:634–7.

(9) Peckham GJ, Fox WW. Physiologic factors affecting pulmonary artery pressure in infants with persistent pulmonary hypertension. J Pediatr 1978;93:1005–10.

(10) Fox WW, Duara S. Persistent pulmonary hypertension in the neonate: diagnosis and management. J Pediatr 1983;103:505–13.

(11) Bendixen HH, Eghert LD, Hedley-Whyte, et al. Respiratory Care. St. Louis: CV Mosby Co, 1965.

(12) Coldiron JS. Estimation of nasotracheal tube length in neonates. Pediatrics 1968;41:823–8.

(13) Froese AB, Bryan AC. Effects of anesthesia and paralysis on diaphragmatic mechanics in man. Anesthesiology 1974;41:242–55.

(14) Greenough A, Wood S, Morley CJ, Davis JA. Pancuronium prevents pneumothoraces in ventilated premature infants who actively expire against positive pressure inflation. Lancet 1984; 1:1–4.

(15) Haworth SG, Reid LM. Persistent fetal circulation: newly recognized structural features. J Pediatr 1976;88:614–20.

(16) Murphy JD, Vawter GF, Reid LM. Pulmonary vascular disease in fetal meconium aspiration. J Pediatr 1984;104:758–62.

(17) Furchgott RF, Zawadzki JV. The obligatory role of endothelial cells in the relaxation of arterial smooth muscle by acetylcholine. Nature 1980;288:373–6.

(18) Short BL, Miller MK, Anderson KD. Extracorporeal membrane oxygenation in the management of respiratory failure in the newborn. Clin Perinatol 1987;14:737–48.

(19) Ortiz RM, Cilley RE, Bartlett RH. Extracorporeal membrane oxygenation in pediatric respiratory failure. Pediatr Clin North Am 1987; 34:39–46.

(20) Bergofsky EH, Lehr DE, Fishman AP. The effect of changes in hydrogen ion concentration on the pulmonary circulation. J Clin Invest 1962;41:1492–1502.

(21) Rudolph AM, Yuan S. Response of the pulmonary vasculature to hypoxia and H-ion changes. J Clin Invest 1966;45:399–411.

(22) West JB. Respiratory physiology—the essentials, 3rd ed. Baltimore: Williams & Wilkins, 1985.

(23) Boros SJ. Variation in inspiratory-expiratory ratio and airway pressure wave form during mechanical ventilation: the significance of mean airway pressure. J Pediatr 1979;94:114–17.

(24) Kolobow T, Moretti MP, Fumagalli R, et al. Severe impairment of lung function induced by high peak airway pressure during mechanical ventilation. Am Rev Respir Dis 1987;135:312–15.

(25) Borelli M, Kolobow T, Spatola R, Prato P, Tsuno K. Severe acute respiratory failure managed with continuous positive airway pressure and partial extracorporeal carbon dioxide removal by an artificial membrane lung. Am Rev Respir Dis 1988;138:1480–7.

(26) Goetzman BW, Sunshine P, Johnson JD, et al. Neonatal hypoxia and pulmonary vasospasm: response to tolazoline. J Pediatr 1976;89:617–21.

(27) Stevenson DK, Kasting DS, Darnall RA, et al. Refractory hypoxemia associated with neonatal pulmonary disease. The use and limitations of tolazoline. J Pediatr 1979;95:595–9.

(28) Stevens DC, Schreiner RI, Bull MJ, et al. An analysis of tolazoline therapy in the critically ill neonate. J Pediatr Surg 1980;15:964–70.

(29) Marron M-J, Crisafi MA, Driscoll JM, et al. Hearing and neurodevelopmental outcome in survivors of persistent pulmonary hypertension (PPHN) of the neonate. Pediatr Res 1990;27:248A.

(30) Sell EJ, Gaines JA, Gluckman C, Williams EA. Persistent fetal circulation: neurodevelopmental outcome. Am J Dis Child 1985;139:25–8.

(31) Hendricks-Munoz KD, Walton JP. Hearing loss in infants with persistent fetal circulation. Pediatrics 1988;81:650–6.

(32) Bifano EM, Pfannenstiel A. Duration of hyperventilation and outcome in infants with persistent pulmonary hypertension. Pediatrics 1988;81:657–61.

(33) Bartlett RH, Roloff DW, Cornell RG, Andrews AF, Dillon P, Zwischenberger JB. Extracorporeal circulation in neonatal respiratory

(34) O'Rourke PP, Crone RK, Vacanti JP, et al. Extracorporeal membrane oxygenation and conventional medical therapy in neonates with persistent pulmonary hypertension of the newborn: a prospective randomized study. Pediatrics 1989;84:957–63.

(35) Kety SS, Schmidt CF. The effects of active and passive hyperventilation on cerebral blood flow, oxygen consumption, cardiac output and blood pressure of normal young men. J Clin Invest 1946;25:107–19.

(36) Haggendahl E, Johansson B. Effects of arterial carbon dioxide tension and oxygen saturation on cerebral blood flow and autoregulation in dogs. Acta Physiol Scand 1965;66:27–53.

(37) Ferrara B, Johnson DE, Chang PN, Thompson TR. Efficacy and neurologic outcome of profound hypocapneic alkalosis for the treatment of persistent pulmonary hypertension in infancy. J Pediatr 1984; 105:457–61.

(38) John E, Roberts V, Burnard ED. Persistent pulmonary hypertension of the newborn treated with hyperventilation: clinical features and outcome. Aust Paediatr J 1988;24:357–61.

(39) Ballard RA, Leonard CH. Developmental follow-up of infants with persistent pulmonary hypertension of the newborn. Clin Perinatol 1984;11:737–43.

failure: a prospective randomized study. Pediatrics 1985;76:479–87.

6

Alternative Therapies for Respiratory Failure

❖

J. Devn Cornish, M.D.
Reese H. Clark, M.D.

Acute respiratory failure continues to be one of the leading causes of death in the neonatal period and the third most frequent cause of death among children thereafter (1). It is also a significant cause of death and disability among adult patients; hundreds of thousands of adults require ventilator support in the United States each year. Although a variety of insults may lead to acute, severe pulmonary dysfunction, therapeutic alternatives once the disease has progressed have basically been limited to endotracheal intubation and mechanical ventilation. The emergence in recent years of several new therapies for acute respiratory failure, of which ECMO is only one, substantially expands the physician's options. However, prudent selection among these alternatives requires a working knowledge of each. In this chapter, we will review many of the newer therapies for acute respiratory failure to place them, along with ECMO, in their proper perspective.

"UNCONVENTIONAL" USE OF MECHANICAL VENTILATORS

First and most obvious among the alternatives to "conventional" mechanical ventilation might be some minor modification of this technique which either reduces the risks or amplifies the benefits of using existing respirators. Approaches that have been proposed for use in adult patients include synchronized intermittent mandatory ventilation (2–6), pressure support ventilation (7–10), mandatory minute volume ventilation (11), airway pressure release ventilation (12–16), and inverse ratio ventilation (17). Constant flow ventilation (18–21) and a variant of this mode called tracheal insufflation of oxygen (22–24) have been proposed based on animal studies but have not yet been shown to be of clinical value in humans. Each of these modalities can be applied using a conventional ventilator design to which microprocessor technology has conferred unique interactive capabilities. The resultant devices are intended to provide improved respiratory support for specific types of patients or during specific phases of the mechanical ventilation course. Unfortunately, the consequence of this growing variety of devices and techniques has been increasing confusion about the interface between the device and the disease process. Which, if any, of these new approaches will prove to be clinically important awaits the test of time.

Among neonatal patients, a more limited range of "new" ventilator strategies has been reported. Inverse ratio ventilation was initially proposed for use in neonates with the respiratory distress syndrome (RDS) (25) where it was felt to contribute to alveolar recruitment and stabilization (26). The application of high mean, end-expiratory, and/or peak airway pressures has become commonplace in the management of the severely hypoxic neonate. As might be anticipated, the consequence has often been the appearance of air leak syndromes of all types (pneumothorax, pneumomediastinum, pulmonary interstitial emphysema, etc.). In similar fashion, many neonatologists have used very fast rates (in excess of 100 breaths per minute) in managing their sickest patients, perhaps in partial emulation of the "hyperventilation" strategy proposed by Drummond et al. (27) and by Fox and coworkers (28). Substantial risks are known to be associated with this strategy (29) which has sometimes been mistakenly referred to as "high-frequency ventilation." As with the new adult strategies mentioned previously, apart from subjective impressions, there is no compelling evidence that any one of these strategies has resulted in an improvement in outcomes among respiratory failure patients.

HIGH-FREQUENCY VENTILATION

Unlike the modifications of conventional ventilator function represented by the previous category, high-frequency ventilation (HFV) is a novel respiratory support modality in both mechanical and physiologic terms. HFV has been defined as mechanical ventilation at four times the normal respiratory rate (30) or at two or more times the resting respiratory rate with a tidal volume that is close to or less than the anatomic dead space (31). Other definitions have been proposed, but the essence of the concept is mechanical ventilation at supraphysiologic rates with low tidal volumes.

Although the commercial production of respirators intended to operate at these very high rates is a new phenomenon, the concept that effective ventilation might be accomplished with tidal volumes substantially less than dead space is not new. In 1915, Henderson and colleagues (32) published a series of remarkable observations made on panting dogs and on tobacco smoke blown into long tubes. They concluded that, "there may easily be gaseous exchange sufficient to support life, even when the tidal volume is considerably less than dead space." Interestingly, this paper seems to have had little impact on either the physiologic understanding or clinical practice of mechanical respiratory support. The first mechanical device designed to supply rapid rate, low tidal volume ventilation was patented in 1959 by Emerson who intuitively predicted much of the theory now used to explain this physiologic enigma. In his patent application (33), Emerson speculated, "Vibrating the column of gas doubtless causes the gas to diffuse more rapidly within the airway and therefore aids in the breathing function...." In 1967, Sjostrand and others developed a ventilator with very low internal compliance which could deliver breaths at rates of 60–100/min using small tidal volumes (34). In 1972, Lunkenheimer and colleagues discovered that dogs could be maintained normocapnic by the oscillations of a loudspeaker diaphragm at rates of 23–40 Hz (35,36). Heijman and associates (37) reported the use of high-frequency positive-pressure ventilation during anesthesia and routine surgery in 1972 and employed this approach (38) to treat neonates with the respiratory distress syndrome in 1974. Subsequent research and clinical applications of this concept followed in rapid succession in the late 1970s and early 1980s (39–44). Much of the best research and clinical information on this subject has been reviewed recently (45–47).

Types of High-Frequency Ventilators

Because so many different devices may be encompassed within the broad definition of high-frequency ventilator, it is easy to become confused when reading the literature. Some of the systems described are well advertised, have been manufactured by large companies, and have been subjected to extensive testing; others have been constructed only for research purposes by the interested investigators and are less well characterized or published. Worse yet, the differences among the reported devices in design and function may be substantial from an engineering or physiologic standpoint though totally transparent to the general reader. As a consequence, it may be tenuous to compare results achieved with any given high-frequency ventilator to those obtained with a dissimilar apparatus, even if both are correctly classified as "high-frequency ventilators." Four distinct subdivisions of high-frequency ventilators have been proposed: high-frequency positive-pressure ventilators (HFPPV), high-frequency jet ventilators (HFJV), high-frequency flow interrupters (HFFI), and high-frequency oscillatory ventilators (HFOV). As though the confusion were not already bad enough, there is no universal agreement as to how these subdivisions are to be defined. Some have delineated them on the basis of the maximum achievable respiratory rate, others on the pattern of the pressure wave produced, and still others on the basis of gas flow dynamics.

In a laudable attempt to decrease the confusion, Froese recommended (48) that all HFV systems be classified either as oscillators, jets, flow interrupters, or positive-pressure ventilators (as above) and then subclassified in terms of whether the expiratory phase is active or passive. Thus, ventilators that actively enhance gas egress (including the "oscillators" generally) are called "active" high-frequency ventilators. Those that rely on accumulated gas pressure within the airways and the intrinsic elastic recoil properties of the thoracopulmonary system for gas escape are referred to as "passive." Ventilator systems that have elements of both are referred to as "hybrid." This classification system is important since it may group ventilators not only by their gas egress characteristics but also according to the underlying physical and physiologic principles on which they function and thus, potentially, according to their clinical effects. Although the same author has since demonstrated that low tidal volume, high-frequency ventilators of different types can be successfully used with similar strategies in the management of experimental animals with diffuse alveolar disease (49), physicians considering the use of HFV for severely ill patients should understand the basic characteristics and performance limitations of each HFV type before applying any device in a clinical setting.

Unlike many conventional respirators, high-frequency positive-pressure ventilators (HFPPVs) are designed to have minimal internal compliance and minimal compressible volume in the circuit and can operate at superphysiologic rates. The tidal volumes are generally less than those used during conventional mechanical ventilation. Sjostrand has reported favorable outcomes using lower measured peak and mean airway pressures than during conventional ventilation in the IMV mode (50). HFPPVs have proved useful for bronchoscopy, laryngoscopy, upper airway surgery, and thoracic and upper abdominal surgery. It is critical to recognize that these results and the low complication rate reported may not necessarily be reproduced if one simply turns a conventional ventilator up to a very high rate in an attempt to simulate HFPPV (29,51). In fact, the "inadvertent PEEP" engendered by repeated insufflation of gas volumes that are incompletely exhaled before the onset of the next inflation may result in a heightened risk of gas trapping (52) and of air leak syndromes (not to mention more subtle forms of airway injury), a result that was never intended by those who introduced HFPPV. There is not presently an HFPPV device marketed for clinical use in the United States.

High-frequency jet ventilators (HFJVs) may be thought of collectively as mechanisms that repeatedly interrupt the flow of a humidified, low-caliber, high-velocity gas stream into the distal trachea, the flow generally being delivered through the narrow channel of a double-lumen endotracheal tube. These are "passive" devices, as gas exhalation occurs spontaneously through the larger lumen of the endotracheal airway. HFJVs are commonly used in concert with conventional ventilators that provide continuous positive airway pressure and occasional conventional ("sign") breaths. They have been extensively studied and provide the basis for much of the laboratory and clinical data in the literature. In addition to the generally accepted indications for HFV (e.g., refractory air leak syndromes—especially bronchopleural fistula, ventilatory failure, and refractory hypoxia), these ventilators have been particularly useful in applications where a standard endotracheal airway cannot be introduced because of their unique ability to insufflate through a very narrow channel. Examples of such situations include laryngoscopy, bronchoscopy, laryngeal or tracheal surgery, and emergency transtracheal ventilation. The Bunnell Life Pulse High Frequency Ventilator (Bunnell Inc., Salt Lake City, Utah), a typical HFJV, is one of only three HFVs that have either been approved or are pending approval by the Food and Drug Administration (FDA) for clinical use in neonates in the United States (53).

There are a number of characteristics of HFJV systems that cause concern in clinical applications. Since gas entry and egress occur through different channels, a specialized endotracheal tube with at least two lumens is required, making reintubation of potentially unstable patients necessary. (Most commonly, a triple-lumen tube is used, the third channel allowing airway pressure to be measured at the tip of the tube.) Because of the high velocity of the gas stream and reliance on passive exhalation, the potential for air trapping, hyperinflation, and air leak syndromes is of concern. Also, this gas stream is difficult to effectively humidify and may be particularly damaging to the airway. Debate continues as to whether potentially life-threatening upper airway injury (particularly necrotizing tracheobronchitis [NTB]) is more common with HFJV than with other forms of HFV or even with conventional ventilators (54–59). Though the reported incidence of NTB and HFJV has clearly been high in the past, no controlled clinical comparisons of HFJV and other modes of ventilation have demonstrated a statistically significant difference in the incidence of NTB based on ventilator type. It has been the subjective impression at many centers, including our own, that the frequency of NTB among HFJV patients has decreased with improvements in the humidification systems.

High-frequency flow interrupters (HFFIs) are not widely employed either for clinical or investigational purposes. Conceptually, an HFFI functions much like an HFJV except that the high-velocity gas stream is delivered to a chamber proximal to the endotracheal tube where the caliber of the gas stream expands and its velocity decreases. As with HFJV, gas egress is passive. These devices generally operate at frequencies of 100–200 breaths per minute (bpm) in adults and up to 1,200 bpm in neonates. A specialized endotracheal tube is not required. The Programmable Volumetric Diffusive Ventilator (Percussionaire Inc., Sandpoint, Idaho) has been used in limited trials in neonates, infants, and adults and is currently being marketed in Europe. It is an archetypal example of HFFI, but is not currently a candidate for FDA approval. The HFV Infant Star ventilator (Infrasonics Inc., San Diego, California) may be categorized either as a flow interrupter or as a hybrid device. Using a microprocessor to govern a set of metered pneumatic valves, which control the flow source, and a venturi system on the exhalation valve to facilitate gas egress, it does produce an oscillating pressure wave form. However, the exhalation system does not actively contribute to gas egress, so exhalation is passive. This device is important since it has recently been approved by the FDA for the treatment of infants with air leak and respiratory failure. However, as a matter of practical experience, it is usually not as effective as other HFV devices in the management of larger neonates since the maximum available tidal volume is quite limited.

High-frequency oscillatory ventilators (HFOVs) may be typified by the original high-frequency ventilator, the Emerson Airway Vibrator (J. H. Emerson, Cambridge, Massachusetts), which is now essentially out of use. It is actuated by a motor that moves a piston back and forth on an eccentric cam. Since air is moved in and out of the airway by exactly equivalent positive and negative piston excursions, there is both active inflation and exhalation, but there is no net air movement. Consequently, a secondary source of inspiratory gas flow, generally referred to as "bias flow," must be introduced, usually by entrainment. The humidification of this relatively large caliber gas stream is fairly simple to control. Gas egress occurs during the negative piston stroke out through a conventional endotracheal tube and through a controlled leak or resistor called a "low-pass filter." HFOVs may be operated at the fastest rates of any HFV, ranging up to 40–50 Hz (2,400–3,000 breaths per minute) in some designs. The multicenter controlled trial of HFV sponsored by the National Institutes of Health

(NIH) (see below) utilized an oscillator (the Hummingbird BMO 20N) exclusively. An updated version of this ventilator, the Humming II (Senko Medical Instruments, Tokyo, Japan) has been used in Japan and is scheduled for clinical trials in the United States. It employs a piston driven by a feedback-controlled linear motor and can operate at rates from 0–30 Hz (53). Perhaps most important at present is the SensorMedics 3100, the only HFOV currently licensed by the FDA for clinical use in neonates. This device oscillates the airway by the to-and-fro movement of a small piston in an electromagnetic field. The movements of the piston are amplified by its connection to a diaphragm (not unlike the loudspeaker experiments of Lunkenheimer and colleagues). The 3100 is capable of varying frequency between 3–18 Hz as well as inspiratory/expiratory time ratio and amplitude of piston displacement.

Clinical Results with High-Frequency Ventilation

Users of HFV systems have reported them to be effective in treating bronchopleural fistula, pulmonary interstitial emphysema, refractory pneumothorax, ventilatory failure, and severe hypoxia. For neonatal patients, efficacy in managing the respiratory distress syndrome, meconium aspiration, persistent pulmonary hypertension, pulmonary hypoplasia, and congenital diaphragmatic hernia has also been claimed. There is even some experimental evidence (60) to imply that HFOV may prevent the "initial insult" that leads to the development of the respiratory distress syndrome (RDS) in premature baboons known to be surfactant deficient. In a variety of clinical settings, these devices are able to effect a dramatic reduction in the arterial P_{CO_2}, although their ability to improve arterial oxygenation has been less uniform. A number of studies have concluded that a given HFV achieved equal or better oxygenation than a conventional mechanical ventilator (CMV) at lower inspired oxygen concentrations and lower mean airway pressures. However, these experimental findings, at least in terms of oxygenation, have frequently not proved to be clinically relevant. More commonly, equivalent oxygenation to that achieved with CMV is obtained only at somewhat higher mean airway pressures and/or inspired oxygen concentrations. Without question, there remain several specialized circumstances in which HFV has unique advantages, such as in the case of upper airway surgery, during procedures where pulmonary motion is undesirable, and (potentially) for the establishment of emergency transtracheal ventilation.

The findings of the few controlled clinical trials direct us to rather more restricted conclusions about the efficacy of HFV than the generalizations just presented might suggest. In a large prospective controlled trial of HFJV versus CMV in adult patients with acute, diffuse lung injury, Carlon and others (61) were unable to demonstrate any significant difference in outcome between the two groups.

The largest prospective controlled trial in neonatal patients was the NIH-sponsored multicenter study reported by the "HIFI Study Group" in 1989 (62). This study of 673 newborns with respiratory failure weighing 750–2,000 grams failed to show any difference in the incidence of bronchopulmonary dysplasia (BPD) or in mortality between those patients randomized to receive HFOV and those treated with CMV. There was a significantly higher rate of crossover from HFOV to CMV than the other direction, and the HFOV group experienced greater incidences of high-grade (3 and 4) intracranial hemorrhage, periventricular leukomalacia, and pneumoperitoneum of pulmonary origin. HFOV was not associated with a decreased oxygen requirement or lower mean airway pressures, and there was a higher likelihood of atelectasis following extubation in the HFOV group. This study concluded that there was no advantage of HFOV (as used) over CMV and that HFOV may be associated with undesirable side-effects. Interestingly, Bryan and Froese (63) have recently suggested that the failure of this and other HFV trials to show benefit in terms of diminished lung injury and improved survival may be attributable to the use of a pressure-sparing as opposed to a volume-optimizing strategy.

Subsequent evaluations of the patients treated in the HIFI trial have been reported. Pulmonary function testing (PFT) at nine months corrected age showed no difference in results between groups, though both HFOV and CMV patients had abnormal PFTs, and the incidence of chronic pulmonary changes consistent with the diagnosis of bronchopulmonary dysplasia was 30–40% in both groups (64). This is similar to the findings of Gerhardt and colleagues from their controlled trial of HFOV compared to CMV (65). A subsequent review of the neurodevelopmental status of the same patients at 16–24 months' "postterm age" (66) provided several disconcerting findings: there was a significantly higher incidence of hydrocephalus (12% vs. 6%, $p < 0.05$) in the HFOV group; Bayley index scores greater than 83 were recorded in 57% of the HFOV-treated infants as compared to 66% of the CMV patients; and the proportion of children with a normal neurodevelopmental status at follow-up (i.e., Bayley score greater than 83 and no major neurologic defect) was significantly less in the HFOV as compared to the CMV group (54% vs. 65%, $p < 0.05$). As might have been anticipated, both treatment groups showed a strong association between the development of grade 3 or 4 intraventricular hemorrhage and the later appearance of major neurological or cognitive defects.

Carlo and co-workers (67) summarized the results of their randomized prospective study of 42 infants with severe respiratory distress syndrome who received either HFJV or CMV. Like the larger HIFI trial, this study failed to demonstrate any differences between the two groups in mortality or in the incidence of bronchopulmonary dysplasia. However, unlike the HIFI trial, the incidences of air leaks, intraventricular hemorrhage, and assignment crossovers also did not differ between the two groups. The authors concluded that the early use of HFJV did not alter either morbidity or mortality; however, in the absence of the undesirable side-effects seen in the larger HFOV trial, they suggested further studies of HFJV in selected high-risk neonates.

These results are in contrast to the findings of a smaller prospective randomized comparison of two distinct strategies of HFOV to CMV by Clark and colleagues (68). Eighty-three premature infants with birthweight less than 1,751 grams were assigned to receive either CMV ($n = 26$), HFOV for 72 hours followed by CMV ($n = 27$), or HFOV alone ($n = 30$). There was no difference among the groups in the incidence of air leak syndromes, intraventricular hemorrhage, or mortality. Both of the HFOV groups tended toward lower rates of chronic lung disease than the CMV group as assessed at 30 days of life and at 36 weeks postconceptual age (PCA), but this difference was statistically significant only between the CMV and the HFOV-alone groups (65% vs. 30% at 30 d, $p = 0.008$; 38% vs. 10% at 36 wk PCA, $p = 0.013$). This finding is supported by the work of Frantz (69), who noted a 17% incidence of chronic lung disease among premature neonates managed with HFOV as compared to 47% in those treated with CMV without an associated increase in neurologic morbidity.

The Role of High-Frequency Ventilation in Neonatal ECMO Candidates

Now let us inquire specifically into the possibility that HFV, clearly a less invasive procedure, might forestall or eliminate the need for ECMO among the traditional neonatal ECMO population. No prospective controlled trial comparing neonatal ECMO candidates randomized to receive ECMO as opposed to HFV has been conducted. However, four groups have retrospectively reviewed their experience with potential ECMO patients treated with HFV, ECMO, or both.

Kohelet and co-workers (70) reported their experience using HFOV to treat neonates with persistent pulmonary hypertension of the newborn (PPHN). Forty-one neonatal patients weighing at least 2.0 kg at birth developed PPHN and were offered a trial of HMOV. Thirty-four experienced a significant increase in mean arterial/alveolar oxygen tension ratio within one hour of starting HFOV, all of whom survived. Of the remaining seven patients, four did not improve on HFOV and were returned to CMV (two died, one normal, one BPD). Three patients who showed early improvement on HFOV went on to die. Significantly, one of these was subsequently diagnosed as having "wet lung syndrome" and necrotizing tracheobronchitis. Although the observed incidence of BPD was similar to that reported using CMV alone, these investigators noted that the duration of CMV support preceding HFOV was significantly longer in the 13 neonates who subsequently developed BPD than in the 21 who did not (44.7 ± 32.3 vs. 19.1 ± 15.6 h, $p < 0.002$). Also, the duration of exposure to a mean airway pressure over 15 cm H_2O was longer in the BPD group (31.8 ± 21.3 vs. 9.5 ± 6.0 h, $p < 0.001$). They suggested that earlier use of HFOV in these patients might be associated with a reduced incidence of BPD.

Carter and others (71), building on the results of their previous study (72), reported 50 neonates who met local ECMO criteria after failing conventional therapy. Four were moribund on arrival and died before they could be started on HFOV or before ECMO could be instituted; 21 improved on HFOV and survived to hospital discharge; 25 required ECMO, of whom 22 (88%) survived to discharge. Thus, a large proportion of neonatal ECMO candidates (46%) who had failed to respond to aggressive conventional ventilator and pharmacologic support strategies could be successfully supported using HFOV without recourse to ECMO.

ECMO patients had a higher incidence of bleeding complications, seizures, and renal failure than did those who received HFOV alone. It has been the aggregate experience of several centers that HFOV and HFJV are more effective in patients with "homogeneous" types of pulmonary pathology, such as the respiratory distress syndrome, pneumonia, and pulmonary interstitial emphysema (73); less uniform types of lung pathology such as meconium aspiration syndrome (MAS), persistent pulmonary hypertension, and congenital diaphragmatic hernia (CDH) seem less likely to respond to HFV and more frequently require ECMO. An informal review of 112 neonatal ECMO candidates managed at Wilford Hall USAF Medical Center in San Antonio, Texas (Figure 6.1), demonstrates these trends. A trial of HFOV was offered upon failure to respond to conventional ventilator and pharmacologic support. Patients who in turn did not improve on HFOV were treated with ECMO. Thirty-three percent (15/45) of meconium aspiration, 72% (26/36) of pneumonia and/or acute respiratory distress syndrome (ARDS), 21% (3/14) of congenital diaphragmatic hernia, and 92% (11/12) of respiratory distress syndrome patients responded to HFOV and did not require ECMO. Patients in the "other" category included four with lung hypoplasia syndromes (other than CDH) and one with congenital heart disease and an anomalous airway; one of the patients with lung hypoplasia did not require ECMO.

Vaucher and co-workers (74) documented the pulmonary and neurodevelopmental status of 45 surviving neonates with birthweight over 2.0 kg who were treated for severe respiratory

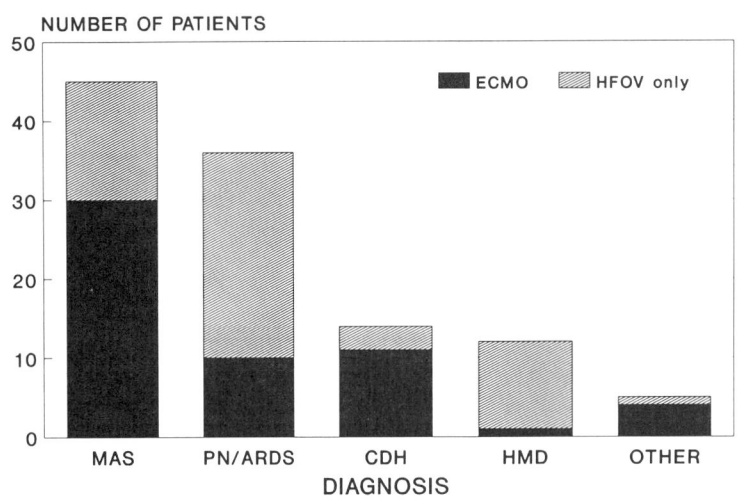

FIGURE 6.1 Neonatal patients with more "homogeneous" lung diseases (such as pneumonia) tend to respond to high-frequency ventilation better than those with "patchy" processes (such as meconium aspiration). MAS = meconium aspiration syndrome, PN/ARDS = pneumonia and/or acute respiratory distress syndrome, CDH = congenital diaphragmatic hernia, HMD = hyaline membrane disease.

failure using HFOV alone ($n = 13$) or ECMO with or without preceding HFOV ($n = 32$) after failing conventional therapy. The risk of chronic lung disease was lower in the ECMO than in the HFOV group (19% vs. 67%), as was the incidence of air leak (77% vs. 41%). Neurologic outcome was similar in both groups, though mental scores were higher in the ECMO-treated group, a difference that was attributable to the lower incidence of chronic lung disease among these patients.

Schwendeman and colleagues (75) have expanded the study of Carter et al. and have evaluated the incidence of chronic lung disease in this larger population. Their review of 48 infants treated with HFOV alone and 46 treated with HFOV and ECMO revealed that 20 of 84 survivors (24%) developed chronic lung disease (CLD), with this finding being more common among those with lung hypoplasia (40% vs. 5%, $p < 0.01$) and among those requiring ECMO as opposed to those receiving only HFOV (38% vs. 11%, $p < 0.01$). However, when infants with lung hypoplasia were excluded from consideration, similar to the exclusion of congenital diaphragmatic (CDH) patients in Vaucher's study, the frequency of CLD became more comparable between the ECMO and the HFOV groups (22% vs. 12%). Among neonates without definable pulmonary hypoplasia, age at initiation of HFOV was higher among those who developed CLD than among those who did not (median 91 vs. 46 h, $p < 0.01$).

These discrepant data on the incidence of CLD among ECMO as opposed to HFOV-treated patients bear further evaluation. The studies of Carter/Schwendeman and of Vaucher differed in the HFOV device and strategy employed, in the definition of chronic lung disease used, and in the ages of patients at follow-up. Removal of CDH patients from the analysis certainly makes the results more comparable. However, evaluation of the raw data for the patients studied by Carter and by Vaucher has convinced the current authors that the much longer period of conventional ventilator support between the moment of meeting ECMO criteria and initiation of ECMO in Carter's group of patients than in Vaucher's may account for the higher demonstrated incidence of chronic lung disease.

Only one study, by Carlo and co-workers (76), has evaluated the use of HFJV for ECMO candidate neonates. Forty-one neonates met rigorous criteria for PPHN and for treatment with ECMO; four were excluded from consideration because they received ECMO; 14 were offered HFJV, generally because of inability to achieve $Paco_2 < 35$ mm Hg using conventional ventilation; and 23 continued on CMV. The 14 treated with HFJV had lower mean airway pressure and $Paco_2$ than previously and than those on CMV. There was no difference between the groups in oxygen gradient, incidence of air leaks, incidence of BPD, duration of ventilator or supplemental oxygen support, or mortality (64% vs. 65%).

What may be said in summary then about the possibility that HFV might decrease the need for ECMO? Kohelet's paper might be taken to imply that the need for ECMO was largely averted by HFOV since 36/41 of his patients survived (88%). However, their patient population may not be comparable to those of the other studies since the criteria for switching from CMV to HFOV were less stringent than usual (arterial/alveolar oxygen ratio < 0.1 with mean airway pressure > 15, $Paco_2 > 45$ mm Hg with ventilator rate > 70 and peak pressure > 30 cm H_2O, and/or "massive air leak"). The study by Vaucher and co-workers did not consider the therapeutic efficacy of HFOV as compared to ECMO but simply evaluated the outcomes among survivors of both techniques. The high mortality rates for both the CMV and HFJV groups in the study by Carlo et al. would easily justify recourse to ECMO where the overall survival rate continues to be 83% (77).

In the study by Carter et al., about half (46%) of the patients who might have been offered ECMO were successfully supported with HFOV. However, most ECMO centers report that a similar proportion of patients referred for ECMO do well almost irrespective of the therapeutic modality or ventilator strategy used. Without prospective controlled trials, it is impossible to determine whether HFV is uniquely effective as an alternative to ECMO (i.e., more so than CMV) and whether, given its risks, HFV is in fact preferable to ECMO in the long run. The question of the comparative risks and benefits of HFV and ECMO will become even more difficult as venovenous ECMO and heparin-free ECMO become more common.

Most advocates of HFV believe it to be acceptably safe and effective in the larger neonate if employed early in the course of respiratory failure and report that improvement on HFV generally occurs within 6–12 hours. The prolonged use of HFV in ECMO candidates who do not show improvement in oxygenation within this time frame is not recommended. This is equivalent to delaying transfer of a qualifying patient to an ECMO center and may increase morbidity and mortality. Use of HFV for stabilization and transport is not practical since transport on HFV is still not well established and is exceptionally difficult. In the patient who meets ECMO criteria, HFV should be offered only if ECMO is readily available, as acute decompensation can and often does occur.

SURFACTANT REPLACEMENT THERAPY

Since the initial report of Avery and Mead (78), the critical role of substances that decrease the surface tension at the alveolar lining has been apparent. The potential therapeutic benefit of replacing missing surfactant in premature infants who are unable to meet their own requirements has likewise been appreciated. In recent years, researchers in this area have been able to identify the individual components of native human surfactant; elucidate the metabolic processes responsible for their production, release, deployment, uptake, and reprocessing; clone and sequence the controlling genes; and even synthesize the constituent lipids and proteins. Natural, synthetic, and semisynthetic surfactant preparations have been developed and tested. The clinical utility of these products in decreasing ventilator support requirements and improving survival for premature infants with surfactant deficiency has been well demonstrated. The potential clinical impact of successful surfactant replacement therapy is substantial since 30,000–40,000 neonates develop the respiratory distress syndrome in the United States and Canada each year (79), and some 300,000–400,000 adults are treated annually for the "adult" or "acute" form of the respiratory distress syndrome (ARDS), some of whom may also benefit from exogenous surfactant.

Artificial Surfactant Preparations

Just as with high-frequency ventilation, there is more than one way to go about replacing deficient surfactant. Three types of surfactant preparations have been tested clinically: totally synthetic mixtures of surfactant-related lipids without accompanying protein moieties, several varieties of surfactant lipids and proteins derived either entirely from animal sources (usually bovine or porcine) or mixed with synthetic additives, and native human surfactant extracted from amniotic fluid. A fourth type of surfactant product that would combine synthetic surfactant lipids with human surfactant proteins produced using recombinant DNA technology is contemplated for the near future. Each of these surfactant types will be discussed so that the potential user may more readily understand the differences in their clinical effects, relative advantages, and hazards.

Two totally synthetic surfactant preparations have been tested. The more extensively studied is Exosurf, a product of the Burroughs Wellcome company (Exosurf Neonatal for Intratracheal Suspension, Burroughs Wellcome Co., Research Triangle Park, North Carolina) that was initially developed by Clements (80). It is composed of dipalmitoyl phosphatidylcholine, cetyl alcohol, and tyloxapol. Both laboratory and clinical evidence support the claim of efficacy for this product (81–83), though, empirically, its onset of action seems to be noticeably slower (on the order of 6–12 hours) than that of other formulations. It is speculated that this may be attributable to the absence of surfactant-associated proteins with the consequent requirement that it be absorbed into pneumocytes, repackaged along with native materials, and secreted in an active form onto the alveolar surface. The European version of a totally synthetic surfactant is known as ALEC (artificial lung-expanding compound). It is composed of dipalmitoyl phosphatidylcholine and unsaturated phosphatidyl glycerol in a 7:3 weight:weight ratio (84). Like Exosurf, its clinical efficacy has also been established (84–86).

A number of extracts of animal surfactant have been tested clinically for the prevention and therapy of RDS in premature infants. Limited experience has been acquired using calf lung surfactant extract (CLSE), a product recovered by bronchoalveolar lavage and chloroform-methanol extraction that contains about 1% protein (87). Clinical trials have also been reported using surfactant prepared from minced porcine lungs by chloroform-methanol extraction and liquid-gel chromatography (Curosurf) that also contains 1% protein (88). More extensive clinical studies have been performed using Surfactant-TA (now known as Survanta in the United States) (89,90). This product is an organic solvent extract of minced bovine lung tissue supplemented with phospholipids (dipalmitoyl phosphatidyl choline, tripalmitin, and palmitic acid). It contains 1–2% hydrophobic apoproteins. Such extracts are devoid of surfactant-associated protein A (SP-A), though they do contain the smaller peptides SP-B and SP-C that are known to impart surfactantlike properties to the phospholipid mixtures and have been shown to be therapeutically effective.

Naturally occurring human surfactant has been isolated by sucrose gradient centrifugation from amniotic fluid obtained aseptically at cesarean section delivery (91). It contains 5% protein, including both large hydrophilic and small hydrophobic apoproteins. The safety of this product is assured by testing the sera of amniotic fluid donors for hepatitis B surface antigen, by heating the surfactant to 56°C to inactivate any HIV particles, and by testing the surfactant for the presence of HIV p24 antigen. Human surfactant has been evaluated in a variety of clinical studies (91–96) and shown to be effective. This finding is of importance principally because a lack of demonstrable clinical benefit using native surfactants would make the study of nonhuman or synthetic surfactants meaningless. However, it is unlikely that human surfactant preparations will ever become commercially available since the requisite processes are not practical in production terms.

Clinical Experience with Surfactant Replacement Therapy

More than three decades of surfactant research have resulted in an abundance of information about the nature of the surface active molecules affecting pulmonary function and their laboratory and clinical effects. As might be expected, given the variety of surfactant preparations available, the results of clinical trials (97–103) using these products are not uniform. However, there have been among the results a number of recurring themes that warrant summary here. First, there is no question that, especially with the protein-containing preparations, surfactant administration results in a rapid improvement (over minutes to hours) in gas exchange and a decrease in ventilator support requirements (81,88,94,102,104,105). Although studies have reported improvements in pulmonary mechanics (106), it is not entirely clear that the clinical changes observed result as much from improvements in compliance and other pulmonary functional parameters as from improved ventilation/perfusion matching and capillary stability with decreased leakage of fluid into the alveoli (107).

Second, a number of individual studies (or the meta-analysis of grouped studies) have shown either a decrease in the incidence of BPD, an improvement in survival, or an improvement in BPD-free survival (81,82,84, 86,88,93,98,108–110). It is of interest that more dramatic improvements in survival have not been demonstrated in most studies, and, in fact, all studies have not shown an improvement in survival (102). There may be several explanations for this phenomenon. Certainly, there are numerous other threats to the survival of premature neonates even if their lung disease has been treated effectively. Perhaps more to the point, virtually none of the studies cited has taken the precaution of testing neonatal study patients prior to surfactant administration to document that they were in fact surfactant deficient. When Merritt and colleagues (96) made this assessment, they found that 20% of the identified study candidates had lung disease other than RDS. However, when they limited their analysis to truly surfactant-deficient recipients, they were able to demonstrate a significant decrease by human surfactant replacement both in total mortality and in deaths caused by RDS or BPD ($p = 0.0001$). Thus, the problem of inconsistent improvements in survival may lie not nearly so much in the efficacy of surfactant therapy as in the precision of the method used in a given study. Similarly, Long and co-workers demonstrated a 50% reduction in overall mortality, but a 66% reduction in deaths attributable to RDS (83).

Third, there is little question that these preparations are safe. Rarely does a study demonstrate any significant difference in the incidence of complications of prematurity (e.g., intracranial hemorrhage, necrotizing enterocolitis, infections, etc.) among treatment groups, much less reveal any unique and untoward effect of the surfactant preparation itself. The intuitive suspicion that these agents might, especially if unevenly distributed, contribute to an increase in the incidence of air leak phenomena has not proved to be the case; in fact, the opposite result has been found repeatedly (81,89,93,98,104). Similarly, it is unusual for a study to show an increased incidence of physiologically significant left-to-right shunting across the ductus arteriosus (95,100). Although one study did show a trend toward more allergic manifestations in survivors treated with surfactant (111), concerns about the potential antigenic consequences of exposure to animal proteins (79) have not been borne out either by clinical experience or by careful testing for antibodies in the blood of treated infants to the foreign surfactant-related proteins known to have been administered (90). One study did show an increased incidence of necrotizing enterocolitis (89) and another an increased incidence of intraventricular hemorrhage (110) in the surfactant-treated group. Even so, the most significant threat to the claim of product safety has come from the anecdotal reports of pulmonary hemorrhage (generally very mild) after surfactant administration. This bleeding may actually be a manifestation of pulmonary edema resulting from early left-to-right shunting across a patent ductus arteriosus that may in turn be amenable to aggressive pharmacologic and surgical management (112).

Obviously, there are more questions remaining than there are ready answers. Benefit has been shown from both "prophylactic" administration of surfactant to premature infants in the delivery room and from "rescue" or "treatment" dosing once clinical evidence of RDS has become manifest (113). The aggregate of available evidence seems to support the conclusion that prophylactic treatment has little or no advantage over administration only to patients with demonstrated disease. It also seems likely from several "multidose" trials (83,94,96,105,106) that repeated administration will become routine. While the intratracheal route of administration is universally accepted, the ideal dosage form and method of dispersal continue to be questioned, with powdered (84) or crystalline preparations being tested and aerosolization at a smaller total dose being considered. As the functional role of the surfactant-associated proteins continues to be delineated, the relative advantage of including specific proteins in the product from human as opposed to animal sources is being debated. This discussion will become all the more exciting as recombinant DNA technology makes the former more available. Ultimately, decisions about dosage form and amount, method and timing of administration, and final composition of the surfactant must take into account the complex interactions between exogenous surfactant and the intrinsic pathways of surfactant production, packaging, secretion, deployment, inhibition, destruction, reuptake, and remanufacture. And consideration will have to be given to the potential risks of perturbing these delicately balanced processes by inadvertent administration of the drug to patients who are not, in fact, surfactant deficient (96).

In view of the demonstrated benefits of exogenous surfactant administration for premature infants with established surfactant deficiency and yet with concern about its potential for untoward consequences, the Committee on the Fetus and Newborn of the American Academy of Pediatrics issued a formal policy statement in April 1991 regarding surfactant replacement therapy (114). In essence, their recommendation was a plea that surfactant be administered (except in emergency circumstances) only in intensive care nurseries where appropriate personnel and facilities are in place to provide comprehensive services to these high-risk patients. Admittedly, pulmonary immaturity is not the only risk to which low-birthweight babies are subjected. Moreover, the restriction of surfactant dosing to competent intensive care facilities seems prudent in view of the incomplete state of our knowledge about the overall effects of this drug.

Exogenous Surfactant in the Neonatal ECMO Candidate

Obviously, the purpose of the foregoing review was largely to set the stage for the question more pertinent to this text: Does surfactant have a role in the treatment of patients with severe respiratory failure who are being considered for ECMO? Although the question is intriguing, and a body of anecdotal experience is already beginning to accumulate, there are, regrettably, very few experimental results available. With regard to neonatal patients, Lotze and colleagues (115) documented an increase in surfactant protein A concentrations in the tracheal aspirates of 23 surviving neonatal ECMO patients as their pulmonary compliance and chest radiographic scores improved. These trends were not seen in two infants who did not survive. Whether this phenomenon was a response to the primary disease process or its preceding therapies, the result of alterations in surfactant kinetics, the effect of ongoing lung maturation during the ECMO course, a reflection of global lung healing, or even a contributor to the observed functional improvement could not be determined from these data.

The fact that the SP-A concentrations from most of the survivors early in the course of their ECMO treatment and from the nonsurvivors at all time points were "comparable with levels of SP-A found in the tracheal aspirates from a population of sick preterm infants with severe hyaline membrane disease" implies that both surfactant deficiency may have contributed to the underlying pulmonary dysfunction that led to the need for ECMO and that intrinsic reconstruction of the functional surfactant pool may have facilitated overall pulmonary recovery. The companion questions as to whether exogenous surfactant therapy might reduce the need for ECMO among neonatal candidates and whether surfactant therapy during the course of ECMO might not shorten the required perfusion support period are intriguing. Results from a small study by Auten and colleagues (116) of 14 term neonates with pneumonia or meconium aspiration imply that surfactant replacement may reduce the need for ECMO, especially if employed before respiratory failure has become advanced. Controlled trials are needed to evaluate these questions further.

Surfactant Therapy for the Treatment of ARDS

The acute respiratory distress syndrome is one of the most common forms of severe respiratory failure outside of the neonatal period (and perhaps among neonates as well). In spite of all of the conventional and novel therapies that have been employed, the mortality rate remains in excess of 50% (87). Independent of which of the manifold insults might lead to ARDS, one of the uniform characteristics of this condition is a "permeability and inflammatory edema with damage and destruction at the air blood interface" (117). In addition to the obvious effects of this edema fluid on gas exchange and lung compliance, fluid obtained from ARDS patients by bronchoalveolar lavage is known to be rich in surfactant inhibitors and to have chemically abnormal surfactant (118), functionally converting ARDS into a surfactant deficiency disease. Limited trials of surfactant replacement therapy in patients with ARDS are beginning to be reported (119,120), though it is too early to draw any conclusions about efficacy. Obviously, the questions of dosage form, route, frequency, and amount become even more pressing in this context. Should the neonatal dose (60–200 mg/kg or 5 mL/kg in the case of Exosurf) be adapted to larger pediatric and adult patients, the total annual requirement for commercial surfactant preparations would be astronomical. (One experienced surfactant researcher estimated that, were the bovine surfactant product to be used, it would require surfactant extract from more than four million cattle per year!) It is conceivable that a different dosing approach, such as the use of an aerosolized surfactant powder, might make surfactant replacement for ARDS more practicable.

LESS CONVENTIONAL THERAPIES FOR ACUTE RESPIRATORY FAILURE

Any implication that high-frequency ventilation and surfactant-replacement therapy are the only novel approaches (besides ECLS) being evaluated for the treatment of life-threatening respiratory failure would be inaccurate. Notable among the many other things being tested are negative-pressure ventilation and liquid ventilation.

Negative-Pressure Ventilation

Negative-pressure ventilation (NPV) is, in fact, one of the oldest forms of mechanical ventilation. Its most publicized application, in the form of the famed "iron lung," was to treat the respiratory distress resulting from polio. Thereafter, NPV was extensively utilized for newborns (121–123). These devices were undeniably effective but made it very difficult to adequately warm the neonatal patient and were rumored to increase the risk of intracranial bleeding due to the requirement for an air seal at the neck. Except for the occasional treatment of patients with neuromuscular disorders (124–126), negative-pressure ventilators have generally been abandoned in favor of positive-pressure ventilation that requires no air locks, specialized heaters, or large pieces of equipment.

However, teleological and intuitive arguments continue to drive the testing of negative-pressure ventilators: namely, since normal inflation of the lungs occurs through the imposition of negative intrathoracic pressure by movement of the thoracic cage, might such an approach to lung inflation not be equally effective for gas exchange (at the same transpulmonary pressure) but less traumatic to the tissues? The neonatology group at the University of California at Irvine has investigated the efficacy of NPV in a number of clinical settings. They reported a 50% survival rate among premature infants (27–34 weeks' gestation) presenting with severe lung disease and PIE (127) when treated with NPV in a nonrandomized fashion. Of note is the fact that the mean age at institution of NPV for survivors was 68.3 hours as compared to 134.3 hours for nonsurvivors. When five neonates with PPHN who met ECMO criteria were treated with NPV (128), each experienced a decrease in ventilatory support requirements and a dramatic improvement in oxygenation; all survived without identified pulmonary or neurologic impairments at discharge. A group of 39 preterm and term newborns with refractory hypoxemia ($PaO_2 < 50$ mm Hg) was treated (129) with a combination of CMV and continuous NPV. A comparison of blood gas values and support requirements prior to and 72 hours after starting NPV showed significant decreases in inspired oxygen concentration (57% vs. 100%), mean airway pressure (5.0 vs. 12.8 cm H_2O), ventilator rate (21 vs. 73 per minute) and peak airway pressure (21 vs. 33 cm H_2O) (all $p < 0.05$). They also showed higher arterial/alveolar oxygen ratio (0.226 vs. 0.057) and PaO_2 (58 vs. 38 mm Hg) and lower oxygen gradient (293 vs. 623) (all with $p < 0.05$). Survival for this group was 32/39 (82%), with eight of the patients developing BPD (24%). These investigators have initiated a randomized controlled trial comparing CMV to this combination of CMV and NPV (130). While their results are yet preliminary, it is possible that the outcome of this study will suggest important innovations in our management of patients with acute respiratory failure.

Speculation as to the physiologic reasons for the observed improvements with NPV is intriguing. It is conceivable that the addition of negative extrathoracic pressure simply increases the effective transpulmonary pressure and consequently the driving pressure forcing oxygen into the blood. If true, this explanation is worrisome since increased transpulmonary pressure may be equivalently damaging to the lungs whether it is achieved by augmenting the positive pressure delivered to the airways or by creating negative pressure around the airways. However, the improvements observed are dramatic enough that this simplistic explanation may not suffice. It is likely that a proportion of the observed hypoxia was attributable to intrapulmonary shunting. Perhaps the addition of NPV reduced intrathoracic pressure and thus improved venous return to the heart, cardiac output, pulmonary blood flow, and ventilation/perfusion matching. While caution must be exercised in drawing conclusions from limited data, these preliminary findings are certainly encouraging and justify further investigation.

Liquid Ventilation

Since the 1920s, efforts have been made to exchange gas in the blood through the lungs by ventilating with a liquid medium. Initial attempts to use saline were unsuccessful in part because of its poor oxygen- and carbon dioxide-carrying capacity (3.0 mL and 55.0 mL/100 mL saline at 1 atm, respectively) and its high surface tension (70 dynes/cm). Perfluorochemicals (PFCs) were shown, by contrast, to have a number of salutary physical chemical properties: at 37°C and 1 atmosphere pressure, these chemicals (specifically FC-80) have an oxygen-carrying capacity of 48.5 mL O_2/100 mL PFC and a carbon dioxide-carrying capacity of 160 mL/100 mL PFC; they have a surface tension of 15 dynes/cm; they are chemically inert and are not biotransformable; they are minimally absorbed by the pulmonary capillaries; because of their high vapor pressure, they are rapidly excreted by the lungs once infused; and they have no known adverse effects in animals (131–137). Moreover, intravenous infusion of the same substances to be used as an artificial blood substitute has caused few adverse effects in humans (138,139). Because of their density (1.76 gm/mL at 25°C), PFCs can easily be administered by gravity drainage from a reservoir into the airway; uniformity of distribution is easily assessed since they are radioopaque.

The first use of normobarically oxygenated fluorocarbon liquid as the respiratory gas exchange fluid in the lungs of mammals was reported in 1966 by Clark and Gollan (140) using FX-80 (now FC-80, 3M Company, St. Paul, Minnesota). They were able to support the respiration of mice, cats, and puppies when totally immersed in oxygenated fluorocarbon. Much of the subsequent research in this area has understandably focused on the undersea, hyperbaric, and aerospace medicine possibilities presented by fluorocarbon ventilation.

Shaffer, a pioneer in this field, along with Wolfson and others (141), showed that, because the low surface tension of PFC "negates the dependency of effective pulmonary gas exchange on surfactant development," the viability of very premature fetal lambs could be substantially extended using liquid ventilation (LV). Lowe and Shaffer also demonstrated that increased pulmonary vascular resistance during PFC ventilation results in more balanced ventilation and perfusion matching within the lungs (142). Additionally, the flux of liquid in and out of the lungs can be used to remove particulate material, adjust body temperature, and deliver drugs. Shaffer's group took advantage of these unique properties by using LV to support four lambs delivered with spontaneously occurring meconium aspiration syndrome (143). (A total of seven meconium-stained lambs were identified, but three developed pneumothoraces and died during a 90-minute "control period" on CMV.) Within 15 minutes of instituting LV, there was a significant improvement in both Pao_2 and arterial/alveolar oxygen gradient. During 90 minutes of LV, dynamic lung compliance increased, alveolar and tracheal peak pressures decreased, and inspiratory elastic work of breathing decreased. When the animals were returned to CMV, they continued to show improvements in oxygenation as compared to the control period.

Based on the foregoing and similarly encouraging results from a wealth of animal testing of LV, the first application of this technique to a human was reported by Greenspan and colleagues in 1989 (144). They reported two 3-min trials of LV separated by 15 minutes of gas ventilation in a 28-week gestation, 980-gram, 12-day-old female with respiratory failure and air leak syndrome who had failed both CMV and HFV. A striking improvement in both oxygenation and ventilation, as well as an increase in lung compliance and a decrease in pulmonary resistance, were achieved and maintained for about two hours after the procedure. Unfortunately, the patient died 19 hours after the return to conventional management techniques. Postmortem examination revealed severe hyaline membrane disease and barotrauma but no evidence of retained PFC. There were no nonpulmonary abnormalities. Subsequently, the same group (145) summarized their experience with LV for a total of three preterm newborns (23–28 weeks' gestation) who had failed conventional therapy (one being the infant who had previously been reported). Lung compliance improved markedly in all three, and oxygenation improved in two. All died after discontinuation of LV.

Several obstacles remain before more generalized application of LV in the clinical arena can be recommended (132). Mild metabolic acidosis is commonly seen in adult animals supported with LV, presumably as a result of the cardiovascular adaptations required. Although relatively simple systems may be employed to provide LV treatment, such systems are neither commercially available nor conceptually familiar to most researchers in the field of pulmonary medicine, much less to clinicians. The extraordinary capability of PFCs to exchange heat may become either an asset or a liability, depending on the amount of attention given to the whole question of thermal equilibrium.

As noted by Fuhrman (146), the feasibility of liquid ventilation as a means of achieving normal gas exchange and impressive improvements in lung compliance in human neonates has been established. Whether this methodology becomes accepted as a therapy for severe respiratory failure will depend on subsequent investigations to document its efficacy, practicality, and safety relative to existing modalities. However, the possibilities seem most exciting.

SUMMARY

Severe acute respiratory failure is a condition of such gravity that the search for effective therapies has been compelling. Unfortunately, until very recently, the only treatment available has been mechanical ventilation. Its relative ease of institution, the limited amount of equipment and monitoring required, and the universal availability of ventilators have guaranteed its wide acceptance. Notwithstanding the undeniable improvements in both mortality and morbidity from acute pulmonary failure attendant upon the wide adoption of respirator therapy, modern medical practitioners have had to confront two unhappy facts: A large proportion of patients still do not survive, and there is an unacceptably high incidence of pulmonary dysfunction (some of which is likely ventilator induced) among those who do.

Six decades of research have demonstrated that the extracorporeal diversion of a patient's blood through an artificial gas exchange device continued over periods as long as eight weeks is an effective and acceptably safe means of increasing survival in humans with refractory respiratory failure. However, it would be naive to believe that, because extracorporeal life support is effective, it is either adequately refined in itself or that it is the only "unconventional" respiratory support modality likely to be effective. We have summarized a number of other candidate therapies whose utility in this context deserves consideration. These include more "conservative" ventilator strategies, as recommended by Drs. Wung and James (see Chapter 5), several innovations on conventional ventilation (e.g., SIMV, PSV, MMV, APRV, IRV), high-frequency ventilation, exogenous surfactant replacement, negative-pressure ventilation, and perfluorochemical (liquid) ventilation.

One would not anticipate the appearance of an ideal or permanent solution to this problem. Rather, it is incumbent upon practitioners who care for patients with life-threatening respiratory failure to become familiar with all of the candidate therapies, to become facile with those that offer reasonable clinical benefit, to balance the use of available approaches in terms of their relative assets, and to seek to develop better technologies for the future. As new therapies are developed, due attention must continue to be given to the prerequisite animal laboratory testing. As they are introduced to the clinical arena, it is critical that investigational modalities not inappropriately delay the institution of known and verified therapies, as such delays may result in avoidable morbidity and mortality by inducing irreversible lung injury. And as each new treatment achieves the status of recognized or "standard" therapy, new and better approaches must be sought to take its place.

REFERENCES

(1) Kleinman JC, Kiely JL. Postneonatal mortality in the United States: an international perspective. Pediatrics 1990;86:1091–7.

(2) Brochard L. Methods in mixed ventilation: advantages, disadvantages and consequences for work of breathing. Schweiz Med Wochenschr 1990;120:1678–80.

(3) Hickling KG, Henderson SJ, Jackson R. Low mortality associated with low volume pressure limited ventilation with permissive hypercapnia in severe adult respiratory distress syndrome. Intensive Care Med 1990;16:372–7.

(4) Marini JJ, Smith TC, Lamb VJ. External work output and force generation during synchronized intermittent mechanical ventilation. Effect of machine assistance on breathing effort. Am Rev Respir Dis 1988;138:1169–79.

(5) Groeger JS, Levinson MR, Carlon GC. Assist control versus synchronized intermittent mandatory ventilation during acute respiratory failure. Crit Care Med 1989;17:607–2,

(6) Kirby RR. Synchronized intermittent mandatory ventilation versus assist control: just the facts, ma'am [editorial]. Crit Care Med 1989;17:706–7.

(7) MacIntyre N, Nishimura M, Usada Y, Tokioka H, Takezawa J, Shimada Y. The Nagoya conference on system design and patient-ventilator interactions during pressure support ventilation. Chest 1990;97:1463–6.

(8) Martin LD, Rafferty JF, Wetzel RC, Gioia FR. Inspiratory work and response times of a modified pediatric volume ventilator during synchronized intermittent mandatory ventilation and pressure support ventilation. Anesthesiology 1989;71:977–81.

(9) MacIntyre NR. Respiratory function during pressure support ventilation. Chest 1986;89:677–83.

(10) Kanak R, Fahey PJ, Vanderwarf C. Oxygen cost of breathing. Changes dependent upon mode of mechanical ventilation. Chest 1985;87:126–7.

(11) Hewlett AM, Platt AS, Terry VG. Mandatory minute volume. A new concept in weaning from mechanical ventilation. Anaesthesia 1977;32:163–9.

(12) Stock MC, Downs JB, Frolicher DA. Airway pressure release ventilation (APRV): a new ventilatory support mode during acute lung injury (ALI). (abstract) Crit Care Med 1986;14:366.

(13) Garner W, Downs JB, Stock MC, Rasanen J. Airway pressure release ventilation (APRV). A human trial. Chest 1988;94:779–81.

(14) Rasanen J, Downs JB, Stock MC. Cardiovascular effects of conventional positive pressure ventilation and airway pressure release ventilation. Chest 1988;93:911–15.

(15) Martin LD, Wetzel RC, Bilenki AL. Airway pressure release ventilation in a neonatal lamb model of acute lung injury. Crit Care Med 1991;19:373–8.

(16) Florete OG Jr, Banner MJ, Banner TE, Rodriguez JC, Kirby RR. Airway pressure release ventilation in a patient with acute pulmonary injury. Chest 1989;96:679–82.

(17) Gurevitch MJ, Van Dyke J, Young ES, Jackson K. Improved oxygenation and lower peak airway pressure in severe adult respiratory distress syndrome. Treatment with inverse ratio ventilation. Chest 1986;89:211–13.

(18) Lehnert BE, Oberdorster G, Slutsky AS. Constant flow ventilation of apneic dogs. J Appl Physiol 1982;53:483–9.

(19) Slutsky AS, Menon AS. Catheter position and blood gases during constant flow ventilation. J Appl Physiol 1987;62:513–19.

(20) Breen PH, Sznajder JI, Morrison P, Hatch D, Wood LK, Craig DB. Constant flow ventilation in anesthetized patients: efficacy and safety. Anesth Analg 1986;65:1161–9.

(21) Perl A, Whitwam JG, Chakrabarti MK, Taylor VM. Continuous flow ventilation without respiratory movement in cat, dog, and human. Br J Anaesth 1986;58:544–50.

(22) Slutsky AS, Watson J, Leith DE, Brown R. Tracheal insufflation of oxygen (TRIO) at low flow rates sustains life for several hours. Anesthesiology 1985;63:278–86.

(23) Mackenzie CF, Barnas G, Nesbitt S. Tracheal insufflation of oxygen at low flow: capabilities and limitations. Anesth Analg 1990;71:684–90.

(24) Burwen DR, Watson J, Brown R, Josa M, Slutsky AS. Effect of cardiogenic oscillations on gas mixing during tracheal insufflation of oxygen. J Appl Physiol 1986;60:965–71.

(25) Lachmann B, Danzmann E, Haendly B, et al. Ventilator settings and gas exchange in respiratory distress syndrome. In: Prakash O, ed. Applied physiology in clinical respiratory care. Boston: Martinus Nijhoff, 1985:141.

(26) Lachmann B, Jonson B, Lindroth M, Robertson B. Modes of artificial ventilation in severe respiratory distress syndrome. Lung function and

morphology in rabbits after washout of alveolar surfactant. Crit Care Med 1982;10:724–32.

(27) Drummond WH, Gregory GA, Heymann MA, Phibbs RA. The independent effects of hyperventilation, tolazoline, and dopamine on infants with persistent pulmonary hypertension. J Pediatr 1981;98:603–11.

(28) Fox WW. Mechanical ventilation in the management of persistent pulmonary hypertension of the neonate (PPHN). Proceedings of the Ross Conference on "Cardiovascular Sequelae of Asphyxia in the Newborn," 1981:102.

(29) Boros SJ, Bing DR, Mammel MC, et al. Using conventional infant ventilators at unconventional rates. Pediatrics 1984;74:487–92.

(30) Slutsky AS, Brown R, Lehr J, Rossing T, Drazen JM. High frequency ventilation: a promising new approach to mechanical ventilation. Med Instrum 1981;15:229–33.

(31) Ackerman NB, Null DM, deLemos RA. High frequency ventilation: history, theory and practice. In: Kirby RR, Smith RA, Desautels DA, eds. Mechanical ventilation. New York: Churchill Livingstone, 1985:307–25.

(32) Henderson Y, Chillingworth FP, Whitney JL. The respiratory dead space. Am J Physiol 1915;38:1–19.

(33) Emerson JH. Apparatus for vibrating portions of a patient's airway. U.S. Patent No. 2,918,917. 1959.

(34) Jonzon A, Oberg PA, Sedin G, Sjostrand U. High-frequency positive-pressure ventilation by endotracheal insufflation. Acta Anaesthesiol Scand Suppl 1971;43:1–43.

(35) Lunkenheimer PP, Frank I, Ising H, Keller H, Dickhut HH. Intrapulmonaler Gaswechsel unter simulierter Apnoe durch transtrachealen, periodischen intrathorakalen Druckwechsel. Anaesthesist 1973;22:232–38.

(36) Lunkenheimer PP, Rafflenbeul W, Keller H, Frank I, Dickhut HH, Fuhrmann C. Application of transtracheal pressure oscillations as a modification of "diffusing respiration." Br J Anaesth 1972;44:627.

(37) Heijman K, Heijman L, Jonzon A, Sedin G, Sjostrand U, Widman B. High frequency positive pressure ventilation during anaesthesia and routine surgery in man. Acta Anaesthesiol Scand 1972;16:176–87.

(38) Heijman K, Sjostrand U. Treatment of the respiratory distress syndrome: a preliminary report. Opusc Med Bd 1974;19:235.

(39) Bland RD, Kim MH, Light MJ, Woodson JL. High-frequency mechanical ventilation of low birthweight infants with respiratory failure from hyaline membrane disease: 92% survival [Abstract]. Pediatr Res 1977;11:531A.

(40) Bland RD, Kim MH, Light MJ, Woodson JL. High frequency mechanical ventilation in severe hyaline membrane disease: an alternative treatment? Crit Care Med 1980;8:275–80.

(41) Butler WJ, Bohn DJ, Bryan AC, Froese AB. Ventilation by high-frequency oscillation in humans. Anesth Analg 1980;59:577–84.

(42) Carlon GC, Miodownik S, Ray C, Kann RC. Technical aspects and clinical implications of high frequency jet ventilation with a solenoid valve. Crit Care Med 1981;9:47–50.

(43) Marchak BE, Thompson WK, Duffy P, et al. Treatment of RDS by high-frequency oscillatory ventilation: a preliminary report. J Pediatr 1981;99:287–92.

(44) Schuster DP, Snyder JV, Klain M, Grevnik A. High-frequency jet ventilation during the treatment of acute fulminant pulmonary edema. Chest 1981;80:682–5.

(45) Froese AB, Bryan AC. High frequency ventilation. Am Rev Respir Dis 1987;135:1363–74.

(46) Slutsky AS. Non-conventional methods of ventilation. Am Rev Respir Dis 1988;138:175–83.

(47) Lunkenheimer PP, Whimster WF, Sykes MK, eds. High frequency ventilation. 20 years of endeavor reviewed: final stress or departure to achievement. An international symposium held in Munster, FRG, Feb 29–30, 1988. Acta Anaesthesiol Scand 1989;33(suppl 90)1–178.

(48) Froese AB, Bryan AC. High frequency ventilation. Am Rev Respir Dis 1987;135:1363–74.

(49) Froese AB. "High frequency ventilation: strategy and device differences." Presented at the Seventh Annual Conference on High-Frequency Ventilation in Infants, Snowbird, Utah, April 1990.

(50) Sjostrand UH. In what respect does high frequency positive pressure ventilation differ from conventional ventilation? Acta Anaesthesiol Scand 1989;33(suppl 90):5–12.

(51) Hird M, Greenough A, Gamsu H. Gas trapping during high frequency positive pressure ventilation using conventional ventilators. Early Hum Dev 1990;22:51–6.

(52) Ackerman NB, deLemos RA. High-frequency ventilation. Adv Pediatr 1984;31:259–93.

(53) Gerstmann DR, deLemos RA, Clark RH.

High frequency ventilation: issues of strategy. Clin Perinatol 1991;18:563–80.

(54) Mammel MC, Ophoven JP, Lewallen PK, Gordon MJ, Sutton MC, Boros SJ. High-frequency ventilation and tracheal injuries. Pediatrics 1986;77:608–13.

(55) Wiswell TE, Clark RH, Null DM, Kuehl TJ, deLemos RA, Coalson JJ. Tracheal and bronchial injury in high-frequency oscillatory ventilation and high-frequency flow interruption compared with conventional positive-pressure ventilation. J Pediatr 1988;112:249–56.

(56) Kercsmar CM, Martin RJ, Chatburn RL, Carlo WA. Bronchoscopic findings in infants treated with high-frequency jet ventilation versus conventional ventilation. Pediatrics 1988;82:884–7.

(57) Hanson JB, Waldstein G, Hernandez JA, Fan LL. Necrotizing tracheobronchitis: an ischemic lesion. Am J Dis Child 1988;142:1094–8.

(58) Polak MJ, Donnelly WH, Bucciarelli RL. Comparison of airway pathologic lesions after high-frequency jet or conventional ventilation. Am J Dis Child 1989;143:228–32.

(59) Muller WJ, Gerjarusek S, Scherer PW. Studies of wall shear and mass transfer in a large scale model of neonatal high-frequency jet ventilation. Ann Biomed Eng 1990;18:69–88.

(60) Meredith KS, deLemos RA, Coalson JJ, et al. Role of lung injury in the pathogenesis of hyaline membrane disease in premature baboons. J Appl Physiol 1989;66:2150–8.

(61) Carlon GC, Howland WS, Ray C, Miodownik S, Griffin JP, Groeger JS. High-frequency jet ventilation: a prospective randomized evaluation. Chest 1983;84:551–9.

(62) HIFI Study Group. High-frequency oscillatory ventilation compared with conventional mechanical ventilation in the treatment of respiratory failure in preterm infants. N Engl J Med 1989;320:88–93.

(63) Bryan AC, Froese AB. Reflections on the HIFI Trial [Editorial]. Pediatrics 1991;87:565–7.

(64) HIFI Study Group. High-frequency oscillatory ventilation compared with conventional mechanical ventilation in the treatment of respiratory failure in preterm infants: assessment of pulmonary function at 9 months of corrected age. J Pediatr 1990;116:933–41.

(65) Gerhardt T, Reifenberg L, Goldberg RN, Bancalari E. Pulmonary function in preterm infants whose lungs were ventilated convention-ally or by high-frequency oscillation. J Pediatr 1989;115:121–6.

(66) HIFI Study Group. High-frequency oscillatory ventilation compared with conventional intermittent mechanical ventilation in the treatment of respiratory failure in preterm infants: neurodevelopmental status at 16 to 24 months of postterm age. J Pediatr 1990;117:939–46.

(67) Carlo WA, Siner B, Chatburn RL, Robertson S, Martin RJ. Early randomized intervention with high-frequency jet ventilation in respiratory distress syndrome. J Pediatr 1990;117:765–70.

(68) Clark RH, Gerstmann DR, Null DM Jr, deLemos RA. Prospective randomized comparison of high-frequency oscillatory and conventional ventilation in respiratory distress syndrome. Pediatrics 1992;89:5–12.

(69) Frantz ID III. Newer methods for treatment of respiratory distress. In: The micropremie: the next frontier. Report of the 99th Ross Conference on Pediatric Research, Columbus, OH. Published by Ross Laboratories, 1990:29–35.

(70) Kohelet D, Perlman M, Kirpalani H, Hanna G, Koren G. High-frequency oscillation in the rescue of infants with persistent pulmonary hypertension. Crit Care Med 1988;16:510–16.

(71) Carter JM, Gerstmann DR, Clark RH, et al. High-frequency oscillatory ventilation and extracorporeal membrane oxygenation for the treatment of acute neonatal respiratory failure. Pediatrics 1990;85:159–64.

(72) Cornish JD, Gerstmann DR, Clark RH, Carter JM, Null DM Jr, deLemos RA. Extracorporeal membrane oxygenation and high-frequency oscillatory ventilation: potential therapeutic relationships. Crit Care Med 1987;15:831–4.

(73) Clark RH, Gerstmann DR, Null DM, et al. Pulmonary interstitial emphysema treated by high-frequency oscillatory ventilation. Crit Care Med 1986;14:926–30.

(74) Vaucher YE, Mannino FL, Cornish JD, Gist K. Adverse pulmonary and developmental outcome following respiratory failure in infants receiving HFOV or ECMO [Abstract]. Pediatr Res 1989;25:266A.

(75) Schwendeman CA, Clark RH, Yoder BA, Null DM Jr, Gerstmann DR, deLemos RA. Frequency of chronic lung disease in infants with severe respiratory failure treated with high-frequency ventilation and/or extracorporeal membrane oxygenation. Crit Care Med 1992;20:372–7.

(76) Carlo WA, Beoglos A, Chatburn RL, Walsh MC, Martin RJ. High-frequency jet ventilation in neonatal pulmonary hypertension. Am J Dis Child 1989;143:233–8.

(77) Extracorporeal Life Support Organization. Report of the Neonatal ECMO Registry. Ann Arbor: University of Michigan, April 1991.

(78) Avery ME, Mead J. Surface properties in relation to atelectasis and hyaline membrane disease. Am J Dis Child 1959;96:517–23.

(79) Reynolds MS, Wallander KA. Use of surfactant in the prevention and treatment of neonatal respiratory distress syndrome. Clin Pharm 1989; 8:559–76.

(80) Taeusch HW Jr, Clements J, Benson B. Exogenous surfactant for human lung disease. Current status [Editorial]. Am Rev Respir Dis 128:791–4.

(81) Bose C, Corbet A, Bose G, et al. Improved outcome at 28 days of age for very low birth weight infants treated with a single dose of a synthetic surfactant. J Pediatr 1990;117:947–53.

(82) Corbet A, Bucciarelli R, Goldman S, et al. Decreased mortality rate among small premature infants treated at birth with a single dose of synthetic surfactant: a multicenter controlled trial. J Pediatr 1991;118:277–84.

(83) Long W, Thompson T, Sundell H, et al. Effects of two rescue doses of a synthetic surfactant on mortality rate and survival without bronchopulmonary dysplasia in 700- to 1350-gram infants with respiratory distress syndrome. J Pediatr 1991;118:595–605.

(84) Morley CJ. Prophylactic treatment of premature babies with artificial surfactant (ALEC). Dev Pharmacol Ther 1989;13:182–3.

(85) Morley CJ, Greenough A, Miller NG, et al. Randomized trial of artificial surfactant (ALEC) given at birth to babies from 23 to 34 weeks gestation. Early Hum Dev 1988;17:41–54.

(86) Morley CJ. The use of artificial surfactant (ALEC) in the prophylaxis of neonatal respiratory distress syndrome. Eur Respir J [Suppl.] 1989;3:81s–86s.

(87) Kwong MS, Egan EA, Notter RH, Shapiro DH. Double-blind clinical trial of calf lung surfactant extract for the prevention of hyaline membrane disease in extremely premature infants. Pediatrics 1985;76:585–2.

(88) Robertson B. European multicenter trials of curosurf for treatment of neonatal respiratory distress syndrome. Lung 1990;168(Suppl):860–3.

(89) Soll RF, Hoekstra RE, Fangman JJ, et al. Multicenter trial of single-dose modified bovine surfactant extract (Survanta) for prevention of respiratory distress syndrome. Ross Collaborative Surfactant Prevention Study Group. Pediatrics 1990;85:1092–102.

(90) Whitsett JA, Hull WM, Luse S. Failure to detect surfactant protein-specific antibodies in sera of premature infants treated with survanta, a modified bovine surfactant. Pediatrics 1991; 87:505–10.

(91) Hallman M, Merritt TA, Schneider H. Isolation of human surfactant from amniotic fluid and a pilot study of its efficacy in respiratory distress syndrome. Pediatrics 1983;71:473–82.

(92) Hallman M, Merritt TA, Jarvenpaa AL, et al. Exogenous human surfactant for treatment of severe respiratory distress syndrome: a randomized prospective clinical trial. J Pediatr 1985; 106:963–9.

(93) Merritt TA, Hallman M, Bloom BT, et al. Prophylactic treatment of very premature infants with human surfactant. N Engl J Med 1986;315: 785–90.

(94) Lang MJ, Hall RT, Reddy NS, Kurth CG, Merritt TA. A controlled trial of human surfactant replacement therapy for severe respiratory distress syndrome in very low birth weight infants. J Pediatr 1990;116:295–300.

(95) Heldt GP, Pesonen E, Merritt TA, Elias W, Sahn DJ. Closure of the ductus arteriosus and mechanics of breathing in preterm infants after surfactant replacement therapy. Pediatr Res 1989;25:305–10.

(96) Merritt TA, Hallman M, Berry C, et al. Randomized, placebo-controlled trial of human surfactant given at birth versus rescue administration in very low birth weight infants with lung immaturity. J Pediatr 1991;118:581–94.

(97) Fujiwara T, Maeta H, Chida S, Morita T, Watabe Y, Abe T. Artificial surfactant therapy in hyaline-membrane disease. Lancet 1980;1:55–9.

(98) Enhorning G, Shennan A, Possmayer F, Dunn M, Chen CP, Milligan J. Prevention of neonatal respiratory distress syndrome by tracheal instillation of surfactant: a randomized clinical trial. Pediatrics 1985;76:145–53.

(99) Gitlin JD, Sol RF, Parad RB, et al. Randomized controlled trial of exogenous surfactant for the treatment of hyaline membrane disease. Pediatrics 1987;79:31–7.

(100) Raju TNK, Vidyasagar D, Bhat R, et al. Double-blind controlled trial of single-dose treatment with bovine surfactant in severe hyaline membrane disease. Lancet 1987;1:651–6.

(101) Kendig JW, Notter RH, Cox C, et al. Surfactant replacement therapy at birth: final analysis of a clinical trial and comparisons with similar trials. Pediatrics 1988;82:756–62.

(102) Horbar JD, Soll RF, Sutherland JM, et al. A multicenter randomized, placebo-controlled trial of surfactant therapy for respiratory distress syndrome. N Engl J Med 1989;320:959–65.

(103) Horbar JD, Soll RF, Schachinger H, et al. A European multicenter randomized controlled trial of single dose surfactant therapy for idiopathic respiratory distress syndrome. Eur J Pediatr 1990;149:416–23.

(104) Fujiwara T, Konishi M, Chida S, et al. Surfactant replacement therapy with a single postventilatory dose of a reconstituted bovine surfactant in preterm neonates with respiratory distress syndrome: final analysis of a multicenter, double-blind, randomized trial and comparison with similar trials. Pediatrics 1990;86:753–64.

(105) Dunn MS, Shennan AT, Possmayer F. Single- versus multiple-dose surfactant replacement therapy in neonates of 30 to 36 weeks' gestation with respiratory distress syndrome. Pediatrics 1990;86:564–71.

(106) Couser RJ, Ferrara TB, Ebert J, Hoekstra RE, Fangman JJ. Effects of exogenous surfactant therapy on dynamic compliance during mechanical breathing in preterm infants with hyaline membrane disease. J Pediatr 1990;116:119–24.

(107) Bhat R, Dziedzic K, Bhutani VK, Vidyasagar D. Effect of single dose surfactant on pulmonary function. Crit Care Med 1990;18:590–5.

(108) Gortner L, Bernsau U, Hellwege HH, Hieronimi G, Jorch G, Reiter HL. A multicenter randomized controlled clinical trial of bovine surfactant for prevention of respiratory distress syndrome. Lung 1990;168(Suppl):864–9.

(109) Hennes HM, Lee MB, Rimm AA, Shapiro DL. Surfactant replacement therapy in respiratory distress syndrome. Meta-analysis of clinical trials of single-dose surfactant extracts. Am J Dis Child 1991;145:102–4.

(110) Collaborative European Multicenter Study Group. Surfactant replacement therapy for severe neonatal respiratory distress syndrome: an international randomized clinical trial. Pediatrics 1988;82:683–91.

(111) Ware J, Taeusch HW, Soll RF, McCormick MC. Health and developmental outcomes of a surfactant controlled trial: follow-up at 2 years. Pediatrics 1990;85:1103–7.

(112) Martin RJ. Neonatal surfactant therapy—where do we go from here? [Editorial]. J Pediatr 1991;118:555–6.

(113) Dunn MS, Shennan AT, Zayack D, Possmayer F. Bovine surfactant replacement therapy in neonates of less than 30 weeks gestation: a randomized controlled trial of prophylaxis versus treatment. Pediatrics 1991;87:377–86.

(114) Committee on Fetus and Newborn 1990–1991. Surfactant replacement therapy for respiratory distress syndrome. AAP News, April 1991: 13.

(115) Lotze A, Whitsett JA, Kammerman LA, Ritter M, Taylor GA, Short BL. Surfactant protein A concentrations in tracheal aspirate fluid from infants requiring extracorporeal membrane oxygenation. J Pediatr 1990;116:435–40.

(116) Auten RL, Notter RH, Kendig JW, Davis JM, Shapiro DL. Surfactant treatment of full-term newborns with respiratory failure. Pediatrics 1991;87:101–7.

(117) Petty TL. Acute respiratory distress syndrome (ARDS). Dis Mon 1990;36:1–58.

(118) Merritt TA, Hallman M, Spragg R, Heldt GP, Gilliard N. Exogenous surfactant treatments for neonatal respiratory distress syndrome and their potential role in the adult respiratory distress syndrome. Drugs 1989;38:591–611.

(119) Lachmann B. Animal models and clinical pilot studies of surfactant replacement in adult respiratory distress syndrome. Eur Respir J [Suppl] 1989;3:98s–103s.

(120) Richman PS, Spragg RG, Robertson B, Merritt TA, Curstedt T. The adult respiratory distress syndrome: first trials with surfactant replacement. Eur Respir J [Suppl] 1989;3:109s–111s.

(121) Stern L, Ramos AD, Outerbridge EW, Beaudry PH. Negative pressure artificial respiration: use in treatment of respiratory failure of the newborn. Can Med Assoc J 1970;102:595–601.

(122) Fanaroff AA, Cha Chul Choon, Sosa R, et al. Controlled trial of continuous negative pressure in the treatment of severe respiratory distress syndrome. J Pediatr 1973;82:921–8.

(123) Chernick V, Vidyasagar D. Continuous negative chest wall pressure in hyaline membrane disease: one year experience. Pediatrics 1972;49:753–60.

(124) Woolam CH. The development of apparatus for intermittent negative pressure respiration. Anaesthesia 1976;31:537–47.

(125) Woolam CH. The development of apparatus for intermittent negative pressure respiration

1919–1976, with special reference to the development and uses of cuirass respirators. Anaesthesia 1976;31:666–85.

(126) Amitani H, Sakashita I, Jyounosono M, Kitajima I, Fukunaga H. The effect of body respirator on the desaturation during the night in Duchenne muscular dystrophy. Rinsho Shinkeigaku—Clinical Neurology 1989;29:871–5.

(127) Cvetnic WG, Waffarn F, Martin JM. Continuous negative pressure and intermittent mandatory ventilation in the management of pulmonary interstitial emphysema. J Perinatol 1989;9:26–32.

(128) Sills JH, Cvetnic WG, Pietz J. Continuous negative pressure in the treatment of infants with pulmonary hypertension and respiratory failure. J Perinatol 1989;9:43–8.

(129) Cvetnic WG, Ingram A, Banks JL. Reintroduction of continuous negative pressure ventilation (CNPV)—two year experience [Abstract]. Pediatr Res 1989;25:306A.

(130) Cvetnic WG, Shoptaugh M, Sills J. Randomized trial of intermittent mandatory ventilation (IMV) vs. continuous negative pressure (CNP) for neonatal respiratory failure—preliminary results [Abstract]. Pediatr Res 1990;27:298A.

(131) Wolfson MR, Shaffer TH. Liquid ventilation during early development: theory, physiologic process and application. J Dev Physiol 1990;13:1–12.

(132) Shaffer TH. A brief review: liquid ventilation. Undersea Biomed Res 1987;14:169–79.

(133) Sargent JW, Seffl RJ. Properties of perfluoronated liquid. Fed Proc (Fed Am Soc Exp Biol) 1970;29:1699–703.

(134) Holaday DA, Fiserova-Bergerova V, Modell JH. Uptake, distribution, and excretion of fluorocarbon FX-80 (perfluorobutyl perfluorotetrahydrofuran) during liquid breathing in the dog. Anesthesiology 1972;37:387–94.

(135) Patel MJ, Syanto P, Yates B, Long DM. Survival and histopathologic changes in lungs of hamsters following synthetic liquid breathing. Fed Proc 1970;29:1740–5.

(136) Forman D, Bhutani VK, Hilfer SR, Shaffer TH. A find structure study of the liquid-ventilation newborn rabbit. Fed Proc 1984;43:647.

(137) Calderwood HW, Ruiz BC, Tham MK, Modell JH, Hood CI. Residual levels and biochemical changes after ventilation with perfluorinated liquid. J Appl Physiol 1975;139:603–7.

(138) Mitsuno T, Ohyanagi H, Naito R. Clinical studies of a perfluorochemical whole blood substitute (Fluosol-DA): summary of 186 cases. Ann Surg 1982;195:60–9.

(139) Ohyanagi H, Toshima K, Sekita M, et al. Clinical studies of perfluorochemical whole blood substitutes: safety of Fluosol-DA (20%) in normal human volunteers. Clin Ther 1979;2:306–12.

(140) Clark LC, Gollan F. Survival of mammals breathing organic liquids equilibrated with oxygen at atmospheric pressure. Science 1966;152:1755–6.

(141) Wolfson MR, Tran N, Bhutani VK, Shaffer TH. A new experimental approach for the study of cardiopulmonary physiology during early development. J Appl Physiol 1988;65:1436–43.

(142) Lowe CA, Shaffer TH. Pulmonary vascular resistance in the fluorocarbon-filled lung. J Appl Physiol 1986;60:154–9.

(143) Shaffer TH, Lowe CA, Bhutani VK, Douglas PR. Liquid ventilation: effects on pulmonary function in distressed meconium-stained lambs. Ped Res 1984;18:47–52.

(144) Greenspan JS, Wolfson MR, Rubenstein SD, Shaffer TH. Liquid ventilation of preterm baby [letter]. Lancet 1989;2:1095.

(145) Greenspan JS, Wolfson MR, Rubenstein SD, Shaffer TH. Liquid ventilation of human preterm neonates. J Pediatr 1990;117:106–11.

(146) Fuhrman BP. Perfluorocarbon liquid ventilation: the first human trial. J Pediatr 1990;117:73–4.

7

Physiology of Extracorporeal Life Support

❖

Robert H. Bartlett, M.D.
Robert E. Cilley, M.D.

Extracorporeal life support (ECLS) is achieved by draining venous blood, removing carbon dioxide (CO_2) and adding oxygen through an artificial lung, and returning the blood to the circulation via a vein (venovenous) or artery (venoarterial). When used in the venoarterial mode, most of the venous blood is diverted from the central circulation, hence the term "cardiopulmonary bypass." In venoarterial bypass (VA), the functions of both heart and lungs are replaced by artificial organs, either totally or partially. The term "extracorporeal membrane oxygenation" (ECMO) has come to mean prolonged partial venoarterial bypass achieved via extrathoracic cannulation. During partial VA bypass, perfusate blood mixes in the aorta with left ventricular blood which has traversed the lungs. Hence, the content of oxygen and CO_2 in the patient's arterial blood represents a combination of blood from these two sources, and the total systemic blood flow is the sum of the extracorporeal flow plus the amount of blood passing through the heart and lungs.

Much has been written about the physiology and pathophysiology of total VA bypass for cardiac surgery (1,2). While the principles of gas exchange and blood flow are the same, there are several important differences between the conduct of ECLS and operating room bypass. These differences are discussed in detail (3,4). This chapter will focus on the physiology of prolonged partial bypass for life support.

In venovenous bypass (VV), the perfusate blood is returned to the venous circulation and mixes with venous blood coming from the systemic organs, raising the oxygen content and lowering CO_2 content in the right atrial blood. Some of this mixed blood is returned to the extracorporeal circuit ("recirculation"), and some of it passes into the right ventricle, the lungs, and into the systemic circulation. Since the volume of blood removed is exactly equal to the volume of blood reinfused, there is no net effect on central venous pressure, right or left ventricle filling, or hemodynamics. The content of oxygen and CO_2 in the patient's arterial blood represents that of right ventricular blood modified by any pulmonary function that might exist. The systemic blood flow is the native cardiac output and is unrelated to the extracorporeal flow.

Arteriovenous (AV) extracorporeal circulation is commonly used for hemodialysis or hemofiltration but not for cardiac or pulmonary support. The AV route could be used for gas exchange, provided the arterial blood was desaturated, and the cardiovascular system could tolerate the arterial venous fistula with a large enough flow to achieve adequate gas exchange. This is, after all, the mechanism of gas exchange in the placenta and fetus. Because of the blood flow requirements for gas exchange support, the arteriovenous route is not a reasonable approach to total extracorporeal life support, except perhaps for the premature infant (5,6).

OXYGEN KINETICS AND TISSUE RESPIRATION

Management of extracorporeal life support requires thorough understanding of normal and abnormal physiology, particularly those aspects of physiology related to respiration at the tissue level. Oxygen consumption (Vo_2) is controlled by tissue metabolism, hence is decreased by rest, paralysis, and hypothermia and increased during muscular activity, infection, hyperthermia, and increased levels of catecholamine and thyroid hormones. The metabolic rate is defined as the Vo_2, or calculations based on the Vo_2. (Volume of oxygen consumed times 5 cal/L estimates the energy expenditure expressed in calories.) The value for oxygen consumption in normal resting humans is 5 to 8 cc/kg/min in newborn infants, 4 to 6 cc/kg/min in children, and 3 to 5 cc/kg/min in adults (7). Although Vo_2 may increase up to 10 times with exercise, sepsis and catecholamines increase Vo_2 by about 50% (8). The amount of oxygen absorbed across the lung in the process of pulmonary gas exchange is exactly equal to the amount of oxygen consumed by peripheral tissues during metabolism (the Fick principle) (9) regardless of the status of pulmonary function. Hence, Vo_2 can be measured at the airway or calculated as the product of arterial venous oxygen content difference times cardiac output (the Fick equation).

Systemic Oxygen Delivery (Do_2)

Do_2 is the amount of oxygen delivered to peripheral tissues each minute, or the product of arterial oxygen content times cardiac output. Oxygen delivery is controlled by cardiac output, hemoglobin concentration, hemoglobin saturation, and dissolved oxygen, in that order. The normal value for Do_2 is four to five times Vo_2 regardless of size, since the oxygen content of normal arterial blood is the same for all ages and sizes of patients (20 cc O_2/dL). Variations in oxygen delivery for patients of different size and metabolic activity are caused by variations in cardiac output. The oxygen content is rarely measured directly for clinical applications, and we are accustomed to describing blood oxygenation in terms of Pao_2 or hemoglobin saturation. However, oxygen content is the most important measurement in the physiologic management of critically ill patients. The relationship of Pao_2, saturation, and oxygen content is described in Figure 7.1. Typical values for venous and arterial blood at different levels of hemoglobin are identified. Notice that there is more oxygen in normal blood with a Po_2 of 40 than in anemic blood with a Po_2 of 100. A unique aspect of cardiorespiratory homeostasis is the tendency to maintain systemic oxygen delivery at the normal level. In anemia, the cardiac output will increase until Do_2 is normalized. In hypoxia, the cardiac output increases, and in chronic hypoxia, red cell mass increases under the influence of erythropoietin until systemic

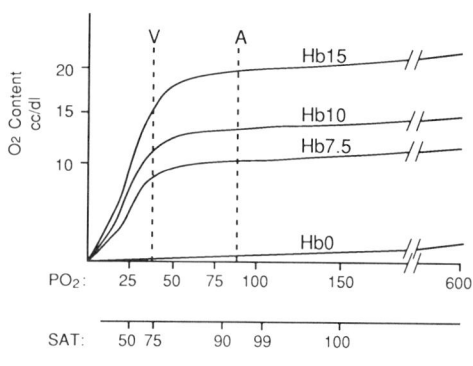

FIGURE 7.1 The relationship of oxygen content, Pao_2, and saturation. Dotted lines identify typical values for arterial and venous blood. In the physiologic range oxygen content is controlled primarily by hemoglobin concentration, rather than Po_2 or saturation.

oxygen delivery is again normalized. We should recognize and assist these compensatory mechanisms in the critically ill patient. For example, the best treatment for a ventilated patient who is hypoxic, anemic, tachycardic, hypotensive, and hypermetabolic is usually red cell transfusion (rather than using inotropic drugs or increasing Fio_2).

The normal relationship between Do_2 and Vo_2 is shown in Figure 7.2. The normal ratio is 5:1, and when Vo_2 changes secondary to variations in metabolism, Do_2 readjusts by increasing or decreasing cardiac output to maintain the normal ratio. If systemic oxygen delivery is moderately decreased, there is no change in oxygen consumption; hence the amount of oxygen extracted from each deciliter of arterial blood is greater. One could imagine a situation in which the rate of tissue metabolism exceeded the rate of oxygen delivery, which would result in anaerobic metabolism, limitation of Vo_2 based on decreased oxygen supply, and oxygen "debt." In theory, this would occur whenever the ratio of delivery to consumption is less than 1:1. In practice, this situation occurs when the ratio is less than 2:1 (10). (The difference is explained by the fact that some of the systemic oxygen delivery goes to tissues that consume very little oxygen like skin, fat, and tendons.) Between this critical point at a Do_2/Vo_2 ratio of 2:1 and the normal ratio of 5:1, decreased delivery is compensated for by increased extraction, maintaining normal hemodynamic and respiratory stability. Since mixed venous blood oxyhemoglobin saturation reflects this ratio exactly, it is the most important monitor for managing critically ill patients (11). If the arterial blood is fully saturated, the venous saturation decreases proportionate to the amount of oxygen extracted from arterial blood. Thus, if the oxygen extraction ratio is 20%, the venous saturation will be 80%; if the oxygen extraction ratio is 33%, the venous saturation will be 67%, etc. These levels of venous saturation corresponding to various Do_2/Vo_2 ratios are identified in Figure 7.2.

Carbon Dioxide Production

The amount of CO_2 produced during systemic metabolism each minute (Vco_2) is approximately equal to the amount of oxygen consumed. The ratio of CO_2 production to oxygen consumption is known as the respiratory quotient, and, depending on the energy substrate, it varies from 0.7 for fat to 0.8 for protein to 1.0 for carbohydrate. Under normal conditions, the rate and depth of breathing are controlled to maintain the arterial Pco_2 at 40 mm Hg. Even a slight increase in metabolically produced CO_2 will result in a proportionate increase in alveolar ventilation, just enough to increase CO_2 excretion so that the arterial

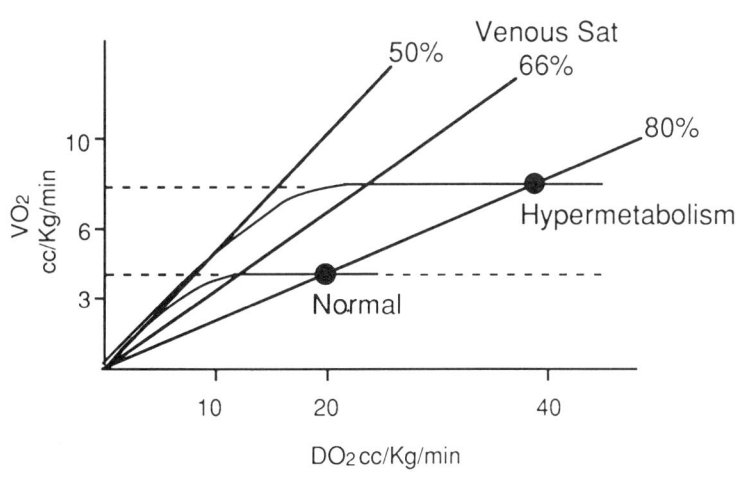

FIGURE 7.2 The relationships between oxygen consumption and delivery are shown for normal and hypermetabolic states. Normally, the ratio of delivery to consumption is 5:1, and the venous blood is 80% saturated. When the ratio is 2:1, the venous saturation is 50%. When the ratio is lower than that, consumption becomes dependent upon delivery.

Pco₂ will remain at 40. Unlike systemic oxygen delivery, CO_2 excretion is not affected by hemoglobin or blood flow but is very sensitive to changes in ventilation. For this reason, and because CO_2 excretion is much more efficient than oxygenation in the lung, CO_2 removal can be maintained at normal levels even during severe lung dysfunction.

GAS EXCHANGE IN EXTRACORPOREAL LIFE SUPPORT

Oxygen Delivery

During ECLS, oxygen delivery is controlled by the combinations of blood oxygenation in the membrane lung, flow through the extracorporeal circuit, oxygen uptake through the native lung, and cardiac output through the native heart.

Blood oxygenation in the membrane lung is a function of the geometry, the thickness of the blood film, the membrane material and thickness, the Fio_2, the residence time of red cells in the gas exchange area, the hemoglobin concentration, and the inlet saturation (the latter two defining the oxygen uptake capacity of each deciliter of blood) (4). All of these factors are included in a single descriptor of membrane lung function called "rated flow" (12). Rated flow is the amount of normal venous blood that can be raised from 75% to 95% oxyhemoglobin saturation in a given period. This concept is illustrated in Figure 7.3. In this example, typical data for the SciMed 0.8 m² and 1.5 m² membrane lungs are shown. The geometry of the 0.8 membrane lung is such that the rated flow is 1,000 cc/min, corresponding to an actual oxygen transfer of 50 cc/min. We use this information to plan which membrane lung to use for ECLS and to evaluate membrane lung performance during perfusion.

As long as the extracorporeal blood flow is less than the rated flow of the membrane lung, the blood leaving the lung will be fully saturated, and the amount of systemic oxygen delivery via the extracorporeal circuit is controlled by blood flow and the oxygen uptake capacity. The amount of oxygen that can be taken up in each deciliter equals gmHb/dL ×

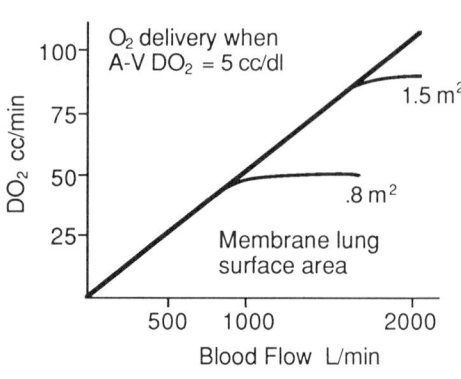

FIGURE 7.3 The concept of "rated flow." Oxygen uptake through a membrane lung is limited by the oxygen carrying capacity of the blood and the amount of blood flow. This relationship for normal venous blood (AvDo₂ = 5) is shown in the solid line. An additional limitation is imposed by the geometry of the membrane lung. The blood flow at which this limitation is reached is called the rated flow, shown here for membrane lungs 0.8 and 1.5 m² surface area.

unsaturated fraction × 1.36 cc/gm. When the outlet blood is 100% saturated, the uptake capacity is the same as the AvDo₂. If the hemoglobin concentration is low or the venous blood saturation is high, the amount of oxygen that can be bound in the membrane lung is decreased. We can compensate for decreased oxygen-binding capacity by increasing blood flow. Conversely, we can achieve oxygen delivery at low blood flow by increasing oxygen-binding capacity. These phenomena are demonstrated in Figure 7.4. Oxygen delivery for venoarterial and venovenous bypass in a typical newborn infant are demonstrated. The oxygen requirement for this infant is 20 cc/min. All of the oxygen requirement can be supplied by venoarterial bypass at a flow of 400 or by venovenous bypass at a flow of 660.

The resulting systemic Po₂ and systemic oxygen delivery are a function of oxygen delivery through the extracorporeal circuit and through the native heart and lung. In planning the size of the circuit and extracorporeal flow rate, it is assumed that there will be no gas exchange across the native lung. With this assumption, in venovenous bypass the arterial

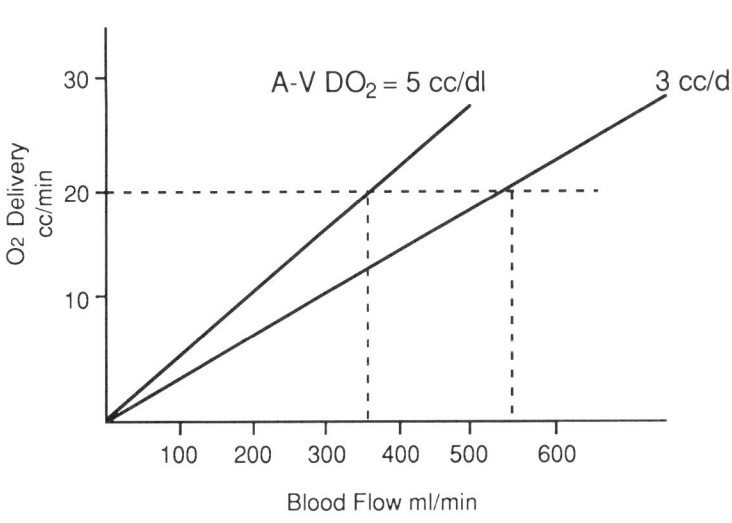

FIGURE 7.4 Oxygen delivery is a function of Avo_2 difference and blood flow. In this example, 20 cc O_2 can be delivered by 400 cc of blood flow when the Avo_2 difference is five (typical VA bypass), or by 660 cc of flow when the Avo_2 difference is three (typical VV bypass).

Po_2 and saturation will be identical to the values in the mixed right atrial blood. Because of the nature of venovenous bypass, this saturation will never be higher than 95%, and typically will be closer to 80% saturation with a Po_2 of approximately 40 mm Hg. Consequently, it is common for a patient on venovenous ECLS to be cyanotic and hypoxic. Systemic oxygen delivery is perfectly adequate as long as there is a compensatory increase in cardiac output.

Improvement in native lung function results in increasing arterial oxygenation, and the amount of native lung function during VV bypass can be identified as a step up from venous to arterial saturation. In venoarterial bypass, the interpretation of arterial blood gases is more complicated. The perfusate blood is typically 100%, saturated with a Po_2 of 500 mm Hg. When the lung is not functioning, the left ventricular ejectate blood is identical to right atrial blood, typically with a saturation of 75% and a Po_2 of 35. In this example, if the hemoglobin is 15 gm/dL, the perfusate oxygen content is 22 cc/dL, and the right atrial and left ventricular oxygen contents are both 15 cc/dL. The resultant arterial blood gases reflect the relative amounts of perfusate and native lung flow. For example, if 50% of the venous return is routed through the extracorporeal circuit, the oxygen content of systemic arterial blood will be 18.5 cc/dL, corresponding to a saturation of 90% and a Po_2 of 55. The systemic oxygen content is determined by the formula:

$$\text{Perfusate content} \times \frac{\text{ECC flow}}{\text{Total flow}} + \text{LV blood content} \times \frac{\text{Lung flow}}{\text{Total flow}}$$

Thus, during VA bypass, an increase in systemic Po_2 may signify improving lung function at constant flows, decreasing native cardiac output at constant extracorporeal flow, or increasing extracorporeal flow at constant native cardiac output.

Carbon Dioxide Removal

The amount of CO_2 eliminated in extracorporeal circulation is a function of the membrane lung geometry, material, surface area, blood Pco_2, and, to a lesser extent, blood flow and membrane lung ventilating gas flow (commonly called "sweep" flow) (13). Usually, the ventilating gas contains no CO_2, so the gradient for CO_2 transfer is the difference between the blood Pco_2 and zero (when the gas flow rate is high). As the Pco_2 drops during the passage of blood through the membrane lung, the gradient decreases, so CO_2 excretion is less at the blood outlet end of the device than at the inlet end. Consequently, the amount of CO_2 transfer is relatively independent of blood flow and only moderately dependent on inlet

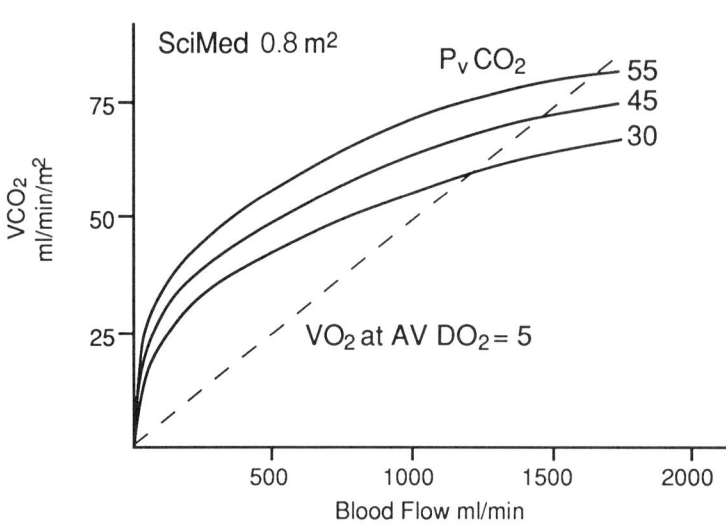

FIGURE 7.5 CO_2 clearance through a membrane lung is dependent primarily on CO_2 gradient and surface area, less dependent on blood flow. CO_2 gradients of 30, 45, and 55 mm Hg are shown. Oxygen transfer is related to oxygen-carrying capacity and blood flow. The normal value is shown on the dotted line. Within the usual range of blood flow, CO_2 transfer is always higher than oxygen transfer.

P_{CO_2}, with the major determinant of CO_2 elimination being total surface area and flow rate of the sweep gas. This is illustrated in Figure 7.5. Characteristics of removal of CO_2 for the 0.8 SciMed membrane lung at different levels of P_{CO_2} are shown over a range of blood flows. Notice that the capacity for CO_2 removal is considerably greater than the capacity for oxygen uptake at the rated flow (see Figure 7.3). For any silicone rubber or microporous membrane oxygenator, CO_2 clearance will always be more efficient than oxygenation when the oxygenator is well ventilated and functioning properly.

The extracorporeal circuit is generally designed to supply total oxygen requirements. For this reason, the membrane lung will be capable of removing an excess of CO_2. Carbon dioxide transfer (but not oxygen delivery) can be selectively increased by increasing sweep flow and the total surface area of the membrane lung in the extracorporeal circuit.

Following the rationale advanced above with regard to oxygen delivery, assuming that there is no gas exchange across the native lung, the arterial P_{CO_2} will be the same as venous P_{CO_2} in venovenous bypass; it will be a function of mixing perfusate and cardiac output blood in venoarterial bypass. However, because of the efficiency of extracorporeal CO_2 removal, the systemic P_{CO_2} can be "set" at any level by matching the membrane lung surface area and gas flow with systemic production of CO_2. In practice, the system is overdesigned for CO_2 removal, and if bypass is run to supply total oxygen requirements, CO_2 removal will be excessive, resulting in major respiratory alkalosis. This situation is controlled by adding CO_2 to the sweep gas, thus decreasing the gradient and decreasing the amount of CO_2 transfer.

If the native lung can supply some oxygen absorption and the intent of extracorporeal circulation is primarily CO_2 removal, this can be accomplished with venovenous access and relatively low blood flow ($ECCO_2R$) (14).

HEMODYNAMICS

Blood flow through the extracorporeal circuit is limited by the size of the venous drainage catheter. Resistance to blood flow varies directly with the length of the catheter and inversely with the fourth power of the radius of the catheter. Consequently, the shortest and largest internal diameter catheter that can be placed in the right atrium will allow the highest rate of extracorporeal blood flow. The superior vena cava allows the most direct access to the right atrium, and the right internal jugular vein usually has a large diameter. A catheter placed in the right internal jugular vein will usually permit venous drainage equivalent to the normal resting cardiac output of patients of all ages and sizes. Blood drains through the venous tubing to a pump that provides pressure that directs the blood through the membrane lung and back into the patient. There is significant resistance to flow through the membrane lung and across the reinfusion catheter, so the pressure on the arterial side of the circuit increases with increasing blood flow. In practice, the pump is set to deliver the desired flow, and the postpump pressure is simply monitored. Pressures as high as 300 mm Hg are safe, although the higher the pressure, the higher the likelihood of blood leaks or circuit disruption.

Some measures must be taken to assure that the pump does not apply suction to the venous catheter; i.e., the pump should be a passive-filling pump. There are two reasons for this: 1) even a small amount of negative pressure will cause major hemolysis, and 2) the right atrium and superior vena cava may become sucked into the catheter, causing endothelial damage. In cardiac surgery, these problems are avoided by including a large blood reservoir into which the venous line drains. A large reservoir is unacceptable for ECLS because the stagnant blood may thrombose and because the extracorporeal circuit must be maintained at essentially a constant volume. The occlusive roller pumps, which are usually used for extracorporeal support, could generate direct suction on the venous catheter. In practice, this problem is avoided by the inclusion of a small collapsible bladder positioned at the lowest point of the venous line. The bladder (or a transducer directly in the venous line) is attached to an electrical switch that slows or stops the roller pump whenever the bladder collapses, then restarts the pump instantly when the bladder fills again.

This system has two important advantages. Whenever the bladder collapses or the pump stops, the suction effect of the syphon between the patient and the level of the bladder stops, avoiding any direct suction on the right atrium. Second, because the pump motor is turned off whenever the bladder is collapsed, the pump cannot generate negative pressure in the blood between the pump and the bladder. Thus, this bladder and electrical switching mechanism provides servoregulation and some measure of safety for prolonged perfusion with a roller pump. The pump is adjusted to provide the desired level of gas exchange or cardiac support. As long as the venous drainage is adequate, the bladder remains distended, and the desired flow is delivered. If venous drainage is impeded for any reason (hypovolemia, pneumothorax, kinking of the venous catheter), the pump stops and an alarm sounds. Flow resumes as soon as venous drainage is reestablished. Early in the course of extracorporeal circulation, flow is increased to the point at which the bladder collapses, thus identifying the physical limitation of venous drainage for the system. This flow rate is usually considerably greater than the flow actually required for extracorporeal support. However, if maximal flow through the system is inadequate after optimizing volume status and increasing the distance between patient and pump, another venous catheter must be added to gain more flow.

A pumping system with all the advantages of the servoregulated roller pump but without the extra bladder and hardware is the passively filling Rhone Poulenc pump, now marketed by Collin Cardio of Paris and used by Durandy et al. (15) for extracorporeal support (as well as for cardiac surgery). This unique pump uses a flaccid but distensible silicone rubber tube that is stretched over rollers without a raceway to push against. The pumping chamber fills passively, allowing the generation of flow and pressure. However, if the venous drainage is inadequate, the pumping chamber simply collapses without generating negative pressure. As the pumping chamber becomes more round, the amount of pressure generated reaches a plateau at about 400 mm Hg, so flow decreases above this pressure and arterial line blowouts cannot occur.

Centrifugal pumps, in which a spinning rotor generates flow and pressure, should be ideal for prolonged extracorporeal circulation (16). At low flow, centrifugal pumps work very well, but these pumps can generate significant negative pressure whenever the venous drainage is impaired, causing extensive hemolysis. Although centrifugal pumps have been used for prolonged support, the potential for hemolysis makes them less desirable.

From the foregoing discussion, it can be seen that both building and monitoring the ECLS circuit requires a knowledge of the pressure, flow, and resistance characteristics of each of the blood conduit components. Although these relationships can be calculated for straight tubes of known diameters, most access catheters have irregular diameters and side holes that require individual characterization. Our group (17) recently described a standard system for describing pressure–flow relationships in blood access devices, which we have called the M number. If the M number for a specific catheter is known, the pressure and flow over the full range of use can be determined from the nomogram (see Figures 7.6 and 7.7). If a given combination of pressure and flow is required, then reference to the nomogram will identify the corresponding M number. Any catheter or combination of catheters with a smaller M number will be capable of meeting the conditions. M numbers for some typical devices used for ECLS are listed in Table 7.1.

The effect of venoarterial bypass on systemic perfusion is reflected in the pulse contour and pulse pressure (Figure 7.8). The extracorporeal pump creates a flow that is essentially nonpulsatile. Consequently, as more blood is routed through the extracorporeal circuit, the systemic arterial pulse contour becomes flatter, then intermittent, then is stopped altogether when total bypass is reached. At total bypass, the left ventricle gradually distends with bronchial and thebesian flow and ejects when it is full, leading to an occasional pulsatile beat. In practice, it is unusual to reach total bypass for any sustained period with extrathoracic cannulation as long as there is cardiac function. Typically, venoarterial ECLS is run at about 80% of resting normal cardiac output, which allows 20% or more of the blood to pass through the lungs and left heart, resulting in a diminished but discernible pulse contour. As

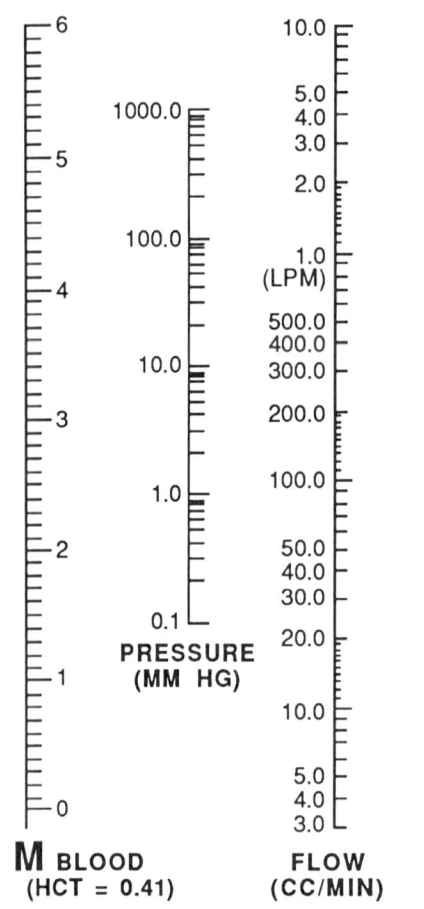

FIGURE 7.6 The M number describes pressure–flow characteristics in vascular access catheters. With this nomogram, the pressure and flow can be determined if the M number is known.

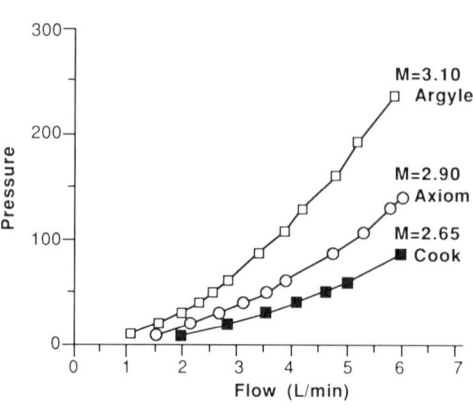

FIGURE 7.7 Pressure–flow characteristics for a range of M numbers.

TABLE 7.1 The M number of catheters and tubing commonly used for ECLS

Catheter	Size	M number
Tubing, 1 m	3/16 in., 4.45 mm ID	4.2
Tubing, 1 m	1/4 in., 6 mm ID	3.1
Tubing, 1 m	3/8 in., 9 mm ID	2.0
Elecath arterial	10 F	4.1
Biomedicus arterial	10 F	4.0
Cook arterial	20 F	3.25
DLP arterial	21 F	2.65
Elecath venous	14 F	3.7
Biomedicus venous	12 F	3.55
Cook venous	28 F	2.65
DLP venous	21 F	3.05

long as total blood flow is adequate, the presence of a pulse contour is not important physiologically (4,18,19).

Venovenous bypass has no effect on hemodynamics. Blood is drained from and returned to the venous circulation at the same rate because the extracorporeal circuit is noncompliant. This is true whether venovenous bypass is achieved with two separate catheters or with a single double-lumen catheter. An interesting variation on venovenous bypass proposed by Kolobow et al. (20) and used by Durandy et al. (15) is the tidal flow system. In tidal flow VV extracorporeal circulation, a single venous catheter in the right atrium is used. Venous blood is drained for approximately 1 s, a valve changes the access, and oxygenator blood is reinfused through the same catheter in a shorter time, typically 0.5 s. This system results in some significant fluctuations in right atrial pressure, but these do not interfere with right ventricular or left-sided hemodynamics. VV and VA bypass are further compared in Table 7.2.

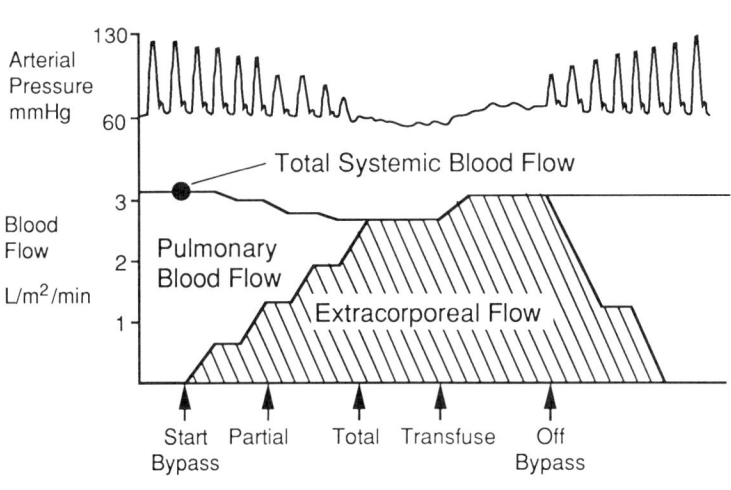

FIGURE 7.8 Arterial pulse contour at different levels of venoarterial bypass. During near-total bypass, the pulse pressure is approximately 10 mm Hg and most of the flow is extracorporeal.

TABLE 7.2 Major differences between venoarterial and venovenous bypass

Hemodynamics	VA	VV
Systemic perfusion	Circuit flow and cardiac output	Cardiac output only
Arterial blood pressure	Pulse contour damped	Pulse contour full
Central venous pressure volume	Not too helpful	Accurate guide to status
Pulmonary artery pressure	Decreased in proportion to ECC flow	Not affected by flow
Effect of R-L shunt	Mixed venous into perfusate blood	None
Effect of L-R (PDA) shunt	Pulmonary hyperperfusion may require increased flow	No effect on ECC flow, usual PDA physiology
Selective R arm, brain perfusion	Occurs	Does not occur
Gas exchange		
Typical blood flow for full gas exchange	80–100 cc/kg/min	100–120 cc/kg/min
Arterial oxygenation	Saturation controlled by ECC flow	80%–95% saturation common at maximum flow
CO_2 removal	Depends on sweep gas and membrane lung size	Same as VA
Oxygenator	0.4 or 0.6	0.6 or 0.8
Decrease initial vent settings	Rapidly	Slowly

ECC = extracorporeal circulation; PDA = patent ductus arteriosus.

COAGULATION CONTROL

Whenever blood contacts a prosthetic surface, the physiologic mechanism of thrombosis begins. Blood proteins adhere instantly to the prosthetic surface, creating a molecular protein layer which forms the blood surface interface for the rest of the period of exposure. The proteins in this layer affect subsequent events. Some proteins like albumin "pacify" or "passivate" the surface, minimizing subsequent cellular or protein interactions. Other proteins, notably fibrinogen, activate factor 12, complement, and platelets. The thrombogenicity of prosthetic surfaces is related to the amount of fibrinogen that adheres during blood exposure. Platelets adhere to fibrinogen on an artificial surface and are stimulated to release platelet granule material, attracting other platelets and stimulating the formation of fibrin. If no anticoagulant is present in the blood and the flow is slow or absent, a platelet fibrin mesh grows in seconds, trapping red cells and white cells in the process and leading to a blood clot. If there is no anticoagulant in the blood but the flow is very fast, there is insufficient time for the growth of a clot before the aggregated platelets are washed away, so gross clotting does not occur.

When fibrin formation is inhibited by heparin, the growth of the clot is impeded even in areas of slow flow, so aggregates of platelets and white cells grow in stagnant zones without the fibrin glue that leads to solid thrombosis. When the platelet/white cell aggregate extends into the stream of rapidly flowing blood, it grows until it waves in the stream and then breaks off. This platelet/white cell aggregate embolizes into the patient and disaggregates in the first capillary bed; the effete platelets recirculate until they are removed by the reticuloendothelial system (21,22). Although it has been shown that extracorporeal circulation can be conducted for long periods without systemic anticoagulation as long as high flow is maintained with no stagnant areas (23), in clinical practice the state of the art is to give systemic heparin continuously in whatever dose is required to maintain the whole blood activated clotting time at around 200 s (approximately one and one half times normal). This generally requires 30 to 60 units of heparin/kg/h. Heparin is bound to platelets and excreted in the urine, so higher heparin doses are required during diuresis and platelet transfusion, lower heparin doses are required in renal failure and thrombocytopenia. Obviously, the heparin effect, rather than the exact heparin level, is the important parameter. Heparin effect must be measured in whole blood (whole blood activated clotting time (ACT)) rather than in plasma (such as partial thromboplastin time or thrombin time).

For the reasons mentioned above, platelets will be consumed during extracorporeal circulation at a steady and continuous rate (24). If new platelets can be made by megakaryocytes rapidly enough to balance this platelet loss, the platelet count remains stable. In most children and newborn infants, the rate of platelet generation does not match the rate of platelet loss, and platelet transfusions are necessary to maintain normal hemostasis. When the platelet count is maintained greater than 75,000/mm^3 and the activated clotting time is less than 200 s, the risk of bleeding is relatively small and the risk of major clotting in the circuit is negligible as long as blood flow continues.

There have been few studies of the effect of prolonged extracorporeal circulation on white cell numbers and function (25). In general, the white blood count and differential count are normal during extracorporeal circulation. Since preexisting bacterial infections usually resolve during ECLS, it is reasonable to think that neutrophil phagocytosis is adequate; however, this has not been studied in detail.

The effect of prolonged extracorporeal circulation on red cells is negligible as long as there is no direct exposure of blood to gas or to negative pressure. The roller pump is adjusted so that it is almost completely occlusive, using the servo-regulation mechanism described above to avoid negative pressure surges. With these precautions, the plasma-free hemoglobin level should be routinely less than 40 mg/dL and the urine should be clear. If plasma hemoglobin levels exceed 40 mg/dL, some cause of hemolysis should be sought.

PHYSIOLOGY OF OTHER ORGANS DURING ECLS

Fluids and electrolytes are managed as they would be in any patient. The generalized edema seen following cardiac surgery is usually related to hemodilution and should not occur during ECLS. Capillary permeability is normal during ECLS, so capillary leakage is indicative of patient disease rather than extracorporeal circulation. If edema occurs, it should be treated with diuresis since many organs, including the lung, malfunction when edematous. Renal function is normal during ECLS. The volume and composition of urine is a good marker of the adequacy of systemic perfusion. The kidney responds to osmotic and loop diuretics, which are often necessary to treat fluid overload.

Energy and protein metabolism are normal during ECLS. When properly managed, the level of catecholamine secretion is normal (unlike cardiac surgery in which catechol secretion is stimulated by hypothermia, hemodilution, and borderline systemic oxygen delivery) (3). As in any critically ill patient, it is general practice to give enteral or parenteral feeding to match caloric and protein requirements. Temperature is regulated by a heat exchanger in the circuit.

Liver function is normal during the early phases of ECLS. After a period of several days, a pattern of cholestatic jaundice and hepatomegaly without liver enzyme elevation may be seen. (M. Reynolds, personal communication, 1989). This is apparently due to the accumulation of platelets and other debris in the reticuloendothelial system of the liver and concomitant limitation of conjugated bile excretion (22).

Cardiac physiology is affected differently by VV extracorporeal circulation than it is by VA extracorporeal circulation. As left atrial pressure drops during VA bypass, left ventricular filling also drops, leading eventually to a decrease in pulse contour, followed by intermittent left ventricular ejection when the ventricle becomes full. If the heart stops beating during venoarterial bypass, the left atrium will gradually fill from bronchial and thebesian flow, leading within minutes or hours to high left atrial pressure, high pulmonary hydrostatic pressure, and cardiogenic pulmonary edema. This situation may be exacerbated by increased afterload due to systemic vasospasm, volume overload, or perfusate flow directed toward the aortic valve. Consequently, if extracorporeal support is used for cardiac failure and the ventricle does not empty, the left side of the circulation must be decompressed to avoid pulmonary edema. This is usually accomplished by the creation of an atrial septal defect via a blade or balloon septostomy. Experimentally, Kolobow et al. (26) have devised a system for cannulating the pulmonary artery to decompress the left side of the heart during VA bypass.

The nervous system and musculoskeletal system should be normal during extracorporeal circulation. Patients are alert and awake and can be managed with minimal to moderate sedation.

Microembolization occurs constantly during ECC. The platelet/white cell emboli referred to earlier can be found regularly in the perfusate (21). In addition, small fibrin/red blood cell (RBC) particles form in stopcocks, bridges, and other stagnant zones and embolize. Since organ function generally remains normal during a month or more of ECC, and since tissue infarcts are not found at autopsy, we assume that this microembolization has no functional significance. However, it is worth noting that any systemic effects of microembolization will be less with VV access than with VA access, indicating that there is a theoretical advantage to using VV for long perfusion.

PHYSIOLOGIC PRINCIPLES IN THE MANAGEMENT OF EXTRACORPOREAL LIFE SUPPORT

Based on an understanding of the physiology of extracorporeal circulation and of the pathophysiology of the patient's primary disease, it is obvious that the goal of extracorporeal life support is to maintain systemic oxygen delivery and CO_2 removal in the proper proportion to systemic metabolism. This is achieved at low ventilator or inotropic drug settings which could not otherwise be tolerated. This process should eliminate any further ventilator-induced lung injury and improve systemic perfusion, allowing time for the native lung or heart to recover from the acute illness.

Planning and Priming the Circuit

Although total support may never be necessary, the circuit must be planned with total support in mind. The tubing, connectors, and pump must be capable of adequate blood flow (typically 100 cc/kg/min for newborn infants, 75 cc/kg/min for children, and 50 cc/kg/min for adults). If venovenous access is used for respiratory support, these estimates of blood flow should be increased by 20%, since higher blood flow will be required for adequate oxygenation because of recirculation. The venous access catheter should be large enough to deliver this amount of blood flow with the assistance of 100 cm of syphon, and the arterial or reinfusion catheter should be large enough to permit this level of blood flow at line pressures less than 300 mm Hg proximal to the membrane lung. The membrane lung must have a rated flow higher than the maximal anticipated blood flow. At present, the spiral coil membrane lung designed by Kolobow and manufactured by the SciMed Corporation of Minneapolis is the only membrane lung used for ECLS in the United States. The sizes of SciMed lungs, along with rated flow, oxygen transfer at rated flow, and CO_2 transfer, are listed in Table 7.3.

Once the circuit components have been selected and assembled in sterile fashion, the system is ready for priming. First the system is filled with CO_2 gas to displace any nitrogen which would form bubbles. Then a saline clear prime is used to displace CO_2. The system is debubbled during circulation through a priming reservoir. A small amount of albumin is then added to decrease subsequent fibrinogen adsorption, and the clear prime is displaced with blood. The blood is recirculated through the priming reservoir until the temperature is 37°C and the electrolytes and blood gases are near normal. Then the circuit is ready for connection to the patient.

TABLE 7.3 Circuit design requires matching the membrane lung to the patient's size (typical values for some SciMed lungs)

Patient size (kg)	SciMed membrane lung surface area size	Rated flow* (L/min)	Gas exchange† (cc/min)
	0.4	0.5 L	30
3–10	0.8	1 L	60
	1.5	2 L	120
10–30	2.5	3 L	180
	3.5	4 L	240
30+	4.5	5 L	300

*Rated flow = maximal flow of 75% saturated venous blood which can be fully oxygenated.
†O_2 + CO_2 exchange at $AvDo_2$ 6 vol % and RQ 1.0. Potential CO_2 exchange is higher.

Cannulation

While the circuit is being primed, vascular access cannulas are placed. For the reasons outlined above, we always use the right internal jugular vein as the location of choice for venous access. The largest internal diameter, shortest catheter that can be placed into the jugular vein usually permits the desired blood flow. A smaller catheter is preferable if the M number is less than that dictated by the desired flow characteristics. If venoarterial circulation is to be used, the right common carotid artery is the vessel of choice because it is large enough to accept a large arterial catheter and provides flow directly into the aortic route. Both the jugular vein and carotid arteries are ligated distally. Both arterial and venous collateral circulations are adequate in almost all patients. The carotid provides excellent access in children and adults. The adequacy of brain collateral circulation is tested by observing left-sided motor and sensory function during temporary occlusion. If venovenous access is used for respiratory support, perfusate blood can be returned directly to the jugular vein catheter using the tidal flow system or a double-lumen catheter. Alternatively, the perfusate can be returned to any large systemic vein. Usually, the femoral vein is catheterized via the saphenous bulb. It is tempting to use the umbilical vein in neonates, but this usually results in portal hypertension and ascites in full-term newborn infants.

Monitoring

ECLS requires several monitors in addition to patient vital signs, blood gases, and ventilator settings. Blood flow is monitored continuously, usually by counting rotations per minute on the roller pump. Although routinely used, this method of measuring flow can be grossly in error if the rollers are not occlusive or if the tubing is not round. Pressure should be monitored on the arterial side of the circuit, preferably before and after the membrane lung. An increasing pressure gradient across the membrane lung suggests thrombosis. The expected postoxygenator pressure should be predicted for any given flow based on the M number of the return catheter. If the pressures are higher than expected, the arterial line or catheter is kinked or occluded. The most important parameter is continuous monitoring of mixed venous saturation (Figure 7.9). This is measured by placing an Oximetrix fiberoptic catheter through a Touhy Borst adapter into the venous line. Since venous drainage blood represents a mixture of blood from the superior vena cava, the inferior vena cava, and the coronary sinus, the SVo_2 is an accurate representation of the Do_2/Vo_2 ratio during venoarterial bypass (10). As long as the SVo_2 is in the range of 75% and all aspects of perfusion are going well, it is not necessary to measure systemic or circuit blood gases more frequently than approximately every eight hours. If the system includes a transcutaneous oximeter and

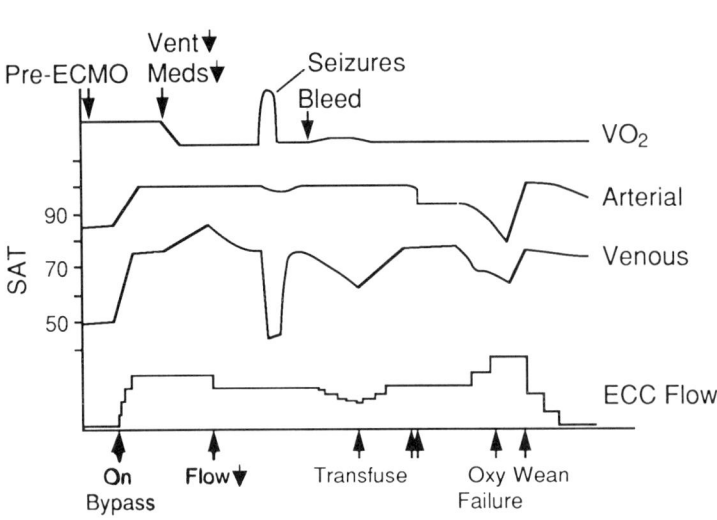

FIGURE 7.9 Venous saturation monitors the ratio of oxygen delivery to oxygen consumption. As shown in this diagram, venous saturation increases when oxygen consumption drops secondary to decreased medications and ventilator settings. Venous saturation decreases when oxygen consumption increases because of seizures. Venous saturation decreases when oxygen delivery decreases due to bleeding and both increase during transfusion.

an on-line P_{CO_2} monitor, sampling of blood for gas analysis is rarely necessary. During venovenous bypass, the mixed venous saturation is elevated because of recirculation. With VV bypass, the intent is to maintain the venous saturation as high as possible, usually between 85% and 90%. If the cardiac output is normal, this level of saturation will be sufficient to maintain normal systemic oxygen delivery. When SVO_2 is combined with transcutaneous oximetry in a patient on VV bypass, the adequacy of extracorporeal support and the amount of lung function can be assessed simultaneously. Measurement of end tidal CO_2 at the airway is another helpful monitor of native lung function. During the early days of an ECLS run, end tidal CO_2 may be 5% or less. As functioning lung units resume ventilation or as pulmonary blood flow to ventilated units increases, end tidal CO_2 will increase. When end tidal CO_2 is near normal (over 35 mm Hg), a trial of weaning should be considered. The status of anticoagulation is monitored by measuring whole blood activated clotting time hourly. Platelet count is measured every 8 to 12 hours.

Managing the Patient on ECLS

The blood flow is set at a level that will provide total oxygen and CO_2 exchange, and mechanical ventilation is reduced to minimal or lung rest settings. Patient arterial blood gases are checked, and continuous monitors are calibrated. Thereafter, venous saturation is maintained at the desired level by increasing or decreasing extracorporeal blood flow. $Paco_2$ is maintained at about 40 mm Hg by adjusting the flow rate and composition of sweep gas. Systemic blood pressure is maintained at the desired level by adjusting blood volume. Hemoglobin is maintained between 14 and 15 g%. Platelet count is maintained at greater than 75,000 and activated clotting time is maintained at approximately 200 s. A major decrease in venous saturation with no change in the other settings is usually caused by an increase in metabolic rate, which may be transient (during crying or seizures) or sustained. A sustained increase in metabolic rate can be matched by an increase in blood flow or can be treated with sedation, paralysis, and/or hypothermia. A major increase in venous saturation with no change in other settings is usually caused by a decrease in metabolic rate or the onset of native lung function. A sudden decrease in venous drainage may be caused by hypovolemia, catheter kinking or malposition, pneumothorax, or pericardial tamponade. A gradual decrease in systemic oxygenation or an increase in $Paco_2$ may be a sign of deteriorating membrane lung function. Membrane lung function is assessed by measuring oxygen and

CO_2 transfer and comparing the results to the expected transfer at that level of blood flow and CO_2 gradient. If the membrane lung is deteriorating, a new lung should be inserted. This is rarely necessary.

Weaning and Decannulation

Indicators of lung recovery include: increasing Pao_2 or decreasing $Paco_2$ without changing ventilator or ECLS settings, increased Vo_2 or Vco_2 measured via the airway, increasing compliance, and a clearing chest x-ray. Indicators of cardiac recovery include: increasing Svo_2 with no change in Vo_2 or other parameters, increasing pulse contour, and improving contractility detected by echocardiography.

When native lung or cardiac function improves, extracorporeal flow is gradually decreased, allowing the native lung to carry more of the load. When 70% to 80% of the gas exchange is occurring via the native lung (i.e., the extracorporeal flow rate is 20% to 30% of the initial flow rate), the patient should be tried off bypass at moderate ventilator settings. In venoarterial bypass, the tubing leading to the patient is clamped, permitting continuing circulation through a bridge. If gas exchange and perfusion are adequate, the catheters can be removed, usually after another period of low flow bypass, to be sure that lung function will be maintained. In venovenous bypass, a trial off bypass consists of capping off gas flow to the membrane lung but continuing extracorporeal flow. With this arrangement, the venous saturation monitor becomes a useful guide to the adequacy of systemic oxygen delivery during the trial.

Using these simple physiologic principles of management, extracorporeal circulation can be maintained in the absence of pulmonary function for one to six weeks.

REFERENCES

(1) Galletti PM, Brecher GA. Heart-lung bypass. New York: Grune & Stratton, 1962.

(2) Ionescu MI, Wooler C. Current techniques in extracorporeal circulation, 2nd ed. London: Butterworth, 1980.

(3) Bartlett RH, Gazzaniga AB. The physiology and pathophysiology of extracorporeal circulation. In: Ionescu M, Wooler C, eds. Current techniques in extracorporeal circulation, 2nd ed. London: Butterworth, 1980.

(4) Bartlett RH, Gazzaniga AB. Extracorporeal circulation for cardiopulmonary failure. Current problems in surgery. Vol. 15, No. 5. Chicago: Year Book Medical Publishers, 1978.

(5) Schmidt S, Dudenhausen JW, Langner K, Laiblin C, Saling EZ. A new perfusion circuit for the newborn with lung immaturity: extracorporeal CO_2 removal via an umbilical arteriovenous shunt during apneic O_2 diffusion. Artif Organs 1984;8:478–80.

(6) Kuwabara Y, Okai T, Kozuma S, et al. Artificial placenta: long term extrauterine incubation of isolated goat fetuses. Artif Organs 1981; 13:527–31.

(7) Kleiber M. The fire of life, 3rd ed. Malabor FL: Robert Krieger Company, 1987.

(8) Bartlett RH, Dechert RE, Mault J, Ferguson S, Kaiser AM, Erlandson EE. Measurement of metabolism in multiple organ failure. Surgery 1982;92:771–8.

(9) Fick A. On the measurement of the blood quantity in the ventricles of the heart. Proceedings of the Physiological Medical Society of Wurzburg, July 9, 1870.

(10) Bartlett RH. Extracorporeal oxygen delivery and life support in neonatal respiratory failure. In: Eyrich K, Reinhart K, eds. Clinical aspects of O_2 transport and tissue oxygenation. Proceedings of the 4th International Steglitz Symposium. Berlin: Springer-Verlag, 1989.

(11) Eyrich K, Reinhart K, eds. Clinical aspects of O_2 transport and tissue oxygenation. Proceedings of the 4th International Steglitz Symposium. Berlin: Springer-Verlag, 1989.

(12) Galletti PM, Richardson PD, Snider MT. A standardized method for defining the overall gas transfer performance of artificial lungs. Trans ASAIO 1972;18:359–68.

(13) Kolobow T. Gas exchange with membrane lungs. In: Gille JP, ed. Neonatal and adult respiratory failure. Paris: Elsevier, 1989.

(14) Pesenti A, Gattinoni L, Kolobow T, Damia G. Extracorporeal circulation in adult respiratory failure. Trans ASAIO 1988;34:43–7.

(15) Durandy Y, Chevalier JY, Lecompte Y. Single cannula venovenous bypass for respiratory membrane lung support. J Thorac Cardiovasc Surgery 1990;99:404–9.

(16) Palder SB, Shaheen KW, Whittlesey GC, Nowlen TT, Kundu SK, Klein MD. Prolonged extracorporeal membrane oxygenation in sheep with a hollow-fiber oxygenator and a centrifugal pump. Trans ASAIO 1988;34:820–2.

(17) Montoya JP, Merz SI, Bartlett RH. A standardized system for describing flow/pressure relationships in vascular access devices. Trans ASAIO 1991;37:4–8.

(18) Rudy LW, Heyman MA, Edmunds LH. Distribution of systemic blood flow during cardiopulmonary bypass. J Appl Physiol 1973; 34:194–200.

(19) Bernstein EF, Cosentino LC, Reich S, et al. A compact low hemolysis non-thrombogenic system for nonthroacotomy prolonged left ventricular bypass. Trans ASAIO 1974;20:643–52.

(20) Kolobow T, Borell M, Spatola R, Tsumo K, Prato P. Single catheter venovenous membrane lung bypass in the treatment of experimental ARDS. Trans ASAIO 1988;34:35–8.

(21) Hicks RE, Dutton RC, Ries CA, Price DC, Edmunds LH Jr. Production and fate of platelet aggregate emboli during venovenous perfusion. Surg Forum 1973;24:250–2.

(22) Dutton RC, Edmunds LH Jr, Hutchinson JC, Roe BB. Platelet aggregate emboli in patients during cardiopulmonary bypass with membrane and bubble oxygenators and blood filters. J Thorac Cardiovasc Surg 1974;67:258–65.

(23) Whittlesey GC, Kundu SY, Salley SO, Nowlen TT, Klein MD. Is heparin necessary for extracorporeal circulation? Trans ASAIO 1988; 34:823–6.

(24) Anderson HL, Cilley RE, Zwischenberger JB, Bartlett RH. Thrombocytopenia in neonates after extracorporeal membrane oxygenation. Trans ASAIO 1986;32:534–7.

(25) Neveceral D, Mackert M, Wauters JP. Neutrophil behavior during hemodialysis: role of membrane contact. Trans ASAIO 1988;34: 564–7.

(26) Kolobow T, Rossi F, Borellim M, Foti G. Long term closed chest partial and total cardiopulmonary bypass by peripheral cannulation for severe right and/or left ventricular failure including ventricular fibrillation. Trans ASAIO 1988; 34:485–9.

8

Interactions of Blood and Artificial Surfaces: In Search of "Heparin-free" Cardiopulmonary Bypass

❖

Robert C. Eberhart, PH.D.

From the beginning, it was realized that blood reacts with the surfaces of a heart-lung machine and that the reaction products are a significant cause of morbidity. Destruction of blood cells, sublethal damage to these elements with sequestration in various organs, fat- and platelet-derived microthrombi, and blood sludging were significant events in these early days, predisposing to postperfusion lung syndrome and regional ischemia (1). As the technology of cardiopulmonary bypass was improved, the blood damage, especially red cell destruction, fat emboli, and sludging, was significantly reduced (2). Problems remained, especially perfusion-induced platelet and leukocyte depletion and difficulties with heparin titration. But various means were used to control, if not eliminate, these problems, for example, routine use of activated clotting time for heparin titration, arterial filtration of microemboli, etc. (3). Reduced blood injury permitted introduction of extracorporeal membrane oxygenation (ECMO), the use of a specially modified heart-lung machine for prolonged periods in cases of adult respiratory distress syndrome. The equipment maintained pulmonary oxygenation and perfusion, buying time while other therapies were applied (4).

ECMO exacerbated the blood damage problems that had been controlled in open heart procedures. Thrombocytopenia, leukopenia, bleeding, and occasional consumption coagulopathies were observed in the original ECMO studies (5,6). This led to concerted efforts to improve the technology of ECMO, culminating in its successful clinical use in the neonatal population (7). Perhaps more importantly, improvements in ECMO materials and a better understanding of blood-material interactions have unmasked a broadly based activation of host defenses (8); indeed, such processes had long been suspected by workers in membrane oxygenator development (9). Complement activation by cardiopulmonary bypass, hemodialysis, and leukapheresis equipment is well documented (10,11). This has been linked to foreign surface-induced transient leukopenia (12) and dysfunction of neutrophils (13). Several pathways contribute (8), but the discovery of the C5a receptor site on the neutrophil membrane, known to induce chemotaxis (14), is the most compelling evidence. A generalized inflammatory response to cardiopulmonary bypass has been proposed (15), but this may relate primarily to contamination (8). Recently, a surface-induced immune reactivity for plasmapheresis equipment has been postulated (16). There is also a documented preference for bacterial colonization on foreign surfaces (17).

In summary, the foreign surfaces of blood-contacting devices, especially the large-surface-area ECMO circuits, may induce thromboembolic damage, a host-defense reaction organized around the neutrophil, the macrophage, and the immune system, and may predispose to bacterial colonization. All such processes must be eliminated if the ECMO system is to be optimally passivated.

PASSIVATION METHODS

Morton and Cumming (18) classified the factors governing foreign surface thrombus formation according to Virchow's classic triad of the initiators of intravascular thrombosis: blood chemistry, (foreign) surface chemistry, and hemodynamics. It is convenient to generalize this classification to include host-defense responses and thus to organize the approaches to surface passivation. Table 8.1 follows this classification for strategies that have been or may be applied to ECMO circuitry. Thus, *infused drugs* may favorably alter blood chemistry, *immobilized biological and other polymer surface and bulk treatments* may improve the foreign surface chemistry, and, interestingly, *hemodynamics* may also be used to advantage. Subsequent discussion is based on this scheme.

Infused Drugs

Heparin To paraphrase Mortensen, "systemic heparin has made ECMO possible; the American Society for Artificial Internal Organs owes its existence to heparin; and yet that chapter in the practice of ECMO may be coming to a close" (unpublished remarks, Symposium on Clinical Applications of ECMO and $ECCO_2R$, 36th Annual Meeting, American Society for Artificial Internal Organs,

TABLE 8.1 Methods to improve the blood compatibility of ECMO circuits

Method	Action	Reference
Infused drugs		
Heparin	Anticoagulant	21
PGI_2, Iloprost	Antiplatelet	33, 34
Piperidine	Antiplatelet	38
Disintegrin	Antiplatelet	44
PPACK	Synthetic antithrombin	47
Aprotonin, FUT175	Serine protease inhibitor	48, 49
Immobilized biologicals		
Heparin	Anticoagulant	50
Urokinase, streptokinase	Fibrinolytic	51
Polymer surface treatment		
Alkylation, hydroxylation	Albumin passivation	81, 90
Polyethylene oxide	Decrease interfacial energy	91
Plasma discharge	Decrease interfacial energy	99
Polymer bulk treatment		
Amphiphilic additive	Modify protein adsorption	101
Silicone rubber film	Coat porous membranes	65, 103
Polyalkylsulfone	Modify protein adsorption	104
Polyphosphazene	Modify protein adsorption	106
Sulfonated polymers	Synthetic heparin	107
Replace plasticizer	Reduce toxic leachables	113
Hemodynamics		
Smooth, contoured surfaces	Reduce flow disturbances	114, 117
Low MW dextran	Fluidity, antiplatelet	118–120
Increase wall shear rate	Endothelial cell release of TPA, PGI_2	30, 121

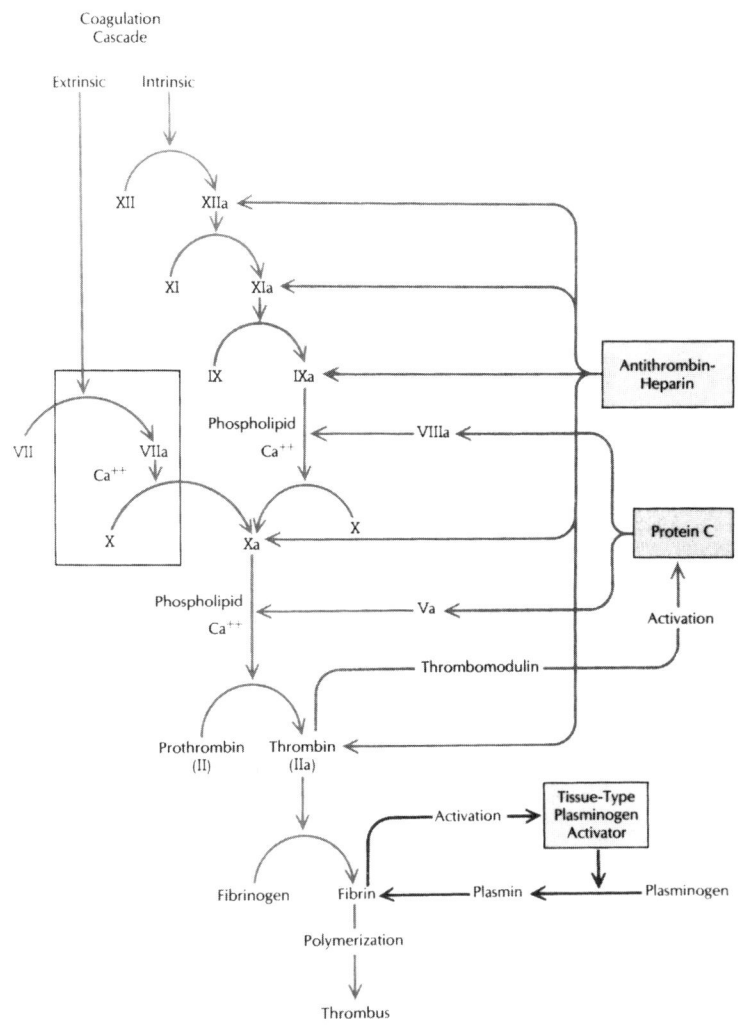

FIGURE 8.1 The coagulation cascade is now viewed as a regulating system in which the powerful mechanisms that drive the cascade are offset by equally potent mechanisms for keeping it in check. Three principal mechanisms appear to govern this negative side of the cascade. 1) The antithrombin-heparin mechanism acts early in the cascade to neutralize the activity of factors XIIa, XIa, IXa, Xa, and IIa (thrombin). 2) The protein C mechanism is activated only in the presence of thrombin and its cofactor thrombomodulin and is accelerated by protein S. Activated protein C inactivates factors VIIIa and Va and thereby slows down further production of thrombin. 3) Tissue plasminogen activator, which requires the presence of fibrin for its activity, converts plasminogen to plasmin, an enzyme that proteolyzes fibrin. (Reprinted with permission from Rosenberg RD, Bauer KA. New insights into hypercoagulable states. Hosp Pract 1986;21:131–7.)

Washington, D.C., April 26, 1990). By virtue of its complexation with antithrombin III, heparin blocks or otherwise interferes with several major steps in the coagulation enzyme cascade (Figure 8.1) (19). No one would question the importance of heparin in preventing these unacceptable events. But systemic heparinization in extracorporeal circulation is not an unmixed blessing. Problems with hemostasis and heparin titration complicate its use (19–24) and may limit the indications for ECMO (21,24). The actions of heparin on the other blood elements are not totally predictable. Heparin frequently induces thrombocytopenia in humans (25). Competing pro- and antiaggregant actions of human heparin compounds on platelets have been reported (26). Heparin may inhibit the activation of the alternate complement pathway (27). Thus, while anticoagulation of ECMO circuits by heparin administration is the obvious method of choice, it may create other problems, and its titration is an intricate task.

Other methods might achieve the anticoagulation gained by heparin administration without some of its undesirable side-effects. For example, the rate of coagulation is modulated by proteins C and S (19,28). It appears possible to slow the rate of coagulation rather than block it and to inhibit platelet activity as well by administration of activated protein C (29). This would conceivably protect tissues prone to bleed while avoiding coagulation and host-defense activation in the extracorporeal circuit. Alternatively, it may be possible to manipulate hemostasis by the extracorporeal blood flow without anticoagulant drugs, or at least with substantial reductions in amount. Murphy and colleagues showed that an anticoagulant effect of endogenous origin could be generated in an arteriovenous extracorporeal circuit of general features, in which the sole requirement was to maintain a blood flow rate greater than 300 mL/min in a ¼-in.-diameter tube with a roller pump (30). Recent evidence in support of this remarkable finding has emerged and will be discussed.

For the time being, these are merely interesting speculations which await experimental confirmation. But they have captured the attention of students of the art and science of extracorporeal circulation and are beginning to be seriously explored.

PGI_2, Iloprost The most critical period for platelet activation occurs at the first exposure of the foreign material to blood (31). But the platelet reactivity of foreign surfaces does not cease after the initial blood contact. Platelet survival following vascular prosthesis implantation in humans and other species is sharply reduced and does not return to normal for several months (32), whereas fibrinogen and plasminogen survival are unchanged. These findings suggest that continued platelet reactivity with ECMO circuitry may be expected, prompting study of the preservation of circulating platelets by drug infusion.

Prostacyclin (PGI_2) and prostaglandin E_1 inhibit platelet aggregation by increasing the intracellular level of cyclic adenosine monophosphate (AMP). Addonizio et al. have demonstrated the ability of prostacyclin (33) and the stable prostacyclin analogue, Iloprost (34), to temporarily control platelet function in vitro. Interestingly, the preservation of circulating platelet numbers and function persists long after the drug-induced inhibition is reversed, and this extended influence is also observed in vivo (35). The effect is reversible, an attractive feature by comparison with cyclooxygenase inhibitors such as aspirin, which impair the platelet for the duration of its lifetime. On the other hand, there are pressor responses of Iloprost and prostacyclin to consider (36). It has also been reported that low doses of PGI_2 and PGE_1 rapidly stimulate the release from human platelets of a protease or proteases that activate factor X (37). It is not known whether Iloprost has the same effect. Actions of these drugs on other elements of host defense in the context of ECMO are unknown. Further study of these drugs appears most favorable in surface-immobilized form, in which the first phalanx of platelets may attach to the treated surface but are inhibited from aggregation, conditioning the surface and improving its passivation.

Piperidine Lasslow et al. have developed a series of carbamolypiperidine and quinoline derivatives with potent antiplatelet characteristics and low toxicity (38). These agents stabilize the platelet membrane, increasing the threshold for platelet aggregation and release of serotonin and platelet factor 4 (39). These substances are thought to act on the prostaglandin metabolic pathway prior to arachidonic acid formation. The most promising congener strikingly lowered the size of platelet thrombi on collagen-coated glass flow surfaces (40) and showed effects on platelets similar to the thrombasthenic state observed with ticlopidine in a baboon model of platelet-dependent thrombosis (41). The influence of these compounds on the cyclooxygenase and lipooxygenase systems has not been investigated. They do not inhibit adenosine diphosphate (ADP)-induced aggregation. The duration of action is very short, which might be beneficial in ECMO applications. The drugs are relatively new, and some routine studies remain to be completed, such as binding to membrane receptors, proteins, and enzymes, and exhaustive analysis of toxic side-effects (42).

Disintegrins Rapid progress has been made in understanding the molecular interactions that result in cell adhesion to substrates (43). The tripeptide sequence arginine-glycine-aspartic acid (RGD), common to many adhesion proteins, has been isolated from several of these proteins, and the class of materials so formed, called integrins, is under intensive investigation in many laboratories. Certain forms have been immobilized successfully on the surfaces of polymers, where they have markedly improved the adhesion, if not the spreading and function, of various cells. Infusion or immobilization of the RGD peptide sequence should not be expected to reduce cell-surface interactions in cardiopulmonary bypass; in fact, only a mild inhibition of the normal loss of circulating platelets from pump oxygenator circuits has been observed. Musial et al. have reported preliminary studies with a series of RGD-containing, low-molecular-weight (MW), cysteine-rich peptides, isolated from various viper venoms, which they term disintegrins (44). Four of these compounds, exhibiting a significant degree of homology, have been shown to markedly inhibit platelet loss and reduce secretion of beta-thromboglobulin during extracorporeal circulation. At concentrations that equally preserved circulating platelets, the disintegrins exhibited varying inhibition of ADP-induced platelet aggregation in vitro. Echistatin, the lowest-MW agent, provided the highest inhibition of platelet aggregation. Two higher-MW agents, albolabrin and flavoridin, were less potent in this test. None of the disintegrins prevented loss of alpha granules and beta-thromboglobulin in thrombin-stimulated, standard platelet aggregometry, nor did they inhibit platelet shape change and pseudopod formation. Disintegrins appear to have transient inhibitory effects on platelet function in vivo, and a short half-life. They appear to have no detrimental effect on blood pressure or core temperature. They may thus be preferable, for extracorporeal circulation and ECMO, to Iloprost, PGE_1, and PGI_2, all of which may cause hypotensive episodes. The disintegrins are in an early investigative phase. Much remains to be learned prior to recommendation for clinical studies.

PPACK Kettner and Shaw described a series of synthetic peptides of arginine chloromethyl ketone that selectively inactivate thrombin (45). At least one agent, D-phenylalanyl-L-prolyl-L-arginyl-chloromethyl ketone (PPACK), apparently mimics the cleavage sites of one of the physiological substrates of thrombin, high-affinity heparin-antithrombin III (ATIII) complex (46). This synthetic antithrombin, infused in micromolar amounts per minute, abolished platelet deposition and release of platelet granule contents and inhibited thrombin-induced blood clotting in vascular graft-bearing baboons (47). Its combined actions on clotting factors and platelets are of great interest. Surface immobilization of such a potent synthetic drug is an attractive possibility.

Aprotonin, FUT175 Serine proteases involved in coagulation and platelet activation are released and/or activated by cardiopulmonary bypass equipment. Serine protease inhibitors may block the activation of proteases and improve thromboresistance during ECMO treatment. Van Oeveren et al. studied this approach in otherwise healthy patients undergoing elective cardiopulmonary bypass (CPB) (48). The serine protease inhibitor, aprotonin, was administered (150 kallikrein inactivator units/mL blood). Kallikrein and plasmin are effectively inhibited at this dose; platelet numbers were virtually unaffected, and thromboxane B2 release by the platelet was suppressed, in contrast to results with untreated controls. Postoperative bleeding was reduced. Tissue plasminogen activator activity was similar in both groups, suggesting that the platelet preservation function of aprotonin was clinically effective. Fibrinogen degradation products, a sign of plasmin activity, were also substantially reduced. No influence of serine protease inhibition was seen in complement activation by the classical and alternate pathways: C4a and C3a rose equally in both groups. Likewise, polymorphonuclear leukocyte numbers were reduced equally during CPB but elevated postoperatively for both groups, and neutrophil elastase levels were similar although the treated group was favored slightly upon release of the aortic cross-clamp.

Tatsumi et al. (49) studied the serine protease inhibitor, FUT175, in a high-flow, venovenous goat model of ECMO therapy. A film-coated, hollow-fiber oxygenator was coupled with a ventricular assist device, both situated between the right atrium and the pulmonary artery. Bleeding tendencies were not observed while fibrinogen and platelet levels were preserved in four-day runs. Dosages in this study were high: a continuous infusion at 40 to 60 mg/h was maintained at the inlet port of the oxygenator. These early results of serine protease inhibition in the context of ECMO are promising, in that they may permit improvement of circuit blood compatibility while preserving hemostatic potential. Additional work is required; careful evaluation of embolization, removal/reduction of the continuous infusion requirement, and possible drug interactions should be studied. Surface immobilization of the drug appears useful in this case as well.

IMMOBILIZED BIOLOGICALS

Attachment of a drug to a polymer surface in order to maintain local drug action is especially attractive for improving the biocompatibility of ECMO circuits. Drugs with known actions can be employed; the dose necessary to modify the circuit is small and applied only at the site of desired action. Complications due to systemic dosage and drug interactions can be avoided. In many applications, the flexibility of the attached drug must be ensured to allow proper interaction with circulating molecules. Thus the technique has come to be called surface immobilization, spacer arm attachment, or end point attachment. This mode of attachment seems to improve the potency of a number of surface immobilized drugs (Figure 8.2). Two reviews of drug immobilization methods have appeared (50,51). Many of the methods cited in these reviews are applicable to ECMO devices. Several infusible drugs are candidates for ultimate application in surface-immobilized form.

Heparin

Many have investigated surface immobilization of heparin. Kim and Feijen (50) classify these methods according to the immobilization scheme (Figure 8.2). Early workers employed quaternary ammonium ion to bind heparin, in turn linking the ionic complex to the polymer substrate by a graphite coat (52) or by a nonspecific, hydrophobic bond involving long-chain fatty acids (53). Heparin is slowly leached from the surface, where it binds with antithrombin III to form the agent active in anticoagulation. This approach has been useful for short-term procedures requiring aortic shunting and is currently being reintroduced for short-term cardiopulmonary bypass. It is less desirable for prolonged ECMO perfusion since the heparin supply may be depleted by the leaching process. Direct binding of heparin to the polymer surface is also less desirable since the rigidly attached heparin does not bind well with antithrombin III. Schmer discovered that spacing the heparin molecule at a distance from the polymer surface improved its potency (55). Kim et al. confirmed this property, using alkyl spacer arms of varying length (56). This method allows the covalently bound heparin molecule to flex, improving its conjugation with antithrombin III. Recent work from this group demonstrates that reductions in protein adsorption and platelet adhesion can be obtained with a few hydrophobic intermediate arms, polyethylene oxide (57). The same research group has recently used the polyethylene oxide spacer arm to immobilize heparin to silicone rubber (58). This is an attractive approach, since multiple actions may be achieved in theory, e.g., anticoagulation and antiplatelet activity, without promoting protein adsorption. But the surface they have created is complex. Physical and chemical analysis indicates the outer (0.5 nm) surface layer is essentially pure silicone rubber, yet preliminary compatibility studies are more

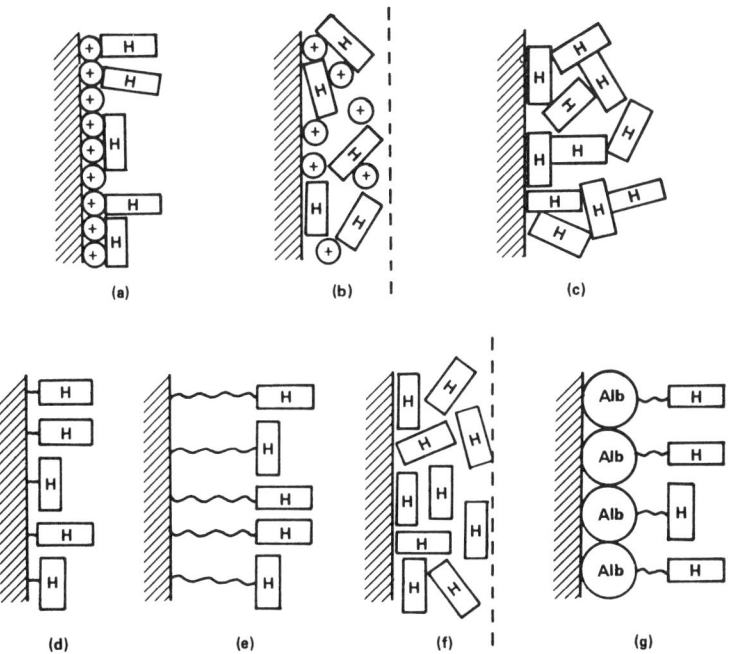

FIGURE 8.2 Various methods for attachment of heparin to surfaces. (A) Heparin bound ionically on a positively charged surface. (B) Ionically bound heparin polymer as a coating on a substrate polymer. (C) Heparin cross-linked surface. (D) Heparin-immobilized surface. (E) Heparin immobilized via spacer arms, the current method of choice. (F) Heparin dispersed in a hydrophobic polymer and slowly released into the bloodstream. (G) Heparin-albumin conjugate surface. Method (G) is not the same as the separate immobilization of heparin and albumin suggested in the text. (Reprinted with permission from Kim SW, Feijen J. Surface modification of polymers for improved blood compatibility. In: Williams DF, ed. Critical reviews of biocompatibility, Vol 1. Boca Raton: CRC Press, 1984:221–60.)

favorable than would be expected with silicone rubber (59). Further study is required in order to link the putative actions of the modified surface groups to observed results.

Perhaps the most carefully investigated heparin attachment method relevant to ECMO is the end point heparin attachment method developed by Larm et al. (60). A mixture of high- and low-affinity nitrite-degraded heparin fragments are attached to aminated surfaces of silicone rubber, polyvinyl chloride (PVC), or other materials. Anticoagulation of surfaces is obtained, consistent with immobilized heparin with ATIII on the surface. Both thrombin and factor Xa are inhibited by the high-affinity, ATIII-immobilized heparin sites. The total amount of ATIII on the surface determines this inhibitory capacity (61). Tests in low- and high-velocity (wall shear rate) segments of arteriovenous fistulas in dogs indicated that thrombin and Xa inhibitory capacities were similar in low shear regions but thrombin inhibition was reduced in high shear regions. Possible explanations for the reduced effectiveness at high fluid shear rate include 1) enhanced platelet activity provoking an excess thrombin-generating capacity (62), 2) conformational alteration of the heparin/ATIII complex to a less potent form, and 3) convection-enhanced leaching of heparin from the surface. Silicone rubber catheters treated by this method have been compared with other surfaces in a randomized 17-week implant trial in canines, with somewhat disappointing results (63). However, it is thought that the attachment technique was not perfected in this series (Lubin M, personal communication). Improved results have been reported recently (Olsson P, unpublished remarks, Symposium on Clinical Applications of ECMO and ECco$_2$R, 36th Annual Meeting, American Society for Artificial Internal Organs, Washington, D.C., April 26, 1990). A preliminary report of reduction of complement activation in pigs by this heparin immobilization process has appeared recently (64). No mechanism explaining this effect is hypothesized.

A novel intracorporeal oxygenator has been developed that provides a thin, continuous silicone rubber film over a microporous substrate (65). The silicone film is treated with a proprietary coating, thought to include immobilized heparin. This coating is used in conjunction with moderate systemic heparinization (Hemochron ACT of 200 s and PTT 80–90 s) to provide thromboresistance protection of the implanted device. The combined treatment was reported to produce neither gross nor microscopic thromboemboli in the pulmonary arterial bed in seven-day implants in sheep (Winter S, unpublished remarks, Symposium on Clinical Applications of ECMO and ECco$_2$R, 36th Annual Meeting, American Society of Artificial Internal Organs, Washington, D.C., April 26, 1990). However, small, localized fibrin thrombi have been found on portions of most intravenacaval oxygenator (IVOX) devices. Phase I clinical trials of safety have begun.

A proprietary heparin surface immobilization treatment for a polypropylene microporous oxygenator system has been announced (66). The entire blood-contacting surface, including all circuit elements, is coated in this process. The coating is a modification of the quaternary ammonium-heparin coating process (53), in which the alkyl is a precisely defined C18 chain-length alkyl. The coated circuit was evaluated in four-hour perfusion in calves, using partial venoarterial bypass with moderate systemic anticoagulation (67). Less thrombus formation and fibrin split products, less platelet depletion, and better-preserved platelet function were observed in the coated group than in controls. In vitro studies supported the platelet results: fewer adherent platelets were found during 60-min loop circulations with heparinized bovine blood of treated hollow fibers (68). These results, obtained with treated hollow fibers, appear similar to those obtained with solid membrane oxygenators. However, water vapor condensation occurs in the gas space of some hollow-fiber membrane oxygenators, reducing gas exchange capacity during prolonged procedures. This must be kept in mind when specifying hollow-fiber equipment for ECMO procedures.

In summary, studies now suggest that inhibition of coagulation in ECMO circuits can be obtained by surface heparin immobilization. A number of attachment methods have been developed, of which one of the covalently bound, intermediate arm methods, which permits heparin flexure and improved complexing with ATIII, is preferred on theoretical grounds. The anticoagulant potency of surface-bound heparin varies with polymer, wall shear rate, and the quality of the heparin. Protection against white thrombus formation by heparin immobilization is less certain. Combined treatment with polyethylene oxide immobilization may provide this broader protection.

Fibrinolytic Agents

Urokinase (UK) converts plasminogen to plasmin to initiate fibrinolysis and thrombus dissolution, preferably at an early stage in thrombus development. UK has been immobilized to nylon, polyester, polyvinyl chloride, polyurethane, agarose, and silicone copolymers (69). Thrombus formation was inhibited to varying degrees for a number of treated materials. Kim et al. (50) demonstrated that the enzymatic activity of UK-bound alkylated agaroses varies with the alkyl spacer arm length, supporting the principle of decreasing flexural rigidity (increasing potency) of the immobilized drug by extending the spacer arm. Fibrinolytic activity was variable in this study. Clinical studies of UK-immobilized nylon and polyester elastomer surgical drains and intravascular catheters have been reported (70). In 125 clinical cases, 91% of treated tubes remained patent for periods as long as 66 days, compared to 5% for PVC controls. Scanning electron microscopy (SEM) revealed neither fibrin accumulation nor platelet adhesion or aggregation on the UK-immobilized tubes.

Mercer et al. (71) studied streptokinase (SK), another plasminogen activator, bound to nylon films. Since plasminogen and plasmin are free to diffuse between circulating blood and interstitial fluid, the authors chose not to place the immobilized enzyme in direct contact with blood, implanting the material instead in the rabbit dorsum. They observed a threefold increase of blood clotting time, maintained for 150 days, which returned to normal upon removal of the implant. The immobilized enzyme lost little activity, no evidence of antibody formation was found, and growth of fibrous tissue was prevented.

Tissue plasminogen activator immobilization onto polymeric substrates has not been reported. Given the promising results with UK and SK immobilization and development of synthetic supplies of the drugs, it appears worthy of study.

In summary, immobilization of UK, SK, or other fibrinolytic enzymes to the surfaces of ECMO circuitry has not yet been accomplished. Promising results have been reported for other applications, and the method is worthy of study for ECMO.

Polymer Surface Treatments

There is a widely held hypothesis concerning the initial steps in the interaction of blood with foreign materials which has provided a convenient general pathway for understanding blood-material interactions. According to this hypothesis, the first step in the surface interaction process is the adsorption and conformational alternation of plasma proteins, especially fibrinogen and certain gamma globulins (72,73). These elements are activated by contact with the foreign surface and, in turn, trigger various blood reactions, including blood coagulation (74) and platelet adhesion (75,76). In high shear regions, von Willebrand factor also promotes platelet adhesion. Adsorbed fibrinogen activates platelets initially, but, when "conditioned" by as-yet unknown processes, it loses this property. Complement-dependent processes may be triggered in like manner (77). This process is called "protein preconditioning" of the surface.

A number of means have been devised to favorably influence protein preconditioning by altering the normal sequence of protein-polymer-blood interactions. Interruption or prevention of the usual protein adsorption and conformational alteration pattern deprives the system of the triggers by which the blood reactions are initiated. Such techniques are advantageous, since the shelf life of the treated material is unrestricted, in contrast to immobilized drugs, and quality control is simplified.

Albumin films Albumin contains none of the peptide sequences that code for cell adhesion and is a bystander in coagulation, platelet adhesion, and other host-defense reactions. Thus, albumin coatings are desirable in theory as surface-passivating films. Reports of successful precoating of albumin on surfaces prior to blood contact have appeared from time to time. However, these reports have been largely anecdotal, and controlled studies have yielded disappointing results (78–80,34). We have developed a series of promising alternative methods by which surfaces are chemically modified so that, in theory, albumin can be adsorbed directly from circulating whole blood (81–83). This eliminates the need for albumin precoating and requires no alteration of clinical routine. In theory, the passivating albumin layer can be maintained indefinitely.

One of these methods takes advantage of the high affinity of albumin for circulating free fatty acids. Straight-chain C16 and C18 hydrocarbons mimic circulating free fatty acids and are readily attached to many polymers by a variety of convenient surface alkylation reactions (81). Polyurethane conduits treated in this fashion bind albumin rapidly at the alkyl site (81,84). Both short-term (85) and long-term (86) improvement in surface-induced thrombus formation have been obtained. The techniques have been partially verified in other laboratories (87,88) (Jakobsen R, personal communication from Battelle-Columbus Labs; FTIR analysis of C16-acylated cellulose and C18 alkylated Biomer films gave a 70/30 ratio of albumin to fibrinogen binding from plasma vs. 10/90 ratio for controls). Perhaps the most interesting results, from the ECMO perspective, came from a randomized, double-blind trial of six different surface treatments of Pellethane 2363-80A pacemaker insulators implanted in dogs for 17 weeks (63,86). The end points were 1) accumulation of thrombus, fibrin, or other biological material, 2) calcification, 3) hemolysis, and 4) circulating platelet counts. Results showed that C16 acylated catheters and those treated by the Mercor process (vide infra) were both significantly better than four other surface treatments: Hydromer (poly N-vinyl pyrrolidone), Carmeda (surface heparinization), and two microphase-altered poly-ether-urethane (PEU) surface layers (Figure 8.3). This study was flawed since no untreated control was used, one process required a special extrusion, and another process replaced polyurethane with a silicone rubber substrate. Nevertheless, the study demonstrated that significant differences in blood compatibility were obtained with different surface treatments and pointed out the utility of a simple endogenous albumin coating process in situ.

A modification of the surface alkylation process was applied to cellulose acetate, a filtration material (82), and Cuprophan, a modified cellulose used in hemodialyzers which activates complement by the alternate pathway (89). Albumin bound avidly to the treated materials and significantly inhibited complement activation by Cuprophan.

Recently, we developed a modified silicone rubber by another process that also substantially increases the binding of albumin (83). A silicone compound with pendant OH^- groups is formed that can be readily cross-linked to silicone rubber and other methylated polymers or bound to other polymers, metals, and ceramics. It is possible to coat entire devices, including oxygenators, with this film. The OH^- coating increases the albumin affinity of the base material substantially and does not reduce the gas exchange capacity of oxygenators. Three versions of the film are under study for ECMO applications: a hydroxylated siloxane, a C16 acylated siloxane, and a C2 acylated siloxane. All have very high albumin affinity and demonstrate reductions in blood clotting but have varying ability to inhibit complement activation. Simple OH^- treatment is the best in this regard (unpublished data of the author). Figure 8.4 demonstrates the improvements in the albumin-binding capacities of silicone rubber obtained by the OH^- and C16 treatments (90). Only 5% conversion of residual vinyls to OH^- or C16 is necessary to achieve significant

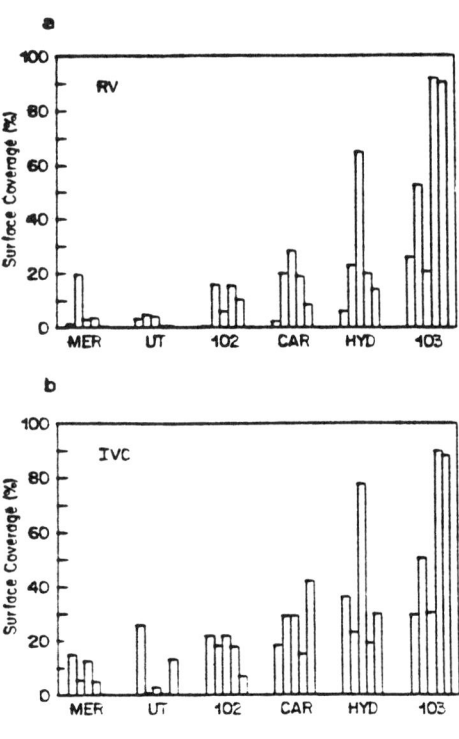

FIGURE 8.3 (A) Surface coverage of polyurethane catheters implanted in the right ventricle for 17 weeks. (B) Surface coverage of polyurethane catheters implanted in the inferior vena cava for 17 weeks. Biological material coverage was determined by planimetry of enlarged photographs. MER = Mercor surface-modifying additive; UT = C16 acylation; 102 = microphase separation of hard/soft segments; CAR = surface heparinization (silicone rubber substrate); HYD = poly(n-vinyl pyrrolidone); 103 = altered formulation of 102 type. (Reprinted with permission from Lubin M, Nappholz T, Miller CW, Wrigley R, Clubb JF Jr. Chronic antithrombogenic materials screen. Pace 1986;9:1154–9.)

results. Albumin-binding kinetics and adsorption isotherms indicate impressive accumulations of albumin. At 400 mg/dL (10% plasma albumin concentrations), the adsorbate is greater than 100 $\mu g/cm^2$, equivalent to a layer 500 molecules thick. Treatment with a protein eluant (0.3% sodium dodecyl sulfate) simulating denaturation of the surface removed less than 5% of this layer, attesting to its durability.

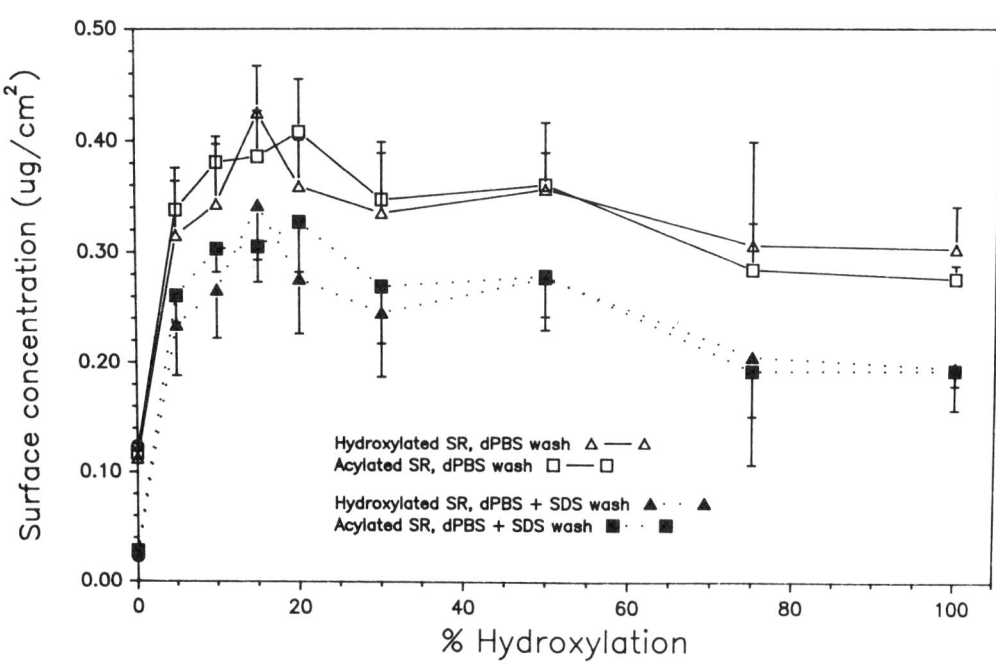

FIGURE 8.4 Influence of the degree of hydroxylation reaction (triangles) and C16 acylation reaction (squares) on albumin binding (0.15 mg/mL albumin solution, incubation for 1 min). Closed symbols indicate results following denaturation with 0.3% sodium dodecyl sulfate. (Reprinted with permission from Tsai CC, Huo HH, Kulkarni PV, Eberhart RC. Biocompatible coatings with high albumin affinity. Trans Am Soc Artif Intern Organs 1990;36:M307–M320.)

Competitive albumin-fibrinogen binding studies suggest that albumin dominates the surface. Conversion of the typical fibrinogen-rich surface to one rich in albumin would indicate, on the basis of the protein preconditioning hypothesis, that the surface becomes passivated. Hydrogen bonding appears to be the most likely explanation for the creation of the albumin multilayer. This technique is currently under development for ECMO applications.

Polyethylene oxide Polyethylene oxide (PEO) has been studied widely as a biocompatible material in various forms: in PEO cross-linked networks, in segmented polyurethanes, copolymerized with siloxane blocks, and as side chains on acrylate polymers (91). The interest relates to the high water content of PEO, which ensures low interfacial energy when a PEO film is properly interposed between blood and synthetic surfaces. Another way of looking at it is that, in essence, PEO and other hydrogels present a "waterlike" surface that is unremarkable to the elements in blood, which are normally bathed in dilute aqueous solution (water). Thus, the PEO film with its trapped water does little to activate blood elements. Protein adsorption and platelet activation are low on surfaces rich in polyethylene oxides (92–95). These desirable properties depend on the presence of other molecular entities (59,93) and the molecular weight distribution of the PEO (93,95). The mechanical strength of pure PEO networks is low; therefore, stabilization is required. This can be done by radiation cross-linking (96) or by creation of an interpenetrating network of PEO and silicone rubber (93). The latter material is attractive for ECMO applications since the silicone rubber can improve the gas exchange characteristics of the thin film.

Plasma discharge There is great interest in treating polymers by ionized gas plasma discharge as a means of increasing biocompatibility. There are two general techniques (97–99). The first seeks to reduce unsatisfied binding capacity of the polymer surface, thus reducing its reaction potential with blood elements, by functionalizing all possible chemical groups through bombardment with energetic ionized species of a dilute inert gas. The second approach is to create a very thin layer of an inert polymer on the surface of interest, usually a fluorocarbon, by excitation of a dilute fluorocarbon monomer gas in a plasma reactor. Both means have essentially the same effect, to reduce the driving potential for activation of molecular elements in the blood. The methods are quite controllable when handled properly and appear to work well for simple devices. Considerable development of these methods for biomaterials applications has been reported, although applications to ECMO-relevant materials such as silicone rubber are rather sparse. Yasuda has a brief report of plasma treatment of silicone rubber tubes with a thin perfluorocarbon layer that improves blood compatibility (100). Application to complex devices such as oxygenators and heat exchangers has not been reported. Control of the discharge process in narrow, tortuous channels, such as those found in oxygenators, heat exchangers, and knitted vascular prostheses, is difficult.

Other Polymer Treatments

Bulk additives Trace amounts of various additives are included in most medical polymers at formulation. This is done for various reasons: to stabilize the material against oxidation or ultraviolet irradiation, to provide lubrication during extrusion or handling, etc. Bulk additives have also been developed that improve blood compatibility, as does the Mercor process (101,102). Additions to bulk materials to modify surface properties become possible because of preferential migration of the additive to the surface of the polymer. By this means, the mechanical properties of the material are partially uncoupled from the properties governing biocompatibility. The chemical structures of biocompatible additives are at present proprietary but are thought to consist of relatively small molecules containing hydrophobic silicone groups with hydrophilic tails of various types. Such molecules, with well-defined hydrophilic and hydrophobic regions, are termed amphiphilic, signifying their ability to conform to the local environment. The additive is dispersed in bulk prior to fabrication, following which it is free to migrate to the surface of the polymer where it is sequestered in a hydrophilic, tail-outward orientation (Figure 8.5). Upon contact with blood, the hydrophilic region is thought to reduce fibrinogen and gamma globulin adsorption, perhaps in a manner similar to that of polyethylene oxide, so that contact-activated biological processes are diminished. One of the most successful surface treatments in the study described by Lubin et al. (63) was of this type. Retention of the additive on the surface of the device has not been described in the literature but is thought to be quite adequate for the purposes of intermediate-term blood contact. Such formulations are commercially available for pump tubing and vascular access devices and theoretically could be developed for ECMO equipment.

Film coatings for microporous oxygenators
Microporous membranes for oxygenators overcome one disadvantage of solid membranes: They substantially reduce the resistance to diffusion of O_2 and CO_2 through the membrane, thereby increasing the efficiency of gas exchange. However, this advantage carries with it the cost of increased diffusion of water vapor and its condensation in the gas space and denaturation of plasma proteins at the gas-blood interface within the micropores. These limit use of the microporous membrane oxygenator to relatively short-term procedures. Dantowitz and Borsanyi proposed coating the microporous membranes of the oxygenator with an ultrathin solid film of silicone rubber or other highly gas-permeable polymer (103). This technique largely preserves the advantages of the microporous oxygenator, while it reduces water vapor permeation and condensa-

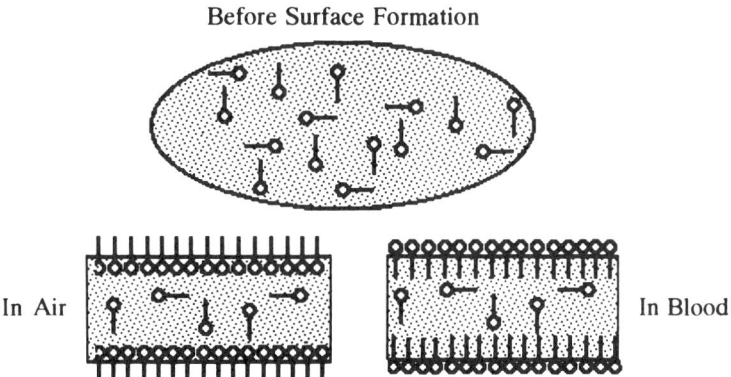

FIGURE 8.5 Surface-modifying additives (SMA) are uniformly distributed throughout the base polymer prior to surface formation. Once the surface is formed, the SMA migrates to the surface, where the environment to which it is exposed determines the orientation of the concentrated SMA. A simplified SMA structure is shown for clarity. ○ = polar; | = nonpolar block. (Reprinted with permission from Ward RS. Surface modifying additives for biomedical polymers. IEEE Eng Med Biol 1989;8:22–5.)

tion, and avoids the protein-denaturing gas-blood interface. The hydroxylated and alkylated silicone rubber films described previously (90) are designed for this purpose. Such technology, suitable for ECMO procedures, has recently been applied to the indwelling vena caval oxygenator (65). The gas exchange capacity of this interesting device has been prolonged by this means. Clinical assessment, including ECMO applications, is currently under way.

Other gas-permeable membranes Ketteringham et al. investigated polyalkylsulfone membranes for oxygenator applications (104). The material has adequate O_2 and CO_2 permeabilities and mechanical strength and potentially favorable blood compatibility. Huo compared the blood compatibility and albumin-binding characteristics of polyalkylsulfone films, synthesized specifically with 16 carbon alkyl chains, with those of the hydroxylated silicone rubber film described above (105). A 2.6-fold increase in Lee-White clotting time was observed for the polyalkylsulfone, identical to the results by Ketteringham et al., versus a twofold increase for the OH silicone rubber. Albumin binding was much lower for the polyalkylsulfone. While the mechanical strength and biocompatibility of the polyalkylsulfones may be superior to silicone rubber, the O_2 and CO_2 permeabilities of this new material are lower. Thus, overall improvement in membrane performance does not appear to warrant conversion of oxygenator construction to this new material.

Allcock and Lampe have proposed a new series of polyphosphazenes as biomedical polymers (106). Stable elastomers with high molecular weight and elastic modulus are synthesized, which permits formation of very thin flexible films. Organic side group substitution permits formation of films that are very resistant to hydrolysis. The phosphorus-nitrogen polymer backbone confers flexibility, while the side groups control hydrophobicity, water stability, and biocompatibility. Attachment of anticoagulants, antibacterial agents, or proteins can be accomplished via the organic side groups. The material appears promising, but no oxygenator-specific development has been reported.

Fougnot et al. (107) and Jozefowicz et al. (108) have created polymers with sulfonated appendages that mimic active portions of the heparin molecule. This "synthetic heparin" is theoretically appealing, since it can be precisely formulated at polymer synthesis, it is durable, its heparinlike activity continues to evolve at the surface as polymer chains turn over, and it may not be subject to the usual restriction of heparinized materials (shelf life, sterilization, etc.). Good results have been obtained with segmented polyether polyurethanes (109). Oxygenator membranes with this property have not been developed but are an attractive prospect for future work.

Plasticizing and stabilizing bulk additives

Bulk additives can improve the biocompatibility of medical polymers, as previously described (101). But other bulk additives in medical polymers, used for other purposes (flexibility, stability, etc.), can leach into the bloodstream and induce low-level toxic effects. The problem has not been perceived to be significant in the context of short-term heart-lung bypass procedures, owing to the high doses of additive necessary to produce measurable effects. But long-term or chronic exposures to leachable toxic additives, which include ECMO, may produce a more significant toxic burden for the patient.

An important focus of this discussion concerns plasticizers for PVC tubing, bags, etc. These articles contain up to 40 wt% plasticizer oil to improve flexibility. The most common PVC plasticizer in current medical use is di(2-ethylhexyl)phthalate (DEHP). DEHP has an extremely high oral LD_{50}, 30 g/kg in rats and rabbits, and is nontoxic in usual applications. However, DEHP has been linked to disturbances in rat brain, altered reticuloendothelial function, microaggregation of platelets, hemolysis, and disturbances of replication in embryonic tissue (110,111). The National Toxicology Program has revised thinking on the toxicity of DEHP, now recognizing a finite risk associated with its use (112). DEHP leaches from PVC tubing into the bloodstream. It has been detected in human lung tissue in microgram amounts after cardiopulmonary bypass and blood transfusion. It has been shown that up to 70 mg of plasticizer is absorbed by the patient in each hemodialysis treatment. The problem is recognized by industry, and development of less toxic plasticizers is under way (113).

Other additives found in medical plastics are used to provide thermal and ultraviolet stability. Heat stabilizers for medical-grade PVC include alkaline earth and heavy metal organics. Toxic effects from these stabilizers have also been reported.

In summary, additives to some polymers used in ECMO circuits are toxic in large doses. The contribution of these additives to blood and tissue damage in the context of ECMO may be small but is unknown. A fresh look at the safety and stability of polymer compositions for ECMO circuits may be in order.

Hemodynamics

Reduction of flow disturbances The science of fluid mechanics teaches that smooth surfaces, gradual contouring of bends and bifurcations, and elimination of sudden changes in diameter reduce fluid flow resistance. This is important in medical device applications, not only for the reduction in conduit pressurization, but also for reductions in blood damage and thromboembolism. Karino and Goldsmith have demonstrated that flow separation, i.e., breakaway of the streamlines that entrain the fluid flow, occurs at rough spots, steps, and bifurcations in conduits, with frequent formation of eddies (114). Figure 8.6 demonstrates the stable trapped eddies that can form. While red cells are shown recirculating in this experiment, platelet recirculation and aggregation have been demonstrated in vitro (115) and in vivo (116). Smooth surfaces are important for other reasons as well. Vroman has shown that fibrinogen is preferentially adsorbed in microscopic surface crevices (117). Given this foothold, fibrinogen can interact with receptors associated with the glycoprotein IIb/IIIa complex, initiating platelet adhesion, as previously described.

Smooth surfaces are produced by solvent polishing, use of lubricants and special extrusion dies, and other means in industrial practice. While ideally smooth surfaces cannot be obtained throughout perfusion circuits, practitioners should be wary of excessive use of connectors, abrupt changes in channel diameter, and similar flow-disturbing circuit design practices.

Fluidity enhancement Fluid flow resistance is reduced in industrial practice by the injection of long-chain, linear polymer molecules,

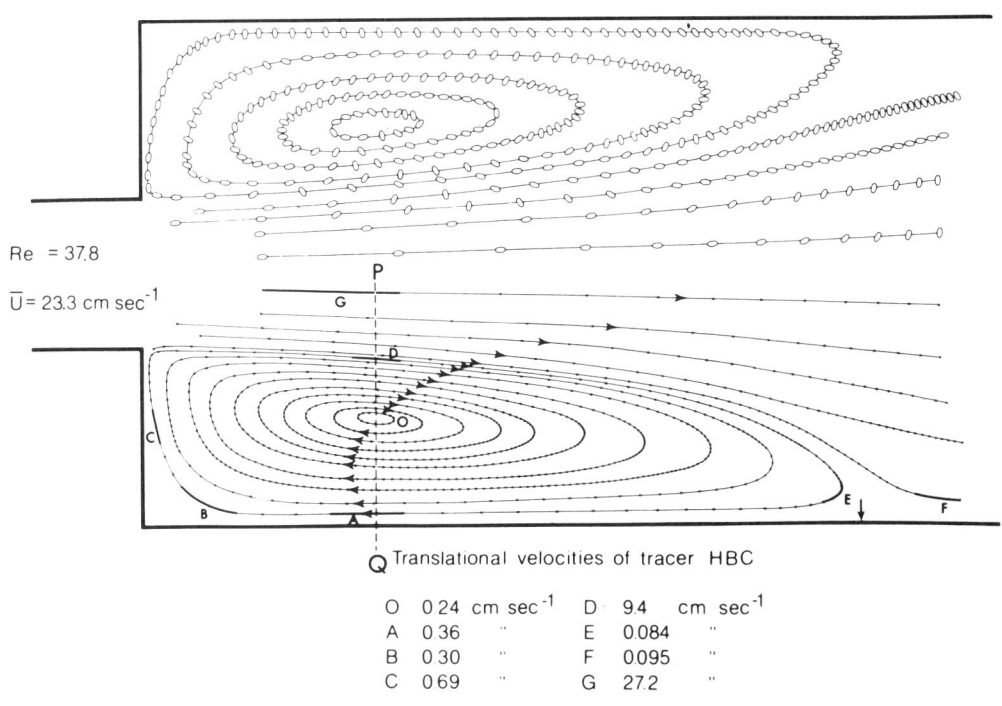

FIGURE 8.6 Flow patterns in the median plane of an annular vortex formed downstream of a 150-μm glass tube into a 500-μm glass tube at Reynolds number = 37.8. The orientation of the red cells is drawn on the orbits of the upper portion of the diagram. The arrows indicate the velocity distribution in the vortex and the adjacent mainstream. The letters A to G and O indicate the positions at which the particle velocities were measured. HBC = hardened blood cells. (Reprinted with permission from Karino T, Goldsmith HL. Flow behaviour of blood cells and rigid spheres in an annular vortex. Phil Trans Roy Soc 1977;B279:413–45.)

which depress the tendency to turbulence and stabilize the flow. Low-molecular-weight dextran, a linear polymer, has been administered at the initiation of ventricular assistance, during vascular grafting procedures (118), and for prevention of deep venous thrombosis (119). Reductions in thromboembolism have been observed which, while perhaps due in part to antiplatelet and anticoagulant activities of polysaccharides (120), may also be attributable to flow stabilization (reduction in flow disturbance). Administration of low-molecular-weight dextran at the institution of ECMO may likewise be beneficial under appropriate circumstances.

Flow-modulated release of TPA It may be possible to manipulate the extracorporeal flow regime to take advantage of the liberation of endogenous heparin, antiplatelet, and fibrinolytic agents triggered by fluid shear-induced effects on endothelial cell membranes. Fluid shear-induced stresses may interact with endothelial cells in a profound way. Diamond et al. (121) have demonstrated a well-defined threshold for viscous flow-induced shear stresses, above which tissue plasminogen activator (TPA) is released from cultured endothelial cells. The rate of TPA release is proportional to the elevation of the applied wall shear stress above this threshold. It has been speculated that endothelial cells may respond as well by release of prostacyclin and heparin. Phasic and steady compression of limbs may induce anticoagulant release by similar means (122). Such phenomena may be used to advantage in ECMO. Fluid shear stresses are elevated at least in the vicinity of cannulation sites and perhaps elsewhere as well, since data suggest that venous return is mobilized by partial venoarterial and venovenous bypass (123). If this is true, there may be a partial endogenous anticoagulation of the subject induced by a fluid mechanical effect.

It is interesting in this regard to recall reports of successful extracorporeal perfusion without systemic or surface heparinization (124,125). It was suggested at the time that, while blood contact with the foreign surface might activate coagulation and other host defenses, the level of that activation might be tolerable. The suggestion was met with skepticism, but the idea was revived years later in a somewhat different form. Murphy et al. (30) showed that extracorporeal circulation might trigger the release of a heparinlike substance from the liver. The active agent was postulated to be an as-yet unknown circulating substance which was activated by interaction with the extracorporeal circuit. Activation of this substance was dependent upon the blood velocity but not upon the material of the extracorporeal circuit. The activated substance appeared to stimulate the release of heparin from the liver, providing a perfusion-induced "endogenous heparinization." In other words, heparin appeared to be released in order to enhance the fluidity of blood under high-flow conditions. It was thought that this endogenous heparinization might explain the earlier results, but, again, work was discontinued.

The discovery of fluid shear-dependent modulation of TPA release from the endothelial cell may integrate and explain these controversial early findings. One or more inhibitors of thrombus formation, possibly including heparin, PGI_2, and TPA, may be released naturally into the bloodstream in response to the mobilization of blood flow induced by extracorporeal circulation. Thus, ECMO patients may be anticoagulated by two externally induced means: 1) the infusion of heparin and 2) the cannulation route and rate of extracorporeal blood flow. The effect of the latter means may be significant yet undetectable by usual assays during ECMO. It may be possible to reduce the administration of systemic heparin during ECMO if this flow-induced anticoagulation effect is verified and reproducible. In view of the compelling reasons for reducing heparinization, this topic deserves further investigation.

SUMMARY

Many factors influence the formation of thrombi and the activation of host defenses during extracorporeal circulation. One drug, heparin, is used for mitigation of all these influences. Systemic heparin therapy is a mixed blessing in the setting of neonatal ECMO. Many alternatives to its use are being investigated, with the primary intent being passivation of the surfaces of the extracorporeal circuit. No single passivation strategy has yet yielded proof of clinical effectiveness. But a combination of treatments appears worthy of note, including 1) combined surface immobilization of heparin and endogenous albumin, 2) infusions of other drugs with antiplatelet or serine protease inhibitory actions, 3) polymer treatments to reduce the reactivity of the surface, and 4) improved surface contouring the other means to reduce flow disturbance and control the stress on endothelial cell membranes. Studies to carefully separate and characterize the effects of these treatments are required—a difficult task. But the prospects for improved passivation of extracorporeal circuits are bright, and the goal is well worth the effort. Heparin is still the drug of choice, but the day is approaching when systemic heparinization may no longer be indicated for passivation of the ECMO circuit.

REFERENCES

(1) Gans H, Krivit W. Problems in hemostasis during open-heart surgery. IV. On the changes in the blood clotting mechanism during cardiopulmonary bypass procedures. Ann Surg 1962; 155:353–9.

(2) Osborn JJ, MacKenzie R, Shaw A, Perkins H, Hurt R, Gerbode F. Cause and prevention of hemorrhage following extracorporeal circulation. Surg Forum 1955;6:96–100.

(3) Hicks RE, Edmunds LH. Microembolus pro-

duction and blood filtration during extracorporeal perfusion. In: Zapol WM, Quist J, eds. Artificial lungs for acute respiratory failure. New York: Academic Press, 1976:157–67.

(4) Hill JD, O'Brien TG, Murray JD, Dontigny L, Bramson MH, Osborn JJ, Gerbode F. Prolonged extracorporeal oxygenation for acute post-traumatic respiratory failure (shock-lung syndrome). N Engl J Med 1972;286:629–34.

(5) Heiden D, Mielke CH Jr, Rodvien R. Platelets, hemostasis and thromboembolism during treatment of acute respiratory insufficiency with extracorporeal membrane oxygenation. J Thorac Cardiovasc Surg 1975;70:644–55.

(6) Rodvien R. Hematologic observations made in patients with acute respiratory distress syndrome in the cooperative ECMO project. Artif Organs 1978;2:12–18.

(7) Bartlett RH, Andrews AF, Toomasian JM, Haiduc NJ, Gazzanigo A. Extra corporeal membrane oxygenation (ECMO) for newborn respiratory failure: 45 cases. Surgery 1982;92:425–33.

(8) Van Oeveren W. Alterations in host defense mechanisms during cardiopulmonary bypass. [Proefschrift (Ph.D. Dissertation)]. Groningen University, 1988.

(9) Kusserow B, Larrow R, Nichols J. Metabolic and morphologic alterations in leukocytes following prolonged blood pumping. Trans Am Soc Artif Intern Organs 1969;15:42–4.

(10) Craddock PR, Fehr J, Brigham KL, Kronenberg RS, Jaub HS. Complement and leukocyte-mediated pulmonary dysfunction in hemodialysis. N Engl J Med 1977;296:769–74.

(11) Chenoweth DE, Cooper SE, Hugli TE, Stewart RH, Blackstone FH, Kirklin JW. Complement activation during cardiopulmonary bypass: evidence for generation of C3a and C5a anaphylatoxins. N Engl J Med 1981;304:497–502.

(12) Hammarschmidt DE, Stroncek DF, Bowers TK, Lammi-Keefe CJ, Kurth DM, Ozalius A. Complement activation and neutropenia during cardiopulmonary bypass. J Thorac Cardiovasc Surg 1981;81:370–7.

(13) Wachtfogel YT, Kucich U, Greenplate J, Guszko P, Abrams W, Weinbaum G. Human neutrophil degranulation during extracorporeal circulation. Blood 1987;69:324–30.

(14) Craddock PR, Hammarschmidt D, White JG, Dalmosso AP, Jacob HS. Complement (C5a) induced granulocyte aggregation in vitro. A possible mechanism of complement mediated leukostasis and leukopenia. J Clin Invest 1977; 60:260–4.

(15) Kirklin JK, Westaby S, Blackstone EH, Kirklin JW, Chenoweth EE, Pacifico AD. Complement and the damaging effects of cardiopulmonary bypass. J Thorac Cardiovasc Surg 1983; 86:845–57.

(16) Malchesky PS, Nosé Y. Biomodulation effects of extracorporeal circulation in apheresis. Semin Hematol 1989;26 (Suppl 1):42–51.

(17) Gristina AG. Biomaterial-centered infection: microbial adhesion versus tissue integration. Science 1987;237:1588–95.

(18) Morton WR, Cumming RD. A technique for the elucidation of Virchow's triad. Ann NY Acad Sci 1977;283:477–93.

(19) Rosenberg RD, Bauer KA. New insights into hypercoagulable states. Hosp Pract 1986;21(3): 131–7.

(20) Bick RL, Schmalhorst WR, Arbegast NR. Alterations in hemostasis associated with cardiopulmonary bypass. Thromb Res 1976;8:285–302.

(21) Coagulation and anticoagulation. In: Bartlett RH, ed. ECMO technical specialist manual, 7th ed. University of Michigan Department of Surgery, 1984.

(22) Hill JD, Dontigny L, de Laval M, Mielke CN Jr. A simple method of heparin management during prolonged extracorporeal circulation. Ann Thorac Surg 1974;17:129–34.

(23) Green TP, Isham-Schopf B, Steinhorn RH, Smith C, Irmiter RJ. Whole blood activated clotting time in infants during extracorporeal membrane oxygenation. Crit Care Med 1990;18: 494–8.

(24) Hill JD, Ratliff JL, Fallat RJ, et al. Prognostic factors in the treatment of acute respiratory insufficiency with long-term extracorporeal oxygenation. J Thorac Cardiovasc Surg 1990;68: 905–17.

(25) Gollob S, Ulin AW. Heparin-induced thrombocytopenia in man. J Lab Clin Med 1962; 59:430–5.

(26) Jacques LB. Heparin: an old drug with a new paradigm. Science 1979;206:528–36.

(27) Kazatchkine MD, Fearon DT, Metcalfe DD, Rosenberg RD, Austen KF. Structural determinants of the capacity of heparin to inhibit the formation of the human amplification C3 convertase. J Clin Invest 1981;67:223–8.

(28) Walker FJ. Regulation of activated protein C by a new protein. J Biol Chem 1980;255:5521–4.

(29) Gruber A, Griffin JH, Harker LA, Hanson SR. Inhibition of platelet-dependent thrombus formation by human activated protein C in a primate model. Blood 1989;73:639–42.

(30) Murphy TL, Walker FJ, Taylor FB III, et al. Endogenous anticoagulation during extracorporeal perfusion: generation of a heparinlike inhibitor. Am J Physiol 1980;239:H742–750.

(31) Clagett GP. Artificial devices in clinical practice. In: Colman RW, Hirsh J, Marder VJ, Salzman EW, eds. Hemostasis and thrombosis, 3rd ed. Philadelphia: J.B.Lippincott, 1991.

(32) Harker LA, Schlichter SJ. Platelet and fibrinogen consumption in man. N Engl J Med 1972;287:999–1005.

(33) Addonizio VP, Macarak EJ, Nicolau KC, Edmunds LH Jr, Colman RW. Effects of prostacyclin and albumin on platelet loss during in vitro simulation of extracorporeal circulation. Blood 1979;53:1033–41.

(34) Addonizio VP, Fisher CA, Jenkin BK, Straus JF III, Musial JF, Edmunds LH Jr. Iloprost (ZK36374), a stable analogue of prostacyclin, preserves platelets during simulated extracorporeal circulation. J Thorac Cardiovasc Surg 1985;89:926–33.

(35) Cottrell ED, Kappa JR, Stenach N, Fisher CA, Tuszynski GP, Switalska, et al. Temporary inhibition of platelet function with iloprost (ZK36374) preserves canine platelets during extracorporeal membrane oxygenation. J Thorac Cardiovasc Surg 1988;96:535–41.

(36) Malpass TW, Amory DW, Harker LA, Ivey TD, Williams DB. The effect of prostacyclin infusion on platelet hemostatic function in patients undergoing cardiopulmonary bypass. J Thorac Cardiovasc Surg 1984;87:550–5.

(37) Dutta-Roy AK, Ray TK, Sinha AK. Prostacyclin stimulation of the activation of blood coagulation factor X by platelets. Science 1986;231:385–8.

(38) Lasslo A, Quintana RP, Meyer AE. Development of novel surface-active compounds for prophylaxis against and treatment of thromboembolic complications. ASAIO J 1983;6:47–59.

(39) Dillingham EO, Lasslo A, Carter-Burks G, Bond SE, Gollamadi R. Relationships between chemical structure and inhibition of ADP-stimulated human thrombocyte release of serotonin and platelet factor 4. Biochim Biophys Acta 1989;99:128–32.

(40) Folie BJ, McIntire LV, Lasslo A. Effects of a novel antiplatelet agent in mural thrombogenesis on collagen coated glass. Blood 1988;72:1393–400.

(41) Hanson SR, Harker LA. Studies on suloctidil in experimental thrombosis in baboons. Thromb Haemost 1985;53:423–7.

(42) Lawrence WH, Tisdelle PA, Turner JE, et al. Some novel inhibitors of platelet aggregation: acute toxicity in mice and its relationship to in vitro activity and toxicity. Fund Appl Toxicol 1988;10:499–505.

(43) Ruoslahti E, Pierschbacher MD. New perspectives in cell adhesion: RGD and integrins. Science 1987;238:491–7.

(44) Musial J, Niewarowski S, Rucinski B, et al. Inhibition of platelet adhesion to surfaces of extracorporeal circuits by disintegrins: RGD-containing peptides from viper venoms. Circulation 1990;82:261–73.

(45) Kettner C, Shaw E. D-Phe-Pro-ArgCH$_2$Cl. A selective affinity label for thrombin. Thromb Res 1979;14:969–73.

(46) Collen D, Matsuo O, Stassen JM, Kettner C, Shaw E. In vivo studies of a synthetic inhibitor of thrombin. J Lab Clin Med 1982;99:76–83.

(47) Hanson SR, Harker LA. Interruption of acute platelet-dependent thrombosis by the synthetic antithrombin D-phenylalanyl-L-prolyl-L-arginyl chloromethyl ketone. Proc Natl Acad Sci 1988;85:3184–8.

(48) Van Oeveren W, Kazatchkine MD, Descamps-Latscha B, Wildevuur C. Effects of aprotonin on hemostatic mechanisms in cardiopulmonary bypass. Ann Thorac Surg 1987;44:640–5.

(49) Tatsumi E, Taenaka Y, Nakatani T, et al. A VAD and novel high performance compact oxygenator for long term ECMO with local anticoagulation. Trans Am Soc Artif Intern Organs 1990;36:M480–M483.

(50) Kim SW, Feijen J. Surface modification of polymers for improved blood compatibility. In: Williams DF, ed. Critical reviews of biocompatibility, Vol 1. Boca Raton: CRC Press, 1984:221–60.

(51) Sefton MV, Cholakis CH, Llanos G. Preparation of nonthrombogenic materials by chemical modification. In: Williams DF, ed. Blood compatibility, Vol 1. Boca Raton: CRC Press, 1987:151–98.

(52) Gott VL, Whiffen JD, Dutton RC. Heparin bonding on colloidal graphite surfaces. Science 1963;142:1297–301.

(53) Leininger RI, Epstein MM, Falb RD, Grode GA. Preparation of nonthrombogenic plastic surfaces. Trans Am Soc Artif Intern Organs 1966;12:151–4.

(54) Salzman EW, Silane M, Lindon J. Thromboresistance of heparin-coated surfaces. In: Lundblad RL, Brown WV, Mann KG, Roberts HR, eds. Chemistry and biology of heparin. Amsterdam: Elsevier, 1981;435–47.

(55) Schmer G. The biological activity of covalently immobilized heparin. Trans Am Soc Artif Intern Organs 1972;18:321–4.

(56) Kim SW, Ebert CD, Lin JY, McRea JC. Nonthrombogenicpolymers: pharmaceutical approaches. ASAIO J 1983;6:76–87.

(57) Park KD, Okano T, Nojiri C, Kim SW. Heparin immobilization onto segmented polyurethaneurea surfaces—effect of hydrophilic spacers. J Biomed Mater Res 1988;22:977–92.

(58) Grainger DW, Kim SW. Poly(dimethylsiloxane)-poly(ethylene oxide)-heparin block copolymers. I. Synthesis and characterization. J Biomed Mater Res 1988;22:231–49.

(59) Grainger DW, Okano T, Kim SW, et al. Poly(dimethylsiloxane)-poly(ethylene oxide)-heparin block copolymers. III. Surface and bulk compositional differences. J Biomed Mater Res 1990;24:547–71.

(60) Larm O, Larsson R, Olsson P. A new nonthrombogenic surface prepared by selective covalent binding of heparin via a modified reducing terminal residue. Biomater Med Dev Artif Organs 1983;11:161–73.

(61) Kodama K, Pasche B, Olsson P, Swedemborg J, Adolfsson J, Larm O. Antithrombin III binding to surface immobilized heparin and its relation to F Xa inhibition. Thromb Haemost 1987;58:1064–7.

(62) Turitto VT, Weiss HJ, Baumgartner HR, Badimon L, Fuster V. Cells and aggregates at surfaces. In: Leonard E, Turitto V, Vroman L, eds. Blood in contact with natural and artifical surfaces. Ann NY Acad Sci 1987;516:453–67.

(63) Lubin M, Nappholz T, Miller CW, Wrigley R, Clubb JF Jr. Chronic antithrombogenic materials screen. Pace 1986;9:1154–9.

(64) Nilsson L, Storm KE, Thelin S, Bagge L, Hultman J, Thorelius J, Nilsson U. Heparin-coated equipment reduces complement activation during cardiopulmonary bypass in the pig. Artif Organs 1990;14:46–8.

(65) Mortensen JD, Berry G. Conceptual and design features of a practical, clinically effective, intravenous mechanical blood oxygen/carbon dioxide exchange device (IVOX). Int J Artif Organs 1989;12:384–9.

(66) Segesser LK, Turina M. Cardiopulmonary bypass without systemic heparinization. J Thorac Cardiovasc Surg 1989;98:386–96.

(67) Toomasian JM, Hsu LC, Hirschl RB, Heiss KF, Hultquist KA, Bartlett RH. Evaluation of Duraflo II heparin coating in prolonged extracorporeal membrane oxygenation. Trans Am Soc Artif Intern Organs 1988;34:410–14.

(68) Tong SD, Rolfs MR, Hsu LC. Evaluation of Duraflo II heparin immobilized cardiopulmonary bypass circuits. Trans Am Soc Artif Intern Organs 1990;34:M654–M656.

(69) Sugitachi A, Takagi K, Imaoka S, Kosaki G. Immobilization of plasminogen activator, urokinase, on nylon. Thromb Haemost 1978;39:426–32.

(70) Sugitachi A, Tanaka M, Kawahara T, Takagi K. Antithrombogenicity of UK-immobilized polymer surfaces. Trans Am Soc Artif Intern Organs 1980;26:274–8.

(71) Mercer LC, Everse KE, Holmes AW, Everse J. Immobilization of the plasminogen activator streptokinase and its fibrinolytic effects in vivo. Thromb Res 1978;13:931–40.

(72) Horbett TA, Brash JL. Proteins at interfaces: current issues and future prospects. In: Brash JL, Horbett TA, eds. Proteins at interfaces: physicochemical and biochemical studies. Washington, DC: Am Chem Soc Symposium Series 343, 1987:1–33.

(73) Brash JL. Protein adsorption at the solid-solution interface in relation to blood-material interactions. In: Brash JL, Horbett TA, eds. Proteins at interfaces: physicochemical and biochemical studies. Washington D.C.: Am Chem Soc Symposium Series 343, 1987:490–506.

(74) Colman RW, Scott CF, Schmaier AH, Wachtfogel YT, Pixley RA, Edmunds LH. Initiation of blood coagulation at artificial surfaces. In: Leonard E, Vroman L, Turitto V, eds. Blood in contact with natural and artificial surfaces. Ann NY Acad Sci 1987;516:253–67.

(75) Salzman EW, Lindon J, McManama G, Ware JA. Role of fibrinogen in activation of platelets by artificial surfaces. In: Leonard E, Vroman L, Turitto V, eds. Blood in contact with natural and

artificial surfaces. Ann NY Acad Sci 1987;516: 184–95.

(76) Gluszko P, Rucinski B, Musial J, et al. Fibrinogen receptors in platelet adhesion to surfaces of extracorporeal circuits. Am J Physiol 1987;252:H615–H621.

(77) Chenoweth DE. Complement activation in extracorporeal circuits. In: Leonard E, Vroman L, Turitto V, eds. Blood in contact with natural and artificial surfaces. Ann NY Acad Sci 1987;516: 306–13.

(78) Chang TMS. Removal of endogenous and exogenous toxins by a microencapsulated adsorbent. Can J Physiol Pharm 1969;4:10–43.

(79) Lyman DJ, Metcalf LC, Albo D Jr, Richards KF, Lamb J. The effect of chemical structure and surface properties of synthetic polymers on the coagulation of blood: in vivo adsorption of proteins on polymer surfaces. Trans Am Soc Artif Intern Organs 1974:20-B:474–8.

(80) Guidoin RG, King MW, Awad J, et al. Albumin coated and critical point dried polyester prostheses as substitutes in the thoracic aorta of dogs. Trans Am Soc Artif Intern Organs 1983; 29:290–5.

(81) Munro MS, Quattrone AJ, Ellsworth SR, Kulkarni P, Eberhart RC. Alkyl substituted polymers with enhanced albumin affinity. Trans Am Soc Artif Intern Organs 1981;27:499–503.

(82) Frautschi JR, Munro MS, Lloyd DR, Eberhart RC. Alkyl derivatized cellulose acetate membranes with enhanced albumin affinity. Trans Am Soc Artif Intern Organs 1983;29:242–4.

(83) Tsai CC, Frautschi JR, Eberhart RC. Enhanced albumin affinity of silicone rubber. Trans Am Soc Artif Intern Organs 1988;34:559–63.

(84) Eberhart RC, Munro MS, Williams GB, et al. Albumin adsorption and retention on C-18 alkyl derivatized polyurethane vascular grafts. Artif Organs 1987;11:375–82.

(85) Munro MS, Eberhart RC, Maki NJ, Brink BE, Fry WJ. Thromboresistant alkyl derivatized polyurethanes. ASAIO J 1983;6:65–75.

(86) Eberhart RC, Munro MS, Frautschi JR, et al. Influence of endogenous albumin binding on blood-material interactions. In: Leonard E, Vroman L, Turitto V, eds. Blood in contact with natural and artificial surfaces. Ann NY Acad Sci 1987;516:78–95.

(87) Grasel TG, Pierce JA, Cooper SL. Effects of alkyl grafting on surface properties and blood compatibility of poly urethane block copolymers. J Biomed Mater Res 1987;21:815–42.

(88) Edelman PG, Ratner BD. Surface properties of polyurethanes with C18 pendant groups attached to the hard segments by two different routes. ACS Polym Mater Sci Eng 1988;59:253–7.

(89) Frautschi JR, Eberhart RC. Improved blood compatibility of alkylated Cuprophan. Trans Soc Biomater 1987;13:125.

(90) Tsai CC, Huo HH, Kulkarni PV, Eberhart RC. Biocompatible coatings with high albumin affinity. Trans Am Soc Artif Intern Organs 1990;36:M307–M320.

(91) Merrill EW, Salzman EW. Polyethylene oxide as a biomaterial. ASAIO J 1983;6:60–64.

(92) Merrill EW, Rempp P, Lutz P, Sagar A, Connolly R, et al. PEO hydrogels from star polymers by radiation-cross linking as model biomaterials. Trans Biomater Soc 1990;13:11.

(93) Chaikoff E. Polyethylene oxide/polysiloxane networks for blood contact [Ph.D. Thesis]. MIT, 1989.

(94) Nagaoka S, Mori Y, Takiuchi H, Yokota K, Tanzawa H, Nishiumi S. Interaction between blood components and hydrogels with poly(oxyethylene)chains. In: Shalaby SW, Hoffman AS, Ratner BD, Horbett TA, eds. Polymers as biomaterials. New York: Plenum Press, 1984: 361–74.

(95) Desai NP, Hubbell JA. Surface modifications of polymeric materials for reduced thrombogenicity. Trans Biomater Soc 1990;13:270.

(96) Merrill EW, Salzman EW, Dennison KA, et al. Nonadsorptive hydrogels for blood contact. Prog Artif Organs 1985;9:909–12.

(97) Yasuda H, Bumgarner MO, Mason RG. Lindholm blood coagulation tests on glow discharge polymer surfaces. Biomater Med Dev Artif Organs 1976;4:307–12.

(98) Chawla AS. Plasma polymerization and plasma modification of surfaces for biomaterial applications. In: Piskin E, Hoffman AS, eds. Polymeric biomaterials. Dordrecht: M. Nijhoff, 1986:221.

(99) Gombotz WR, Hoffman AS. Gas discharge techniques for biomaterials modification. In: Williams DF, ed. Critical reviews of biocompatibility, Vol 4. Boca Raton: CRC Press, 1987:1–42.

(100) Yasuda HK, Matsuzawa Y, Hanson SR, Hanson SR, Harker LA. Blood surface interaction investigated with ultrathin coatings of glow discharge polymers applied onto the inner surface

of small diameter Silastic tubing. Trans Biomater Soc 1984;7:338.

(101) Ward RS, White KA, Hu CB. Use of surface-modifying additives in the development of a new biomedical polyurethane urea. In: Plank H, Egbers G, Syre I, eds. Polyurethanes in biomedical engineering I. Amsterdam: Elsevier, 1984:181–200.

(102) Ward RS. Surface modifying additives for biomedical polymers. IEEE Eng Med Biol 1989; 8:22–5.

(103) Dantowitz P, Borsanyi A. Blood oxygenator with preformed, membrane-lined capillary channels. In: Johnsson-Hegyeli, R, ed. Proceedings, artificial heart program conference. Washington D.C.: U.S. Govt. Printing Office, 1968:339–46.

(104) Ketteringham JM, Zapol WM, Gray DN, et al. Polyalkylsulfone: a new polymer for membrane oxygenators. Trans Am Soc Artif Intern Organs 1973;19:61–71.

(105) Huo HH. Surface modification to enhance the biocompatibility of the Biomedicus pump [M.S. Thesis]. University of Texas Southwestern Medical Center, Dallas, Texas, 1989.

(106) Allcock HR, Lampe FW. Contemporary polymer chemistry. Englewood Cliffs: Prentice Hall, 1981:146–54.

(107) Fougnot C, Jozefonvicz J, Jozefowicz M, Samama M, Bara L. New heparin-like insoluble material: I & II. Ann Biomed Eng 1979;7:429–39, 441–50.

(108) Jozefowicz M, Jozefonvicz J. Antithrombogenic polymers. Pure Appl Chem 1984;56: 1335–44.

(109) Grasel TG, Cooper SL. Properties and biological interactions of polyurethane anionomers: effect of sulfonate incorporation. J Biomed Mater Res 1989;23:311–38.

(110) Rubin RJ, Jaeger RJ. Some pharmacologic and toxicologic effects of Di-2-ethylhexyl phthalate (DEHP) and other plasticizers. Environ Health Perspect Experimental Issue 1973;3:53–9. (This issue is devoted to discussion of the toxicity of phthalate ester plasticizers.)

(111) Kevy SC, Jacobsen MS. Hepatic effects of a phthalate ester plasticizer leached from poly(vinyl chloride) blood bags following transfusion. Environ Health Perspect 1982;45:57–64. (This issue is also devoted to discussion of the toxicity of phthalate ester plasticizers.)

(112) Technical Report on the Carcinogenesis Bioassay of Di(2-ethylhexyl)phthalate. U.S. Department of Health and Human Services, NIH, National Toxicology Program, Research Triangle Park, NC, 1982. DHHS Pub. No. 86-1768.

(113) Hull EH, Mathur KK. High molecular weight citric acid esters as effective plasticizers for medical grade PVC. In: Lee SM, ed. Advances in biomaterials. Lancaster, PA: Technomic Publishers, 1987:186–98.

(114) Karino T, Goldsmith HL. Flow patterns in vessels of simple and complex geometries. Ann NY Acad Sci 1987;516:422–41.

(115) Karino T, Goldsmith HL. Aggregation of human platelets in an annular vortex distal to a tubular expansion. Microvasc Surg Res 1979;17: 217–37.

(116) Litwak RS, Silvay G, Shiang H, Leonard EF. Evaluation of artificial interfaces with in vivo systems. Ann NY Acad Sci 1977;283:542–9.

(117) Vroman L. Methods of investigating protein interactions on artificial and natural surfaces. Ann NY Acad Sci 1987;516:300–5.

(118) Schoen FJ, Clagett GP, Hill JD, Chenoweth DE, Anderson JM, Eberhart RC. The biocompatibility of artificial organs. ASAIO J 1987;10: 824–33.

(119) Clagett GP, Reisch JS. Prevention of venous thromboembolism in general surgical patients. Ann Surg 1988;208:227–40.

(120) Fischer AM, Mauzac M, Tapon-Bretaudiere J, Josefonvicz J. Anticoagulant activity of dextran derivatives. II. Mechanism of thrombin inactivation. Trans Soc Biomater 1985;6:198–202.

(121) Diamond SL, Eskin SG, McIntire LV. Fluid flow stimulates tissue plasminogen activator secretion by culture human endothelial cells. Science 1989;243:1483–5.

(122) Salzman EW, McManama GP, Shapiro AH, et al. Effect of optimization of hemodynamics on fibrinolytic activity and antithrombotic efficacy of external pneumatic calf compression. Ann Surg 1987;206:636–41.

(123) Fallatt RJ, Hill JD, Lamy M, Ratliff J, Dietrich HP, Eberhart RC. Clinical hemodynamics and gas exchange by three ECMO cannulation methods. In: Zapol WM, Qvist J, eds. Artificial lungs for acute respiratory failure. New York: Academic Press, 1976;297–318.

(124) Fletcher JR, McKee AE, Mills M, Herman CM. Twenty-four hour membrane oxygenation in dogs without anticoagulation. Surgery 1976;80: 214–23.

(125) Fletcher JR, McKee AE, Herman CM. Membrane oxygenation in baboons without anticoagulants. J Surg Res 1977;22:273–80.

9

Cardiac Changes During Prolonged Extracorporeal Membrane Oxygenation

❖

Gerard R. Martin, M.D.

Extracorporeal membrane oxygenation (ECMO) has been shown to successfully support infants and young children with life-threatening pulmonary or cardiac diseases (1,2). ECMO has been performed predominantly by the venoarterial technique (3), but the venovenous technique shows promise in many circumstances. This chapter will focus on the cardiac changes associated with venoarterial ECMO in infants (4). It is important to note that ECMO is a form of *partial* cardiopulmonary bypass. In diverting a fraction of systemic venous return to an oxygenator and returning oxygenated blood to the infant, ECMO allows only a portion of cardiac stroke work to continue. Differences in the fraction of total cardiac output that arises from the ECMO circuit and the heart may account for many different changes in cardiac performance.

BEFORE ECMO

The majority of infants treated with ECMO have some form of persistent pulmonary hypertension of the newborn (PPHN). Before instituting ECMO, all infants receive a thorough cardiac evaluation to assess the severity of the PPHN and to exclude structural congenital heart disease. Although clinical history, physical examination, arterial blood gases, and chest roentgenogram are all important in this evaluation, combined m-mode, two-dimensional, and Doppler echocardiography is by far the most conclusive method of cardiac evaluation (5,6).

The manifestations of PPHN are most striking on the right ventricle. In utero, the right ventricle pumps 60% of the combined ventricular output into the main pulmonary artery (7). Pulmonary blood flow accounts for only a fraction of right ventricular output (3%–5%). Since pulmonary vascular resistance is greater than systemic vascular resistance, the majority of right ventricular cardiac output is directed through the ductus arteriosus to the descending aorta. This difference in resistance ratio during fetal life is due to both a high-resistance pulmonary circulation and a low-resistance placental circulation. As a result, the right ventricle of a fetus or a neonate is quite different from the right ventricle of an older child. The fetal right and left ventricles generate the same systolic pressure. The fetal and neonatal right ventricle have end-diastolic chamber dimensions and wall thicknesses similar to those of the left ventricle. The right ventricle pushes the interventricular septum posteriorly in utero as well as during the first week of life (8–11).

During transitional circulation, there is a rapid pulmonary vasodilatation and a decrease in pulmonary vascular resistance. Pulmonary vasodilatation is the result of both physical expansion of the lungs and an increase in arterial oxygen tension. Increases in pulmonary blood flow result in increased pulmonary venous return, increased left atrial pressure, and closure of the foramen ovale. Removal of the placental circulation results in the loss of this low-resistance circuit and thus, in an increase in systemic vascular resistance. If the ductus arteriosus has not fully constricted at this point, the direction of shunting reverses from right-to-left to left-to-right. Ductal constriction occurs in response to the increase in arterial oxygen tension (12); this normally occurs during the first 24 hours after birth. After this initial rapid decrease in pulmonary vascular resistance, there is a slower decrease over the next six to eight weeks due to remodeling and growth of the pulmonary microcirculation.

The normal changes during the transitional circulation have been studied by echocardiography. The ductus arteriosus may remain persistently patent during the first several days after birth in some infants (13–15). The direction of shunting in the ductus arteriosus, however, is from left to right. The right ventricle maintains its thick wall during the first month after birth (16). Interventricular septal morphology stays flattened during the first week after birth, reflecting the high right ventricular pressure (11).

The normal changes in pulmonary circulation can be interrupted by the various perturbations that cause PPHN (17). PPHN has dramatic effects on the transitional circulation and, in particular, right ventricular performance. With PPHN, pulmonary vascular resistance is persistently increased equal to or above systemic levels. Since the low-resistance placental circulation has been removed, the high pulmonary vascular resistance represents an increase in afterload for the right ventricle. In an effort to maintain normal cardiac output, the right ventricle dilates. Tricuspid insufficiency is common during the normal transitional circulation, especially in infants with PPHN (18,19). Right ventricular dilatation may exaggerate the flattening of the interventricular septum and actually compress the left ventricle. The pulmonary valve may close early due to pulmonary hypertension. This can be demonstrated by either m-mode or Doppler echocardiography (20).

The ductus arteriosus and foramen ovale may remain patent and allow right-to-left shunting. The right-to-left shunt can be demonstrated by either pulse Doppler echocardiography, saline contrast echocardiography, or by color flow Doppler echocardiography (21–23). The severity of PPHN can be estimated by the direction of shunting at the ductus arteriosus or by the peak velocity of tricuspid valve insufficiency (24–26). Using the Bernoulli principle, the pressure difference across the tricuspid valve in systole is estimated to be four times (velocity) squared. This pressure difference is added to an estimated right atrial pressure to predict right ventricular systolic pressure. Right atrial pressure is usually estimated to be 5 mm Hg. In the absence of right ventricular outflow tract stenosis, right ventricular pressure is equal to pulmonary arterial systolic pressure.

Cardiac output may be estimated by Doppler echocardiography (27,28). If PPHN is severe, with significant hypoxia and acidosis, left ventricular failure may cause low systemic output. Left ventricular function may also be impaired by positive-pressure ventilation. By combining the information from the clinical condition of the infant with the echocardiographic estimation of severity of PPHN, the management of these sick infants can be improved.

Evaluation of Cardiac Structures

Echocardiography is also important in diagnosing the presence of structural heart disease. The accuracy of echocardiography in evaluating congenital heart disease has been well documented (29). Infants with lung disease present a particular challenge for echocardiography because of limitations in acoustic windows. Ventilators and air leaks make imaging difficult. Total anomalous pulmonary venous drainage has been the most difficult diagnosis to exclude in infants with PPHN. The physiology in obstructed, total anomalous pulmonary venous drainage is very similar to that of PPHN. In both conditions, pulmonary blood flow is obstructed, the difference being that in PPHN the obstruction is at the pulmonary arteriolar level, whereas in total anomalous pulmonary venous drainage the obstruction is at the venous level. Severe hypoxemia is present in both conditions. The chest x-ray may provide some hints to the diagnosis since, in most instances, the heart size is normal to small in obstructed, total anomalous pulmonary venous drainage. In PPHN, heart size may be either normal or increased if hypoxia, acidosis, or both are severe. Echocardiography shows right-to-left shunting across the foramen ovale and ductus arteriosus in both conditions. Since both conditions result in pulmonary hypertension, right ventricular dilatation is common and the left-sided structures may be compressed, making visualization of the pulmonary venous connections difficult. Color flow Doppler echocardiography has been extremely useful in showing the site of drainage of the pulmonary veins (30).

Evaluation of Cardiac Performance

The evaluation of cardiac performance prior to ECMO is particularly important now that venovenous ECMO is being used for infants with PPHN. Systemic hypotension, acidosis, and the need for inotropic support are common in infants with PPHN. This has been considered to be strong evidence for ventricular failure; thus, the conclusion was that venoarterial ECMO would be necessary to support the systemic circulation. It is our impression that ventricular failure is limited to the right ventricle in most circumstances. Analysis of left ventricular function by plotting wall stress and velocity of circumferential fiber shortening (VCFS) (31) shows that these critically ill infants actually have normal contractility (32) for their degree of afterload (Figure 9.1). Thus, most infants may be candidates for venovenous ECMO, since ventricular

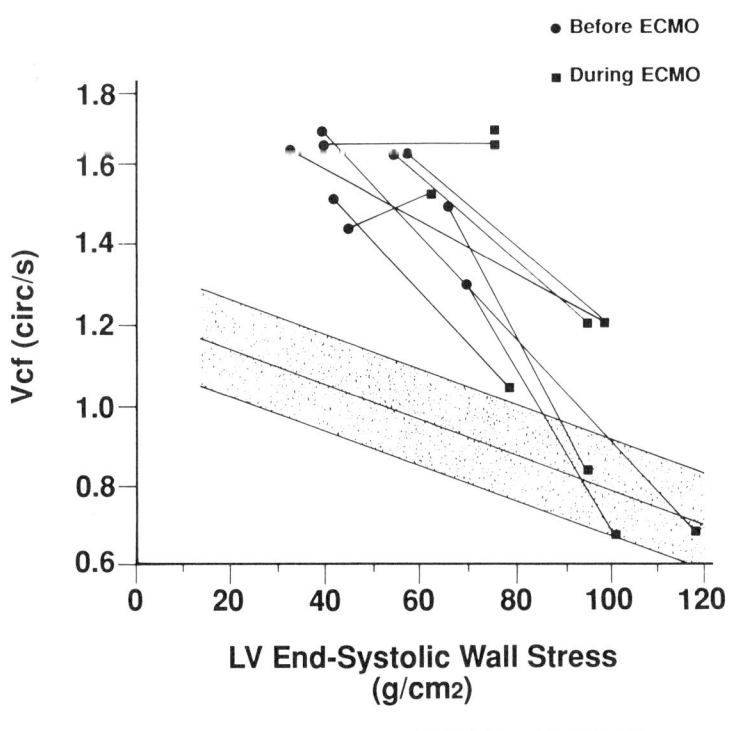

FIGURE 9.1 Velocity of circumferential fiber shortening plotted against wall stress. Before ECMO, contractility (VCFS) is above normal for the level of wall stress (afterload). During ECMO, VCFS decreases but is normal for the level of wall stress.

failure is predominantly a right ventricular phenomenon and left ventricular output can be maintained by right-to-left shunting at the foramen ovale.

An older child being considered for ECMO may be more susceptible to right ventricular failure than a neonate. An older child's right ventricle has not had the benefit of systemic right ventricular pressure prior to the lung injury. Thus, right ventricular failure may play a more important role in determining the need for ECMO than in a neonate. In addition, neither the foramen ovale or the ductus arteriosus is likely to be patent, and important sources of left ventricular filling may be absent.

DURING ECMO

ECMO is *partial* cardiopulmonary bypass. A fraction of systemic venous return is directed away from the heart to a membrane oxygenator and returned to the aorta at systemic pressure. The membrane oxygenator provides oxygen delivery and carbon dioxide removal, and the pump provides blood flow. There are many hemodynamic changes associated with the use of ECMO in infants. Some are the expected changes caused by reduced systemic venous return to the heart, and others are complications of ECMO.

After starting ECMO, a period of adjustment occurs during which the arterial blood gases normalize. Vital signs remain remarkably stable during this time. Heart rate does not change significantly during or after ECMO (Figure 9.2), and, in the majority of infants, normal sinus rhythm is maintained. Blood pressure increases during ECMO and returns to baseline after ECMO (Figure 9.2). The increase in mean arterial blood pressure during ECMO occurs despite a discontinuation of inotropic support used before ECMO in nearly all infants. Both systolic and diastolic pressures increase during ECMO. Since there is less pulsatile flow, aortic pulse pressure decreases during ECMO.

Echocardiographic Changes

We have used echocardiography to evaluate cardiac performance during ECMO. Various m-mode measurements of cardiac performance have been examined (4). Diastolic dimensions of the ventricular and atrial chambers do not change significantly during ECMO. Systolic dimensions of the ventricular chambers increase, indicating a decrease in ventricular shortening fraction (Figure 9.3). Left ventricu-

FIGURE 9.2 Heart rate and blood pressure response to ECMO. Closed circles show no change in heart rate during or after ECMO. Open circles show an increase in mean arterial pressure during ECMO and a return to baseline after ECMO. * = significant difference from before ECMO, $p \leq 0.01$. (Reproduced with permission from Martin GR, Short BL. Doppler echocardiographic evaluation of cardiac performance in infants on prolonged extracorporeal membrane oxygenation. Am J Cardiol 1988;62:929–34.)

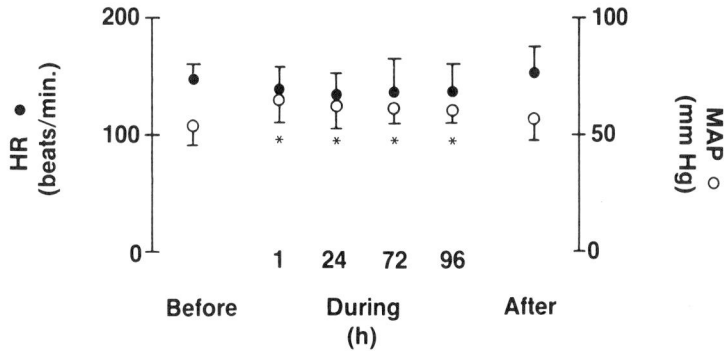

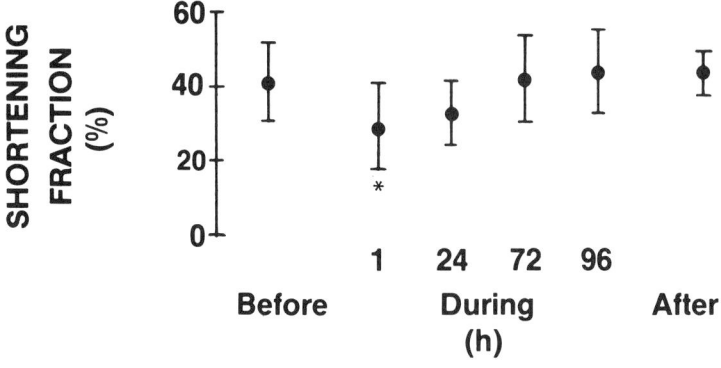

FIGURE 9.3 Left ventricular shortening fraction response to ECMO. Shortening fraction decreased 1 h after beginning ECMO and returned to baseline 72 h after beginning ECMO. * = significant difference from before ECMO, $p \leq 0.01$. (Reproduced with permission from Martin GR, Short BL. Doppler echocardiographic evaluation of cardiac performance in infants on prolonged extracorporeal membrane oxygenation. Am J Cardiol 1988;62:929–34.)

lar velocity of circumferential fiber shortening, an index of contractility, decreases after beginning ECMO. Ventricular wall stress, an index of afterload, increases during ECMO. These indices of performance return to baseline as the ECMO flow rates decrease.

Peak and mean blood flow velocities are normal before ECMO and decrease 30%–50% after ECMO is begun (Table 9.1). These velocities return to normal after 72 hours of ECMO, concurrent with reductions in ECMO pump flows. Pulmonary blood flow velocities may fail to increase if there is no resolution of the PPHN or if right ventricular failure is present.

Knowledge of normal blood flow velocities during ECMO was useful in detecting congenital heart disease in an infant with coexisting lung disease. A 24-hour-old infant with meconium aspiration was referred for ECMO.

TABLE 9.1 Blood flow velocities (cm/s) in infants undergoing ECMO

Site	Before ECMO	During ECMO				After ECMO
		1 h	24 h	72 h	96 h	
PA*						
Peak	66 ± 20	42 ± 12§	52 ± 17	63 ± 13	70 ± 13	86 ± 16§
Mean	43 ± 13	27 ± 8§	33 ± 12	38 ± 9	44 ± 8	54 ± 10
LVOT†						
Peak	77 ± 26	42 ± 14§	56 ± 20	70 ± 17	67 ± 11	86 ± 12
Mean	46 ± 8	26 ± 8§	34 ± 12	43 ± 11	43 ± 8	53 ± 9
AO‡						
Peak	88 ± 30	47 ± 14§	67 ± 28	78 ± 25	73 ± 17	97 ± 18
Mean	53 ± 20	30 ± 9§	43 ± 19	48 ± 17	46 ± 10	59 ± 13

Note: Data are mean ± standard deviation.
*PA = pulmonary artery.
†LVOT = left ventricular outflow tract.
‡AO = aorta.
§Significant difference from before ECMO, $p \leq 0.01$.

Right ventricular failure and decreased right ventricular cardiac output were noted. During ECMO, right ventricular performance improved, and a pulmonary arterial systolic velocity of 200 cm/s was present. This was immediately recognized as being out of the range of normal blood flow velocities on ECMO. Critical valvular pulmonic stenosis was suspected. The infant developed an intracranial hemorrhage during ECMO and died. The cardiac diagnosis was confirmed at autopsy.

In proportion to the velocity measurements, there is a similar reduction in the estimated ventricular stroke volumes during ECMO (Figure 9.4). Right and left ventricular stroke volumes are nearly identical during ECMO and increase in an inverse relationship to ECMO pump flow. This increase in stroke volume occurs when there is a decrease in pulmonary arterial pressure and thus indicates the resolution of PPHN. If ventricular output fails to increase, or if pulmonary arterial systolic pressure fails to decrease, it is likely that chronic lung disease has developed.

Because heart rate does not change during or after ECMO, left ventricular cardiac output has a similar trend. Total aortic flow (pump flow plus ventricular cardiac output) does not

FIGURE 9.4 Left and right ventricular stroke volume response to ECMO. Left and right ventricular stroke volume decreased after beginning ECMO. Stroke volume returned to baseline 72 h after beginning ECMO. * = significant difference from before ECMO, $p \leq 0.01$. (Reproduced with permission from Martin GR, Short BL. Doppler echocardiographic evaluation of cardiac performance in infants on prolonged extracorporeal membrane oxygenation. Am J Cardiol 1988;62:929–34.)

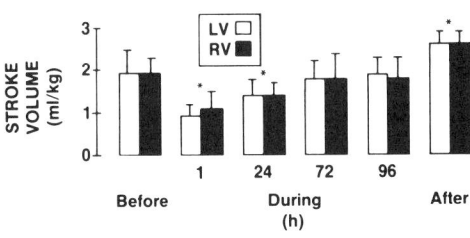

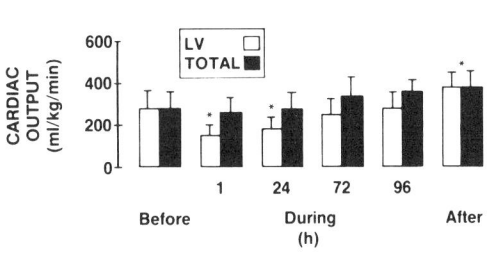

FIGURE 9.5 Left ventricular and total aortic blood flow response to ECMO. Left ventricular blood flow decreased after beginning ECMO and returned to baseline 72 h after beginning ECMO. Total aortic blood flow (left ventricular blood flow plus ECMO pump flow) did not change during ECMO. * = significant difference from before ECMO, $p \leq 0.01$. (Reproduced with permission from Martin GR, Short BL. Doppler echocardiographic evaluation of cardiac performance in infants on prolonged extracorporeal membrane oxygenation. Am J Cardiol 1988;62:929–34.)

change during ECMO, indicating an inverse relationship between cardiac performance and pump flow (Figure 9.5).

Shortening fraction, velocity of circumferential fiber shortening, wall stress, and stroke volume are all estimates of cardiac performance. They are influenced by heart rate, preload, afterload, and contractility. Heart rate does not play a role in the changes of cardiac performance during ECMO. Preload is the parameter most affected during ECMO (33). Preload is decreased at high ECMO flow rates, thereby contributing to the decreased blood flow velocities and stroke volumes. Afterload and contractility are also affected. The mechanisms behind increases in afterload are not understood, but changes in renin-angiotensin-aldosterone system are suspected. Changes in both afterload and preload may account for the decreases in contractility seen during ECMO.

In an attempt to ascertain the importance of an increase in afterload on the decrease in cardiac performance, we have given hydralazine to a group of infants immediately after beginning ECMO (34). The anticipated decrease in cardiac performance was seen in each of the infants, and hydralazine did not result in improved indices of cardiac performance. This is consistent with the finding that contractility (VCFS) normalized for afterload (wall stress) is normal in infants on ECMO (Figure 9.1). Thus, it would appear that the majority of changes in cardiac performance may be attributed to decreases in preload alone. Understanding that there is an expected decrease in cardiac performance during ECMO is important so that potentially deleterious therapies are not undertaken. In contrast to these normal decreases in cardiac performance, cardiac "stun," the total absence of cardiac contribution to cardiac output, may occur (35). This will be discussed later in the chapter.

Doppler echocardiography has been used to document and follow the course of pulmonary hypertension in infants on ECMO. Pulmonary arterial pressure usually remains increased throughout the first 48 hours on ECMO and subsequently decreases into the normal range by the time the infant is ready to be taken off ECMO (Figure 9.6). We have had several patients with persistently elevated pulmonary artery pressure. These infants have had chronic ventilator requirements after ECMO or have expired from cor pulmonale. We believe that the routine estimation of pulmonary arterial pressure is important in determining the prognosis of infants on ECMO.

In addition to the noninvasive evaluation of infants on ECMO, we have performed cardiac catheterization in eight infants. The hemodynamic measurements made at catheterization are shown in Figure 9.7. Atrial and ventricular pressures are comparable to those found in a similar group of infants with PPHN who were not on ECMO. Surprisingly, atrial pressure was normal to slightly elevated in the setting of venous return partially directed away from the heart. Oxygen saturations were in the normal range in both the systemic venous and arterial circulations. The arteriovenous (AV) oxygen difference calculated on the basis of these measurements showed normal oxygen delivery. Varying pump flow rates and determining the most optimal flow rates for oxygen delivery have not yet been accomplished.

ECMO flow rates must be taken into account in the estimation of pulmonary artery pressure. Figure 9.8 shows the effect of weaning ECMO flow rate in an infant with congeni-

FIGURE 9.6 Pulmonary arterial and aortic systolic pressure and pulmonary arterial to aortic pressure ratio response to ECMO. Pulmonary arterial systolic pressure and pulmonary-to-aortic pressure ratio decrease after 48 h on ECMO. * = significant difference from before ECMO, $p \leq 0.05$. (Reproduced with permission from Martin GR, Short BL. Doppler echocardiographic evaluation of cardiac performance in infants on prolonged extracorporeal membrane oxygenation. Am J Cardiol 1988;62:929–34.)

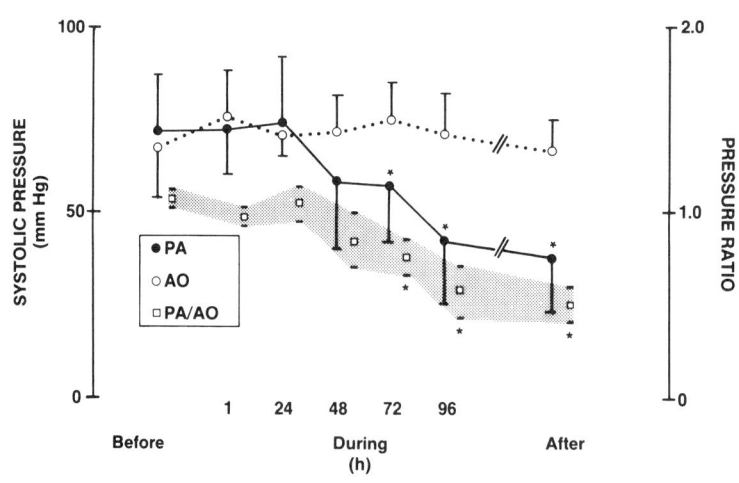

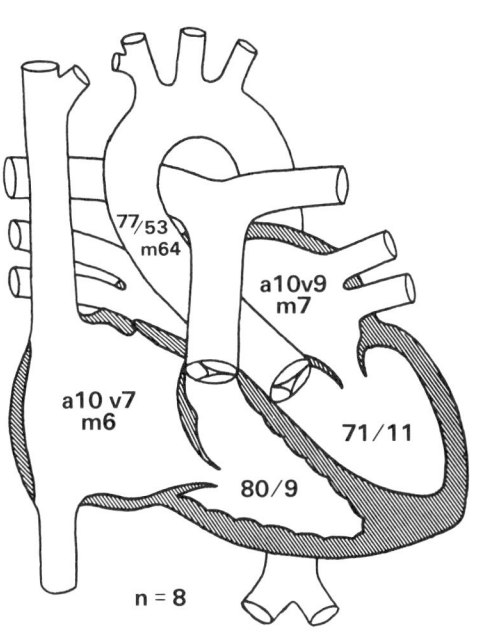

FIGURE 9.7 Intracardiac pressures obtained during cardiac catheterization in infants on ECMO.

TABLE 9.2 Abnormal cardiac changes during ECMO

Hypertension
Hypotension
Arrhythmia
Errant cannula placement
Patent ductus arteriosus
Cardiac stun

tal diaphragmatic hernia. At high ECMO flow rates, the pressure in the pulmonary artery was 50% of systemic values. When ECMO flow rate was decreased and there was an increase in right ventricular cardiac output, the pulmonary artery pressures increased to systemic levels. This indicated a fixed, increased pulmonary vascular resistance, whereby pressure was dependent only on flow. Therefore, if pulmonary artery pressure is to be used as a prognostic factor during ECMO, pump flow rates must be taken into consideration.

The normal changes in cardiac performance have been described. Understanding these normal changes is important, since they may be associated with changes in other organ systems during ECMO or may affect survival. Taylor et al. (36) have shown that these normal decreases in cardiac performance alter cerebral blood flow during ECMO. A possible association between these changes and the high incidence of intracranial defects documented by neuroimaging techniques is speculative. In addition to normal cardiac changes during ECMO, a number of abnormal cardiac changes have been observed (Table 9.2).

Pressure Abnormalities

Blood pressure abnormalities occur frequently at the beginning of ECMO. Systemic hypertension is the most common blood pressure abnormality during ECMO. The diagnosis of hypertension is made when the mean blood pressure in a infant is greater than 65 mm Hg. The cause of hypertension is unknown, but it is thought to be neurohormonally mediated. The first step in the management of hypertension is to wean the patient off of all inotropic agents. Because of the risk of intracranial hemorrhage, hypertension is treated aggresively if it does not resolve spontaneously. We have used hydralazine (0.15 mg/kg/dose), Labetalol (1.0 mg/kg/dose), and/or nitroprusside (0.25–8.0 μg/kg/min) to treat hypertension. Phentolamine (0.10 mg/kg/dose) has been effective when other drugs have failed to lower blood pressure.

Hypotension occurs much less often than hypertension. Given that the aortic flow is adequate on ECMO, it would appear that hypotension is caused by inadequate peripheral vascular tone. This has been a problem more often in infants with septic shock. Vasoactive agents with alpha effect are required to support the blood pressure in this setting.

Documentation of Catheter Position

The cardiac rhythm that predominates during the ECMO course is sinus rhythm. During the cannulation process, however, a myriad of arrhythmias have been detected. Sinus bradycardia has occurred during cannulation. This

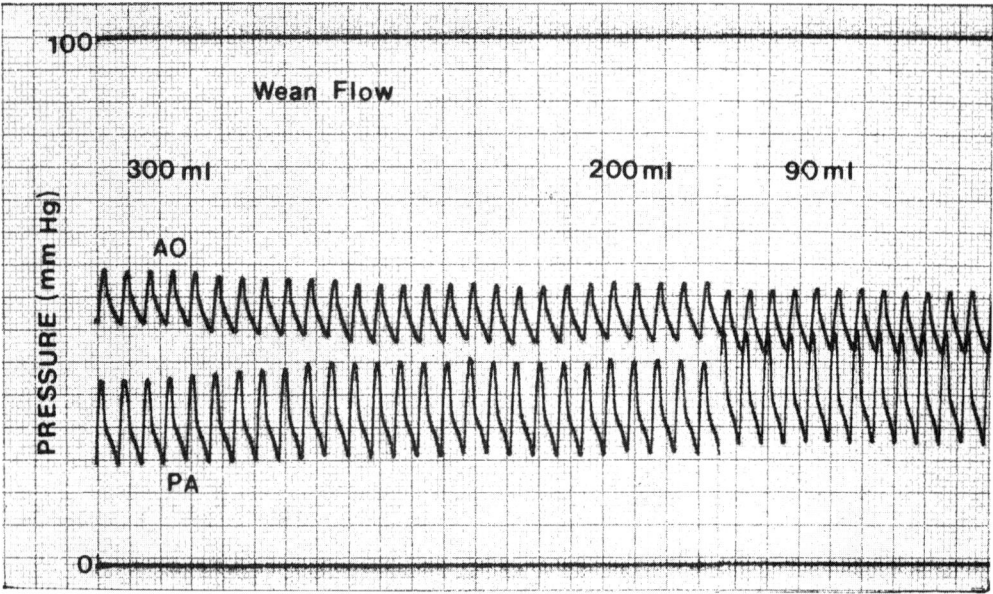

FIGURE 9.8 Increase in pulmonary arterial pressure to systemic levels as ECMO flow rate is decreased from 300 to 90 cc/min.

may be due to stimulation of the vagus nerve or as a result of hypoxia and acidosis which may be present in critically ill infants when ECMO is begun. Atrial or ventricular ectopy, occurring as a result of mechanical stimulation of the right atrium or ventricle by the venous cannula, is common during ECMO. Less commonly, atrial flutter or supraventricular tachycardia have occurred. These arrhythmias are best treated by simply repositioning the venous cannula. During the first hour after ECMO, serum potassium and calcium levels may be deranged, resulting in ventricular ectopy. A rhythm strip with T-wave or QT-interval abnormalities may alert the ECMO team to these possibilities. Treatment of the electrolyte disturbance usually results in normal sinus rhythm. As a rule, the treatment of rhythm disturbances during ECMO is no different from treatment in any other setting.

The positions of cannulas have been checked routinely by a chest x-ray. More recently, we have noticed that, in infants who have mediastinal shift, it is particularly difficult to determine cannula position by chest x-ray. In these infants, echocardiography has been useful. Low arterial cannula placement may interfere with aortic valve opening and has resulted in transient cardiac stun. High arterial cannula placement may result in damage to the head and neck vessels, causing hematoma or dissection of the vessels. Low venous cannula placement may result in arrhythmias, and a high venous cannula may result in inadequate venous drainage to the pump.

Patent Ductus Arteriosus

Patent ductus arteriosus is common during ECMO (Table 9.3). The shunting patterns of the patent ductus change, as do lung disease and pulmonary vascular resistance. We find it particularly useful to follow the ductal shunting as a sign of clinical improvement. Left-to-right shunting through the ductus commonly occurs in an infant on ECMO and usually is not significant enough to impair weaning from the ECMO circuit. We treat infants with patent ductus arteriosus with furosemide and fluid restriction. It is rare that a patent ductus arteriosus requires ligation during ECMO. The ductus arteriosus usually closes spontaneously and only occasionally remains patent after discharge from the hospital.

TABLE 9.3 Ductus arteriosus patency and shunting patterns in infants on ECMO

Time	R to L*	Bidirectional	L to R†
Before ECMO	6	7	0
During ECMO			
1 h	5	4	5
24 h	4	2	3
72 h	1	2	2
96 h	1	0	4
After ECMO	0	0	0

*R to L = right-to-left.
†L to R = left-to-right.

Cardiac Stun

Cardiac stun is the complete or near-complete absence of ventricular contribution to cardiac output during ECMO (35). This results in a marked decrease in aortic pulse pressure (≤ 5 mm Hg) and a marked increase in the patient's Pao_2, almost equaling that of the membrane lung (350–450 mm Hg) (Figure 9.9). Cardiac stun occurs infrequently (5% of infants at this institution) and is only transient, lasting between 1 and 64 hours (mean 33 h). Although the infants who develop stun appear sicker before ECMO, the cause of stun is not known. We hypothesize that it is due to either a reperfusion abnormality or a mismatch between afterload and contractility during ECMO. Stun appears to be an important phenomenon since mortality is higher in these infants than in those without stun. More work is necessary to better define this observation.

Finally, a number of infants with structural congenital heart disease have been treated by ECMO. The majority of these have resorted to ECMO because of diagnostic errors in patients with coexistent lung disease. In some instances, infants with known congenital heart disease and coexistent lung disease have been placed on ECMO for a period of stabilization prior to correction of the heart disease. The timing of cardiac surgery is based on resolution of the lung disease. The transition of an infant from ECMO to cardiopulmonary bypass can be made easily at the time of median sternotomy. The ECMO cannulas are clamped at the time of cardiopulmonary bypass and left in the neck until reversal of heparin is achieved at the end of the heart surgery. Rarely, cardiac support may be necessary after repair of the structural defect.

Not much is known about the effects of venovenous bypass on cardiac performance. An important finding of the work on venoarterial ECMO is that left ventricular performance appears to be adequate during ECMO, and, in most infants, the left ventricle would likely support the systemic circulation if oxygenation is provided by venovenous bypass. In some instances, particularly in severely acidotic or asphyxiated infants, the support of the systemic circulation with venovenous bypass

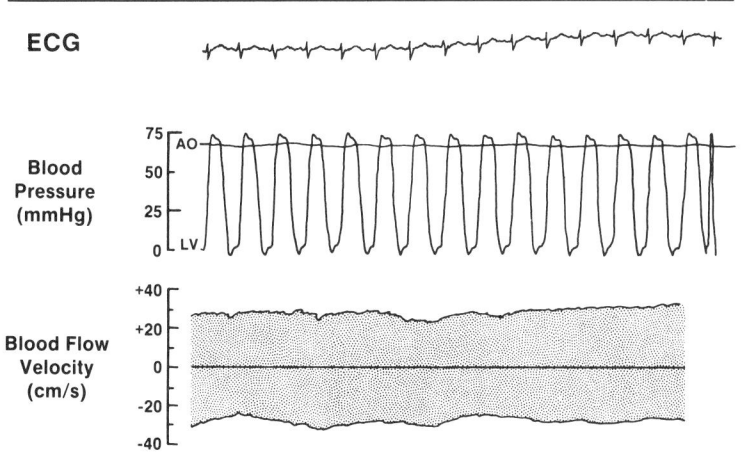

FIGURE 9.9 Cardiac hemodynamics in cardiac stun. Despite normal sinus rhythm and ventricular pressure at systemic levels, there is no aortic pulsatility. Blood flow velocity in the ascending aorta is nonpulsatile and bidirectional as blood from the arterial cannula swirls in the aorta above the aortic value.

alone may be difficult. Preliminary studies in healthy lambs have shown that preload to the ventricular chambers and cardiac output can be maintained during the rapid removal and return of blood adequate to achieve systemic oxygenation (37,38).

SUMMARY

In conclusion, cardiac performance has been shown to be significantly changed by ECMO. Decreases in preload alone may account for the majority of cardiac changes observed. Most changes are transient and well tolerated by the infant. Whether or not any of the cardiac changes associated with ECMO adversely affect the outcome of the infant has yet to be shown. More work on the evaluation of cardiac performance and correlation of performance with outcome may indicate the need to alter cardiac performance during ECMO. Venovenous ECMO should be evaluated extensively before any recommendations are made regarding its use in PPHN.

REFERENCES

(1) Bartlett RH, Roloff DW, Cornell RG, Andrews AF, Dillon PW, Zwischenberger JB. Extracorporeal circulation in neonatal respiratory failure: a prospective randomized study. Pediatrics 1985;76:479–87.

(2) O'Rourke PP, Crone RK, Vacanti JP, Ware JH, Lillehei CW, et al. Extracorporeal membrane oxygenation and conventional medical therapy in neonates with persistent pulmonary hypertension of the newborn: a prospective randomized study. Pediatrics 1989;84:957–63.

(3) Short BL, Pearson GD. Neonatal extracorporeal membrane oxygenation: a review. J Intensive Care Med 1986;1(1):54.

(4) Martin GR, Short BL. Doppler echocardiographic evaluation of cardiac performance in infants on prolonged extracorporeal membrane oxygenation. Am J Cardiol 1988;62:929–34.

(5) Fox WW, Duara S. Persistent pulmonary hypertension in the neonate: diagnosis and management. J Pediatr 1983;103:505–14.

(6) Linday LA, Ehlers KH, O'Loughlin JE, LaGamma EF, Engle MA. Noninvasive diagnosis of persistent fetal circulation versus congenital cardiovascular defects. Am J Cardiol 1983;52:847–51.

(7) Rudolph AM. Distribution and regulation of blood flow in the fetal and neonatal lamb. Circ Res 1985;57:811–21.

(8) Hagan AD, Deely WJ, Sahn D, Friedman WF. Echocardiographic criteria for normal newborn infants. Circulation 1973;48:1221–6.

(9) Cyr DR, Guntheroth WG, Mack LA, Shuman WP. A systematic approach to fetal echocardiography using real-time/two-dimensional sonography. J Ultrasound Med 1986;5:343–50.

(10) St John Sutton MG, Raichlen JS, Reichek N, Huff DS. Quantitative assessment of right and left ventricular growth in the human fetal heart: a pathoanatomic study. Circulation 1984;70:935–41.

(11) Rein AJJT, Sanders SP, Colan SD, Parness IA, Epstein M. Left ventricular mechanics in the normal newborn. Circulation 1987;76:1029–36.

(12) Heymann MA, Iwamoto HS, Rudolph AM. Factors affecting changes in the neonatal systemic circulation. Ann Rev Physiol 1981;43:371–83.

(13) Takenaka K, Waffarn F, Dabestani A, Gardin JM, Henry WL. A pulsed Doppler echocardiographic study of the postnatal changes in pulmonary artery and ascending aortic flow in normal term newborn infants. Am Heart J 1987;113:759–66.

(14) Freund M, Wranne B. Ultrasound assessment of ductal closure, pulmonary blood flow velocity, and systolic pulmonary arterial pressure in healthy neonates. Pediatr Cardiol 1986;6:233–7.

(15) Mahoney LT, Coryell KG, Lauer RM. The newborn transitional circulation: a two-dimensional Doppler echocardiographic study. J Am Coll Cardiol 1985;6:623–9.

(16) Roge CLL, Silverman NH, Hart PA, Ray RM. Cardiac structure growth pattern determined by echocardiography. Circulation 1978;57(2):285–90.

(17) Tiefenbrunn LJ, Riemenschneider TA. Persistent pulmonary hypertension of the newborn. Am Heart J 1986;111:564–72.

(18) Reller MD, Rice MJ, McDonald RW. Tricuspid regurgitation in newborn infants with respiratory distress: echo-Doppler study. J Pediatr 1987;110:760–4.

(19) Martin GR, Silverman NH, Soifer SJ, Lutin

WA, Scagnelli SA. Tricuspid regurgitation in children: a pulsed Doppler, contrast echocardiographic and angiographic comparison. J Am Soc of Echocardiography 1988;1:257–63.

(20) Turkevich D, Groves BM, Micco A, Trapp JA, Reeves JT. Early partial systolic closure of the pulmonic valve relates to severity of pulmonary hypertension. Am Heart J 1988;115:409–18.

(21) Van Hare GF, Silverman NH. Contrast two-dimensional echocardiography in congenital heart disease: techniques, indications and clinical utility. J Am Coll Cardiol 1989;13:673–88.

(22) Ritter SB. Two-dimensional Doppler color flow mapping in congenital heart disease. Clin Cardiol 1986;9:591–6.

(23) Liao PK, Su WJ, Hung JS. Doppler echocardiographic flow characteristics of isolated patent ductus arteriosus: better delineation by Doppler color flow mapping. J Am Coll Cardiol 1988;12:1285–91.

(24) Musewe NN, Smallhorn JF, Benson LN, Burrows PE, Freedom RM. Validation of Doppler-derived pulmonary arterial pressure in patients with ductus arteriosus under different hemodynamic states. Circulation 1987;76:1081–91.

(25) Yock PG, Popp RL. Noninvasive estimation of right ventricular systolic pressure by Doppler ultrasound in patients with tricuspid regurgitation. Circulation 1984;70:657–62.

(26) Currie PJ, Seward JB, Chan K, et al. Continuous wave Doppler determination of right ventricular pressure: a simultaneous Doppler-catheterization study in 127 patients. J Am Coll Cardiol 1985;6:750–6.

(27) Walther FJ, Siassi B, Ramadan NA, Ananda AK, Wu PYK. Pulsed Doppler determinations of cardiac output in neonates: normal standards for clinical use. Pediatrics 1985;76:829–3.

(28) Walther FJ, Siassi B, Ramadan NA, Wu PYK. Cardiac output in newborn infants with transient myocardial dysfunction. J Pediatr 1985;107:781–5.

(29) Gutgesell HP, Huhta JC, Latson LA, Huffines D, McNamara DG. Accuracy of two-dimensional echocardiography in the diagnosis of congenital heart disease. Am J Cardiol 1985;55:514–18.

(30) Kimball TR, Weiss RG, Meyer RA, Daniels SR, Ryckman FC, Schwartz DC. Color flow mapping to document normal pulmonary venous return in neonates with persistent pulmonary hypertension being considered for extracorporeal membrane oxygenation. J Pediatr 1989;114:433–7.

(31) Colan SD, Borow KM, Neumann A. Left ventricular end-systolic wall stress-velocity of fiber shortening relation: a load-independent index of myocardial contractility. J Am Coll Cardiol 1984;4:715–24.

(32) Karr SS, Martin GR, Short BL. Cardiac performance in infants referred for extracorporeal membrane oxygenation. J Pediatr 1991;118(3):437–42.

(33) Kimball TR, Daniels SR, Weiss RG, et al. Changes in cardiac function during extracorporeal membrane oxygenation for persistent pulmonary hypertension in the newborn infant. J Pediatr 1991;118:431–6.

(34) Martin GR, Chauvin L, Short BL. Effects of Hydralazine on cardiac performance in infants on ECMO. J Pediatr 1991;118:944–8.

(35) Martin GR, Short BL, Abbott C, O'Brien AM. Cardiac stun in infants undergoing extracorporeal membrane oxygenation. J Thorac Cardiovasc Surg 1991;101:607–11.

(36) Taylor GA, Martin GR, Short BL. Cardiac determinants of cerebral blood flow during extracorporeal membrane oxygenation. Invest Radiol 1989;24:511–16.

(37) Moront MG, Keszler M, Analouei A, Cox C, Milewski M, Visner MS. The effect of variable preload on left ventricular function in a single cannula system for extracorporeal membrane oxygenation. Surg Forum 1988;38:291–3.

(38) Koul B, Wetterberg T, Sjoberg T, Kimblad PO, Kugelberg J, Steen S. Veno-right ventricular bypass as total extracorporeal lung assistance. J Thorac Cardiovasc Surg 1991;101:719–23.

10

ECMO and the Brain

Christine A. Gleason, M.D.

Patients who require extracorporeal membrane oxygenation (ECMO) for temporary pulmonary and/or cardiac support are often the most critically ill patients in the neonatal, pediatric, or adult intensive care units. They may already have sustained brain injuries prior to the initiation of ECMO therapy. ECMO has effects on brain blood flow, metabolism, and function—some primary effects of the procedure itself, some secondary to its effects on systemic blood pressure, oxygenation, and carbon dioxide levels. These ECMO effects may ameliorate or potentiate further brain injury.

In this chapter, basic principles of the regulation of cerebral blood flow and metabolism are discussed first, to provide a framework for subsequent discussion of the effects of pre-ECMO therapies on the neonatal brain and the effects of ECMO on normal and injured brains. Current markers of cerebral injury are then described and evaluated. Finally, modifications of ECMO technology that could optimize neurologic outcome are discussed, including measures currently being developed.

REGULATION OF CEREBRAL BLOOD FLOW AND ENERGY METABOLISM

Cerebral blood flow (CBF) is regulated by many systemic and local factors, including 1) arterial blood pressure, 2) intracranial pressure, 3) arterial O_2 content, 4) hematocrit, and 5) arterial CO_2 tension. Cerebral O_2 consumption (CMR_{O_2}) is an important determinant of CBF; these variables are said to be "tightly coupled." Responsivity of the cerebral circulation to the stimuli listed above is also determined, in part, by CMR_{O_2}.

Cerebral blood flow is normally regulated to maintain adequate oxygen and substrate delivery to the brain. When blood flow regulatory limits and oxygen extraction capabilities of the brain are exceeded, the brain suffers hypoxic damage. When abnormally low cerebral blood flow is the primary abnormality, then the brain suffers ischemic damage. In most clinical situations, both hypoxic and ischemic damage occur, although one type may predominate.

In this section, normal physiologic principles of CBF regulation and energy metabolism will be discussed, along with responses to pathophysiologic conditions commonly encountered in ECMO patients.

Autoregulation

Cerebral autoregulation refers to the maintenance of constant cerebral blood flow despite changes in cerebral perfusion pressure (1). The autoregulatory range has both upper and lower limits; above or below these limits, CBF changes passively with changes in perfusion pressure. Cerebral autoregulation has been demonstrated in several species and across developmental stages but the mechanism of this important phenomenon remains elusive. Possibilities include 1) myogenic mechanisms, with changes in vascular tone responding to alterations in transmural pressure (1); 2) metabolic mechanisms, in which vasoactive substances are released in response to tissue hypoxia or hyperoxia that accompanies an initial change in perfusion pressure (2); and 3) local mechanoreceptors initiating a local reflex arc (3).

Autoregulation of CBF is of great interest because of the many clinical circumstances under which it may be impaired, resulting in tissue hypoxia, hemorrhage, or both. Asphyxia, hypoxia, head trauma, and hypercapnic acidosis, even when relatively mild, have been shown to attenuate or even abolish autoregulation (4–6).

The Cushing's response is characterized by increasing systemic arterial pressure, enough to maintain cerebral perfusion pressure when intracranial pressure rises. Harris et al. (7) have shown that this response is highly developed in fetal sheep, possibly as an adaptation to the rigors of head compression during labor. If the newborn human Cushing's response is similarly well developed, then the newborn brain may be better able to preserve cerebral perfusion pressure when intracranial pressure (ICP) is elevated (as with postasphyxial cerebral edema).

Hypoxia

When arterial oxygen content (CaO_2) or tension (PaO_2) decreases, the brain responds by increasing CBF. Increased CBF preserves cerebral oxygen transport ($= CaO_2 \times CBF$) and cerebral O_2 consumption $[= (CaO_2 - CvO_2) \times CBF]$. There is a limit beyond which CBF cannot increase, and then O_2 transport falls. The brain must then increase O_2 extraction to maintain $CMRO_2$. There is a limit to this also (cerebral venous PO_2), and when this is reached, $CMRO_2$ falls and brain tissue hypoxia results.

Jones et al. (8) studied hypoxic hypoxia in neonatal sheep and found that CBF correlates best with CaO_2; CBF first increases, then decreases as CaO_2 decreases. Studies have shown similar cerebral hypoxic responses in newborn and adult sheep (9). Developmental differences have been noted, however, in the regional brain blood flow responses to hypoxia. Ashwal and associates (10) have demonstrated a hierarchy of responsivity in fetal sheep in which the brain stem is more responsive than the subcortex or cortex. Such a hierarchy has not been noted in more mature sheep. The fetal sheep brain is relatively mature near term. Studies in immature fetal sheep (11) have shown that cerebral O_2 transport is not maintained during hypoxic hypoxia, and therefore, fractional O_2 extraction must increase to maintain $CMRO_2$. This suggests that important regulatory mechanisms are not fully developed in the immature brain, and the brain may be more vulnerable to hypoxic injury.

Cerebral hypoxic responses have been studied almost exclusively in an acute setting: 15–60 min of hypoxic hypoxia, with PaO_2 generally 30–40 mm Hg. Of more interest to clinicians, however, are the cerebral circulatory responses to more prolonged hypoxia. Bender et al. (12) have demonstrated a sustained increase in CBF and no change in $CMRO_2$ during four hours of hypoxic hypoxia in newborn sheep, and Bocking et al. (13) have demonstrated similar findings during 48 hours of hypoxic hypoxia in fetal sheep.

Anemic hypoxia produces an equivalent rise in CBF so that oxygen delivery is maintained despite reduced CaO_2 (8). Arterial PaO_2 changes little, if at all, in anemic hypoxia, and changes in blood viscosity alone are not sufficient to account for the increase. Patchy areas of tissue hypoxia, with some areas receiving only plasma, could produce vasodilation of the cerebral circulation (6,14). This theory supports the concept that increased CBF during either anemic or hypoxic hypoxia actually reflects a relationship between tissue PO_2 and CBF. The connection between CaO_2

and CBF may be an indirect one, because at moderate and severe levels of hypoxia, CaO_2, PaO_2 and tissue PO_2 are at approximately the same position on the steep portion of the oxyhemoglobin dissociation curve (6).

Hyperoxia

Several studies have demonstrated a decrease in cerebral blood flow when PaO_2 is raised to relatively hyperoxic levels. Gleason et al. (15) raised fetal PaO_2 from 20 to 73 mm Hg in fetal sheep and noted a 46% drop in CBF. Kennedy et al. (16) showed a 20%–30% decrease in CBF with extreme hyperoxia (PaO_2 = 349 mm Hg) in neonatal puppies; this CBF response disappeared by age three weeks. Rahilly (17) demonstrated a 33% drop in cranial blood flow in term infants breathing 100% O_2, and Leahy et al. (18) showed a 15% drop in CBF in preterm infants treated similarly. These results are not surprising when the CBF response to hyperoxia is placed along the inverse hyperbolic hypoxic response curve previously described by Jones et al. in fetal sheep (19). It is certainly an important point to consider with regard to placing a hypoxemic newborn on ECMO, where the carotid PaO_2 may be as high as 500 mm Hg.

Polycythemia/Hyperviscosity

Arterial O_2 content increases when hemoglobin concentration rises, as does whole blood viscosity. An increase in CaO_2 alone results in decreased CBF, as noted above. The independent effect of hyperviscosity on decreasing CBF in polycythemic infants has been studied by Massik et al. (20) In this study, methemoglobin was used to dissociate the effects of hematocrit and CaO_2 as the hematocrit was raised in lambs. The results indicated that approximately 50% of the decrease in CBF during polycythemia could be attributed to hyperviscosity and the remainder to changes in CaO_2.

Alterations in Cerebral Oxygen Consumption

Cerebral blood flow is normally coupled with $CMRO_2$, so when clinical conditions alter $CMRO_2$, CBF is regulated appropriately (21). For example, barbiturate coma lowers $CMRO_2$, and, therefore, CBF is comparably reduced. Donegan et al. (22) studied CBF autoregulation and hypoxic responses during pentobarbital-induced coma in newborn lambs. The CBF response to hypoxia (30%–50% reduction in CaO_2) was attenuated during coma, but only in proportion to the decrease in $CMRO_2$. Cerebral vascular reactivity to CO_2 may also be altered by decreasing $CMRO_2$. Fujishima et al. (23) noted reduced CO_2 reactivity in adult patients with hypothermia, deep anesthesia, or brain trauma; the one common denominator for these conditions was decreased $CMRO_2$.

Cerebral O_2 consumption increases during neuronal excitation (24,25). Increased CBF mirrors the increased $CMRO_2$ but may not be enough to supply adequate O_2 so that tissue PO_2 may fall. However, Leniger-Follert and Lubbers (26) reported that increased local CBF during electrical stimulation was not *secondary* to local tissue hypoxia. In this study, local PO_2 always increased with increased microflow (26). If seizure activity is sustained, the high metabolic rate and possibly maximal CBF may increase the brain's susceptibility to hypoxic-ischemic injury for superimposed stresses such as hypotension or hypoxia (27). Current research indicates that adenosine may contribute to the coupling of CBF and $CMRO_2$. In the brain, adenosine is a potent pial artery dilator. Increases in adenosine level during seizures temporally parallel the changes in CBF (28).

CARBON DIOXIDE REACTIVITY

Carbon dioxide is a potent cerebral vasodilator. Cerebrovascular $PaCO_2$ response curves are sigmoid, with the steep portion in the normocapnic range (30–50 mm Hg); the plateau portions include the upper vasodilator limit (70–80 mm Hg) and the lower vasoconstrictor limit (20–25 mm Hg). Temporal responses of CBF to changes in $PaCO_2$ are rapid. Pial arterial diameter changes are apparent within 1–2 min, and steady-state responses are reached within 8–12 min (4). Mechanisms of CO_2-induced cerebral vascular reactivity may be several, including activation of neural pathways and vascular prostaglandin reactivity, but the primary mechanism is alteration of brain interstitial fluid pH by CO_2, which easily and rapidly crosses the blood-brain barrier (4). Metabolic acidosis or alkalosis does not alter CBF unless there are coincident changes in $PaCO_2$, because H^+ and HCO^-_3 do not easily pass the blood-brain barrier.

Hypocapnia is often induced clinically by hyperventilation. Numerous studies have demonstrated a 30%–40% reduction in CBF after 15–30 min of moderately severe hypocapnia ($PaCO_2$ = 15–25 mm Hg). A gradual increase in CBF during prolonged hypocarbia has been shown by Gleason et al. (29) in newborn lambs and Hanson et al. (30) in newborn piglets; CBF returns to baseline after six hours of hyperventilation in lambs. In hyperventilated lambs (29), and in a similar study of adult goats (31), significant cerebral hyperemia is noted after abrupt discontinuation of hyperventilation.

Hypercapnia is often encountered clinically in pre-ECMO patients and may be acute (e.g., pneumothorax, accidental extubation) or chronic. Acute CO_2 responsivity increases with brain maturation (32). The decreased responsivity in the immature brain could be explained by lower $CMRo_2$, but in lambs, $CMRO_2$ almost doubles at birth, with no corresponding change in CO_2 responsivity. Regional CO_2 sensitivity during development does seem to correlate with regional $CMRo_2$; brain stem CO_2 sensitivity is highest in immature brain, which has a correspondingly high metabolic rate (32). Prolonged hypercapnia has been evaluated by Levasseur et al. in adult rabbits (33). They noted decreased pial arteriolar CO_2 responsivity after six days of hypercarbia, presumably due to increased cerebrospinal fluid (CSF) bicarbonate concentration.

The combined effects of hypocapnia and hypoxia, a common pre-ECMO clinical situation, have been explored in several animal models. MacMillan et al. (34) showed that the combination of hypoxia (Pao_2 = 30) and moderately severe hypocapnia ($Paco_2$ = 18) causes deterioration in brain cellular energy state in rats. Gregory et al. (35) hyperventilated anesthetized, paralyzed lambs for two hours and then added hypoxia for an additional hour. They found that, despite hypocapnia, CBF increased during hypoxemia to a level just above the baseline normocapnic value. They noted no rebound hyperemia or "luxury perfusion" when the hypoxemic hyperventilated lambs were made abruptly normocapnic.

Studies by Delivoria-Papadopoulos and associates (36) have suggested that severe hypocapnia ($Paco_2$ < 10) results in tissue ischemia. Others have agreed, pointing to changes in electroencephalograms and in cerebral production of lactate. With regard to the latter point, alkalosis increases phosphofructokinase enzyme activity, resulting in increased glycolysis with lactate production. Increased lactate concentrations are therefore not secondary to increased anaerobic metabolism (21). Furthermore, studies have demonstrated maintenance of stable $CMRo_2$ during prolonged hypocapnia (29), a point that argues against the presence of profound tissue hypoxia.

Brain Energy Metabolism

Oxygen and glucose are the brain's primary energy substrates. While the requirement for oxygen is absolute, other substrates can replace or augment glucose during special circumstances such as hypoglycemia or anoxia (37).

When oxygen delivery to the brain is impaired, and oxygen extraction capability is exceeded, tissue hypoxia ensues, and brain damage is the result. The issue of decreased vulnerability of the immature brain or "resistance" to anoxic insult continues to be debated. Increased survivability after prolonged anoxia has been demonstrated in immature animals, such as newborn rats, and there have been occasional anecdotal reports in newborn infants, but whether or not such increased survivability reflects resistance of the *brain* to anoxia is debatable. Nevertheless, immature animals do have better survival, and this has been variously attributed to 1) lower cerebral O_2 consumption, 2) predominance of anaerobic metabolism as an energy source, or 3) circulatory adaptations in immature animals, such as greater stores of cardiac glycogen that enable the heart to sustain the cerebral circulation. None of these possible mechanisms accounts for increased survival in all species, and none has been definitely proven to be important exclusively in immature animals (37).

Hypoglycemia occurs quite commonly in sick newborn infants, although the associated physiologic conditions vary considerably. Poor glycogen stores, increased glucose demands, hyperinsulinism, and poor glucose intake are among the more common of these conditions. Cerebral effects of hypoglycemia may depend in part on the cerebral effects of the associated physiologic conditions. Alternative oxidative substrates are available to the brain, including ketone bodies, lactate, amino acids, and lipids. Owen et al. (38) showed that cerebral ketone body consumption accounts for 50% of cerebral O_2 consumption in obese adults who are starved for five to six weeks. Availability and utilization of these alternative substrates depend in part on the corresponding clinical conditions, as well as the species and brain maturity. Hypoglycemia is associated with decreased cerebral glucose consumption but no change in cerebral O_2 consumption (37). Whether this response is adaptive or pathologic is not known.

Cerebral Ischemia

Complete cerebral ischemia or absence of cerebral blood flow is an uncommon clinical occurrence; partial ischemia, such as may occur with a tight nuchal cord or severe perinatal asphyxia, is more commonly seen in newborns. Revival time is inversely correlated with completeness of the ischemic injury. Even a trickle of blood flow (without hyperglycemia) may improve outcome (21).

Animal research models of cerebral ischemia abound. When interpreting results from these studies, it is important to consider the unique features of the particular insult, the anatomical differences between the species used, and the developmental variability.

The Levine rat model (39) is often discussed in relation to ECMO patients because, in this model, rats undergo unilateral carotid artery ligation, combined with anoxic anoxia, and sustain extensive ipsilateral neuronal loss. The hippocampus is the most vulnerable region. Rats have poor vertebral-occipital collateral circulation, unlike other species including humans, sheep, and dogs, thus making the rat brain particularly vulnerable to this type of insult.

The cat model of middle cerebral artery occlusion is another popular cerebral ischemia model, producing a reproducible anatomic infarction lending itself to pharmacologic and physiologic interventions before, during, and after the insult.

Lastly, compression ischemia, induced by infusion of CSF into the ventricular system to raise ICP above systemic blood pressure, has been used in dog and sheep models. This model allows control of the timing and severity of the insult (partial ischemia = raise ICP to mean arterial blood pressure (BP); complete ischemia = raise ICP above systolic BP).

Both complete and partial ischemia are followed initially by excessive hyperemia or "luxury perfusion" (40) and subsequently by a delayed hypoperfusion (21). During the latter period, there is generally an uncoupling of CBF and metabolism. The "no-reflow" phenomenon does exist (41), but is not of much clinical importance because it describes an initial hindrance to reperfusion following complete ischemia. Metabolic cascades during and following ischemia have been described in detail by Siesjo and others. These cascades have provided the framework for pharmacologic and metabolic interventions before, during, and after cerebral ischemia, designed to prevent or ameliorate neuronal death or injury. For example, studies have shown that nutritional state prior to ischemia influences recovery; hyperglycemia prior to complete ischemia results in worse recovery, attributed to enhanced tissue lactic acidosis (42). Fed or glucose-infused rats exposed to incomplete ischemia have poorer recovery compared to fed animals exposed to complete ischemia (43).

Selective vulnerability to ischemic injury of pyramidal cells in the hippocampus and Purkinje cells in the neocortex has been demonstrated, although the mechanisms are unknown. One theory is that calcium influx into cells, stimulated by excitatory amino acids, triggers a series of reactions, including production of oxygen free radicals, leading to cell death. Selective vulnerability may relate to selective cell membrane permeability of these cells to calcium. Antagonists of the excitatory amino acid neurotransmitters (e.g., glutamate and aspartate) have been advocated as possible therapies for ischemic cerebral injuries (44). Alternatively, therapies with calcium antagonists or oxygen free radical scavengers have been suggested. A Swedish group devised a "cocktail" of oxygen free radical scavengers and a calcium channel blocker which was administered intravenously to exteriorized fetal sheep *after* an acute asphyxial insult (umbilical cord tied). Treated sheep demonstrated better neurologic recovery and CBF than untreated sheep two hours following the insult (45). Administration of such a "cocktail" after an asphyxial insult certainly has significant clinical potential.

EFFECTS OF PRE-ECMO THERAPIES ON THE NEONATAL BRAIN

Neonatal ECMO patients have often been run through a full arsenal of therapies devised to treat pulmonary hypertension and neonatal respiratory failure. These therapies themselves have specific effects on the brain or may induce conditions such as hypocarbia which, in turn, have specific effects on the brain. In this section, the cerebral effects of the following pre-ECMO therapies will be discussed:

1. Hyperventilation
2. Hypercapnia and hypoxia
3. Metabolic alkalosis/acidosis
4. Drug therapies
   a. Pancuronium
   b. Sedatives
   c. Vasoactive agents
      Fentanyl
      Morphine
5. Positive-pressure ventilation
6. Volume support

Hyperventilation

Hyperventilation, with resulting hypocapnic alkalosis, is often used to induce pulmonary vasodilation in babies with pulmonary hypertension. Although studies have shown that it is the pH, not the $PaCO_2$, that influences pulmonary vascular resistance (46), it is often faster to induce and easier to maintain a desired level of alkalosis via hyperventilation than by alkali infusion, so the former is attempted more commonly.

Hypocapnia decreases CBF, but the response is variable, depending on the degree of hypocapnia, the level of systemic oxygenation, brain maturity, and $CMRO_2$. During prolonged hypocapnia, CBF gradually returns towards baseline normocapnic values, probably due to normalization of CSF pH secondary to an accumulation of metabolic acids, such as lactate. Lactate production is not secondary to tissue hypoxia/anaerobic glycolysis but reflects alkalotic stimulation of glycolytic enzymes.

Certain clinical conditions and the institution of ECMO may result in abrupt normalization of $PaCO_2$ after hyperventilation. Studies have shown that if prolonged hyperventilation is abruptly discontinued after six hours in newborn lambs, significant cerebral hyperemia develops and persists for at least 90 min (29). This response most likely reflects relative acidosis of CSF and perivascular tissues and probably takes a few hours to normalize. Posthypocapnia hyperemia might contribute to development of an intracranial hemorrhage in an ECMO patient who has been hyperventilated for hours and who is suddenly made normocapnic.

Hyperventilation is often combined with hypoxemia, sometimes for many hours. Few studies have looked at the cerebral responses to this combination. The reports of Gregory et al. (35) and of MacMillan et al. (34) summarizing this relationship have been cited previously.

Hypercapnia and Hypoxia

Although not exactly considered a "therapy" for neonatal pulmonary hypertension, respiratory failure, or both, many neonatologists today are reevaluating the detrimental effects of hyperventilation and aggressive ventilator settings aimed at maintaining $PaO_2 > 80-100$ mm Hg. They are opting more often for a "kinder, gentler" approach to ventilation, accepting higher $PaCO_2$ and lower PaO_2, often for many hours or even days. The cerebral effects of prolonged hypoxia have been outlined in the previous section, as have the cerebral effects of hypercapnia. Several studies have examined the cerebral effects of combined hypoxia and hypercapnia. Adult human data have suggested an additive vasodilatory effect, implying that hypoxic cerebral vasodilatory limits are not maximal (48). However, McPherson et al. (49), in a study of adult dogs, concluded that if hypoxia is sufficiently severe to impair $CMRo_2$, then superimposed hypercapnia has a detrimental influence due to decreasing blood pressure associated with decreasing CBF and O_2 delivery.

Data from animal studies have been conflicting. Gardiner et al. (50) found that hypoxia in newborn sheep does not increase CBF beyond the level achieved with hypercapnia alone ($Paco_2$ range 34–56 mm Hg). They also noted a reduction in $CMRo_2$ with combined hypoxia and hypercapnia. On the other hand, Massik et al. (51) showed that the magnitude of the hypoxic vasodilatory response in newborn sheep was not altered by coexisting hypercapnia; the vasodilatory effects were additive. In addition, they found no change in $CMRo_2$ and no evidence that hypercapnia causes a reflex increase in sympathetic tone which interferes with hypoxic vasodilation.

Metabolic Alkalosis/Acidosis

Cerebrovascular resistance is thought to be directly related to the brain interstitial pH (52). Biological membranes are highly permeable to CO_2, so a change in $Paco_2$ has an almost immediate effect on interstitial pH and, consequently, on CBF. In contrast, hydrogen and bicarbonate ions do not diffuse as easily through membranes. Therefore, induction of acute metabolic acidosis or alkalosis during normocapnia has not been shown to change CBF or autoregulation (53,54). During hypocapnia, addition of metabolic alkalosis does not alter CBF. However, during hypercapnia, bicarbonate infusion causes a significant decrease in CBF (55) bicarbonate concentration, suggesting that hypercapnia alters the blood-brain permeability to ions. Such alterations in the blood-brain barrier may also be associated with hypoxic/ischemic brain insult.

Sodium bicarbonate may be used clinically to correct metabolic acidosis in neonates. Its use has been limited by the reported associations of hypernatremia, intracranial hemorrhage (56), and acute changes in arterial CO_2.

Clinical studies like these are difficult to interpret if bicarbonate is given because of metabolic acidosis that may be secondary to perinatal asphyxia, itself a major risk factor for intracranial hemorrhage. Laptook (57) evaluated the cerebral effects of sodium bicarbonate (2 mEq/Eg over 3 min) administered to paralyzed newborn piglets to correct metabolic acidosis associated with hypoxemia. They noted no alterations in brain blood or O_2 delivery. Constant $Paco_2$ was maintained by increasing the ventilator rate during the bicarbonate infusion.

Drug Therapies

Pancuronium Several clinical and animal research studies have attempted to evaluate the cerebral effects of nondepolarizing muscle relaxants. Peabody (58) studied preterm infants paralyzed with pancuronium and reported increased cerebral blood flow velocity by the Doppler technique, but this could have been secondary to hypoxia and/or hypercapnia. Belik et al. (59) studied unanesthetized newborn lambs paralyzed with pancuronium and reported no alterations in CBF and metabolism. However, the animals did show a transient increase in systolic blood pressure (average 32%) immediately following paralysis. This may have represented a response to a brief episode of hypoxia caused by transient ventilation/perfusion mismatch.

Sedatives In appropriate clinical doses, the most common neonatal sedatives, fentanyl and morphine, induce their effects by binding to opiate receptors in the brain. Their use is not associated with changes in cerebral blood flow or oxygen metabolism (29,60). However, at higher doses, both drugs have systemic vasodilatory effects and may cause hypotension and, in the presence of impaired autoregulation, decreased CBF.

Vasoactive drugs Dopamine, dobutamine, isoproterenol, and tolazoline are four vasoactive drugs commonly used in pre-ECMO neonatal patients. They are used to increase systemic blood pressure and cardiac output (dopamine, dobutamine) and to dictate the vasculature (isoproterenol and tolazoline). Isoproterenol also increases cardiac output in newborns, but at the expense of marked tachycardia and, often, decreased systemic blood pressure. Tolazoline is not a selective pulmonary vasodilator, and its use is almost always accompanied by severe systemic hypotension. Any cerebral effects of these drugs probably relate primarily to their effects on systemic blood pressure and cardiac output.

Positive-pressure ventilation

Pre-ECMO patients require significant positive-pressure ventilation. Some of these patients have suffered perinatal asphyxia. High mean airway pressure (MAP) may decrease venous return and impair cardiac output, with consequent hypotension. If autoregulation has been impaired by asphyxia/hypoxia or if the autoregulatory limits have been reached, then CBF may decrease. On the other hand, when MAP is quickly decreased, such as when ECMO flow is increased, CBF may increase dramatically.

Both continuous positive airway pressure (CPAP) and positive-pressure ventilation can theoretically impede venous return from the head insofar as the positive pressure is transmitted to the pleural space. The effect is similar to that of superior vena caval obstruction, leading to intracerebral venous and capillary engorgement and consequent hemorrhage (61). The effects of CPAP and intermittent positive-pressure ventilation on cerebral venous pressure appear to be additive. Furthermore, maximal venous stasis is caused when high airway pressure is used with prolonged inspiratory time and high frequency (61). The least stasis is seen at low mean airway pressure, short inspiratory time, and slow ventilatory rates, a combination rarely, if ever, used in pre-ECMO patients.

Hill et al. (62) have used transcutaneous Doppler technique in preterm infants to demonstrate marked increases in flow velocity in the anterior cerebral arteries (ACA) in association with the development of a pneumothorax. Subsequently, each of nine studied babies developed an intracranial hemorrhage. It was proposed that pneumothorax leads to decreased venous return and cardiac output, with increased systemic blood pressure, causing increased ACA flow velocity in a pressure-passive cerebral circulation that is exacerbated by hypercarbia.

Volume Expansion

Pre-ECMO patients may begin life hypovolemic secondary to acute hemorrhage, or they may develop hypovolemia because of septic shock or continued fluid losses. Additionally, cardiac output may be low because of myocardial insufficiency or decreased venous return secondary to high mean airway pressures. In each of these clinical conditions, volume expanders are often needed and administered repeatedly to maintain systemic blood pressure and adequate filling pressures. Because it is difficult to measure filling pressures accurately or to know precisely what contribution hypovolemia is making to systemic hypotension, patients often become "volume overloaded." The cerebral effects of volume expansion following asphyxia have been evaluated by Laptook et al. (63) in newborn piglets. They found significantly lower arterial blood pressure and CBF in piglets that did not receive plasmanate volume expansion (15 mL/kg). Rapid or slow infusion rates did not influence the pattern of brain blood flow, and no intracranial bleeding was observed. It is notable, however, that newborn piglets have relatively mature brains. In a retrospective study, Goldberg et al. (64) noted an association between rapid volume expansion (with blood or colloid) in the first 24 hours of life and intracranial hemorrhage in preterm infants.

Goddard-Finegold et al. (65) examined the cerebral effects of volume expansion alone and after hypovolemic hypotension in newborn puppies. The puppies subjected to volume expansion (15% increase) alone had increased jugular venous pressure and microscopic subependymal germinal matrix hemorrhages. Puppies undergoing hypotension followed by volume reexpansion had significant increases in blood pressure (above baseline) during reexpansion, and several of these animals had significant intracranial hemorrhages.

EFFECTS OF ECMO ON NORMAL AND INJURED BRAIN

From the earliest applications of ECMO, there has been serious concern about its effects on the brain. Many descriptive studies have been published. These include reports of intracranial hemorrhage and infarction during ECMO, high-sided brain lesions linked to carotid ligation, cerebral venous congestion, Doppler flow studies demonstrating alterations in carotid blood flow and cerebral blood vessel pulsatility, and neurodevelopmental outcome in both newborns and adults. Several studies have been done evaluating the cerebral effects of ECMO in normal animal models and, more recently, in hypoxic and hyperventilated animals. Preliminary results are available from these studies.

In this section, clinical reports relating to the cerebral effects of ECMO will be summarized, and preliminary results from research using animal ECMO models will be reviewed.

Clinical Reports

Glass et al. (66) have reported neurodevelopmental follow-up at age one year for 100 infants treated with ECMO at Children's Hospital, Washington, D.C. There was a high incidence of intracranial hemorrhage (29% total, 12% major) and nonhemorrhagic CNS abnormalities (12%). In spite of this and in spite of the severity of their illnesses prior to ECMO, the majority (60%) of infants had normal neurodevelopmental progress at one year. However, the presence of intracranial hemorrhage significantly worsened the neurodevelopmental prognosis.

Taylor et al. (67) reported neuroimaging results from the first 207 ECMO patients at Children's Hospital in Washington, D.C. Intracranial abnormalities were found on head ultrasound and/or computed tomography scan in 46% of infants. One-half of these infants had hemorrhages only. Preterm (< 37 wk) infants were at higher risk of developing these intracranial abnormalities than their more mature counterparts.

Schumacher et al. (68) reported right-sided CNS lesions in eight of 69 ECMO patients, implicating right carotid artery ligation, jugular vein ligation, or both in the pathogenesis of these lesions. This study was potentially biased by small numbers and by no comparative data from patients with left-sided or bilateral lesions. However, it was notable that the infants with right-sided lesions were profoundly hypoxic and hypotensive upon initiation of ECMO. Intracranial Doppler flow studies have shown that blood flow to the right cerebral hemisphere is preserved after right carotid artery ligation by collateral circulation via the anterior communicating artery of the circle of Willis (69). Carotid artery Doppler flow studies have further demonstrated that collateral flow to the carotid artery distal to the ligation is established rapidly (70). Campbell et al. (71) reported a higher incidence of left-sided focal seizures in ECMO patients, but they found no lateralizing predominance in EEG activity. In contrast, Zak and Donn (72) found that 79% of ECMO patients having only EEG evidence of seizures had increased right-hemisphere activity.

Lott et al. (73) used Doppler vascular studies to evaluate internal carotid artery (ICA) flow in four ECMO survivors 4–11 years of age. They found that the ICA was patent, and forward flow was achieved by retrograde channeling through the external carotid artery; the size and volume of flow in the right ICA was about 50% of that in the left. Although no clinical symptoms of right hemisphere dysfunction were noted, 60% of children had asymmetric brain stem auditory evoked responses (BAERS), with right-sided predominance in the majority. Raju et al. (74) recently used similar techniques to study middle cerebral artery flow before, during, and after ECMO in three neonates. Within 15 min of carotid artery ligation, blood flow was detected in each infant's right middle cerebral artery; in one infant, this flow was only 50% of pre-ECMO flow and remained lower than normal during ECMO. The vertebrobasilar and contralateral ICA systems were the major sources of reperfusion of the right cerebral hemisphere via the circle of Willis. By 2–10 weeks after ECMO, flow velocities in the left cerebral arteries were 116%–217% of the right-sided flow velocities.

Voorhies et al. (75) measured regional cerebral blood flow by Xenon inhalation in 12 ECMO survivors 24 hours after decannulation. They noted no significant interhemispheric differences in cerebral blood flow. Ten infants also underwent digital intravenous angiography; in each case, there was prompt bilateral filling of both middle cerebral arteries.

The literature on adult acute cardiopulmonary bypass reports several observations of interest, but the results must be interpreted and extrapolated carefully because of the considerable differences in clinical conditions and bypass techniques. Lundar et al. (76) used transcranial Doppler flow evaluation and measurement of cerebral perfusion pressure (utilizing epidural ICP) to evaluate cerebral autoregulation and CO_2 reactivity during bypass in adult patients. They noted loss of cerebral autoregulation but maintenance of CO_2 reactivity. Henriksen (77) used Xenon injection in adult bypass patients and demonstrated a significant increase in CBF after the initiation of bypass with evidence of excessive hyperemia (luxury perfusion). Johnsson et al. (78) used similar techniques and found no change in CBF while on bypass, but noted a significant increase in CBF after bypass was discontinued. Finally, Stump et al. (79) used Xenon clearance techniques to monitor CBF during adult bypass and reported a spontaneous decline in CBF during bypass with no changes in $PaCO_2$ or temperature noted during the period of decline. The same group further reported cerebrovascular responsiveness to hyperoxia (80) and impairment of autoregulation (81) while on bypass. Differences in results among these studies may be due in part to variations in temperature and blood gas regulation during bypass. A recent study (82) showed that CBF during adult bypass is directly related to body temperature, with decreased CBF and impaired autoregulation noted only with deep hypothermia. Sotaniemi et al. (83) reported long-term (five years) cerebral outcome after open heart surgery in 44 adult patients who underwent valve replacement. They found a strong correlation between the clinical outcome immediately postoperatively and the long-term neuropsychological outcome, even if recovery had been rapid initially. They also observed that a long duration of perfusion impaired neuropsychological performance independent of the clinical outcome. Finally, Nevin et al. (84) found an association between hypocapnia and consequent cerebral hypoperfusion during adult bypass and neurologic deficits postoperatively.

Animal Research

Several studies have been published evaluating the cerebral effects of acute cardiopulmonary bypass in adult animal models. Results from these studies are difficult to extrapolate to neonates undergoing ECMO because the methodology differs substantially (bubble oxygenators, fibrillated heart, hypothermia, etc.) and because adult animals are used at different stages of brain development and with variations in vascular anatomy. Nevertheless, several important observations warrant mention. Rudy et al. (85) measured organ blood flow by the microsphere method during cardiopulmonary bypass in adult rhesus monkeys. At initiation of bypass, brain blood flow decreased and remained low during bypass. In this study, there were on changes in $PaCO_2$, cardiac output, temperature, or systemic blood pressure to explain the decrease in cerebral blood flow. Santillan et al. (86) used adult cats to study cerebral effects of cardiopulmonary bypass; they measured CBF by the microsphere method and regional CBF by direct visualization (using a microtransilluminator) of the microcirculation. During bypass, CBF increased by 80%, and dilatation of cerebral cortical arterioles was observed. They concluded that these findings were reminiscent of the "luxury perfusion syndrome." In addition, they observed a direct correlation (but $r = 0.42$) between blood pressure and CBF during bypass when data points from individual animals were pooled. No such relationship was noted before bypass. Although this implies that cerebral autoregulation was impaired during bypass, true autoregulatory experiments must determine the changes in CBF, if any, in response to stepwise alterations in blood pressure in individual animals.

Microemboli have been implicated as a cause of neurologic complications following cardiopulmonary bypass. Clark et al. (87) detected microemboli using a continuous-wave ultrasound device located immediately distal to the roller pump head. Two 30-min perfusions, using a bubble oxygenator and hemodilution were performed in dogs. A large number of microemboli were noted during the first 10–15 min of perfusion. The microemboli decreased with time. Use of an arterial filter significantly decreased the number of emboli. Physical disturbance of the oxygenator increased the rate of microemboli. Anderson et al. (88) subjected adult pigs to three hours of nonpulsatile cardiopulmonary bypass and measured brain blood flow and glucose consumption (using labeled deoxyglucose). They noted that, while blood flow remained normal, glucose consumption declined, indicating perfusion in excess of metabolic demand. Such findings were not noted during pulsatile bypass.

Recently, research efforts have been directed towards the effects of ECMO as it is used clinically on the neonatal brain. Short et al. (89) used a newborn lamb model of venoarterial ECMO and the radioactive microsphere technique to measure CBF and $CMRO_2$ during the initiation of bypass. They found no significant changes in either CBF or $CMRO_2$ after 30 min and after two hours of bypass, at flow rates commonly used initially in newborn infants. In addition, no right/left cerebral blood flow differences were observed. Walker et al. (90) used the same model to demonstrate normal CO_2 responsivity by the newborn brain during ECMO. The findings of both studies have been corroborated anecdotally by Doppler flow studies in newborn infants. However, the animal findings cannot be readily extrapolated to newborn infants without consideration of the differences in cerebrovascular anatomy between lambs and humans. Lambs have a well-developed vertebrobasilar arterial system, allowing for adequate collateral circulation to the right internal carotid artery following bilateral carotid artery ligation. Although newborn infants also have vertebral artery collaterals to the carotid arteries, the system is not sufficiently developed to allow for bilateral carotid ligation. An additional consideration with regard to extrapolating results from the lamb studies is that these newborn lambs were healthy, without the pre-ECMO hypoxia, acidosis, hypotension, and perinatal asphyxia common to ECMO patients. Preliminary results are available from a recent study addressing one of these issues. Bender et al. (12) subjected newborn lambs to prolonged (four hours) hypoxemia (PaO_2 33 mm Hg) and then unilateral carotid artery and jugular vein ligation. CBF remained increased (by 127%) after four hours of hypoxemia and was unchanged by vessel ligation. $CMRO_2$ was unaltered by hypoxemia and remained unaltered following vessel ligation. Finally, no right/left differences in CBF were noted after vessel ligation.

Markers of Cerebral Injury

For years, neonatologists have sought markers of cerebral injury in order to give parents a prognosis and to evaluate appropriate therapies. This quest continues today for ECMO patients; such markers are essential before, during, and after ECMO therapy. Current markers may be separated into the following categories:

1. Neuroimaging

    a. Cranial ultrasound

    b. Computed tomography (CT) scan

    c. Magnetic resonance imaging (MRI)

2. Electroencephalogram (EEG) and stimulus-evoked potentials

3. Brain metabolism

    a. Nuclear magnetic resonance (NMR) spectroscopy

    b. Positron emission tomography (PET) scan

4. Brain blood flow techniques

    a. Doppler

    b. Xenon

    c. PET scan

5. Neurodevelopmental assessment

These categories necessarily overlap in order to provide more accurate markers; for example, descriptions of intracranial hemorrhages by cranial ultrasound need matching neurodevelopmental follow-up data.

Neuroimaging Cranial ultrasound is usually used to screen ECMO candidates for intracranial hemorrhage prior to initiation of ECMO. Many ECMO centers consider a significant intracranial hemorrhage a contraindication to ECMO because of the likelihood of progressive hemorrhage. Although ultrasound is a sensitive imaging tool for the detection of major intracranial abnormalities in neonates, it is not as sensitive as CT scan in detecting smaller but still clinically significant lesions such as focal atrophy, subarachnoid hemorrhages, small parenchymal hemorrhages, and/or infarcts. The latter is especially relevant to the pre-ECMO patient. Klesch et al. (91) reported that 47% of infants with pulmonary hypertension and EEG abnormalities had cerebral infarction documented by sonograms, CT scan, or autopsy. Placing such infants on ECMO may result in conversion of a previously nonhemorrhagic infarction to a hemorrhagic one, which may therefore be labeled as an ECMO complication.

Taylor et al. (67) have reported imaging (CT and cranial sonogram) results from a large group ($n = 207$) of infants treated with ECMO. Forty-six percent had intracranial abnormalities; 50% had hemorrhage only, 28% had nonhemorrhagic only, and 22% had both conditions combined. There was no lateralizing predominance of injury. Neuroimaging CT abnormalities obtained three weeks after discontinuation of ECMO were correlated with developmental outcome at one year by Taylor et al. (92) Imaging abnormalities were associated with an increased risk of developmental delay at one year, but the sensitivity and specificity of normal imaging in predicting normal outcome was low.

MRI of the brain is being utilized in some centers now to follow post-ECMO patients. The advantages of MRI over CT scan include 1) lack of ionizing radiation; 2) greater sensitivity to blood flow, edema, hemorrhage, and, of particular importance, myelination (93); 3) lack of beam-hardening artifacts; and 4) easier differentiation between gray and white matter.

EEG and evoked potentials EEGs have been performed by some centers during ECMO, but interpretation of results has been difficult and conflicting. Recently, Campbell et al. (71) and Schumacher et al. (68) have used EEG following ECMO to evaluate potential lateralizing effects of right common carotid artery ligation. Campbell et al. (71) noted no increased incidence of right hemisphere EEG abnormalities in a select group of post-ECMO patients in whom EEGs were obtained "as clinically indicated." However, there was a predominance of left-sided focal seizures compared to right-sided seizures. Schumacher et al. (68) selected a group of post-ECMO patients with clinical indications for EEG study and noted a predominance of abnormal right-sided findings. However, these findings were in a small, select group, and it is difficult to extrapolate the results to all ECMO patients.

Evoked potentials (EPs) are electrographic brain responses to an environmental stimulus. Stimulus-evoked potentials can evaluate auditory, visual, and somatosensory functions. Because asphyxiated infants and/or infants with pulmonary hypertension have been identified as being at high risk for hearing loss (94), auditory EPs have been measured in many post-ECMO patients as a hearing screen prior to discharge; abnormal results are followed up.

Brain metabolism NMR was initially used for clinical spectroscopy to measure the concentration of adenosine triphosphate (ATP), phosphocreatine (PCr), and inorganic phosphate (Pi), as well as the intracellular tissue pH. These metabolites are intimately involved in the regulation of cellular energy. Alterations in CBF and metabolism produce energy changes that can be assessed noninvasively with NMR and phosphorus. A distinctive "NMR signature" can be noted over an area of localized hemispheric infarct, and spectroscopy is very sensitive to changes in tissue oxygenation (95).

PET has recently been introduced as a clinical and research tool by which cerebral oxygen and glucose extraction may be measured. The potential diagnostic and prognostic value of this tool has not yet been realized. Doyle et al. (96) used intravenous ^{18}F-2-fluoro-2-deoxy-D-glucose (^{18}FDG) to assess regional cerebral glucose metabolism by positron emission tomography in five neonates with structural brain abnormalities. Decreased glucose metabolism was identified in regions of the brain shown by CT scan to be structurally abnormal.

Brain blood flow studies Alterations in cerebral blood flow and distribution, impairment of CBF autoregulation, and changes in CBF pulsatility may all represent markers of CNS insult before, during, and after ECMO. There has been, therefore, a major clinical effort to apply basic techniques of CBF measurement to neonates at risk for CNS injury and, more recently, to ECMO patients. Three CBF techniques are currently being utilized; ^{133}Xenon clearance, Doppler flow velocities, and PET. In addition, digital intravenous angiography (DIVA) has been used to demonstrate bilateral filling of middle cerebral arteries (75) following ECMO. Younkin et al. (97) used ^{133}Xenon by inhalation in 21 term newborns "at risk for" (but without definite) neurologic problems. Regional flow differences were noted; flow was lowest in the frontal cortex and highest in the temporal and occipital regions, distinctly different from adult brain blood flow distribution. This group hopes to utilize this methodology to measure localized disturbances in regional CBF caused by focal neurologic problems.

Taylor et al. (69) have used transcutaneous Doppler ultrasound to study cerebral hemodynamics in infants at the onset of ECMO and during an ECMO run. The set onset of ECMO was associated with decreased pulsatility, more marked in the right middle cerebral artery (MCA) than in the left. In addition, the origin of blood to the right cerebral hemisphere was altered, with retrograde flow in the right internal carotid artery observed in over one-half of patients. As bypass flow was decreased, pulsatility increased. The investigators speculated that, at the onset of ECMO, altered MCA pulsatility may impair the capacity for autoregulation. Myers et al. (98) used serial Doppler ultrasound to monitor cerebral blood flow velocity in preterm infants; they reported dynamic changes in cerebral blood flow velocity in one infant during and after cardiac tamponade secondary to a pneumopericardium. They recommended utilizing this technique to "probe CNS autoregulatory pathophysiology and to evaluate the effects of therapeutic interventions" (98).

Volpe et al. (99) have used PET with intravenous injection of ^{15}O-labeled water to measure regional CBF in preterm infants with severe intracranial hemorrhage. They found that focal areas of parenchymal hemorrhage were actually small central components of much larger ischemic lesions. They speculated that this "tip of the iceberg" phenomenon accounted for the significantly poorer neurodevelopmental outcome of infants with parenchymal hemorrhages.

Neurodevelopmental outcome It is absolutely essential that findings from neuroimaging studies, EEG, evoked potentials, PET scans, and Doppler or Xenon flow studies be correlated with neurodevelopmental outcome. Without such correlations, study results may be of academic interest only. One study (52) retrospectively reviewed neuroimaging studies, developed a "neuroimaging score," and then correlated this score with Bayley scales at approximately 12 months. Although individual outcomes could not be predicted accurately with neuroimaging, the score was a potentially useful adjunct in assigning post-ECMO babies to neurodevelopmental risk categories.

MODIFICATIONS IN ECMO TECHNOLOGY TO OPTIMIZE CNS OUTCOME

Measures to protect the brain from injury prior to and during ECMO must continue to be undertaken. It appears that prior cerebral injury significantly increases the patient's risk of further CNS injury while on ECMO. Protective measures must start with prevention of perinatal asphyxia, which begins with good prenatal care and ends with skilled neonatal resuscitation. Once a newborn becomes critically ill with pulmonary hypertension, meconium aspiration, sepsis, etc., clinical measures designed to protect the brain pre-ECMO should include the following:

1. Stabilization of blood pressure. Hypotension is clearly detrimental, but rapid increases in blood pressure should also be avoided in a potentially pressure-passive cerebral circulation.

2. Correction of acidosis.

3. Avoidance of severe hypoxemia ($Pa_{O_2} < 30$ mm Hg).

4. Avoidance of sudden changes in Pa_{CO_2}.

5. Correction of significant anemia or polycythemia.

6. Normalization of coagulation factors.

While initiating and then maintaining ECMO support, the following measures are recommended to optimize CNS outcome:

1. Avoid rapid alterations in $PaCO_2$, particularly at the initiation of ECMO in a patient who has had prolonged hypocarbia.

2. Avoid hypertensive surges.

3. Avoid emboli.

4. Minimize cerebral venous stasis.

The following potential measures to protect the brain are currently being developed and tested in ECMO patients:

1. Heparin-bonded tubing to eliminate the need for systemic heparinization.

2. Reanastomosis of the carotid artery and the internal jugular vein after ECMO.

3. Proximal venous drainage to maintain stable intracranial venous pressure despite ligation of the jugular vein.

4. Microemboli arterial filters.

REFERENCES

(1) Lassen NA. Cerebral blood flow and oxygen consumption in man. Physiol Rev 1959;39:183.

(2) Kontos HA, Wei EP, Raper AJ, Rosenblum WI, Navari RM, Patterson JL. Role of tissue hypoxia in local regulation of cerebral microcirculation. Am J Physiol 1978;234(5):H582–H591.

(3) Mchedlishvili GI, Nikolaishvili LS, Antia RV. Are the pial arterial responses dependent on the direct effect of intravascular pressure and extravascular and intravascular PO_2, PCO_2, and pH? Microvasc Res 1976;10:298.

(4) Busija DW, Heistad DD. Factors involved in the physiological regulation of the cerebral circulation. Rev Physiol Biochem Pharmacol 1984;101:161–211.

(5) Tweed A, Cote J, Lou H, Gregory G, Wade J. Impairment of cerebral blood flow autoregulation in the newborn lamb by hypoxia. Pediatr Res 1986;20:516–9.

(6) Jones MD Jr, Koehler RC, Traystman RJ. Regulation of cerebral blood flow in the fetus, newborn, and adult. In: Guthrie RD, ed. Neonatal intensive care. New York: Churchill Livingstone Inc, 1988.

(7) Harris AP, Koehler RC, Gleason CA, Jones MD Jr, Traystman RJ. Cerebral and peripheral circulatory responses to intracranial hypertension in fetal sheep. Circ Res 1989;64:991–1000.

(8) Jones MD Jr, Traystman RJ, Simmons MA, Molteni RA. Effects of changes in arterial O_2 content on cerebral blood flow in the lamb. Am J Physiol 1981;240:H209–H215.

(9) Koehler RC, Traystman RJ, Zeger S, Rogers MC, Jones MD Jr. Comparison of cerebrovascular response to hypoxic and carbon monoxide hypoxia in newborn and adult sheep. J Cereb Blood Flow Metab 1984;4:115–22.

(10) Ashwal S, Majcher JS, Longo LD. Patterns of fetal lamb regional cerebral blood flow during and after prolonged hypoxia: studies during the posthypoxic recovery period. Am J Obstet Gynecol 1981;139:365–72.

(11) Gleason CA, Hamm C, Jones MD Jr. Effect of acute hypoxemia on brain blood flow and oxygen metabolism in immature fetal sheep. Am J Physiology (in press.)

(12) Bender KS, Short BL, Walker LK, Gleason CA, Solca ME, Traystman RJ. Effects of hypoxemia, carotid artery (CA) and jugular vein (JV) ligation on cerebral blood flow (CBF) and oxygen consumption ($CMRO_2$) in newborn lambs [Abstract]. Pediatr Res 1989;25:208A.

(13) Bocking AD, Gagnon R, Richardson BS, Homan J, White SE. Cerebral blood flow during prolonged hypoxemia in fetal sheep [Abstract]. Society for Gynecologic Investigations Annual Meeting, Baltimore MD, Scientific abstracts 1988;183.

(14) Jones MD Jr, Traystman RJ. Cerebral oxygenation of the fetus, newborn, and adult. Semin Perinatol 1984;8:205–16.

(15) Gleason CA, Jones MD Jr, Traystman RJ, Notter RH. Fetal cerebral responses to ventilation and oxygenation in utero. Am J Physiol 1988;255:R1049–R1054.

(16) Kennedy C, Grave GD, Jehle JW. Effect of hyperoxia on the cerebral circulation of the newborn puppy. Pediatr Res 1971;5:659–67.

(17) Rahilly PM. Effects of 2% carbon dioxide, 0.5% carbon dioxide and 100% oxygen on cranial blood flow of the human neonate. Pediatrics 1980;66:685.

(18) Leahy FAN, Cates D, MacCallum M,

Rigatto H. Effect of CO_2 and 100% O_2 on cerebral blood flow in preterm infants. J Appl Physiol: Respir Environ Exercise Physiol 1980; 48(3):468–72.

(19) Jones MD Jr, Sheldon RE, Peeters LL, Meschia G, Battaglia FC, Makowski EL. Fetal cerebral oxygen consumption at different levels of oxygenation. J Appl Physiol: Respir Environ Exercise Physiol 1977;43(6):1080–4.

(20) Massik J, Tang Y-L, Hudak ML, Koehler RC, Traystman RJ, Jones MD Jr. Effect of hematocrit on cerebral blood flow with induced polycythemia. J Appl Physiol 1987;62(3):1090–6.

(21) Siesjo BK. Cerebral circulation and metabolism. J Neurosurg 1984;60:883–908.

(22) Donegan JH, Traystman RJ, Koehler RC, Jones MD Jr, Rogers MC. Cerebrovascular hypoxic and autoregulatory responses during reduced brain metabolism. Am J Physiol 1985; 249:H421–H429.

(23) Fujishima M, Scheinberg P, Busto R, Reinmuth OM. The relation between cerebral oxygen consumption and cerebral vascular reactivity to carbon dioxide. Stroke 1971;2:251–7.

(24) Metzger H. Effects of direct stimulation on cerebral cortex oxygen tension level. Microvascular Res 1979;17:80–89.

(25) Plum F, Duffy TE. The couple between cerebral metabolism and blood flow during seizures. In: Ingvar DH, Lassen NA, eds. Brain work. Proceedings of the Alfred Benzon Symposium VIII. Copenhagen. Munksgaard, 1975.

(26) Leniger-Follert E, Lubbers DW. Behavior of microflow and local PO_2 of the brain cortex during and after direct electrical stimulation. Pflugers Arch 1976;366:39–44.

(27) Meldrum BS, Nilsson B. Cerebral blood flow and metabolic rate early and late in prolonged epileptic seizures induced in rats by bicuculline. Brain 1976;99:523–42.

(28) Winn HR, Welsh JE, Rubio R, Berne RM. Changes in brain adenosine during bicuculline-induced seizures in rats. Circ Res 1980;47:568–77.

(29) Gleason CA, Short BL, Jones MD Jr. Cerebral blood flow and metabolism during and after prolonged hypocapnia in newborn lambs. J Pediatr 1989;155:309–14.

(30) Hansen NB, Nowicki PT, Miller RR, Malone T, Bickers RG, Menke JA. Alterations in cerebral blood flow and oxygen consumption during prolonged hypocarbia. Pediatr Res 1986; 20:147–50.

(31) Albrecht RF, Miletich DJ, Ruttle M. Cerebral effects of extended hyperventilation in unanesthetized goats. Stroke 1987;18:649–55.

(32) Rosenberg AA, Jones MD Jr, Traystman RJ, Simmons MA, Molteni RA. Response of cerebral blood flow to changes in PCO_2 in fetal, newborn, and adult sheep. Am J Physiol 1982;242:H862–H866.

(33) Levasseur JE, Wei EP, Kontos HA, Patterson JL Jr. Responses of pial arterioles after prolonged hypercapnia and hypoxia in the awake rabbit. J Appl Physiol: Respir Environ Exercise Physiol 1979;46(1):89–95.

(34) MacMillan V. The effect of combined hypocapnia and hypoxemia upon the energy metabolism of the brain. Can J Physiol Pharmacol 1974;52:1136–46.

(35) Gregory GA, Ong W, Tweed A, Wade JG. The effects of severe alkalosis and hypoxemia on cerebral metabolism in the newborn lamb. Anesthesiology 1982;57:A424–35.

(36) Delivoria-Papadopoulos M, Wagerle LC, Cahillane G, Goplerud JM, Mishra OP. Cerebral oxygenation and membrane dysfunction following hyperventilation in newborn (NB) piglets [Abstract]. Pediatr Res 1988;23:231A.

(37) Jones MD Jr. Energy metabolism in the developing brain. Sem Perinatol 1979;3(2):121–9.

(38) Owen OE, Morgan AP, Kemp HG, Sullivan JM, Herrera MG, Cahill GF Jr. Brain metabolism during fasting. J Clin Invest 1967;46(10):1589.

(39) Levine S. Anoxic-ischemic encephalopathy in rats. Am J Pathol 1960;36:1–13.

(40) Lassen NA. The luxury-perfusion syndrome and its possible relation to acute metabolic acidosis localised within the brain. Lancet 1966;2:1113–5.

(41) Ames A III, Wright RL, Kowada M, et al. Cerebral ischemia. II. The no-reflow phenomenon. Am J Pathol 1968;52:437–53.

(42) Rehncrona S, Rosen I, Siesjo BK. Brain lactic acidosis and ischemic cell damage. 1. Biochemistry and neurophysiology. J Cereb Blood Flow Metab 1981;1:297–311.

(43) Rehncrona S, Rosen I, Siesjo BK. Excessive cellular acidosis: an important mechanism of neuronal damage in the brain? Acta Physiol Scand 1980;110:435–7.

(44) Meldrum B. Possible therapeutic applica-

tions of antagonists of excitatory amino acid neurotransmitters. Clin Sci 1985;68:113–22.

(45) Thiringer K, Hrbek A, Karlsson K, Rosen KG, Kjellmer I. Postasphyxial cerebral survival in newborn sheep after treatment with oxygen free radical scavengers and a calcium antagonist. Pediatr Res 1987;22:62–6.

(46) Schreiber MD, Heymann MA, Soifer SJ. Increased arterial pH, not decreased $PaCO_2$, attenuates hypoxia-reduced pulmonary vasoconstriction in newborn lambs. Pediatr Res 1986;20:113–7.

(47) Wung J-T, James LS, Kilchevsky E, James E. Management of infants with severe respiratory failure and persistence of the fetal circulation, without hyperventilation. Pediatrics 1985;76:488–94.

(48) Shapiro W, Wasserman AJ, Patterson JL. Human cerebrovascular response to combined hypoxia and hypercapnia. Circ Res 1966;29:903.

(49) McPherson RW, Eimerl D, Traystman RJ. Interaction of hypoxia and hypercapnia on cerebral hemodynamics and brain electrical activity in dogs. Am J Physiol 1987;253:H890–H897.

(50) Gardiner RM. Cerebral blood flow and oxidative metabolism during hypoxia and asphyxia in the new-born calf and lamb. J Physiol 1980;305:357–76.

(51) Massik J, Jones MD Jr, Miyabe M, et al. Hypercapnia and response of cerebral blood flow to hypoxia in newborn lambs. J Appl Physiol 1989;66(3):1065–70.

(52) Kontos HA, Raper AJ, Patterson JL. Analysis of vasoactivity of local pH, PCO_2 and bicarbonate on pial vessels. Stroke 1977;8:358–60.

(53) Hermansen MC, Kotagal UR, Kleinman LI. The effect of metabolic acidosis upon autoregulation of cerebral blood flow in newborn dogs. Brain Res 1984;324:101–5.

(54) Harper AM, Bell RA. The effect of metabolic acidosis and alkalosis on the blood flow through the cerebral cortex. J Neurol Neurosurg Psychiat 1963;26:341–4.

(55) Arvidsson S, Haggendal E, Winso I. Influence on cerebral blood flow of infusion of sodium bicarbonate during respiratory acidosis and alkalosis in the dog. Acta Anaesth Scand 1981;25:146–52.

(56) Simmons MA, Adcock EW III, Bard H, Battaglia FC. Hypernatremia and intracranial hemorrhage in neonates. N Engl J Med 1974;291:6–10.

(57) Laptook AR. The effects of sodium bicarbonate on brain blood flow and O_2 delivery during hypoxemia and acidemia in the piglet. Pediatr Res 1985;19:815–9.

(58) Peabody JL. Muscle relaxants—a potential danger to infants at risk for intraventricular hemorrhage. Pediatr Res 1981;15:709A.

(59) Belik J, Wagerle LC, Delivoria-Papadopoulos M. Cerebral blood flow and metabolism following pancuronium bromide in newborn lambs. Pediatr Res 1984;18:1305–8.

(60) Yaster M, Koehler RC, Traystman RJ. Effects of fentanyl on peripheral and cerebral hemodynamics in neonatal lambs. Anesthesiology 1987;66:524–30.

(61) deLemos RA, Tomasovic JJ. Effects of positive pressure ventilation on cerebral blood flow in the newborn infant. Clin Perinatol 1978;5(2):395–409.

(62) Hill A, Perlman JM, Volpe JJ. Relationship of pneumothorax to occurrence of intraventricular hemorrhage in the premature newborn. Pediatrics 1982;69:144–9.

(63) Laptook A, Stonestreet BS, Oh W. The effects of different rates of plasmanate infusions upon brain blood flow after asphyxia and hypotension in newborn piglets. J Pediatr 1982;100(5):791–6.

(64) Goldberg RN, Chung D, Goldman SL, Bancalari E. The association of rapid volume expansion and intraventricular hemorrhage in the preterm infant. J Pediatr 1980;96(6):1060–3.

(65) Goddard-Finegold J, Armstrong D, Zeller RS. Intraventricular hemorrhage following volume expansion after hypovolemic hypotension in the newborn beagle. J Pediatr 1982;100(5):796–9.

(66) Glass P, Miller M, Short B. Morbidity for survivors of extracorporeal membrane oxygenation: neurodevelopmental outcome at 1 year of age. Pediatrics 1989;83(1):72–8.

(67) Taylor GA, Short BL, Fitz CR. Imaging of cerebrovascular injury in infants treated with extracorporeal membrane oxygenation. J Pediatr 1989;114(4):635–9.

(68) Schumacher RE, Barks JDE, Johnston MV, et al. Right-sided brain lesions in infants following extracorporeal membrane oxygenation. Pediatrics 1988;82(2):155–60.

(69) Taylor GA, Short BL, Glass P, Ichord R. Cerebral hemodynamics in infants undergoing extracorporeal membrane oxygenation: further observations. Radiology 1988;168:163–7.

(70) Ichord R, Short BL, Davis R. Carotid artery

(71) Campbell LR, Bunyapen C, Holmes GL, Howell CG, Kanto WP. Right common carotid artery ligation in extracorporeal membrane oxygenation. J Pediatr 1988;113:110–13.

(72) Zak LK, Donn SM. Association of extracorporeal membrane oxygenation (ECMO) and neonatal seizures [Abstract]. Clin Res 1988;36:900A.

(73) Lott IT, Towne BM, McPherson DM. Permanent ligation of the right common carotid artery at birth: 18 cases. Pediatr Res 1985;19:392A.

(74) Raju TNK, Kim SY, Meller JL, Srinivasan G, Ghai V, Reyes H. Circle of Willis blood velocity and flow direction after common carotid artery ligation for neonatal extracorporeal membrane oxygenation. Pediatrics 1989;83:343–7.

(75) Voorhies TM, Tardo CL, Starrett AL, et al. Evaluation of the cerebral circulation in neonates following extracorporeal membrane oxygenation. Ann Neurol 1985;18:380.

(76) Lundar T, Lindegaard K-F, Froysaker T, Aaslid R, Grip A, Nornes H. Dissociation between cerebral autoregulation and carbon dioxide reactivity during nonpulsatile cardiopulmonary bypass. Ann Thorac Surg 1985;40:582–7.

(77) Henriksen L. Brain luxury perfusion during cardiopulmonary bypass in humans. A study of the cerebral blood flow response to changes in CO_2, O_2 and blood pressure. J Cereb Blood Flow Metab 1986;6:366–78.

(78) Johnsson P, Messeter K, Ryding E, Nordstrom L, Stahl E. Cerebral blood flow and autoregulation during hypothermic cardiopulmonary bypass. Ann Thorac Surg 1987;43:386–90.

(79) Stump DA, Rogers AT, Prough DS, Gravles GP, Wallenhaupt SA. Spontaneous decline of cerebral blood flow during hypothermic cardiopulmonary bypass. Anesth Analg 1988;67:S223.

(80) Rogers AT, Stump DA, Prough DS, Angert KC, Wallenhaupt SA. Cerebrovascular responsiveness to PaO_2 is preserved during hypothermic cardiopulmonary bypass. Anesthesiology 1987;87:12.

(81) Rogers AT, Gravles GP, Prough DS, Stump DA, Angert KC. Cerebral autoregulation is impaired during cardiopulmonary bypass. Anesthesiology 1988;65:A12.

(82) Greeley WJ, Ungerleider RM, Smith LR, Reves JG. The effects of deep hypothermic cardiopulmonary bypass and total circulatory arrest on cerebral blood flow in infants and children. J Thorac Cardiovasc Surg 1989;97:737–45.

(83) Sotaniemi KA, Mononen H, Hokkanen TE. Long-term cerebral outcome after open-heart surgery. Stroke 1986;17:410–6.

(84) Nevin M, Adams S, Colchester ACF, Pepper JR. Evidence for involvement of hypocapnia and hypoperfusion in aetiology of neurological deficit after cardiopulmonary bypass. Lancet 1987;2:1493–5.

(85) Rudy LW Jr, Heymann MA, Edmunds LH Jr. Distribution of systemic blood flow during cardiopulmonary bypass. J Appl Physiol 1973;34(2):194–200.

(86) Santillan GG, Chemnitius JM, Bing RJ. The effect of cardiopulmonary bypass on cerebral blood flow. Brain Res 1985;345:1–9.

(87) Clark RE, Dietz DR, Miller JG. Continuous detection of microemboli during cardiopulmonary bypass in animals and man. Cardiovasc Surg 1976;54(Suppl 3):III74–III78.

(88) Anderson K, Waaben J, Husum B, et al. Nonpulsatile cardiopulmonary bypass disrupts the flow-metabolism couple in the brain. J Thorac Cardiovasc Surg 1985;90:570–9.

(89) Short BL, Walker LK, Gleason CA, et al. The effect of extracorporeal membrane oxygenation (ECMO) on cerebral blood flow and cerebral oxygen metabolism in the newborn sheep. Pediatr Res 1990;28:50–3.

(90) Walker LK, Short BL, Gleason CA, et al. Cerebrovascular response to CO_2 during ECMO. Pediatr Res 1988;23:429A.

(91) Klesch KW, Murphy TF, Scher MS, Buchanan DE, Maxwell EP, Guthrie RD. Cerebral infarction in persistent pulmonary hypertension of the newborn. Am J Dis Child 1987;141:852–7.

(92) Taylor GA, Glass P, Fitz CR, Miller MK. Neurologic status in infants treated with extracorporeal membrane oxygenation: correlation of imaging findings with developmental outcome. Radiology 1987;165:679–82.

(93) Gooding CA, Brasch RC, Lallemand DP, Wesbey GE, Brant-Zawadzki MN. Nuclear magnetic resonance imaging of the brain in children. J Pediatr 1984;104(4):509–15.

(94) Hendricks-Munoz KD, Walton JP. Hearing loss in infants with persistent fetal circulation. Pediatrics 1988;81(5):650–6.

(95) Delivoria-Papadopoulos M, Chance B. ^{31}P NMR spectroscopy in the newborn. In: Guthrie

RD, ed. Neonatal intensive care. New York: Churchill Livingstone, 1986.

(96) Doyle LW, Nahmias C, Firnau G, Kenyon DB, Garnett ES, Sinclair JC. Regional cerebral glucose metabolism of newborn infants measured by positron emission tomography. Dev Med Child Neurol 1983;25:143–51.

(97) Younkin D, Delivoria-Papadopoulos M, Reivich M, Jaggi J, Obrist W. Regional variations in human newborn cerebral blood flow. J Pediatr 1988;112:104–8.

(98) Myers TF, Patrinos ME, Muraskas J, Caldwell CC, Lambert GH, Anderson CL. Dynamic trend monitoring of cerebral blood flow velocity in newborn infants. J Pediatr 1987;110:611–6.

(99) Volpe JJ, Herscovitch P, Perlman JM, Raichle ME. Positron emission tomography in the newborn: extensive impairment of regional cerebral blood flow with intraventricular hemorrhage and hemorrhagic intracerebral involvement. Pediatrics 1983;72:589–601.

11

Pre-ECMO Considerations for Neonatal Patients

Billie L. Short, M.D.

Over the 10-year period from 1973, when the first neonatal patient was entered into the Neonatal Registry data base, until 1983, only 99 infants had been treated with extracorporeal membrane oxygenation (ECMO) in only three ECMO centers in the United States. Following those initial years, the development and expansion of ECMO therapy have been explosive; more than 4,000 infants have been treated in more than 60 new ECMO programs. Although ECMO has become accepted as a rescue therapy offered to an increasing number of newborns, it is still in its infancy regarding its development and potential applications. Current use of ECMO resembles that of ventilator therapy for infants 25 years ago, a time when ventilator therapy was personnel-intensive and physicians stayed in the hospital to take care of infants in respiratory failure. The ventilator itself was designed primarily for adult use and then modified for neonatal applications (1). Although this chapter will describe the clinical procedures currently used in neonatal ECMO, as with any new technology, significant changes in these procedures will occur in the next few years. This chapter will address only the clinical procedures used for venoarterial ECMO in the neonate. Adult, pediatric, and venovenous ECMO are reviewed in Chapters 20, 19, and 18, respectively.

CRITERIA FOR ECMO THERAPY

One of the most controversial topics related to ECMO therapy has been the patient selection criteria (2–9). Because of the invasive nature of ECMO and the potential risks associated with this therapy, ECMO criteria used today attempt to select a population of infants who have a high (80%) mortality risk with conventional therapy. Assumptions about the ability of ECMO to increase survival can only be true if our criteria are specific for this high-risk population. The ultimate test for the efficacy of ECMO and the predictability of ECMO criteria would be a randomized clinical trial. Although two randomized trials have been completed, most centers have used historical controls to develop their criteria (2,8,10). In the prospective randomized trial by O'Rourke et al. (8), the design may have skewed the predictability of their criteria, but it must be noted that the criteria employed in that study, thought to predict an 80% mortality from retrospective data, produced only a 40% mortality when applied prospectively. It is, therefore, imperative that ECMO centers continually evaluate their criteria, particularly as less invasive therapies become available.

The potential risk-producing procedures associated with ECMO include ligation of the carotid artery and jugular vein, prolonged systemic anticoagulation, alterations in pulsatile blood flow patterns, exposure to potential toxins such as aluminum and phthalate esters (plasticizer) from the circuit, and other risks yet to be determined (11–14). With its long-term outcome still unknown, use of ECMO should be limited to the term or near-term infant who has a 20% or less chance of survival with conventional therapy.

Development of patient selection criteria requires an in-depth retrospective review of potential ECMO cases over a period when clinical care was similar to present. This process is laborious but vital. The development of criteria should be undertaken early in an ECMO program's development because of the time needed for this process. For example, at Children's National Medical Center (CNMC), the chart review and statistical analysis took eight months.

Although criteria that have been developed in other centers are available, clinical management and patient populations differ enough to make these criteria invalid in other institutions (4,5,7). What is considered "maximal conventional therapy," such as hyperventilation, in one institution may not be used in others. Also, differences in patient populations, such as the percentage of patients who are inborn versus the percentage of outborn, may significantly alter applicability of criteria from one center to another. Therefore, all ECMO centers should attempt to develop criteria based on their management techniques and patient population.

Inclusion Criteria

Several general "inclusion" criteria for ECMO are based on known complications of the procedure. These are listed in Table 11.1. Each of these inclusion criteria will be discussed separately.

TABLE 11.1 General inclusion criteria for ECMO

Gestational age ≥34 weeks or
Birthweight ≥2,000 grams
No significant coagulopathy or bleeding complications
No major intracranial hemorrhage
Mechanical ventilation < 10–14 days
Reversible lung injury
No major cardiac lesion
No major nonpulmonary pathology
Life-threatening cardiac and/or respiratory failure unresponsive to conventional treatment

Gestational age ≥34 weeks or birthweight ≥ 2,000 grams The requirement for systemic anticoagulation of the ECMO patient places significant limitations on the population treated. Initial use of ECMO in the late 1960s and early 1970s in premature infants weighing <2,000 grams or <34 weeks gestation resulted in significant mortality related to intracranial hemorrhage (14–18). Although some refinement of the procedure occurred in the early 1980s, premature infants continue to experience significantly higher risks of intracranial hemorrhage with ECMO therapy than more mature neonates. This increased risk may result from the combination of systemic anticoagulation and the effect of ECMO on the brain (see Chapter 10) (19). Concerns for an increased rate of intracranial hemorrhage in premature infants are corroborated by findings in infants in the ECMO population at CNMC of 34–36 weeks gestational age. This group of patients has a 50% incidence of intracranial hemorrhage, representing more than 50% of the major intracranial hemorrhages seen in the total population at CNMC (14,20). Therefore, it is recommended that only neonates weighing more than 2,000 grams or older than 33 weeks' gestational age be considered candidates for ECMO. New advances, such as heparin-bonded circuits and a better understanding of the effects of ECMO on the brain, may permit us to lower the gestational age cutoff in the future (21).

Lack of significant coagulopathy or bleeding complications The requirement for systemic anticoagulation also places infants with significant coagulopathies or bleeding complications such as pulmonary hemorrhage at extreme risk. All attempts should be made to correct any coagulopathy prior to the institution of ECMO. If the coagulopathy is severe and cannot be corrected with appropriate blood product replacement, the infant should not be considered for ECMO.

The septic infant is of concern because of commonly associated coagulopathy. Although these infants are at higher risk for bleeding complications on ECMO, correction of their coagulopathies and meticulous heparin management have permitted successful treatment (22).

Many infants have blood-tinged tracheal aspirate fluid before ECMO that can be easily managed with higher peak end-expiratory pressures (PEEP) and lower activated clotting times. An infant with an uncontrolled, massive pulmonary hemorrhage prior to ECMO should not be considered a candidate. Any bleeding that is uncontrolled prior to ECMO will only become "your worst nightmare" after systemic anticoagulation. It should be remembered that almost all deaths on ECMO are related to a bleeding complication (23,24).

No major intracranial hemorrhage (> grade I IVH) As above, heparin therapy precludes the treatment of any infant with a major intracranial hemorrhage. Infants with Grade I intraventricular hemorrhages (IVH) or small parenchymal hemorrhages can be treated if heparin management is monitored closely and activated clotting times are kept between 190 and 210 seconds. At CNMC, 13 infants had a small subependymal or parenchymal hemorrhage prior to ECMO, only five of which extended after ECMO was instituted (14). New centers should not attempt to treat infants with any intracranial hemorrhage until significant experience with ECMO has been attained (at least 10 patients).

Mechanical ventilation less than 10 to 14 days and reversible lung disease The limit of 10 to 14 days of assisted ventilation is related to the development of chronic lung disease after this period of assisted ventilation and the inability of ECMO to reverse permanent pulmonary fibrosis.

The power of ECMO therapy lies in the ability of the infant to reverse the underlying lung disease in a relatively short time. Therefore, the infant must have a disease process that can be improved or completely reversed within 14 to 20 days. After 14 days, the risks of complications related to the ECMO procedure itself, such as clot formation, nosocomial infections (including neck wound infections), and mechanical failures such as tubing rupture, begin to increase. The maximal time on the ECMO circuit is not known, but the above factors have made most centers limit time on the circuit to less than three or four weeks.

Because of the cardiopulmonary support given by this therapy, ECMO has allowed many infants thought to have irreversible lung disease to live. Patients in this category have included some infants with congenital diaphragmatic hernia, renal dysplasia, oligohydramnios, and pulmonary hypoplasia hydrops (25–29).

No major cardiac lesion Cardiac disease should be ruled out before ECMO's institution. However, infants with severe lung disease complicating congenital heart disease may be offered ECMO before repair of their cardiac disease if their clinical status makes them poor candidates for surgery.

Eighty Percent Mortality Criteria

Commonly used criteria are 1) the alveolar-arterial (A-a) oxygen gradient, 2) the oxygen index (OI), and 3) Pao_2 levels <50 mm Hg over a specific time period (3,6,7,30). These are summarized in Table 11.2. The first two may be calculated as follows:

$$A_aDo_2 = P_B - 47 - Paco_2 - Pao_2 \qquad (1)$$

where P_B is the barometric pressure and 47 is the partial pressure of water vapor.

$$OI = \frac{MAP \times Fio_2 \times 100}{Pao_2} \qquad (2)$$

where MAP is the mean airway pressure.

Most centers require that ECMO candidates

TABLE 11.2 The most commonly used neonatal ECMO criteria

A_aDo_2
  Range: 605 to 620 torr × 4 to 12 hours
Oxygen index (OI)
  Range: >35 to >60 × 0.5 to 6 hours
Pao_2
  Range: <35 to <50 mm Hg × 2 to 12 hours
Barotrauma
  pH <7.25 × 2 hours or with hypotension
Acute deterioration
  Range: Pao_2 <30 to <40 mm Hg

Note: 50% of centers use more than one of the above.

---

meet local criteria since these reflect the patient management techniques of each center. In most centers, 30% to 50% of infants transferred for ECMO improve and require no therapy.

Infants are sometimes placed on ECMO using the criterion of "acute deterioration." Generally, this means a Pao_2 of <30 mm Hg with or without hypotension or an infant who is in cardiopulmonary arrest. Data from CNMC have shown that infants who go on ECMO with a Pao_2 of <30 mm Hg have a mortality rate of 50%. Criteria for patients with congenital diaphragmatic hernia (CDH) may differ from criteria for those without CDH in some institutions (see Chapter 17).

ECMO REFERRALS: WHEN TO CALL AND HOW TO TRANSPORT

ECMO is a "high-tech," "people-intensive" therapy treating a relatively small number of infants. To ensure the maintenance of clinical expertise and cost effectiveness of ECMO, centers should be developed to meet demonstrated regional needs. For this to work effectively, regional ECMO centers must be capable of transporting critically ill infants from referral centers to their institution. Most ECMO centers cover a large regional area and use a combination of ground and air (both helicopter and fixed wing) transport.

One of the most difficult tasks in running a successful regional ECMO program is knowing when a patient should be transferred to the ECMO center. Because most infants with disease states treated by ECMO improve without ECMO, the referring physician must attempt to determine which infants are at high risk for failing maximal therapy before they are too sick for transport. Early consultation with the ECMO center allows both teams to participate in determining the appropriate time for referral.

Most ECMO centers require that patients referred for ECMO meet criteria in their institution. Therefore, to decrease the risk of death in transport, infants should be transferred before they meet ECMO criteria. Kanto and others (31,32) found that 12% of their ECMO referrals died prior to the transport team's arrival at the referring center or during the transport. Of these deaths, 32% involved CDH patients, indicating that early referral of these patients is warranted. Data from our center show that approximately 20 infants per year, or 16% of our ECMO referrals, died prior to or during transport. For patients not surviving transport, the average peak inspiratory pressure (PIP) at the time of the referral call was 50 cm H_2O with a Pao_2 of 28 mm Hg, as compared to 45 cm H_2O and 40 mm Hg in our ECMO survivors. It appears that earlier transfer may have increased the survival in these infants.

There are no standard criteria for transfer, but data from the Extracorporeal Life Support Organization (ELSO) Neonatal Registry and from each regional ECMO center characterizing the blood gas data and ventilator requirements typical of ECMO patients before initiation of ECMO can be used to determine minimal criteria for transfer. As can be seen in Table 11.3, the typical ECMO patient is on a PIP of 45.9 cm H_2O with a rate of 96 breaths per minute (bpm), Fio_2 of 1.00, resulting in an average pH of 7.39, $Paco_2$ of 41, and Pao_2 of 41. Consultation for transfer should occur before incurring these ventilator requirements and definitely before reaching a Pao_2 of 40. As noted in Table 11.3, respiratory acidosis was associated with significant increase in mortality. Therefore, any infant in this category should be transferred earlier.

TABLE 11.3 Average ventilator settings and blood gas values at institution of ECMO: survivors vs. nonsurvivors

	Total	Survivors	Nonsurvivors
Rate	97 ± 74	96 ± 74	99 ± 75
Fio_2	1.00	1.00	1.00
PIP*	46 ± 11	46 ± 10	45 ± 12
PEEP†	4 ± 3	4 ± 3	6 ± 3
MAP‡	19 ± 5	19 ± 5	19 ± 5
pH	7.39 ± 0.2	7.41 ± 0.2	7.29 ± 0.2§
Pco_2	42 ± 24	39 ± 21	52 ± 32§
Po_2	41 ± 32	41 ± 31	38 ± 32§

Note: Data from the Extracorporeal Life Support Organization (ELSO) Neonatal Registry, July 1990. Data displayed in mean ± standard deviation.
*PIP = peak inspiratory pressure.
†PEEP = positive end-expiratory pressure.
‡MAP = mean airway pressure.
§$p < 0.05$, survivors vs. nonsurvivors.

Studies Required Prior to Transfer for ECMO

Infants with congenital heart disease are not usually considered candidates for ECMO. If cardiology consultative services exist in the referring hospital, congenital heart disease should be ruled out prior to transfer. The infant with significant pulmonary disease, such as meconium aspiration, in addition to a congenital heart defect may be a candidate for ECMO, but only after consultation with pediatric cardiology and cardiovascular experts. The rationale in treating these infants with ECMO is to supply the time needed for resolution of the lung disease, permitting repair of the cardiac lesion under more controlled conditions. Transfer of the infant from the ECMO circuit to the cardiovascular bypass circuit can be performed easily in the surgical suite.

Other studies that should be obtained before transfer of the ECMO patient include: head ultrasound to rule out a significant intracranial hemorrhage; coagulation studies, including partial thromboplastin time (PTT), prothrombin time (PT), fibrinogen, fibrin degradation products (FDP), and platelet count; calcium and electrolyte levels; white blood cell count with differential; and hemoglobin and hematocrit levels. These studies will help the ECMO center determine whether the patient should be considered for ECMO and, if so, help the treatment team anticipate difficulties.

Transport of the ECMO Candidate

Transport of an ECMO candidate can be extremely difficult, requiring an experienced transport team with appropriate equipment. Equipment and expertise become significant factors when long-distance transports are involved. ECMO candidates generally require a fractional inspired oxygen concentration of 1.00 and ventilator rates and pressures higher than usual. The team must be able to provide appropriate ventilator support with an ample oxygen supply for transport. This becomes even more difficult when air transport is involved. Centers should not try to "put together" the transport of an ECMO candidate. Air transport requires special equipment and a team trained in high-altitude ventilation techniques. The reader is referred to the text on neonatal transport edited by MacDonald and Miller for further details (33).

The Pre-ECMO Evaluation

On admission to the ECMO center, it must be determined whether the patient is an appropriate ECMO candidate. Although studies may have been done prior to admission, most should be repeated before the initiation of ECMO. Ultrasound examination of the head should be repeated to ensure that an intracranial hemorrhage did not occur during transport. The cardiac evaluation should be repeated if there are any questions concerning the possibility of cardiac disease. It is also important to attempt to document the severity of pulmonary hypertension in these infants using Doppler flow techniques. This information can be used later if the infant cannot be weaned from ECMO appropriately (see Chapter 9) (34). The following studies should be obtained on admission to determine if there are any abnormal values requiring correction prior to ECMO: serum electrolyte and calcium levels, hemoglobin and hematocrit, and clotting studies, including fibrinogen, fibrin degradation products, PT/PTT, platelets, and a baseline activated clotting time.

Most ECMO candidates have been pharmacologically paralyzed, making the neurologic status difficult to evaluate. It is, therefore, imperative to obtain a complete prenatal history, including Apgar scores, history of resuscitation, any history of seizure activity, and a description of the neurologic status of the infant prior to paralysis. Infants who have sustained severe neurologic damage should not be considered for ECMO.

ECMO EQUIPMENT

Most equipment used for ECMO therapy is modified cardiopulmonary bypass equipment which was initially designed for short-term bypass. To ensure safe and effective use of ECMO equipment, the limitations of each piece of equipment must be understood and considered before its application to long-term bypass.

There is no one "ECMO machine." Each ECMO center must design an ECMO system using equipment it has evaluated and designed to meet its unique requirements. It is recommended that bioengineering experts and cardiopulmonary perfusionists be consulted in the evaluation and design of the ECMO system. Basic equipment needed for a complete system is listed in Table 11.4, and an example of a complete system is seen in Figures 11.1–11.3. Each piece of equipment will be discussed separately.

TABLE 11.4 Equipment used in neonatal ECMO

Roller occlusion pump
Pump base
Venous return monitor
Heating unit
Coagulation timer
Membrane mounting board
Oxygen blender
Carbon dioxide or carbogen tank
O_2 and CO_2 flow meters
Temperature probes, in-line
Oxygen saturation monitor, in-line

The ECMO System

The ECMO system should be designed with space requirements and the possibility that the ECMO patient may have to be transported taken into consideration. Although these systems are not designed to be transported, occasionally, an infant with suspected heart disease may require a trip to the cardiac catheterization laboratory; furthermore, some major surgical procedures in the operating room may be necessary. The system should be set up on a cart or base that can be moved if necessary. The system at CNMC is placed on the pump base made by the pump company. This approach has the advantage that the pump base provides all the electrical power, which makes it possible to connect the electrical systems of the individual components to the base. Thus, only one electrical cord is needed to supply the entire system. Others have used carts of various designs. A mock unit should be designed and taken to the bedside to ensure its appropriate size before the permanent system is purchased and assembled.

Tubing Packs, Raceway Tubing, and Catheters

After the final design of the equipment has been determined, the disposable tubing packs can be designed to best fit that system. Blood exposure is a significant risk with ECMO; therefore, all efforts should be made to decrease the volume of the circuit. The size of the tubing is dependent on the blood flows

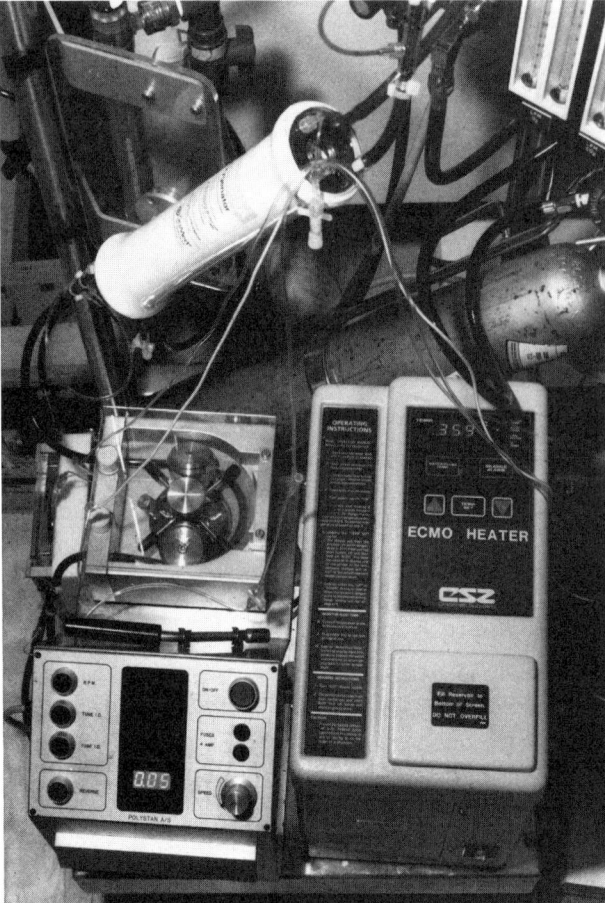

FIGURE 11.1 The complete ECMO system with tubing, membrane lung, and priming bag in place.

needed during the course of ECMO. Because neonatal flow requirements usually are <500 mL/min, ¼-inch internal diameter tubing will offer minimal circuit resistance and volume requirement.

The circuit design should attempt to enhance laminar flow patterns to decrease hemolysis and/or fibrin deposition and the formation of clots. Therefore, changes in tubing diameter, acute angles in the circuit, or stagnant zones are to be avoided. Although Figure 11.4 represents a minimal change in diameter, it exemplifies a stagnant flow area at the ¼-inch × ¼-inch connector/tubing interface. Most circuits have some fibrin formation at these connections after an ECMO run, but if the anticoagulation is not monitored closely and is allowed to decrease to low levels, clots can form at these points.

Tubing Packs

Many companies will custom design tubing packs to meet the requirements of individual ECMO centers. In determining this design, it is sometimes helpful to obtain a tubing pack designed by a center with clinical experience and then discuss the rationale of the design with that center. The perfusion service should be involved in design of the system, not only to take advantage of its expertise, but also to provide the ECMO team access to the company making tubing packs used by the perfusion team. This association will usually enhance the commitment of the supply company to the needs of the ECMO team.

The tubing pack design will have to accommodate needed entry points into the system, but should minimize these to help decrease the

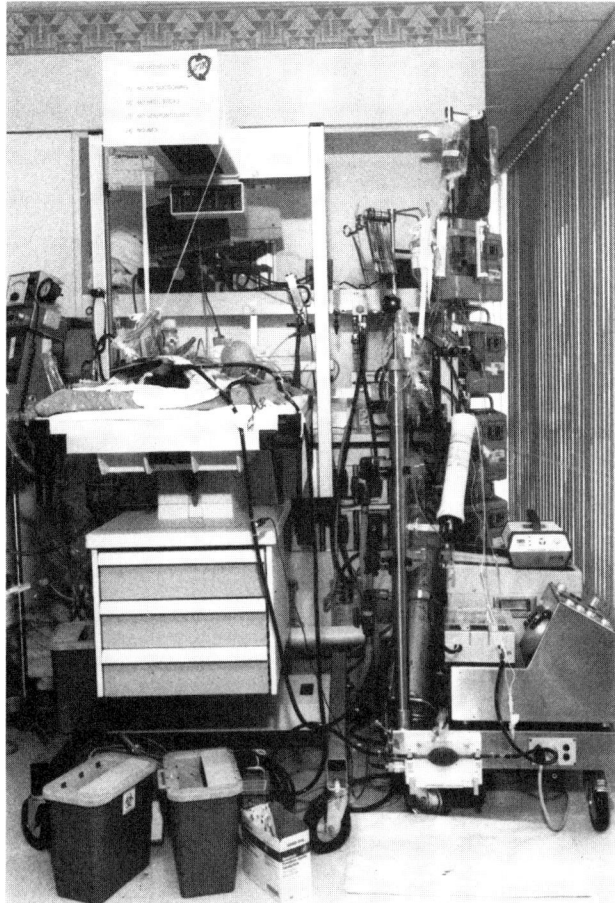

FIGURE 11.2 A side view of the ECMO system showing the venous return monitor and bladder holder at the bottom of the pump (white box).

risk of infection and accidental blood loss. Essential ports are proximal to the bladder for blood sampling, following the bladder for IV fluid infusions, after the pump head but before the membrane for setting pump occlusion, and after the membrane for pressure monitoring, blood sampling, and infusion of platelets. CNMC tubing circuit is shown in Figure 11.3. Other in-line connections can include a ¼-inch × ¼-inch oxygen saturation detector (OTC-0250, American Bentley, Irvine, California) or ¼-inch × ¼-inch connector with Luer-Lok for placement of the oxygen saturation catheter (Oximetrix 3, Abbott Critical Care Systems, Mountain View, California) for venous saturation measurement on the prebladder side of the venous line and a temperature probe on the postheat exchanger side of the arterial line.

Raceway tubing is the tubing that is in the roller head of the pump. If ordinary ¼-inch polyvinyl chloride tubing is used, it must be "walked" out of the raceway every 12 hours to decrease the incidence of raceway rupture. Two types of tubing have been shown to be effective for long-term raceway use and do not require walking: Superygon 65, ¼-inch inside diameter × ¹⁄₁₆-inch wall thickness (Norton Performance Plastics, Akron, Ohio) and Bypass 65, ¼-inch by ³⁄₃₂-inch (American Bentley, Irvine, California). Each of these have been tested in the laboratory for 14 days of use without signs of stress or rupture marks. It must be noted that any tube can rupture when used for long-term runs and should be examined daily for stress marks. At CNMC, the only raceway rupture after changing to "long-term" raceway tubing

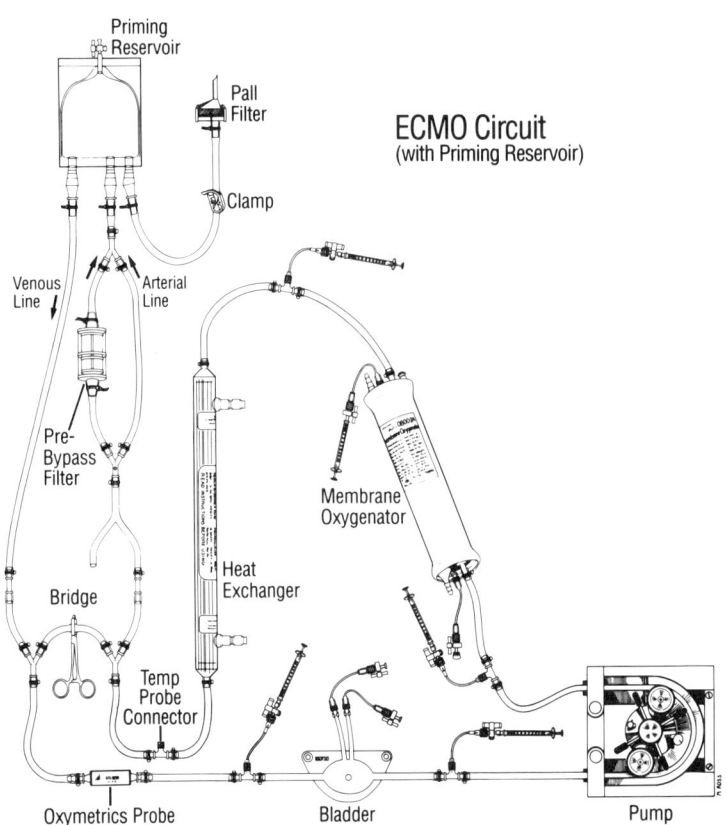

FIGURE 11.3 Schematic of the ECMO circuit with priming reservoir. Important components are labeled. (Drawing by Martha Ross.)

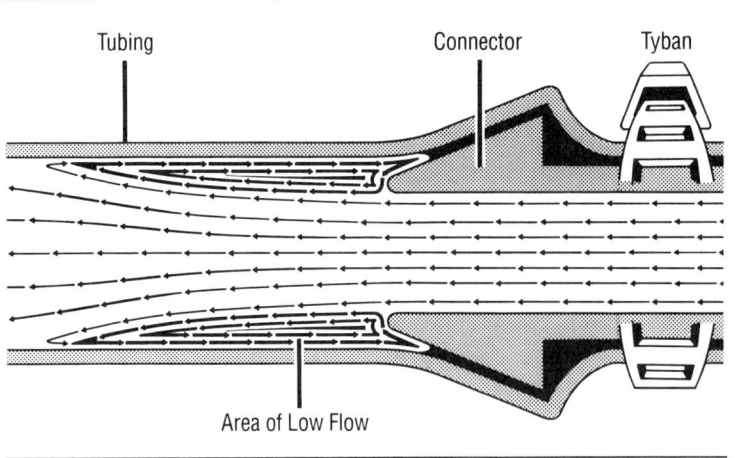

FIGURE 11.4 Schematic of a ¼-inch × ¼-inch connector and tubing interface with "eddy flow" area where fibrin and clots can form. (Drawing by Martha Ross.)

was in an infant managed on ECMO for more than 14 days (1/200 cases).

ECMO Catheters

ECMO catheters consist of the arterial and venous inlet and outlet catheters. The arterial catheter, which returns blood from the circuit into the arch of the aorta, also acts as the major resistance component in the circuit. The arterial catheter can restrict flow, causing significant back-pressure in the circuit. This, in turn, can lead to hemolysis or even rupture of the circuit. The venous catheter is the outflow catheter; it determines the rate at which blood can be taken from the right atrium into the ECMO system. The venous catheter becomes the major limitation on flow and therefore can determine the ability of the ECMO circuit to oxygenate the patient.

Several laws of physics must be reviewed to understand the development and proper design of catheters used in ECMO. Resistance to flow depends on the geometry of the tubing used and the characteristics of the fluid. Poiseuille's law defines those relationships in the following equation:

$$R = \frac{8\mu \, 1L}{\pi r^2}$$

where $8/\pi$ is the constant of proportionality, $1L$ (cm) is the length of the tubing; μ (Poise = dyne-s/cm^2) is the coefficient of viscosity, and r (cm) is the radius of the tubing. Therefore, the longer the tubing, the greater the resistance, or the smaller the radius, the greater the resistance. Thus, the arterial catheter is the highest resistance component of the circuit since it is the element with the smallest diameter. From these relationships, one can see that a short catheter with a large lumen will lead to lower pressures in the circuit (35).

Figure 11.5 describes the pressure–flow characteristics of commonly used arterial catheters

FIGURE 11.5 The pressure–flow relationship of commonly used arterial catheters is shown. Biomed 10F is from Biomedicus, Inc., Eden Prairie, Minnesota; Elecath 10 and 8F, Electro-Catheter Corp., Rahway, N.J.; Argyle 10 and 8F, Argyle/Sherwood, Inc., St. Louis, Missouri.

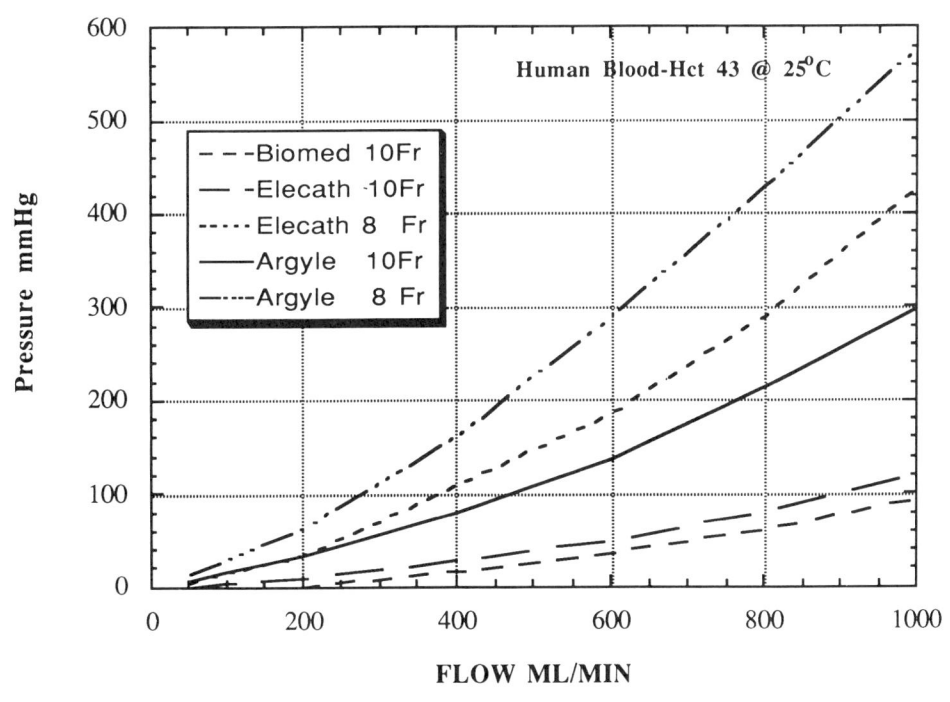

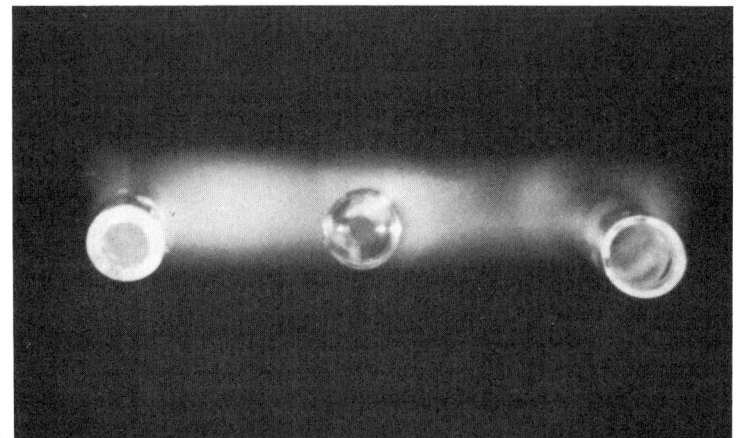
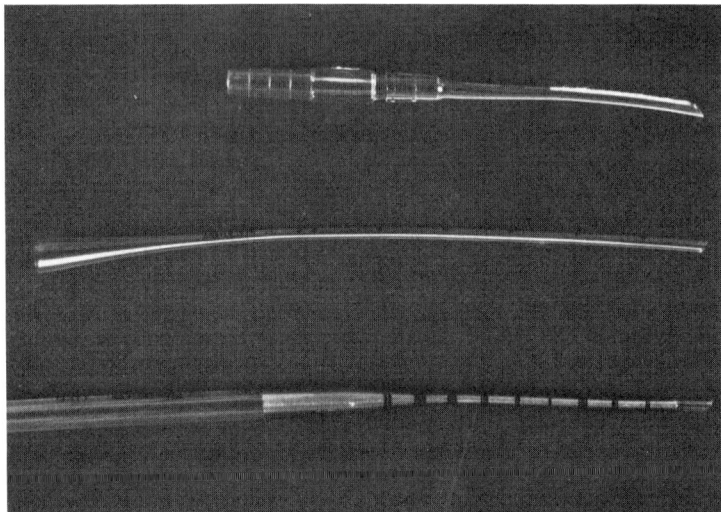
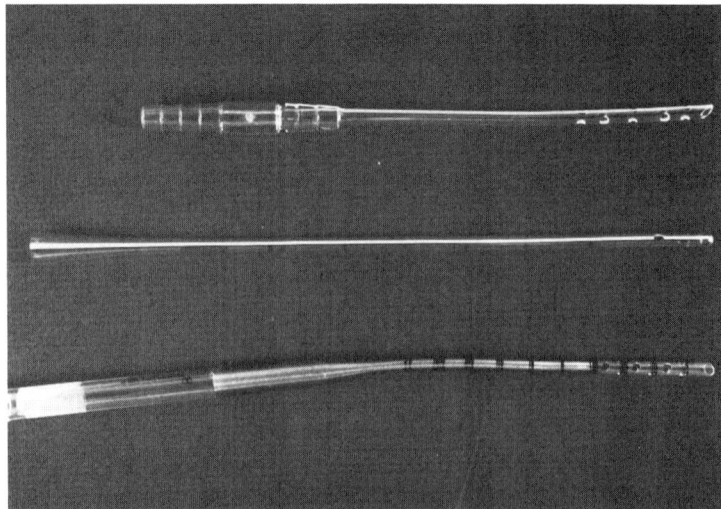

FIGURE 11.6 (A) End-hold picture of (from left to right) Elecath, Argyle, and Biomedicus catheters showing the increased internal diameter in the Biomedicus due to the thin wall design. (B) Commonly used arterial catheters (from top to bottom): Elecath, Argyle, and Biomedicus. (C) Commonly used venous catheters (from top to bottom): Elecath, Argyle, and Biomedicus.

showing the Biomedicus 10 French catheter to be optimal. This can be explained by the large internal diameter depicted in Figure 11.6A, which shows an end-on picture of three catheters. In this figure, the internal diameter of the Biomedicus catheter is seen to be much larger than the other catheter with the same external diameter. When evaluating catheters, the internal diameter, not the external diameter, is the critical factor.

Blood flow rates vary directly as the fourth power of the radius of the tubing and are inversely proportional to the length of the tubing:

$$Q \alpha r^4$$
$$Q \alpha 1/1L$$

Therefore, to maximize flow into the circuit, the venous catheter should be as short and have as large a lumen as possible. See Figure 11.6B and 11.6C for examples of commonly used catheters and Chapter 12 on vascular access for further discussion.

Blood Pumps

Two pump systems have been used most widely for neonatal ECMO: the positive displacement roller pump and the centrifugal pump. Both systems deliver nonpulsatile flow. Pulsatile pumps have not been used for long-term bypass and will not be discussed in this chapter.

The centrifugal pump systems cause significant hemolysis in the neonate, a phenomenon that is not as severe in larger patients placed on these systems. The hemolysis may be related to the low flow rates used for neonatal ECMO with their associated increased heat production and/or significant negative venous pressure in neonatal systems. These pumps have features that could make them safer, including the absence of a raceway (eliminating the risk of tubing rupture in the raceway) and afterload-dependent arterial output, eliminating the possibility of tubing rupture caused by occluding the arterial side of the circuit which eliminates the need for a venous control system and decreases the risk of major air embolus. However, concern over the increase in hemolysis and the need to change the pump head every 48–72 hours has caused most centers to use the roller occlusion pump (36).

Various manufacturers make positive displacement pumps for cardiopulmonary bypass. Because these pumps are designed for short-term bypass, it is important to evaluate each system carefully. Important considerations include reliability, ease and accuracy of use, and minimal maintenance requirements. Pumps are either belt-driven or direct-drive systems. The direct-drive mechanism eliminates the problems sometimes associated with belt-driven pumps, including fraying, stretching, and breaking of the belt. All pump systems require meticulous maintenance to assure reliability.

Roller occlusion pump systems generally calculate rather than directly measure the displayed blood flow rate. Rotational speed of the pump is displayed in revolutions per minute (RPM), and the flow output is displayed in liters per minute (LPM). The control microprocessor takes the RPM value and calculates blood flow based on the size of tubing selected (i.e., ¼ inch versus ⅜ inch). The flow value displayed is mathematically the stroke volume of the pump multiplied by the RPM. The stroke volume is the volume of the fluid delivered by one complete revolution of the pump head. This value varies with size (diameter) of the raceway tubing. Most pumps today calculate a flow that is within ±5% of the actual flow rate.

Although the digital readout on most cardiovascular pumps is quite accurate, the most common factor resulting in an inaccurate value is improper occlusion of the roller head. If occlusion of the pump is lost during long ECMO runs in which the round shape of the tubing becomes flattened, the digital readout, calculated as described above, will not change, but actual flow will be decreased. One of the first signs that this is happening is loss of oxygenation in the patient not explained by change in the clinical state and/or a significant decrease in pre- and postmembrane pressure while at a constant flow rate. The primary cause of loss of occlusion is change in contour of the tubing. Systems today rarely lose occlusion related to movement of the rollers.

ECMO Blood Heater and Extracorporeal Heat Exchanger

The ECMO heater is a microprocessor-based, hyperthermia-only blood warmer. Two units specifically made for ECMO are commercially available (Model 333, Cincinnati Subzero, Cincinnati, Ohio, and SMS-3000, Seabrook Medical Systems, Inc., Cincinnati, Ohio). They are designed and intended for use with an extracorporeal heat exchanger. These units have the capacity to maintain and regulate blood temperature in an ECMO circuit from 25° to 40°C. Each unit has a built-in monitor with high-temperature safety controls designed to shut the unit down in the event of a malfunction.

The extracorporeal heat exchanger used most commonly is made by SciMed Life Systems, Inc. (P-7-14, SciMed Life Systems, Minneapolis, Minnesota). This heat exchanger is a cylindrical countercurrent blood heater consisting of a polycarbonate cylinder with stainless steel tubes inside for blood passage. Hot water from the ECMO blood heater circulates into the cylinder, transferring heat to the stainless steel tubes filled with flowing blood. The countercurrent principle provides maximum heat transfer (Figure 11.7).

The purpose of the heat exchanger is to warm the blood to body temperature before it returns to the patient. The heat exchanger is located after the membrane in the circuit for two reasons. First, because of the heater's geometry, it acts as a bubble trap. Second, the loss of blood temperature is exaggerated at low pump rates as blood flows through the membrane lung which is ventilated with cool gas. Therefore, to maintain normal blood temperature at low blood flow rates, the heat exchanger must be placed after the membrane and close to the patient.

It must be remembered that most heat exchangers are designed for conventional intraoperative cardiopulmonary bypass and not the low-heparin, low-flow states of neonatal ECMO. Therefore, before a new unit is used clinically, it must be tested in the laboratory for heat transfer, flow, and clotting characteristics. Many units tested in our laboratories at CNMC have shown significant fibrin and clot formation at low flow rates and, therefore, would be dangerous to use clinically.

Venous Return Monitor and Bladder Holder

The venous return monitor (VRM) is an electronic device that monitors blood flow from the patient into the system. This system functions as a servoregulator for the ECMO system and is designed to alarm and stop the pump in the event that venous flow from the patient decreases, thus ensuring that input equals output (Figures 11.2, 11.3). If this system is not in place and venous return decreases without servoregulation, the roller pump will continue to pump, developing increasingly more negative pressure and causing "cavitation" of the tubing. Cavitation is a condition in which gas comes out of solution. Also, the extreme negative pressure can pull air into the circuit at loose connection points. This can result in an air embolus. The most common causes of loss of venous return are misplacement of the venous catheter (usually down the inferior vena cava), pneumothorax or pneumopericardium, unrecognized intracranial or intrathoracic bleeding, kinking of the venous catheter, or a narrowed catheter by overtightening the securing ligatures during cannulation.

Three VRM systems exist. The first is a plunger device commercially made by Sea-

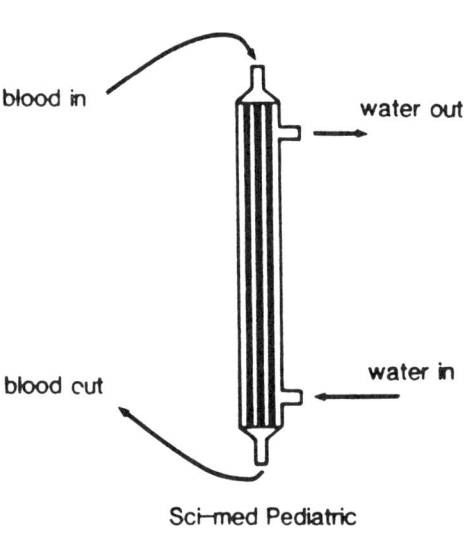

FIGURE 11.7 Schematic of the heat exchanger showing the countercurrent flow characteristics used to increase heat transfer. (Drawing by Martha Ross.)

brook (SMS-3100 Pump Controller and SMS-3200 Bladder Holder, Seabrook Medical Systems, Inc., Cincinnati, Ohio). This system has a plunger that rests behind the venous reservoir bladder, monitoring volume of the bladder. With a drop in volume of 4 to 6 cc, the system will signal an alarm and stop the roller pump until the volume returns to normal. The system used at CNMC has no movable parts and consists of a high-precision electronic proximity sensor to track the distance to the posterior wall of the bladder, which changes with volume changes. The sensor is encapsulated inside the bladder box, employing an electronic beam transmitted through the plastic housing. Very little maintenance is required for this system. Both of these systems incorporate an assembly to hold the venous bladder which contains parts of the venous return monitor. The third system used requires a separate bladder holder. This system uses the pressure monitoring servoregulation system that is an "add-on" to most cardiopulmonary roller pump units. When the pressure monitor is placed before the bladder, this system will measure venous pressure which can be used as an indicator of venous outflow. These systems servoregulate pump flow depending on the venous pressure in the circuit. When using these systems, one must remember that, if the height of the patient is changed, the system needs to be recalibrated.

Venous Reservoir: "The Bladder"

The venous reservoir bag, or "bladder," is a silicone 50- or 30-cc reservoir into which venous blood is drained from the right atrium. The bladder has two functions: 1) it is a very effective bubble trap, and 2) it provides a large compliant "vessel" so that venous return can be monitored safely. The bladder allows the roller pump to pull against the larger volume in the bladder, decreasing the risk that significant negative pressure will be placed on the right atrium when venous return decreases significantly (Figure 11.3).

The major complication associated with the bladder is the development of stagnant flow patterns near the bottom, which allows the development of fibrin and clots at low flow with low activated clotting times (ACT). The development of the 30-cc reservoir has improved these flow patterns. Two companies make the neonatal bladder: SciMed Life Systems, Minneapolis, Minnesota (R-50 and R-30 models) and Gish Biomedical Inc., Santa Ana, California (30-cc ECMO Bladder).

Gas Delivery System

The gas delivery systems used to ventilate the membrane lung are composed of three basic components: a high- and low-flow O_2 flow meter assembly, a low-flow CO_2 flow meter, and an air/oxygen blender. Most oxygen flow meters have a high O_2 flow meter with a range of 0 to 10 LPM in 1-LPM gradations or a low flow meter 0 to 2.2 LPM with 0.05 LPM gradations. The blended gas outlet of the blender is fed to the input of the high/low O_2 flow meter assembly. The type of CO_2 flow meter selected will depend on whether carbogen (5% CO_2 and 95% O_2) or pure CO_2 is used. If pure CO_2 is used, a flow meter with a range of 0 to 1 LPM should be used with 0.02-LPM gradations. (Smaller gradations would be preferred but are not commercially available.) The output of the flow meter assembly is routed to the gas inlet of the membrane lung.

When the gas flow is connected to the membrane lung, it must be remembered that the flow should not exceed the rated flow of the membrane (each membrane has a rated gas flow 3 L/min/m^2 of membrane surface area). The gas outlet should never be blocked. Either situation can result in an air embolus. All gas into the flow meter system should be set at 50 psi.

Membrane Lung

The only membrane lung approved for long-term use is the SciMed Membrane Lung (SciMed Life Systems, Inc., Minneapolis, Minnesota). The membrane sizes used most often are the 0.8 m^2 and the 0.6 m^2 (0800-A or 0600), although the membrane comes in various sizes (ranging from 0.4 m^2 to 4.5 m^2) for use with different-sized patients (Table 11.5). Although the 0.6 m^2 membrane supplies sufficient oxygen transfer for neonatal ECMO, laboratory data indicate that CO_2 transfer is limited. Therefore, most centers use the 0.8 m^2

TABLE 10.5 Membrane oxygenator specifications for neonatal applications*

	Model #		
	0400-2A	0600-2A	0800-2A
Surface area (m²)	0.4	0.6	0.8
Priming volume (mL)	60	90	100
Maximum gas flow rates (L/min)	1.2	1.8	2.4
Maximum blood flow rates (L/min)	0.35	1.0	1.2
Maximum size (kg)	4	10	11

*SciMed, Life Systems, Inc., Minneapolis, MN.

membrane, especially if the patient has a problem with CO_2 retention or it is necessary to lower the $Paco_2$ below 40 mm Hg.

The SciMed membrane lung is a homogenous reinforced silicone rubber membrane envelope with a plastic spacer screen inside (Figure 11.8A,B). The envelope is wound spirally around a polycarbonate spool and encased in a tightly fitted silicone rubber sleeve. Externally manifolded silicone rubber tubes provide access to and from the interior of the membrane envelope for gas flow. Gas flows through the interior of the envelope, separated from the blood phase by the silicone membrane. Countercurrent flow produces maximum gas transfer (Figure 11.9). This transfer

FIGURE 11.8 (A) Schematic of membrane lung showing the countercurrent flow relationships of blood flow and gas flow used to increase gas transfer. (Drawing by Martha Ross.) (B) Schematic of the membrane lung showing the large surface area and the relationship of the gas inlet and outlet ports to the internal envelope. (Drawing by Martha Ross.)

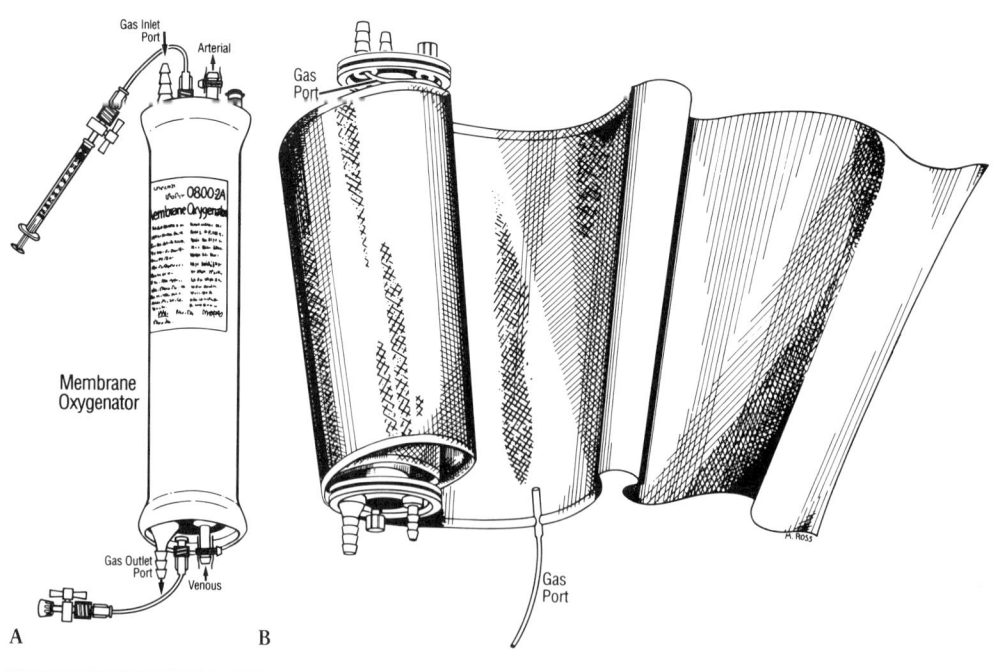

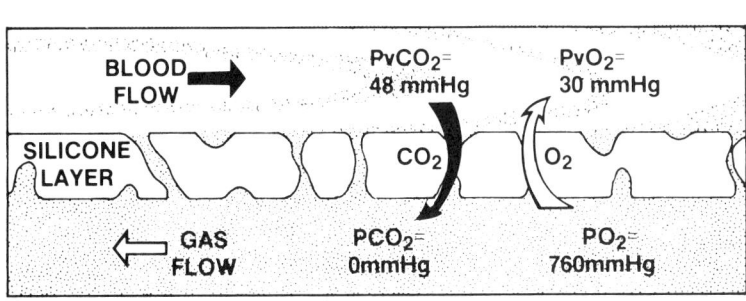

FIGURE 11.9 Schematic of silicone membrane lung showing separation of blood and gas compartments, with transfer of gases across the silicone membrane because of a pressure gradient. (Drawing by Martha Ross.)

occurs through simple diffusion along pressure and concentration gradients.

Gas flow should be maintained within the stated operating range to ensure that blood flow into the membrane has optimal flow characteristics, resulting in use of the maximal surface area of the membrane. Exceeding the membrane gas flow recommendations can result in an air embolus across any pinhole areas in the membrane lung. It also results in shunting of blood to nonventilated areas of the membrane lung, decreasing gas exchange efficiency.

With low blood flow rates (less than 100 mL/min), "supersaturation" of the blood can occur. This is the result of blood with a high dissolved oxygen content leaving the membrane and then being warmed in the heat exchanger. Oxygen that is bound to hemoglobin or dissolved in plasma may be released as fine "bubbles." This risk can be reduced if the oxygen concentration in the sweep gas is decreased as the blood flow decreases. When blood flows of 100 mL/min are reached, the blender should be turned down to 90% oxygen. Flows of 60 mL/min require that the blender be decreased to 60% or less.

In addition to gas flow limitations, each size of the membrane lung has a maximum blood flow rating. Above this flow, the membrane lung will lose its ability to completely oxygenate and ventilate the blood. Most uses of neonatal ECMO do not exceed the blood flow limits of the 0.6 or 0.8 m^2 membrane.

As blood is pumped across the spiral-wound oxygenator, a pressure gradient is produced between the blood inlet and outlet ports (Figure 11.3). It is important to understand the pressure characteristics of the membrane lung for safe use of the ECMO system. The inlet pressure is usually between 200 and 350 mm Hg and must, by definition, be greater than the blood outlet pressure which is usually 100 to 250 mm Hg. These pressures are related to the blood flow rate and the resistance components of the system, i.e., the membrane lung and the arterial catheter. The Silastic membrane lung is a high-resistance membrane, and it is normal to have a 100- to 200-mm Hg pressure drop across the membrane. The arterial catheter is the component of the system with highest resistance; therefore, a catheter with a large internal diameter will have a lower postmembrane pressure than one with a smaller internal diameter, i.e., 10 Fr versus 8 Fr. Postmembrane pressures should be monitored at all times to ensure that complications such as arterial line kinking or clotting will be noted immediately. Circuit pressures above 300 mm Hg over a length of time may result in significant hemolysis, with pressures over 500 mm Hg resulting in circuit rupture. Any increase of over 50 mm Hg in the postmembrane pressures without an increase in blood flow rates should be evaluated. Remember that the arterial catheter can be tied too tightly at cannulation, resulting in pressures high enough to rupture the circuit. Of equal importance is the loss of pressure. If this happens with no change in blood flow rates, occlusion of the pump has been lost and should be checked immediately.

In-Line Oxygen Monitoring

In-line oxygen monitoring has been attractive, but to date only a few of these systems work for extensive periods because of fibrin and protein deposit on the sensors. Two oxygen saturation monitors are currently being used with good results: the OTC-0250 Optical Transmission Cell (American Bentley, Irvine, California) and the Oximetrix 3 System (Abbott Critical Care Systems, Mountain View, California). Interpretation of these systems is reviewed in the Clinical Management section of Chapter 13. Any in-line monitor designed for short-term use should be evaluated in the laboratory before attempting to use it in long-term ECMO. The sensors or probes should be evaluated for clot or fibrin formation, and the validity of the readout should be determined over time. Most in-line systems evaluated by our team have been inaccurate after 12 hours or require constant recalibration involving removal of the patient from bypass. The risks associated with these systems should be weighed against their clinical usefulness.

Blood Coagulation Tester

A bedside test for clotting time is needed. Most centers use an ACT device which measures whole blood coagulation as stimulated by glass beads, other particles, or specific activators in the measurement tubes (see the section on heparin management for further details). The most commonly used system is the Hemachron 400 (International Technidyne, Edison, N.J.). If this device is used, the P214/P215 tubes, which require only 0.4 mL of blood, should be used. Larger tubes require 2 mL of blood and are not as accurate if ACT levels are below 500 seconds.

Bedside Cart

The ECMO specialist cannot leave the pump side to get supplies, especially those needed in an emergency. Therefore, a bedside cart should be provided containing routine supplies (i.e., syringes, needles, etc.) and emergency supplies and equipment (i.e., sterile raceway tubing, ¼-inch × ¼-inch connectors, etc.). Carts used by automobile mechanics are excellent because they have a large number of drawers.

Priming of the ECMO Circuit

The first step in preparing to place an infant on ECMO is to prime the system. This process usually takes 30 to 45 minutes to ensure that all air or particles are removed from the circuit. With proper priming, the hematocrit will be 40% to 45%, with a blood gas of pH 7.50, a Pco_2 of 30 to 35 mm Hg, and a Po_2 of 100 to 150 mm Hg. The precise details of priming are beyond the scope of this chapter, but the concepts will be covered (Figure 11.3). First, the circuit is flushed with pure CO_2. This step will remove air from the circuit and replace it with CO_2, which is highly soluble and will decrease the risk of microbubbles in the circuit. After this flush, the circuit is placed on suction to remove CO_2 and to create negative pressure in the blood path of the circuit. This facilitates filling the circuit with fluid. While on suction, the circuit is flushed with normal saline. At this phase, any bubbles are removed from the membrane lung and heat exchanger by gentle tapping with the palm of the hand. The SciMed membrane lung may require extensive debubbling. This is an extremely important step, and all gas bubbles must be removed from the circuit prior to the albumin/blood flush. The saline is circulated through a prebypass filter to remove any plastic particles in the tubing that may remain from manufacture of the tubing pack. After all gas is removed from the circuit, the normal saline solution is drained from the priming bag and replaced by 25% albumin. The albumin solution is "walked" slowly (50–60 cc/min) through the system which pushes the normal saline solution out. Because a hematocrit of 40% to 45% is required at the end of the prime, packed red blood cells are used instead of whole blood, as in cardiopulmonary bypass. The colloid used in ECMO priming should be 25% albumin to ensure that the infant's protein levels do not decrease. Studies have shown that certain 25% albumin products contain toxic levels of aluminum and should be avoided (11). After the albumin has been circulated, it is drained from the priming bag and replaced with two units of packed red cells (PRBCs). The packed cells are then slowly (50–60 mL/min) "walked" through the circuit. This results in an albumin/PRBC mixture with a hematocrit of 40% to 45%. Reversal of the citrated blood is not required. When reversal is done with calcium, heparin must be placed in the prime to prevent clotting. This can result in abnormally high ACTs at cannulation and can compound the risk of bleeding complications, such as intracranial hemorrhage. Studies in our center have shown that ionized calcium levels do not significantly decrease if citrated blood is used without reversal.

After the PRBCs have been "walked" through the circuit, the suction is left on the membrane with the inlet port open which pulls air through the membrane, oxygenating and removing CO_2 from the bagged blood. Ten to 15 mL of sodium bicarbonate should be added to buffer the blood. After the blood becomes a pink color, the suction should be removed. At this point, the blood gas on the system should be approximately pH 7.50, PCO_2 30 to 35 mm Hg, and PO_2 of 100 to 150 mm Hg. If the suction is not removed, the blood will become extremely alkalotic, with CO_2 as low as 8 mm Hg and pH of 7.80. This should be avoided because of the effects of extreme alkalosis on red cell function. The heat exchanger should be attached, and the blood should be at body temperature before ECMO is initiated. If the circuit is not going to be attached to the patient within 20 minutes, the membrane should be attached to the gas flow system with the blender placed at room air, O_2 at low flow of 1 L/min, and only minimal CO_2. Blood gas values of the circuit should be obtained prior to the initiation of ECMO.

Evaluation of a neonate for ECMO and assembly of the ECMO circuit are now complete. Technical considerations continue in the next two chapters, with discussion of cannulation procedure and management of a neonate while on an ECMO circuit.

REFERENCES

(1) Stahlman MT. Assisted ventilation in newborn infants. In: Smith GF, Vidyasagar D, eds. Historical review and recent advances in neonatal and perinatal medicine, vol. II. Evansville, IL: Mead Johnson Nutritional Division, 1983.

(2) Bartlett RH, Roloff DW, Cornell RG, et al. Extracorporeal circulation in neonatal respiratory failure: a prospective randomized trial. Pediatrics 1985;76:479–87.

(3) Beck R, Anderson KD, Pearson GD, et al. Criteria for extracorporeal membrane oxygenation in a population of infants with persistent pulmonary hypertension of the newborn. J Pediatr Surg 1986;21:297–302.

(4) Cole CH, Jillson E, Kessler D. ECMO: regional evaluation of need and applicability of selection criteria. Am J Dis Child 1988;142:1320–4.

(5) Dworetz AR, Moya FR, Sabo B, Gladstone I, Gross I. Survival of infants with persistent pulmonary hypertension without extracorporeal membrane oxygenation. Pediatrics 1989;84:1–6.

(6) Krummel TM, Greenfield LJ, Kirkpatrick BV, et al. Alveolar-arterial oxygen gradients versus the neonatal pulmonary insufficiency index for prediction of mortality in ECMO candidates. J Pediatr Surg 1984;19:380–4.

(7) Marsh TD, Wilkerson SA, Cook LN. Extracorporeal membrane oxygenation selection criteria: partial pressure of arterial oxygen versus alveolar-arterial oxygen gradient. Pediatrics 1988;82:162–6.

(8) O'Rourke PP, Crone RK, Vacanti JP, et al. Extracorporeal membrane oxygenation and conventional medical therapy in neonates with persistent pulmonary hypertension of the newborn: a prospective randomized study. Pediatrics 1989;84:957–63.

(9) Wung JT, James LS, Kilchevsky E, James E. Management of infants with severe respiratory failure and persistence of the fetal circulation, without hyperventilation. Pediatrics 1985;76:488–94.

(10) Hollenberg NK, Dzau VJ, Williams GH. Are uncontrolled clinical studies ever justified? N Engl J Med 1980;303:1059–60.

(11) Kelly AT, Short BL, Rains TC, May JC, Progar JJ. Aluminum toxicity and albumin. Trans ASAIO 1989;35:674–6.

(12) Schneider B, Schena J, Troug R, Jacobson M, Kevy S. Exposure to di(2-ethylhexyl)phthalate in infants receiving extracorporeal membrane oxygenation (Letter). N Engl J Med 1989;320:1563.

(13) Schumacher RE, Barks JDE, Johnston MV, et al. Right-sided brain lesions in infants following extracorporeal membrane oxygenation. Pediatrics 1988;82:155–61.

(14) Taylor GA, Short BL, Fitz CR. Imaging of cerebrovascular injury in infants treated with extracorporeal membrane oxygenation. J Pediatr 1989;114:635–9.

(15) Callaghan JC, de Los Angeles J. Long-term extracorporeal circulation in the development of an artificial placenta for prematurity and respira-

tory distress syndrome. Surg Forum 1961;12: 215–17.

(16) Rashkind WJ, Freeman A, Klein D, Toft RW. Evolution of a disposable plastic low volume pumpless oxygenator as a lung substitute. J Pediatr 1965;66:94–102.

(17) Dorson W Jr, Baker E, Cohen ML, et al. A perfusion system for infants. Trans ASAIO 1969; 15:155–60.

(18) White JJ, Andrews HG, Risonberg H, Mazur D, Haller JA Jr. Prolonged respiratory support in newborn infants with a membrane oxygenator. Surgery 1971;70:288–96.

(19) Cilley RE, Zwischenferger JB, Andrews AF, et al. Intracranial hemorrhage during extracorporeal membrane oxygenation in neonates. Pediatrics 1986;78:699–703.

(20) Revenis M, Glass P, Sanchez L, Short B. Outcome of low birth weight (LBW) babies on extracorporeal membrane oxygenation (abstract). Pediatr Res 1990;27:254A.

(21) Short BL, Walker LK, Gleason CA, Jones MD, Traystman RJ. Effects of extracorporeal membrane oxygenation on cerebral blood flow and cerebral oxygen metabolism in newborn sheep. Pediatr Res 1990;28:50–53.

(22) McCune S, Short BL, Miller MK, Lotze A, Anderson KA. Extracorporeal membrane oxygenation therapy in neonates with septic shock. J Pediatr Surg 1990;25:479–82.

(23) Short BL, Miller MK, Anderson KA. Extracorporeal membrane oxygenation in the management of respiratory failure in the newborn. Clin Perinatol 1987;14:737–48.

(24) Toomasian JM, Snedecor SM, Cornell RG, Cilley RE, Bartlett RH. National experience with extracorporeal membrane oxygenation for newborn respiratory failure. Trans ASAIO 1988;34: 140–7.

(25) Heaton JFG, Redmond CR, Graves ED, Falterman KW, Arensman RM. Congenital diaphragmatic hernia: improving survival with extracorporeal membrane oxygenation. Pediatr Surg Int 1988;3:6–10.

(26) Langham MR, Krummel TM, Bartlett RH, et al. Mortality with extracorporeal membrane oxygenation following repair of congenital diaphragmatic hernia in 93 infants. J Pediatr Surg 1987;22:1150–4.

(27) Newman KD, Van Meurs KP, Short BL, Anderson KD. Extracorporeal membrane oxygenation and congenital diaphragmatic hernia: should any infant be excluded? J Pediatr Surg 1990;25:1048–52.

(28) Stolar C, Dillon P, Reyes C. Selective use of extracorporeal membrane oxygenation in the management of congenital diaphragmatic hernia. J Pediatr Surg 1988;23:207–11.

(29) Van Meurs KP, Newman KD, Anderson KD, Short BL. Effect of extracorporeal membrane oxygenation on survival of infants with congenital diaphragmatic hernia. J Pediatr 1990; 117:954–60.

(30) Ortiz RM, Cilley RE, Bartlett RH. Extracorporeal membrane oxygenation in pediatric respiratory failure. Pediatr Clin North Am 1987; 34:39–46.

(31) Boedy RF, Howell CG, Kanto WP Jr. Hidden mortality of ECMO. J Pediatr 1990;117: 462–6.

(32) Howell CG, Hatley RM, Boedy FR, et al. Recent experience with diaphragmatic hernia and ECMO. Ann Surg 1990;211:793–8.

(33) MacDonald MG, Miller MK, eds. Emergency transport of the perinatal patient, 1st ed. Boston: Little, Brown, & Co., 1989.

(34) Martin GR, Short BL. Doppler echocardiographic evaluation of cardiac performance in infants on prolonged extracorporeal membrane oxygenation. Am J Cardiol 1988;62:929–34.

(35) Van Meurs KP, Mikesell GT, Seale SR, Short BL, Rivera O. Maximum blood flow rates for arterial cannulae used in neonatal ECMO. Trans ASAIO 1990;36:679–81.

(36) Steinhorn RH, Isham-Schopof B, Smith C, Green TP. Hemolysis during long-term extracorporeal membrane oxygenation. J Pediatr 1989; 115:625–30.

12

Vascular Access for Extracorporeal Life Support

❖

Steven L. Moulton, M.D.
Ralph E. Delius, M.D.
Robert M. Arensman, M.D.

As one traces the history of extracorporeal life support in humans, it is evident that vascular access has played an important role in the remarkable development of this field. Not long ago, vascular access was commonly devised from two or more appropriately sized chest tubes or custom-made cannulas. These cannulas allowed central vascular access using a variety of peripheral routes and cannulation schemes. Over the past several years, cannula design and cannulation techniques have been adapted to meet the physiologic needs of a growing patient population. At the present time, vascular access can be accomplished through a single incision or through the use of percutaneous cannulas to allow rapid resuscitation and early stabilization of critically ill patients.

This chapter outlines the evolution of peripheral vascular access for extracorporeal life support. It is organized into three sections, covering adult, pediatric, and neonatal patient groups. Each section focuses on the history of which veins and arteries have been utilized with greatest success, the routes and techniques in current use, and the problems and controversies that remain to be solved.

ADULT VASCULAR ACCESS

Background

In the early 1950s, both Gibbon (1) and Dennis et al. (2) used extracorporeal circulation for total support of a patient during open heart surgery. Shortly thereafter, Helmsworth et al. (3) employed partial venovenous bypass to alleviate respiratory symptoms in a patient with end-stage cor pulmonale. Venous drainage for the 75-minute trial was obtained with two long, fenestrated catheters that were advanced into the inferior vena cava via the proximal saphenous veins. Blood return was via two right antecubital veins, and gas exchange was provided by a bubble oxygenator. Although the patient reported symptomatic improvement, the short bypass period had little effect on his overall course; he died 24 days later. Further clinical investigation into the development of a lung substitute then waned until the introduction of membrane oxygenators in the late 1950s and early 1960s. These devices provided an efficient means for gas exchange and permitted more extensive study of prolonged extracorporeal life support. Laboratory studies were usually carried out using venovenous bypass since this mode of support allowed investigators to study artificial oxygenation and the effects of prolonged surface exposure without disturbing hemodynamic function (4–6). It is therefore not surprising that most of the early clinical experience with extracorporeal life support was gained using venovenous bypass.

Venovenous extracorporeal life support with a membrane oxygenator was used clinically by Hill and associates (7) beginning in 1966. Vascular access was achieved by placing a large 32 to 36 French wire-reinforced vinyl cannula in a femoral vein, in combination with a large perfusion cannula in the right internal jugular vein (Figure 12.1). This simple arrangement provided flows of 1.2 to 1.9 L/min/m^2; however, recirculation of oxygenated blood from the return cannula back to the extracorporeal circuit limited the bypass flow to about 50% of the cardiac output. As a result, the patient's Fio$_2$ could be reduced to about 60%, but the minute ventilation and mean airway pressure remained at preperfusion levels. Venovenous flow rates were enhanced and recirculation fractions reduced in this and in subsequent clinical trials (8,9) by using larger venous cannulas and adding distal cannulation of the femoral and jugular veins. Yet even with these modifications, none of the patients in these early series survived.

The poor results of these early clinical trials are not surprising, given that venovenous bypass was justifiably limited to moribund patients whose need for cardiopulmonary support far exceeded the capabilities of the technique. All of these patients were in extremis, and all had failed conventional ventilatory support to the extent that hypoxic myocardial depression was either imminent or well established. To overcome these physiologic obstacles, investigators turned to venoarterial bypass. This mode of support offered several advantages, including right ventricular decompression, left ventricular support, an increase in the bypass volume, reduced pulmonary artery pressures, and lower ventilator settings (10).

The question arose as to the optimal location for reinfusion of oxygenated blood into the arterial system (11). Hill and co-workers (12,13) cannulated the femoral artery; Carlson (14) used the axillary artery; and Zapol and associates (8) introduced a long cannula via the femoral artery to the aortic root. The advantages of femoral artery and vein cannulation were self-evident when Hill et al. (15) reported

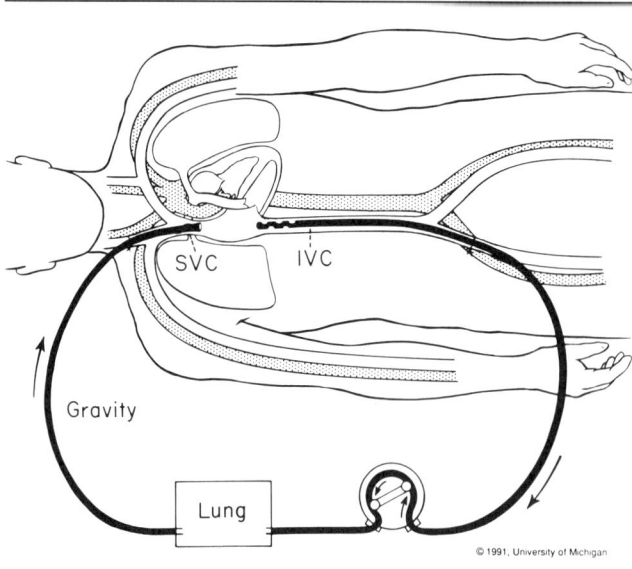

FIGURE 12.1 Low-flow venovenous bypass. (Modified with permission from Bartlett RH. Extracorporeal life support for cardiopulmonary failure. Curr Probl Surg 1990;27:635.)

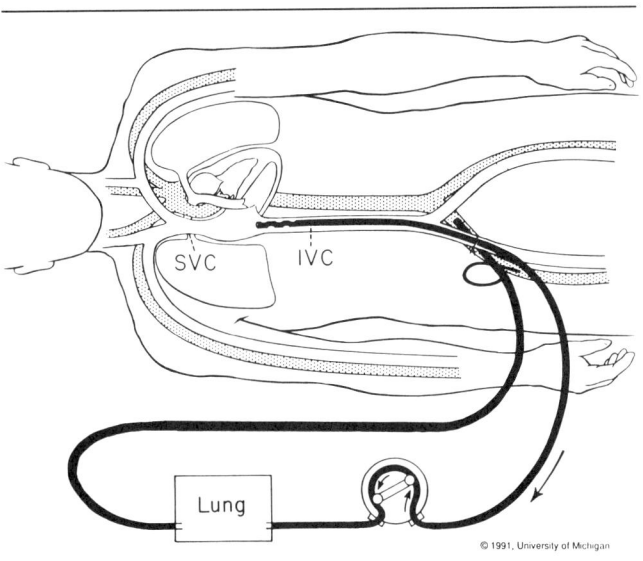

FIGURE 12.2 Venoarterial bypass via the femoral vessels. (Modified with permission from Bartlett RH. Extracorporeal life support for cardiopulmonary failure. Curr Probl Surg 1990; 27:635.)

the first successful use of prolonged extracorporeal oxygenation using this cannulation scheme (Figure 12.2). Diversion of a large proportion (60% to 75%) of the total venous return through the extracorporeal circuit allowed a reduction in the ventilator settings to an FiO_2 of 0.4 to 0.6 and a reduction in peak airway pressures by 15 to 20 cm of water.

Unfortunately, this cannulation scheme precluded perfusion of the thoracic aorta and proximal aortic branches with well-oxygenated blood (15,16).

Perfusion through the brachial or axillary artery was performed to avoid maldistribution of oxygenated blood from the extracorporeal circuit (Figure 12.3). Yet this cannulation

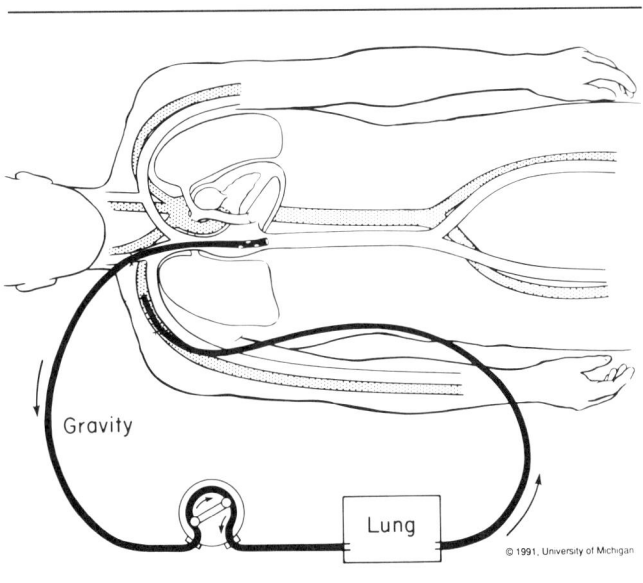

FIGURE 12.3 Venoarterial bypass with reinfusion via the right axillary artery. (Reprinted with permission from Bartlett RH. Extracorporeal life support for cardiopulmonary failure. Curr Probl Surg 1990;27:635.)

scheme was also less than ideal, because: 1) the smaller-caliber cannula necessary for vascular access was limited by its lower flow rate and higher pressure gradient; 2) requisite hemostasis with electrocautery increased the risk of brachial plexus injury; and 3) the use of an arm vessel for reinfusion required two incisions, which increased the potential for bleeding and the complexity of the bypass circuit (17).

Cooper and associates (18) introduced a long, thin-walled polyurethane cannula through the femoral artery to perfuse the aortic root. With this approach, they demonstrated complete mixing of saturated extracorporeal blood with desaturated left ventricular blood to yield uniform dispersion throughout the body (17). This enabled the calculation of right-to-left pulmonary shunt and oxygen consumption (19). Perfusion to the level of the aortic root never gained favor, however, partly because of the greater resistance in the arterial return line introduced by the long cannula. Another concern was incompetence of the aortic valve at high flow rates (>85% bypass) (20).

To overcome the disadvantages of pure venovenous or venoarterial bypass, investigators (21,22) divided the oxygenated perfusate between two reinfusion cannulas, one directed into the right atrium and the other into the axillary or femoral artery (Figure 12.4). Perfusion through the right atrial return cannula was measured by an in-line electromagnetic flow meter and the amount regulated by an externally placed C clamp. This cannulation scheme was termed mixed venovenous-venoarterial bypass. It was used to improve oxygenation of the aortic root and principal branches of the aortic arch. This cannulation scheme fell into disfavor, however, because of its greater complexity and the added risk of bleeding due to two incisions and greater surgical dissection.

By 1974, 150 patients with acute respiratory failure of varying causes and severity had undergone a course of extracorporeal life support, with a survival rate of approximately 10% to 15% (23). Yet which types of acute lung injury managed with extracorporeal life support were associated with an increased incidence of survival remained undefined (21,24). The National Institutes of Health therefore sponsored a randomized multicenter trial of extracorporeal membrane oxygenation versus conventional therapy in adults with acute respiratory failure. Since the majority of survivors treated up until that time had been supported with venoarterial bypass, this mode was utilized for all bypass patients. High-flow venoarterial bypass (approaching 90% of the cardiac output) was established, with arterial return directed to the aortic arch in many but not all

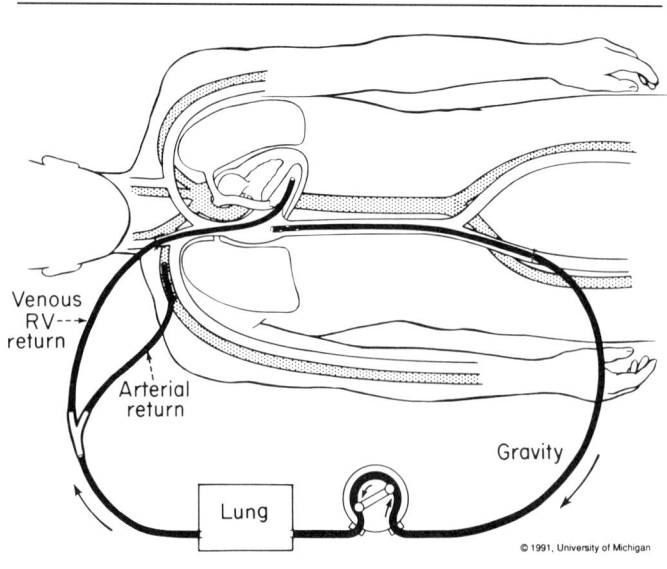

FIGURE 12.4 Mixed venovenous-venoarterial bypass. (Reprinted with permission from Bartlett RH. Extracorporeal life support for cardiopulmonary failure. Curr Probl Surg 1990; 27:635.)

cases (25). Additional ventilatory support was provided using positive end-expiratory pressure (PEEP), supplemental oxygen, and tidal volumes of at least 0.5 L at a rate of 15 breaths per minute (26). The results were discouraging: Patients supported with bypass had no significant increase in survival when compared with patients given standard therapy (27).

This negative study nearly halted the use of extracorporeal life support in adult patients, except in a few centers scattered across the United States, Italy, and West Germany. Kolobow and other investigators at these centers returned to the laboratory and set about studying the basic mechanisms of lung injury and its progression in acute respiratory failure. Their findings led to the hypothesis that extracorporeal carbon dioxide removal ($ECCO_2R$) was fundamentally more important than extracorporeal oxygenation (28). These investigators demonstrated that high ventilatory rates and high peak airway pressures, which are required for CO_2 removal in the adult respiratory distress syndrome (ARDS), are profoundly injurious to any remaining lung that may otherwise be capable of providing sufficient oxygenation (29).

Pesenti, Gattinoni, and others have implemented $ECCO_2R$ using a variety of cannulation schemes, including proximal and distal cannulation of the femoral and internal jugular veins (30), a double-lumen catheter for femoral vein cannulation (31), and saphenosaphenous vein cannulation with reinfusion via the internal jugular vein (32). More recently, percutaneous cannulation has been shown to provide rapid vascular access with a low risk of bleeding (32). Once bypass is established, blood flow is kept relatively low at one-quarter to one-third of the total cardiac output. These low flow rates have essentially eliminated earlier problems associated with recirculation, yet they are sufficient for CO_2 removal.

A subset of adult patients with pulmonary failure are in need of both CO_2 removal and extracorporeal oxygenation. These patients require high flow venovenous or venoarterial bypass. The venous cannula with the largest internal diameter and the shortest length that can be introduced into the jugular vein will usually permit the desired blood flow (33). If venovenous bypass is planned, the perfusate can be returned through the jugular vein cannula using a tidal flow system, or it can be returned to the femoral vein via the saphenous bulb (Figure 12.5). If the patient is hemodynamically compromised and venoarterial bypass is necessary, the perfusate is returned through the right common carotid artery. The right internal jugular vein and right common

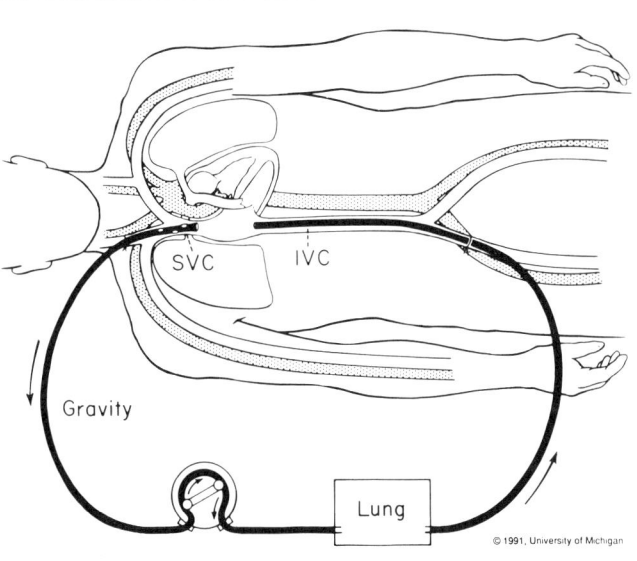

FIGURE 12.5 High-flow venovenous bypass. (Reprinted with permission from Bartlett RH. Extracorporeal life support for cardiopulmonary failure. Curr Probl Surg 1990;27:635.)

carotid artery are ligated during cervical cannulation. The adequacy of cerebral collateral circulation can be tested prior to carotid artery ligation by observing left-sided motor and sensory function during temporary arterial occlusion. If there is concern over whether or not the patient will tolerate common carotid artery ligation, the arterial return can be directed into the common femoral artery, keeping in mind the maldistribution of the oxygenated perfusate associated with this cannulation scheme.

Current Technique

The two methods currently used for vascular access in adult patients are surgical cutdown and percutaneous cannulation. In general, surgical cutdown is more time-consuming and appears to be associated with an increased risk of bleeding from the operative site during the bypass period. Nevertheless, when confronted with the need to place the largest cannulas possible—as for high-flow venovenous or venoarterial bypass—surgical cutdown has the advantage of allowing direct visualization of vessel size and the manner in which the vessel accommodates a given cannula.

Surgical cannulation can be performed at the patient's bedside, provided the patient can be monitored carefully. There must be sufficient space for nursing duties, operating room personnel and equipment, plus the extracorporeal circuit. Arrest medications should be drawn up and ready. The groin is exposed by placing a soft roll beneath the right buttock to extend the hip and abduct the leg. Thorough preparation of the neck and groin with exclusion of the contaminated and potentially infectious perineum is vitally important.

If venovenous bypass is planned, the patient is sedated (morphine sulfate 0.1–0.2 mg/kg) and paralyzed (pancuronium 0.1 mg/kg or succinylcholine 2 mg/kg). The internal jugular vein is cannulated first in order to limit the period during which femoral venous return is disrupted. One percent lidocaine is used for local anesthesia. An oblique or transverse incision is made over the middle third of the right sternocleidomastoid muscle, and dissection is carried down through the platysma muscle using electrocautery. The superficial fascia along the medial border of the right sternocleidomastoid muscle is divided, and the muscle is retracted laterally with a Weitlander retractor. The carotid sheath is exposed, and the internal jugular vein, vagus nerve, and right common carotid artery are identified. The facial vein defines the superior extent of dissection. The patient is anticoagulated (heparin 100 U/kg), and the internal jugular vein is mobilized proximally and distally to allow encirclement with two 2-0 silk ligatures. The distal ligature is tied, and the vessel is occluded proximally with an angled vascular clamp. A transverse or longitudinal venotomy is made, and a prepared venous cannula is passed into the right atrium. The proximal ligature is tied to secure the cannula within the lumen of the vessel, and anchoring skin sutures are placed (Figure 12.6).

Femoral vein cannulation is performed through an oblique or vertical groin incision just medial to the femoral artery below the inguinal ligament. Dissection is carried down through the subcutaneous tissue to the level of the fossa ovalis where the saphenous vein joins the femoral vein. Weitlander or Gelpe retractors are placed, and adequate exposure is obtained. An appropriately sized venous cannula is selected, flushed, and clamped. If the common femoral vein is used for cannulation,

FIGURE 12.6 Cannulation of the right internal jugular vein.

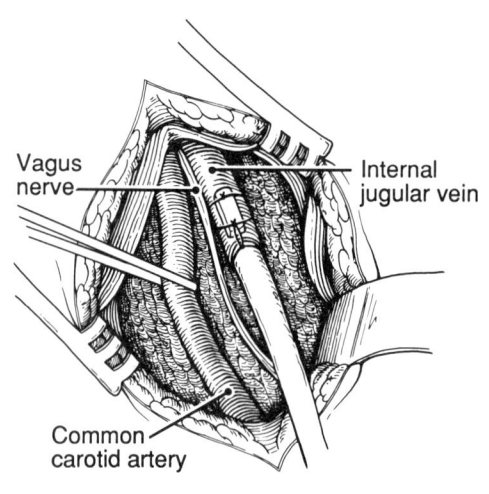

it is necessary to establish distal venous drainage. This can be done by attaching a piece of Luer "IV extension set" tubing to a Luer connector in the venous drainage line and passing the tubing distally into the vessel (33). Femoral vein cannulation via the saphenous bulb alleviates the need to pass a distal venous cannula and simplifies the overall cannulation scheme (Figure 12.7). Proper placement of the femoral vein cannula at approximately L2 (below the renal veins) is confirmed with fluoroscopy. If two groin cannulae are used for venous drainage, they are joined with a Y-connector. The patient is placed on bypass, and the pump flow is gradually increased. Hemostasis is obtained with electrocautery, and the wound is instilled with thrombin glue (10,000 units of thrombin mixed with 500 mg of calcium chloride in one syringe is combined in the wound with an equal volume of cryoprecipitate from a second syringe). The wounds are closed in the usual fashion.

If venoarterial bypass is planned via the cervical vessels, only light sedation should be given at the initiation of the cannulation procedure. This allows the patient's left-sided motor and sensory functions to be tested following temporary occlusion of the right common carotid artery. If there is no apparent neurologic deficit, the common carotid artery is ligated proximal to the carotid artery bifurcation, and the patient is further sedated and paralyzed. A vessel loop is passed around the artery, and a vascular clamp is applied proximal to the distal ligature. A transverse or longitudinal arteriotomy is made, and the intima is tacked against the media with 6-0 monofilament suture to prevent intimal dissection. A 20 French or larger arterial cannula is inserted 6 to 8 centimeters to the origin of the right common carotid artery and secured within the lumen of the vessel. Internal jugular vein cannulation is performed as described previously.

If the patient does not tolerate temporary occlusion of the common carotid artery, the

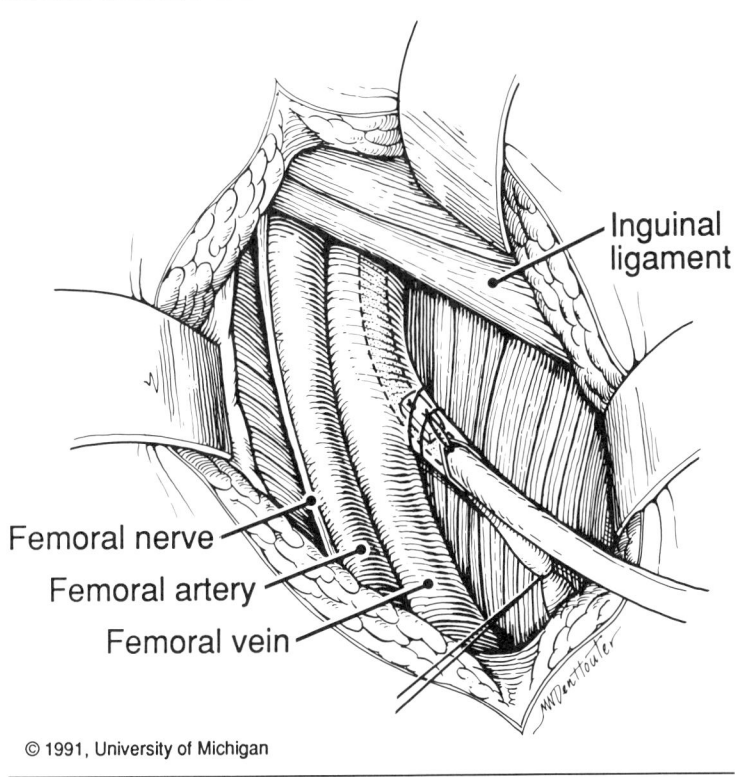

FIGURE 12.7 Femoral vein cannulation via the saphenous bulb.

arterial return from the extracorporeal circuit can be directed into the common femoral artery. The common femoral artery is exposed through a vertical or horizontal groin incision where it is found to course under the middle third of the inguinal ligament. The femoral artery is cannulated with a 20 French or larger arterial cannula; distal perfusion is provided through Luer "IV extension set" tubing (Figure 12.8). The right internal jugular vein is cannulated for venous return. If additional venous return is necessary, the femoral vein can be cannulated as described above.

Percutaneous cannulation for venovenous or venoarterial bypass is performed using the Seldinger technique and standard anatomical landmarks. To begin, a flexible J tip guidewire is passed into the right internal jugular vein. Successively larger dilators are threaded over the guidewire using a rotary motion until the dilator venous cannula assembly is passed. Finally, the dilator and guidewire are removed to leave the cannula in place. Percutaneous femoral vein access is limited to low flow situations due to the risk of hemolysis with long, narrow cannulas (33). Percutaneous arterial access is gained using the femoral artery; the carotid artery is not used because of the risk of distal embolization.

The removal of surgically placed cannulas can be performed at the patient's bedside, provided the practices of close patient monitoring and sterile technique can be followed. Vascular surgical instruments are used, together with surgical loupes and a headlamp. The patient is paralyzed to avoid air embolism when the venous cannula is withdrawn. Heparin is administered to the patient until the procedure is completed. The venotomy sites are exposed, and the vessels are mobilized. Each venous cannula is clamped and carefully removed to ensure that adherent clots are not dislodged. Brisk proximal and distal back-bleeding are confirmed; if absent, back-bleeding is reestablished by gentle passage of an embolectomy catheter. The femoral vessels are repaired in a primary fashion or patched with saphenous vein. Repair of the right internal jugular vein is optional; repair of the right common carotid artery is controversial. Percutaneous cannulas are disconnected from the bypass circuit, gently flushed, clamped, and removed. Manual compression is applied to the cannulation sites for 15 to 30 minutes.

Problems and Controversies

Bleeding from cannulation sites and other operative sites or sites of injury during bypass is one of the major problems that remain to be solved in the coming decade. The impact of this problem dates back to the National Heart, Lung and Blood Institute trial of adult ECMO, in which the marginal benefit obtained from ECMO was nullified by bleeding complications. At present, several thromboresistant surfaces are under development, and a few are undergoing clinical testing. Coating the circuit and bypass cannulas with a thromboresistant surface will reduce the bleeding risks and broaden the indications for extracorporeal life support.

Antibiotic coating of the extracorporeal circuit is another important surface modification currently under development. Antibiotic bonding to an artificial surface is achieved

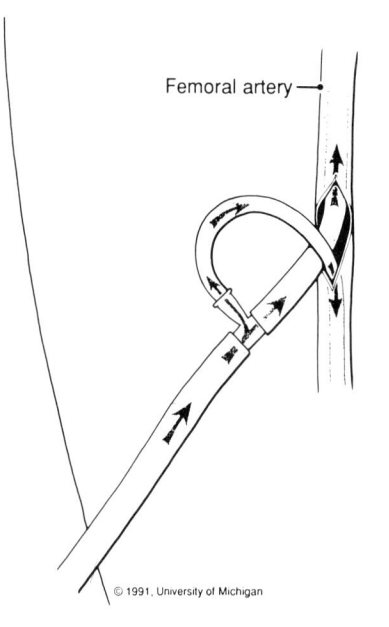

FIGURE 12.8 Femoral artery cannulation with allowance for distal perfusion.

by coating the surface with a cationic (positively charged) surfactant and then immersing the surface in a solution containing an anionic (negatively charged) antibiotic. Although heparin-antibiotic surface combinations have yet to be evaluated, the advantages of such combinations for long-term support are far reaching.

Further refinements in cannula design will include optimizing cannula dimensions, minimizing wall thickness, and streamlining cannula connections. One can expect the development of an adult percutaneous double-lumen venovenous cannula.

PEDIATRIC VASCULAR ACCESS

Background

Severe acute respiratory failure is uncommon in the pediatric age group, so the clinical experience with pediatric extracorporeal life support remains limited. The earliest published report of extracorporeal oxygenation in this age group was that of Rashkind et al. (34) in 1965. These investigators used arteriovenous bypass via the femoral vessels to support four children with cystic fibrosis and severe pulmonary failure for four to eight hours; although each showed some degree of clinical improvement, all succumbed to their underlying disease. In the late 1960s, Hill et al. (7) used venovenous bypass via the jugular and femoral veins to provide temporary but unsuccessful extracorporeal support to a child with an inhalational burn injury. The first successful use of extracorporeal life support for pulmonary failure in a child was published by Schulte et al. (35) in 1972. This report describes a 10-year-old patient who underwent 43 hours of venoarterial bypass after developing fulminant pulmonary edema following repair for tetrology of Fallot. Three years later, Kolobow and co-workers (36) published the first successful use of venovenous bypass for pediatric pulmonary failure. Over the next several years, many adult series included one or two pediatric patients, all of whom were cannulated in much the same fashion as the adults, depending on the latest scheme and most recent success.

In a review of pediatric extracorporeal life support by Anderson et al. (37), 17 of 33 patients were placed on bypass for primary pulmonary failure; the remaining 16 patients had pre- or postoperative cardiac support. Thirteen of the 17 patients with primary pulmonary failure were supported with venoarterial bypass. Venous access was obtained via the right internal jugular vein, the femoral vein, or both, and oxygenated blood was reinfused through the axillary, carotid, or femoral artery. The remaining four patients were placed on venovenous bypass, with return of oxygenated blood by direct cannulation of the saphenofemoral junction or the femoral vein. Carotid artery ligation was routinely performed on patients who were less than three years of age. The authors caution that the neurologic status of older children should be assessed with temporary occlusion of the right common carotid artery before permanent ligation.

The experience in New Orleans has been somewhat different, in that all but one of 32 pediatric patients with primary cardiac (10) or pulmonary (22) failure have been cannulated for venoarterial bypass via the right common carotid artery and internal jugular vein (38). No neurologic sequelae have been reported in these children. Moreover, several patients at this center have undergone repair of the right common carotid artery at the time of decannulation, primarily because of the unknown long-term effects of carotid artery ligation.

Current Technique

Venovenous bypass is gaining wider acceptance in the management of pediatric patients with noncardiac respiratory failure, as this mode of bypass avoids the need to ligate or repair the common carotid artery (37). Cannulation for venvenous bypass using the jugular or femoral veins is performed in much the same fashion as in the adult patient and is described above.

If there is an element of cardiac failure in a pediatric patient with primary pulmonary disease, or if one wishes to minimize the risk of medianstinitis associated with transthoracic cannulation following median sternotomy for repair of a congenital cardiac defect, venoarterial cannulation can be performed using the iliac or cervical vessels. A toddler's iliac vessels are considerably larger than the femoral vessels and are therefore able to provide a higher percentage of bypass flow. Access is via a retroperitoneal approach above the right or left inguinal ligament; distal cannulation of the iliac vessels is usually not necessary (Figure 12.9). The alternative is cervical cannulation of the right internal jugular vein and right common carotid artery, as is routinely performed in neonates and young children (37). Table 12.1 lists suggested pediatric cannula sizes based on the weight of the patient (33).

Problems and Controversies

Advances in pediatric extracorporeal life support will follow developments in adult and neonatal circulatory support, simply because of the greater patient experience in the latter groups. One can expect the development of a

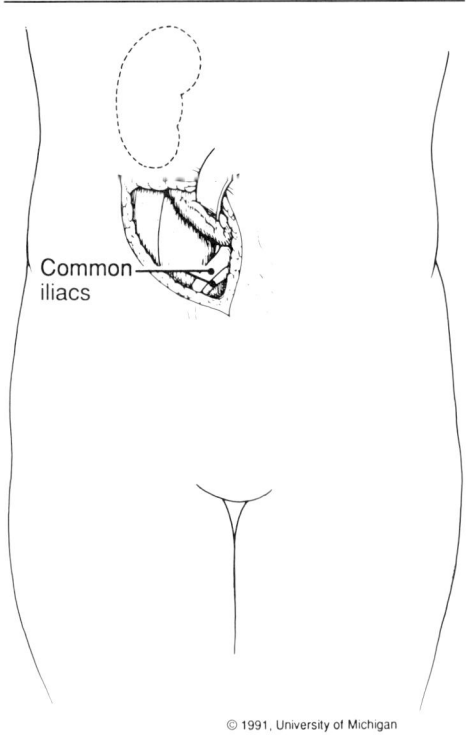

FIGURE 12.9 The common iliac vessels provide sufficient venoarterial access in toddlers.

TABLE 12.1 Cannulas for pediatric venoarterial ECLS

	Weight of patient (kg)			
	8–12	12–20	20–35	35+
Venous (Fr)	16–20	20–24	21–24	>28
Arterial (Fr)	12–16	14–18	16–20	20+

wider variety of pediatric arterial and venous cannulas, including percutaneous and double-lumen cannulas (37).

NEONATAL VASCULAR ACCESS

Background

Neonates present a special problem because of their small size and the limited number of sites available for high-volume vascular access. This was noted by several early investigators, beginning with Enhorning and Westin (39) in 1954 and Westin, Nyberg, and Enhorning (40) in 1958, following their efforts to support "previable" human fetuses for periods of up to 12 hours using umbilical vessel arteriovenous bypass. Dorson et al. (41–43) used larger umbilical catheters and later augmented arterial outflow with a femoral artery cannula. Rashkind et al. (34) used one or both femoral arteries of four critically ill neonates to achieve arteriovenous bypass flows of 40% to 50% of the cardiac output. Although arteriovenous perfusion mimics the placental circulation, it was complicated in these early clinical trials by progressive cardiovascular collapse. Arteriovenous bypass was therefore abandoned in the mid-1960s in favor of venovenous bypass, which at the time appeared to offer promise in the early adult and pediatric clinical trials. By 1970, White and associates (44) were able to support a newborn infant for up to 10 days on venovenous bypass using the right internal jugular vein for venous drainage and the umbilical vein for the return of oxygenated blood. Although this infant died, as did all the others in these early clinical trials, these investigators made important observations regarding potential routes for neonatal vascular access, cannula design, and blood flow; they also gained information on the hematologic effects and gas exchange limitations of the extracorporeal circuit.

The first successful application of extracorporeal life support in a neonate was performed in 1975 by Bartlett and co-workers (45), who used venoarterial bypass. This mode of bypass substantially increased the available bypass flow to allow further reduction in ventilator settings, while providing a means to support the systemic circulation. Vascular access was via the right internal jugular vein and right common carotid artery. These vessels are disproportionately large in neonates, and both proved amenable to distal ligation.

Since this first successful case, the development of neonatal venoarterial extracorporeal life support (ECLS) has enabled survival of an ever-increasing number of newborn infants with severe pulmonary failure. With this success has come the ability to better recognize potential ECLS candidates and thus initiate extracorporeal life support earlier in the course of disease, before the onset of myocardial failure due to prolonged hypoxemia. Simultaneously, investigators have continued to pursue venovenous bypass as a means to avoid ligation of the right common carotid artery and to reduce the risks of air or particle emboli that may emanate from the extracorporeal circuit. Additional theoretical advantages of venovenous bypass include maintenance of normal hemodynamics and improved oxygen delivery to the pulmonary circulation and coronary arteries.

Neonatal venovenous bypass was performed successfully by Andrews and co-workers (46, 47) in the early 1980s using the right internal jugular vein for venous drainage and a femoral vein for the return of oxygenated blood. Their efforts led to a report comparing venovenous and venoarterial extracorporeal life support in newborns with pulmonary failure (48). Their findings indicated that venovenous bypass provides excellent pulmonary support to hemodynamically stable infants whose illnesses are characterized by pulmonary hypertension. Nevertheless, several problems were encountered relating specifically to femoral vein ligation and cannulation. These problems included the added time required for a second surgical incision and groin dissection, persistent leg swelling, and poor wound healing; three of 10 patients developed leg length discrepancies. Three of 11 infants required conversion from venovenous to venoarterial bypass. In one case, this was due to persistent hypoxemia, which resulted from the recirculation of oxygenated blood from the femoral venous return cannula to the atrial drainage cannula. By comparison, no detectable complications were attributed to right internal jugular vein or common carotid artery ligation. Overall, patients on venoarterial bypass required longer perfusion times and had a higher mortality rate than patients on venovenous bypass, but they also had lower birthweights and less favorable diagnoses.

Two different methods of single cannula venovenous bypass via the right internal jugular have solved the problems associated with femoral vein cannulation in the neonate. One method utilizes a tidal flow system with a single-lumen cannula; blood drainage and reinfusion are accomplished by pneumatically occluding either the blood outflow or inflow line in an alternating fashion (49). The other method utilizes a thin-walled polyurethane double-lumen cannula (50). This cannula has an eccentric septum that creates a large lumen with side holes for venous drainage and a small blind-tipped lumen with side holes for the return of oxygenated blood (Figure 12.10). When the cannula is properly oriented in the right atrium, the perfusate side holes are directed toward the tricuspid valve to minimize recirculation of oxygenated blood. Clinical experience with the double-lumen cannula for venovenous bypass appears promising for infants with pulmonary failure who do not have overwhelming myocardial dysfunction (51).

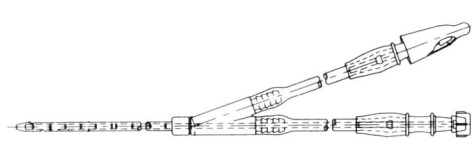

FIGURE 12.10 Neonatal double-lumen venovenous cannula.

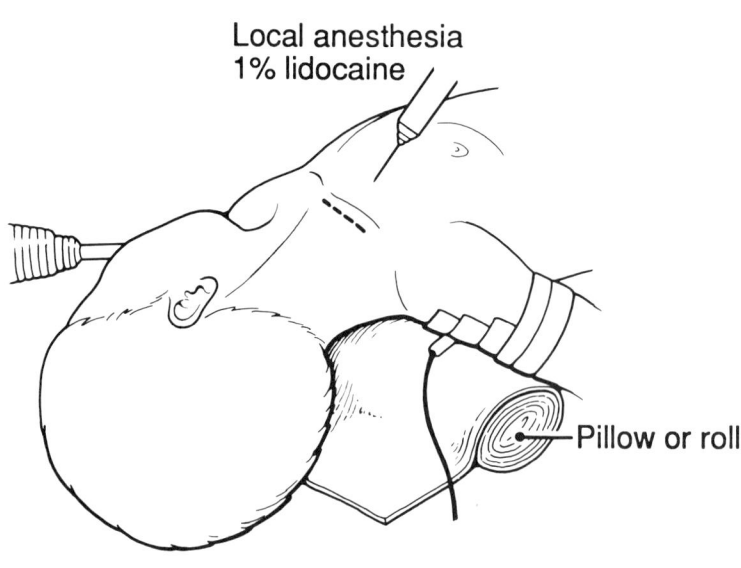

FIGURE 12.11 Positioning for cervical cannulation.

Current Technique

Cannulation and decannulation for neonatal extracorporeal life support are performed in the neonatal intensive care unit. The patient is positioned with the head toward the aisle, a roll is placed beneath the shoulders, and the head is turned to the left (Figure 12.11). The chest, neck, and right side of the head are prepared and draped in a sterile fashion. An

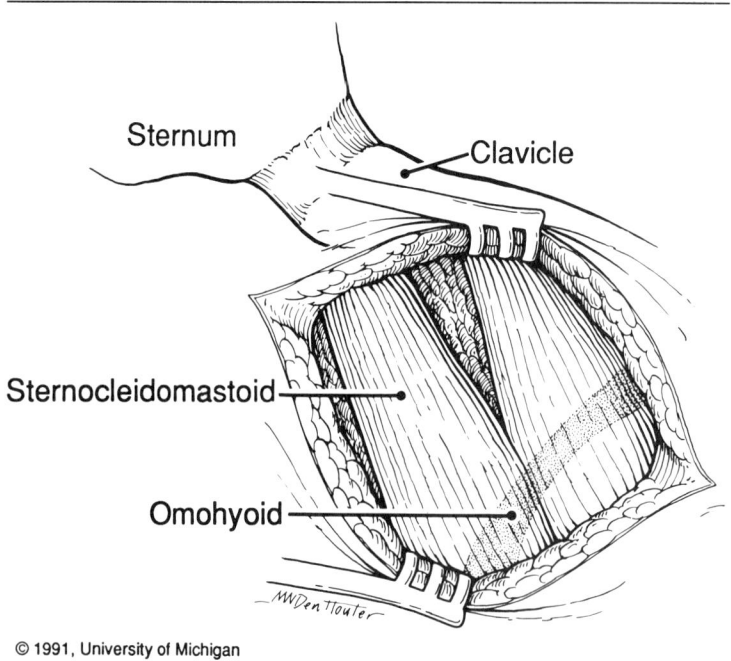

FIGURE 12.12 The two heads of the sternocleidomastoid muscle are encountered through a low transverse cervical incision.

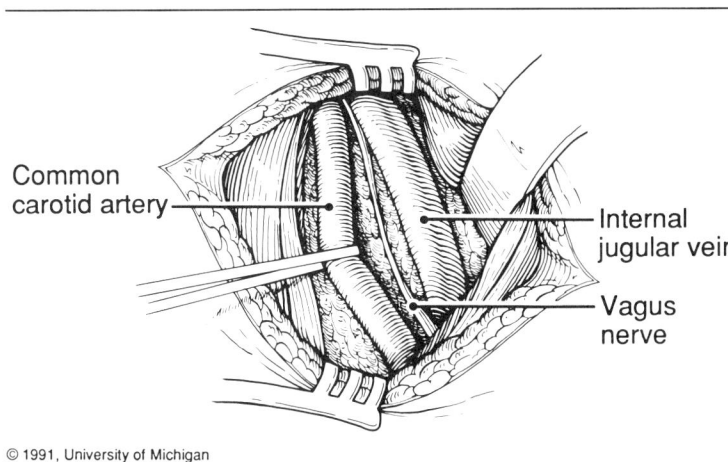

FIGURE 12.13 The right internal jugular vein and common carotid artery are exposed beneath the sternocleidomastoid muscle.

oblique or transverse cervical incision is made over the middle or lower one-third of the right sternocleidomastoid muscle, respectively. The advantage of the oblique incision is its direct approach to the carotid sheath and its ease of extension should rapid central access become necessary. The disadvantage of this incision is the fact that it crosses Langer's lines, which causes it to heal with a fibrous contracture.

The platysma muscle and underlying areolar tissue are divided with electrocautery to expose the sternocleidomastoid muscle (Figure 12.12). Dissection proceeds between the sternal heads of the muscle if a low transverse incision is used, or along the medial edge of the muscle if an oblique incision is made. Sutures or a Weitlander retractor are carefully positioned to retract the wound margins but avoid injury to the recurrent laryngeal nerve (52). The facial vein is often encountered via the oblique incision and should be preserved as a possible site for central venous access at the time of decannulation (53). The tendon of the omohyoid muscle must be cut to expose the carotid sheath if the approach is through a low transverse incision.

The carotid sheath is opened, and the internal jugular vein, common carotid artery, and vagus nerve are identified (Figure 12.13). Heparin (40–100 U/kg) is given intravenously. One percent lidocaine and 20% papaverine are instilled within the wound to promote vascular relaxation.

If venoarterial bypass is planned, the common carotid artery is ligated 5 to 10 mm proximal to the carotid artery bifurcation, well below the superior thyroid artery. Proximal control of the common carotid artery is established with an angled ductus clamp. A transverse or longitudinal arteriotomy is performed adjacent to the distal ligature, and the proximal edge of the arteriotomy is secured with two 6-0 monofilament stay sutures to prevent subintimal dissection (54) during insertion of the arterial cannula (Figure 12.14) (55).

FIGURE 12.14 Fine stay sutures open the right common carotid arteriotomy and fix the intima against the sidewall of the vessel.

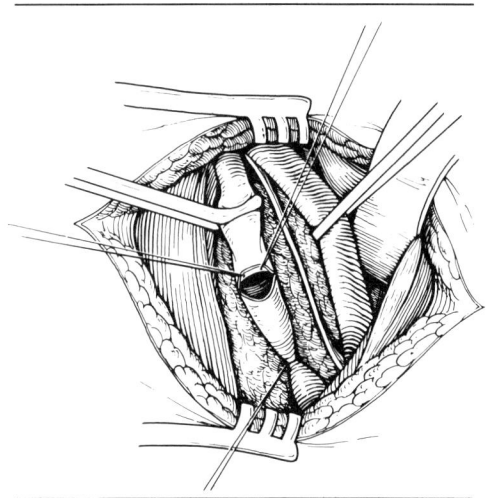

The arterial cannula is passed to a point just proximal to the takeoff of the right common carotid artery from the brachiocephalic artery; this is approximately 1.5 cm via a low transverse incision, versus about 2.5 cm via the oblique incision. The arterial cannula is secured within the vessel lumen, using one or two circumferential ligatures; the knots are buttressed with a small piece of a vessel loop to prevent injury to the vessel wall when these ligatures are removed during decannulation. The arterial cannula is anchored to the skin with monofilament suture.

The vein is cannulated in a similar fashion. It is mobilized and ligated distally; proximal control is established using vascular forceps. A transverse venotomy is made, and the venous cannula is advanced 5.5 to 6.5 cm into the right atrium, depending on the location of the venotomy site and the size of the infant (Figure 12.15). The cannula is secured within the vessel lumen and anchored to the skin. A sterile loop of the extracorporeal circuit is divided, and the cannulas are connected to their recipient neck lines, ensuring that no air bubbles enter the circuit. Bypass is initiated, and pump flow is gradually increased.

The wound is irrigated and hemostasis ob-

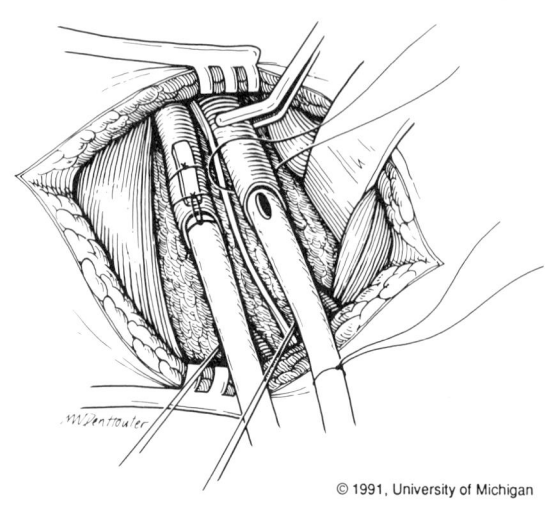

FIGURE 12.15 Cannulation of the right internal jugular vein.

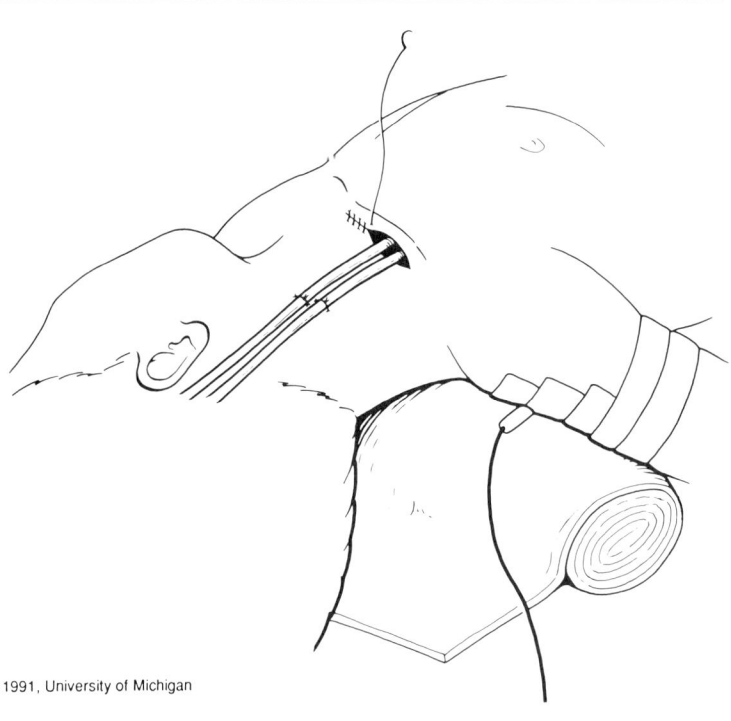

FIGURE 12.16 Closure of the low transverse cervical incision.

tained. Thrombin glue is instilled, and the skin margins are approximated with a running stitch (Figure 12.16). Catheter position is confirmed by x-ray immediately following cannulation and on a daily basis (Figure 12.17). Questions regarding the exact location of the arterial cannula tip in relation to the aortic valve can be answered by echocardiography. A small amount of bleeding from the operative site is not uncommon during bypass, but if it exceeds 30 mL/hour, the site should be explored.

Decannulation is performed at the patient's bedside in much the same fashion as the cannulation procedure described above. The patient is positioned with a roll beneath the shoulders, and the head is turned to the left with care to prevent accidental decannulation. Following sterile preparation and draping, the neonate is anesthetized with intravenous morphine or fentanyl and paralyzed to prevent air embolus (56). Once the ventilator settings have been adjusted to support the patient in a paralyzed state, the neck lines are clamped, and the main bridge is opened to prevent stagnation within the extracorporeal circuit. Both vessels are mobilized, proximal control is achieved, the cannulas are sequentially removed, and each vessel is ligated. A two-layer interrupted closure is performed.

Several centers have reported on the feasibility of carotid artery reconstruction (57–61), but the selection of patients best suited for this operation, the recognition of contraindications, and the best methods for repair are not well understood. Until more information is gained about the relative risks and benefits of carotid artery reconstruction, routine ligation is an accepted form of practice.

Problems and Controversies

Proponents of neonatal extracorporeal life support have for years drawn attention away from the controversy surrounding carotid artery ligation and focused instead on the benefits of the technique. With time, this strategy has proven effective. For although several small series (62–66) have suggested that there is an increased incidence of right-sided brain lesions in neonatal ECLS patients, larger studies (67–69) have failed to show convincing evidence linking carotid artery ligation with adverse developmental outcome. Now, however, as the feasibility and safety of neonatal extracorporeal support became more established, the proponents of ECLS are divided on the issue of whether the carotid artery should be permanently ligated or repaired.

There are four principal arguments against carotid artery reconstruction following neonatal ECLS (61). The first argument contends that there is no need for arterial repair since there is little clinical evidence to suggest that carotid artery ligation is harmful in the neonatal period. This viewpoint is supported by positron emission tomography (70), angiography, and radioisotope studies (71), which demonstrate early symmetrical cerebral blood flow in neonatal ECLS survivors. A more recent, long-term follow-up study by Lott et al. (66) suggests, however, that right-sided cerebral perfusion above the ligated carotid artery may be both asymmetric and insufficient for normal cerebral development. This study showed a significant decrease in the amplitude of the long-latency auditory and somato-

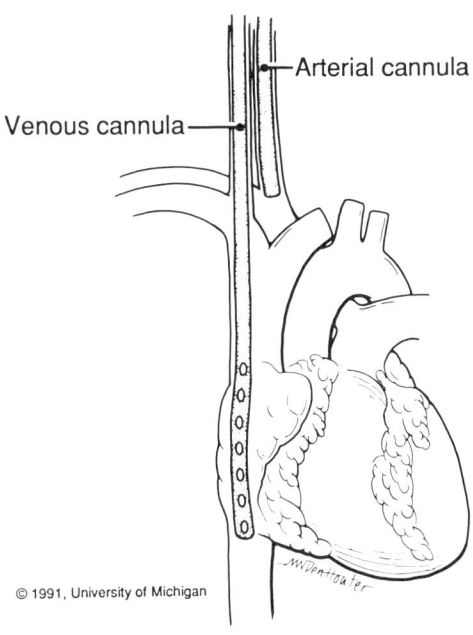

FIGURE 12.17 Cervical cannulation for venoarterial bypass.

sensory evoked potentials over the right versus the left hemisphere of the brain in long-term ECLS survivors.

The second argument against carotid artery reconstruction accepts the finding that carotid artery ligation may alter cerebral development but contends that whatever damage has been done is permanent. Therefore, reestablishing flow through the right common carotid artery simply places the patient at risk for further neurologic injury. The counterargument suggests that these observed changes may be the result of chronic, if not temporary, cerebrovascular insufficiency, and therefore avoidable if early reconstruction is performed. Several studies (72–74) have shown that blood flow in the right internal carotid artery is reversed and directed away from the brain in a majority of neonatal ECLS patients and survivors. This reversed blood flow pattern changes direction several months after common carotid artery ligation, so that blood flow in the right internal carotid artery is once again directed cephalad (66,72). The implication of these findings is that right common carotid artery ligation may yield a cerebral circulatory pattern that is temporarily insufficient to meet the needs of the developing brain. The fact that these changes take place over several months' time may be a reflection of the time needed for the development of collateral flow across the head and neck to supply the right internal carotid artery. Whether or not blood flow to the brain is insufficient during this period could perhaps be answered by a trial of carotid artery reconstruction, followed by a comparison of right- and left-sided auditory and somatosensory evoked potentials.

The third argument against carotid artery reconstruction centers on the issue of reperfusion injury. Reperfusion injury occurs when ischemic tissue is perfused with oxygenated blood, giving rise to free radical formation, cell membrane injury, and ion fluxes. This is most likely to occur shortly after right common carotid artery ligation, when the extracorporeal pump flow is increased and the right hemisphere is reperfused with oxygenated blood derived from collateral vessels. Presumably, then, if extracorporeal support effectively perfuses the cerebrovasculature, reperfusion injury is unlikely at the time of decannulation. The possibility remains, however, that there may be some areas of underperfused cerebral tissue during bypass, which may be reperfused at the time of decannulation and carotid artery repair.

The fourth argument against carotid artery reconstruction in the neonate relates to the risks of embolic phenomena, anastomotic problems, and the potential to produce turbulent flow with plaque formation. Since neurologic injury following carotid surgery in adults is almost always the result of technical error, those who choose to embark on vascular reconstruction in the neonate must be highly skilled and knowledgeable of modern vascular surgery techniques.

The optimal timing of carotid artery reconstruction would appear to be at the time of decannulation while the artery is exposed and isolated. This is particularly true if long-term perfusion imbalances are to be avoided. Occasionally, a patient will be too unstable to undergo vascular repair at the time of decannulation, in which case a delayed repair might be considered. The drawback to this approach is that it may subject the patient to a much larger operation. Proximal control of the right common carotid artery for delayed placement of an autologous vein or prosthetic graft could require a median sternotomy.

Whether or not carotid artery reconstruction will become accepted practice at the time of decannulation for neonatal extracorporeal life support has yet to be determined. In the meantime, we must continue to explore alternative means of vascular access for neonatal venoarterial bypass, including right subclavian artery and umbilical vessel cannulation (75).

SUMMARY

Several parameters must be taken into consideration when the optimal cannulation scheme for an individual patient is determined. These parameters include the patient's age, size, available cannulation sites, and underlying disease processes. Other important considerations include the systemic oxygen tension required to meet the patient's specific needs and whether or not cardiac support is needed. Since simplicity, ease of instrumentation, and hemorrhage are always overriding issues, vascular access techniques using percutaneous methods or a single skin incision are preferred. Thus, venovenous extracorporeal CO_2 removal using percutaneous cannulation of the right internal jugular and femoral veins is currently best suited for adult patients with primary pulmonary dysfunction. Larger cannulas for improved flow and better oxygenation in adult and pediatric patients are best placed by surgical cut-down.

Whereas the adult patient with cardiopulmonary failure can be supported with a ventricular assist device and extracorporeal oxygenation, the absence of a suitable ventricular assist device for children and infants suggests that venoarterial extracorporeal support must become more physiologic, safer, and easier to institute. Until then, venoarterial cannulation for cardiopulmonary failure in children and infants is best performed through a single neck incision using the right internal jugular vein and common carotid artery. These vessels can be ligated if there is no evidence of associated cerebrovascular insufficiency. Alternatively, the common iliac vessels or the right subclavian artery and vein can be used for vascular access. Neonates with primary pulmonary dysfunction can be supported using a tidal flow system or double-lumen venovenous catheter. Whether or not venovenous bypass through a single cannula in the umbilical vein (75) will become feasible, and thereby supplant the need for operative cannulation of the neonate, remains to be determined.

REFERENCES

(1) Gibbon JH Jr. Application of a mechanical heart and lung apparatus to cardiac surgery. Minn Med 1954;37:171–80.

(2) Dennis C, Spring DS, Nelson GE, Karlson KE, et al. Development of a pump-oxygenator to replace the heart and lungs. An apparatus applicable to human patients and application to one case. Ann Surg 1951;134:709–21.

(3) Helmsworth JA, Clark LC Jr, Kaplan S, Sherman RT. Clinical use of extracorporeal oxygenation with oxygenator-pump. JAMA 1952;150:451–3.

(4) Spragg RG, Hill RN, Wedel MK, Masterson A, Moser KM. Platelet kinetics in venovenous membrane oxygenation. Trans ASAIO 1975;21:171–7.

(5) Depp DA, Hughes RK. Venovenous perfusion with a membrane oxygenator. J Thorac Cardiovasc Surg 1971;62:658–68.

(6) Hanson EL, Bartlett RH, Burns NE, et al. The use of a membrane oxygenator in air breathing and hypoxic lambs: venovenous bypass. Surgery 1973;73:824–98.

(7) Hill JD, Fallat R, Cohn K, et al. Clinical cardiopulmonary dynamics during prolonged extracorporeal circulation for acute respiratory insufficiency. Trans ASAIO 1971;17:355–61.

(8) Zapol W, Pontoppidan H, McCullough N, Schmidt V, Bland J, Kitz R. Clinical membrane lung support for acute respiratory insufficiency. Trans ASAIO 1972;18:553–60.

(9) Rea WJ, Eberle JW, Ecker RR, Watson J, Sugg WL. Long-term membrane oxygenation in respiratory failure. Ann Thorac Surg 1973;15:170–8.

(10) Hill JD, Rodvien R, Snider MT, Bartlett RH. Clinical extracorporeal membrane oxygenation for acute respiratory insufficiency. Trans ASAIO 1978;24:753–63.

(11) Leitz KH. Oxygenation in peripheral venoarterial bypass. In: Zapol WM, Qvist J, eds. Artificial lungs for acute respiratory failure. Washington D.C.: Hemisphere Publishing, 1976:319–27.

(12) Hill JD. Extracorporeal oxygenation for acute respiratory insufficiency: clinical experience. Mt Sinai J Med NY 1973;40:189–98.

(13) Hill JD, deLeval MR, Fallat RJ, et al. Acute respiratory insufficiency: treatment with prolonged extracorporeal oxygenation. J Thorac Cardiovasc Surg 1972;64:551–62.

(14) Carlson RG. Discussion. J Thorac Cardiovasc Surg 1972;64:560.

(15) Hill JD, O'Brien TG, Murray JJ, et al. Prolonged extracorporeal oxygenation for acute post-traumatic respiratory failure (shock-lung syndrome). N Engl J Med 1972;286:629–34.

(16) Kanarek D, Zapol W, Ahluwalia B, Qvist J, Hales C, Liland A. Radionuclide imaging of the circulatory distribution of membrane lung perfusion. Trans ASAIO 1974;20:262–8.

(17) McEnany MT, Zapol WM, Seebacher J, et al. Cannulation of the proximal aorta during long-term membrane lung perfusion. J Thorac Cardiovasc Surg 1975;70:631–43.

(18) Cooper JD, Duffin J, Zapol WM. Cannulation of ascending aorta for long-term mem-

(19) Snider MT, Zapol WM. Assessment of pulmonary oxygenation during venoarterial bypass with aortic root return. In: Zapol WM, Qvist J, eds. Artificial lungs for acute respiratory failure. Washington D.C.: Hemisphere Publishing, 1976:257–73.

(20) Secker-Walker JS, Edmunds JF, Spratt EH, Conn AW. The source of coronary perfusion during partial bypass for extracorporeal membrane oxygenation (ECMO). Ann Thorac Surg 1976;21:138–43.

(21) Hill JD, Rattliff JL, Fallat RJ, et al. Prognostic factors in the treatment of acute respiratory insufficiency with long-term extracorporeal oxygenation. J Thorac Cardiovasc Surg 1974;68:905–17.

(22) Zapol WM, Qvist J, Pontoppidan H, Liland A, McEnany T, Laver MB. Extracorporeal perfusion for acute respiratory failure. J Thorac Cardiovasc Surg 1975;69:439–49.

(23) Gille JP. Respiratory support by extracorporeal circulation with a membrane artificial lung. Bull Physiopathol Respir 1974;10:373–410.

(24) Bartlett RH, Gazzaniga AB, Fong SW, Burns NE. Prolonged extracorporeal cardiopulmonary support in man. J Thorac Cardiovasc Surg 1974;68:918–32.

(25) Bartlett RH, Gazzaniga AB. Extracorporeal circulation for cardiopulmonary failure. Curr Probl Surg 1978;15(5):1–96.

(26) Extracorporeal support for respiratory insufficiency: a collaborative study in response to RFP-NHLI-73-20. U.S. Dept. Health Education and Welfare, National Institutes of Health, Bethesda, MD, 1979.

(27) Zapol WM, Snider MT, Hill JD, et al. Extracorporeal membrane oxygenation in severe acute respiratory failure. JAMA 1979;242:2193–6.

(28) Kolobow T, Gattinoni L, Tomlinson T, White D, Pierce J, Iapichino G. The carbon dioxide membrane lung (CDML): a new concept. Trans ASAIO 1977;23:17–21.

(29) Kolobow T, Moretti MP, Fumagalli R, et al. Severe impairment in lung function induced by high peak airway pressure mechanical ventilation: an experimental study. Am Rev Respir Dis 1987;135:312–15.

(30) Gattinoni L, Pesenti A, Rossi GP, et al. Treatment of acute respiratory failure with low-frequency positive-pressure ventilation and extracorporeal removal of CO_2. Lancet 1980;2:292–4.

(31) Pesenti A, Kolobow T, Marcolin R, et al. A double lumen catheter allowing single vessel cannulation for extracorporeal respiratory assistance. Eur Surg Res 1982;14:119.

(32) Pesenti A, Gattinoni L, Kolobow T, et al. Extracorporeal circulation in adult respiratory failure. Trans Am Soc Artif Intern Organs 1988;34:43–7.

(33) Chapman RA, Bartlett RH. Extracorporeal life support manual for adult and pediatric patients. (Unpublished.)

(34) Rashkind WJ, Freeman A, Klein D, Toft RW. Evaluation of a disposable plastic low volume, pumpless oxygenator as a lung substitute. J Pediatr 1965;66:94–102.

(35) Schulte HD, Bircks W, Dudziak R. Erste erfahrungen mit der Bramson-Membrane-Lunge. Thoraxchirurgie 1972;20:54–9.

(36) Kolobow T, Stool E, Sacks K, et al. Acute respiratory failure: survival following ten days support with a membrane lung. J Thorac Cardiovasc Surg 1975;69:947–53.

(37) Anderson HL, Attorri RJ, Custer JR, Chapman RA, Bartlett RH. Extracorporeal membrane oxygenation for pediatric cardiopulmonary failure. J Thorac Cardiovasc Surg 1990;99:1011–21.

(38) Adolph V, Bonis S, Falterman K, Arensman R. Carotid artery repair after pediatric extracorporeal membrane oxygenation. J Pediatr Surg 1990;8:867–70.

(39) Enhorning G, Westin B. Experimental studies of the human fetus in prolonged asphyxia. Acta Physiol Scand 1954;31:359–74.

(40) Westin B, Nyberg R, Enhorning G. A technique for perfusion of the previable human fetus. Acta Pediatr Stockholm 1958;47:339–49.

(41) Dorson WJ, Baker E, Hall H, et al. A long-term partial bypass oxygenation system. Ann Thorac Surg 1969;8:297–311.

(42) Dorson WJ, Baker E, Cohen ML, et al. A perfusion system for infants. Trans ASAIO 1969;15:155–60.

(43) Dorson WJ, Meyer B, Baker E, et al. Response of distressed infants to partial bypass lung assist. Trans ASAIO 1970;16:345–51.

(44) White JJ, Andrews HG, Risemberg H, Mazur D, Haller JA. Prolonged respiratory support in newborn infants with a membrane oxygenator. Surgery 1971;70:288–96.

(45) Bartlett RH, Gazzaniga AB, Huxtable RF, Schippers HC, O'Conner MJ, Jefferies MR. Extracorporeal circulation (ECMO) in neonatal

respiratory failure. J Thorac Cardiovasc Surg 1977;74:826–33.

(46) Andrews AF, Toomasian J, Oram A, Bartlett RH. Total respiratory support with venovenous (VV) ECMO. Trans ASAIO 1982;28:350–3.

(47) Andrews AF, Klein MD, Toomasian JM, et al. Venovenous extracorporeal membrane oxygenation in neonates with respiratory failure. J Pediatr Surg 1983;18:339–46.

(48) Klein MD, Andrews AF, Wesley JR, et al. Venovenous perfusion in ECMO for newborn respiratory insufficiency: a clinical comparison with venoarterial perfusion. Ann Surg 1985;201: 520–6.

(49) Zwischenberger JB, Toomasian JM, Drake K, Andrews AF, Kolobow T, Bartlett RH. Total respiratory support with single cannula venovenous ECMO: double lumen continuous flow vs. single lumen tidal flow. Trans Am Soc Artif Intern Organs 1985;31:610–15.

(50) Otsu T, Merz SI, Hultquist KA, et al. Laboratory evaluation of a double lumen catheter for venovenous neonatal ECMO. Trans ASAIO 1989;35:647–50.

(51) Anderson HL, Otsu T, Chapman R, Bartlett RH. Venovenous extracorporeal life support in neonates using a double lumen catheter. Trans ASAIO 1989;35:650–3.

(52) Schumacher RE, Weinfeld IJ, Bartlett RH. Neonatal vocal cord paralysis following extracorporeal membrane oxygenation. Pediatrics 1989;84:793–6.

(53) Ford EG, Kitagawa H, Atkinson JB. Vascular access in the neonate following extracorporeal membrane oxygenation. J Pediatr Surg 1990;25:594–595.

(54) Bartlett RH, Gazzaniga AB, Jefferies MR, Huxtable RF, Haiduc NJ, Fong SW. Extracorporeal membrane oxygenation (ECMO) cardiopulmonary support in infancy. Trans ASAIO 1976; 22:80–93.

(55) German JC, Worcester C, Gazzaniga AB, et al. Technical aspects in the management of the meconium aspiration syndrome with extracorporeal circulation. J Pediatr Surg 1980;15:378–83.

(56) Krummel TM, Greenfield LJ, Kirkpatrick BV, Mueller DG, Ormazabal M, Salzberg AM. Clinical use of an extracorporeal membrane oxygenator in neonatal pulmonary failure. J Pediatr Surg 1982;17:525–31.

(57) Weinhaus L, Canter C, Noetzel M, McAlister W, Spray TL. Extracorporeal membrane oxygenation for circulatory support after repair of congenital heart defects. Ann Thorac Surg 1989;48:206–12.

(58) Lewin JS, Masaryk TJ, Modic MT, Ross JS, Stork EK, Wiznitzer M. Extracorporeal membrane oxygenation in infants: angiographic and parenchymal evaluation of the brain with MR imaging. Radiology 1989:173:361–5.

(59) Spector ML, Wiznitzer M, Walsh-Sukys MC, Stork EK. Carotid reconstruction in the neonate following ECMO. J Pediatr Surg 1991; 26:357–61.

(60) Crombleholme TM, Adzick NS, deLorimer AA, Longaker MT, Harrison MR, Charlton VE. Carotid artery reconstruction following extracorporeal membrane oxygenation. Am J Dis Child 1990;144:872–4.

(61) Moulton SL, Lynch FP, Cornish JD, Bejar RF, Simko AJ, Krous HF. Carotid artery reconstruction following neonatal extracorporeal membrane oxygenation. J Pediatr Surg 1991;26:794–9.

(62) Towne BH, Lott IT, Hicks DA, Healey T. Long-term follow-up of infants and children treated with extracorporeal membrane oxygenation (ECMO): a preliminary report. J Pediatr Surg 1985;20:410–14.

(63) Schumacher RE, Barks JDE, Johnston MJ, et al. Right sided brain lesions in infants following extracorporeal membrane oxygenation. Pediatrics 1988;82:155–60.

(64) Campbell LR, Bunyapen C, Holmes GL, Howell CG, Kanto WP. Right common carotid artery ligation in extracorporeal membrane oxygenation. J Pediatr 1988;113:110–13.

(65) Schumacher RE, Spak C, Kileny PR. Asymmetric brain stem auditory evoked responses in infants treated with extracorporeal membrane oxygenation. Ear Hear 1990;11:359–62.

(66) Lott IT, McPherson D, Towne B, Johnson D, Starr A. Long-term neurophysiologic outcome following neonatal extracorporeal membrane oxygenation. J Pediatr 1990;116:343–9.

(67) Krummel TM, Greenfield LJ, Kirkpatrick BV, et al. The early evaluation of survivors after extracorporeal membrane oxygenation for neonatal pulmonary failure. J Pediatr Surg 1984; 19:585–90.

(68) Glass P, Miller MK, Short BL. Morbidity for survivors of extracorporeal membrane oxygenation: neurodevelopmental outcome at one year of age. Pediatrics 1989;83:72–8.

(69) Adolph V, Ekelund C, Starret A, Falterman K, Arensman R. Developmental outcome of

neonates treated with extracorporeal membrane oxygenation. J Pediatr Surg 1990;25:43–6.

(70) Perlman JM, Altman DI, Powers WJ, Volpe JJ. Cerebral injury and regional cerebral blood flow in newborn infants undergoing extracorporeal membrane oxygenation. Ann Neurol 1987; 22:421.

(71) Voorhies TM, Tardo CL, Andrea LS, et al. Evaluation of the cerebral circulation in neonates following extracorporeal membrane oxygenation. Ann Neurol 1985;18:380.

(72) Mitchell DG, Merton DA, Graziana LJ, et al. Right carotid artery ligation in neonates: classification of collateral flow with color doppler imaging. Radiology 1990;175:117–23.

(73) Raju TNK, Kim SY, Meller JL, et al. Circle of Willis blood velocity and flow direction after common carotid artery ligation for neonatal extracorporeal membrane oxygenation. Pediatrics 1989;83:343–7.

(74) Wong WS, Tsuruda JS, Liberman RL, et al. Color Doppler imaging of the intracranial vessels in the neonate. AJNR 1989;10:425–30.

(75) Cornish JD, Dudell G, Evans ML, Sweet L, Moulton SL. Use of umbilical vessels for neonatal ECMO cannulation—possibilities and precautions. Trans ASAIO (in press).

13

Clinical Management of the Neonatal ECMO Patient

❖

Billie L. Short, M.D.

This chapter will consider routine and emergency management of the neonatal patient once ECMO has begun. As mentioned before, new approaches to management are continuously being developed and should be incorporated as indicated.

ROUTINE MANAGEMENT

A team approach to the management of the ECMO patient is critical. Duties of the bedside nurse, respiratory therapist, and ECMO specialist should be delineated to ensure that the patient is cared for efficiently and effectively. Most neonatal patients require ECMO support for about five days. For recovery to occur in such a short time, many physiologic changes must take place, making daily care of the infant a fine art. Daily parameters should be recorded and placed at the bedside for use by the ECMO specialist. These should include acceptable ranges for hematocrit, platelet count, activated clotting time (ACT), mean blood pressure, patient Pao_2, patient $Paco_2$, and pump $Ppco_2$. The plan for weaning should be outlined, i.e., whether the ECMO blood flow or Fio_2 to the membrane is to be weaned, and emergency ventilator settings should be specified in case the infant has to be removed from ECMO. These parameters should be reviewed daily and updated as the patient's status changes.

Caution in routine care must be taken because of the use of systemic anticoagulation. A sign should be placed above the infant's bed indicating that no IV punctures, heel sticks, or nasal suctioning should occur. Patient data, including systolic, diastolic, and mean arterial blood pressures, heart rate, urine output, chest tube output, or other tube drainage, should be monitored hourly. Postmembrane pressures should be monitored constantly but recorded hourly. Daily laboratory values should include a white cell count with differential, magnesium, phosphorus, serum osmolality, and creatinine/blood urea nitrogen. If indicated, a bilirubin and serum plasma hemoglobin level should be obtained. Laboratory values monitored every 8 to 12 hours include hemoglobin, hematocrit, calcium, and serum electrolytes. Hourly blood tests include activated clotting times, bedside dextrometer testing for glucose, and arterial blood gases, although in-line venous saturation monitors may permit the collection of fewer blood samples. Postmembrane blood gases should be obtained at least every eight hours to insure proper functioning of the membrane and determine the postmembrane CO_2 level, which can affect the respiratory drive of the patient (see below).

Infection is a great concern on ECMO; therefore, rules used in perfusion should also apply to the ECMO circuit. These include the concept that a port is used for only one thing; either fluid withdrawal or fluid infusion. The only exception to this is the postmembrane port where platelets are infused and arterial samples are taken. Blood withdrawn to clear the line should never be infused back into the system. This should be discarded and considered as "blood out." When a port is used, the stopcock should be cleaned with betadine and/or alcohol, and the stopcock should be changed if it becomes "sticky." The pump and its components should be kept clean, and any blood products spilled should be cleaned with a 5% bleach solution. Gloves should be worn at all times when entering the circuit; mask and protective goggles should be worn if a major procedure such as changing a pigtail is being undertaken. Because of the concern for nosocomial infection, infants are kept on prophylactic antibiotics during the ECMO run.

Intravenous fluids and the heparin drip can be placed into the circuit at various ports. The easiest ports are those between the venous control monitor ("bladder") and the pump. Infusing hyperalimentation fluid or other fluids into the top of the bladder is not recommended because then fluids tend to layer out at the top and become concentrated, causing precipitation or clot formation. This is also true for the heparin drip, because it will layer out and not be distributed in a constant fashion. Drugs given in small boluses, such as antibiotics and fentanyl, should not be injected into the bladder for the same reason. These medications can be given into a prepump port or after the membrane. Blood for laboratory tests and ACTs should be drawn proximal to the heparin drip and any other infusion. The easiest port to use is the one before the bladder.

Platelets *must* be given *after the membrane* to decrease aggregation in the membrane lung. Large-volume infusions such as blood or albumin can be given into the top of the bladder.

Packed red blood cells (PRBCs) are used when 10% of the blood volume has been removed. The use of quad-packs can decrease donor exposure, which is significantly higher than in the routine intensive care patient (1). If the hematocrit is 45% or greater, 5% albumin should be used for transfusion instead of PRBCs. If a bleeding complication occurs and factor replacement is needed, then fresh frozen plasma (FFP) or cryoprecipitate should be considered instead of albumin.

Platelet counts should be kept above $60,000/mm^3$ in the routine ECMO cases or greater than $100,000/mm^3$ in infants with bleeding complications. Concentrated platelets are preferred because of their small volume (8 to 10 mL versus 25 to 30 mL in unconcentrated platelets) (2).

Daily chest x-rays are taken to evaluate the pulmonary status of the patient and to determine whether catheter placement has changed. This importance of daily x-rays is shown in Figure 13.1 in which a routine film showed reherniation postoperatively in a patient with left-sided congenital diaphragmatic hernia (CDH) who was still asymptomatic at the time of the x-ray.

Lung compliance studies can be of help in predicting successful decannulation, especially when the appearance of complications makes it necessary to consider early decannulation (3). An old-fashioned, but very effective, technique for assessing pulmonary improvement is to hand bag the infant daily. When the chest moves easily with a peak pressure of 20 cm H_2O or less, the infant will successfully come off ECMO.

Because of systemic anticoagulation and preexisting hypoxia, the ECMO patient is at risk for developing an intracranial hemorrhage on ECMO, so frequent cranial ultrasounds must be done. Many hemorrhages start small and cause no clinical signs until they have expanded to a lethal size. Knowledge of such a hemorrhage would cause changes in daily care, such as alterations in heparin management or early removal of the patient from ECMO. Late

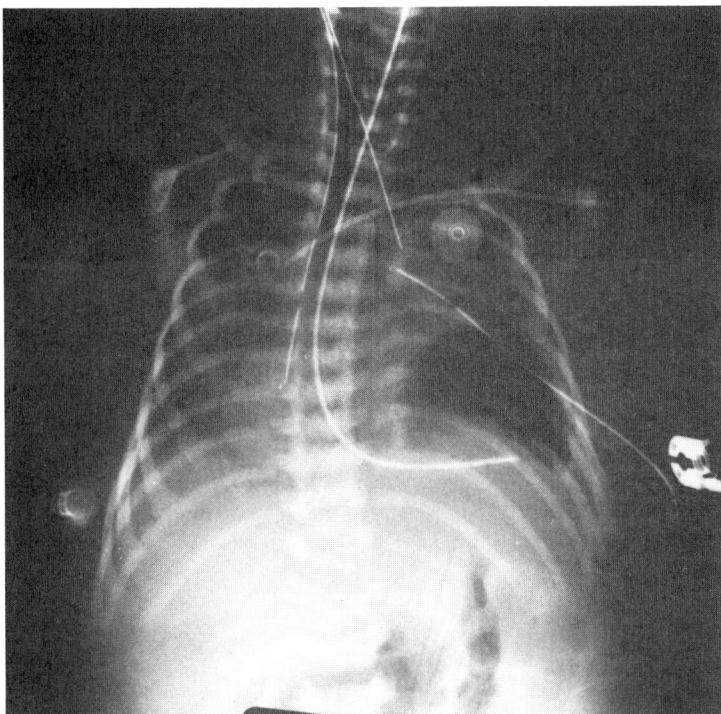

FIGURE 13.1 Daily routine x-ray showing reherniation on the left of a patient with CDH on ECMO. The infant had been repaired pre-ECMO and was asymptomatic at the time of x-ray.

bleeds have occurred in some infants on ECMO, making it necessary to continue ultrasound evaluations even after the high-risk period of the first 24 to 72 hours.

Evaluation of any bleeding source is critical. Significant bleeding from the neck incision is unusual, especially when "thrombin" fibrin glue is employed. If neck bleeding exceeds 5–10 cc/h, the surgical team should reexplore the site. Usually, packing the area with gelfoam and topical thrombin will stop the bleeding. Chest tubes, especially in the patients with CDH, can bleed extensively. This type of bleeding often cannot be stopped; therefore, careful documentation of blood loss and a plan for replacement must be made. If tracheal aspirate fluid becomes blood-tinged, the need for suctioning should be reevaluated and higher peak and expiratory pressures should be considered.

At the other end of the spectrum, clot formation or fibrin formation in the circuit must be evaluated daily. Infants at risk for bleeding will have low ACT levels, which place them at risk for clot formation in low-flow areas of the circuit. The circuit should be changed if clots are noted on the postmembrane side of the circuit. If clot formation is abnormally high, one should consider that the patient may be deficient in antithrombin III, protein C, or protein S and should have blood samples analyzed. Most cases of antithrombin III deficiency at Children's National Medical Center (CNMC) have been transient deficiencies, not of the hereditary form, although this should be considered and a hematology consult should be obtained (4).

FLUID AND NUTRITION

The average age of most infants when placed on ECMO is two or three days. They usually receive routine maintenance fluids (80–100 mL/kg/day). Because of blood pressure instability, many infants may be on pressor drips, thus increasing their fluid intake. Most infants will have received significant fluid boluses for blood pressure instability before being placed on ECMO; albumin is the most commonly used colloid. In a review of patients treated with ECMO at CNMC, it was found that a fluid bolus of 10 mEq/kg of sodium had been administered prior to ECMO. It is not surprising that these infants become edematous when on ECMO and require very little sodium replacement (0–1 mEq/kg/day).

The typical ECMO patient becomes markedly edematous and has decreased urine output for the first two to three days. Most centers give these infants 80–100 cc/kg/day of total fluid. This calculation of maintenance fluids should include lipids and total parenteral nutrition, the heparin drip, fluids for the arterial line, and any blood products given for other than replacement of "blood out." Most infants require furosemide either daily or twice daily in the first three days of ECMO. Routine hemofiltration is not usually warranted unless oliguria or anuria occurs (see the section on ultrafiltration below). Most infants on ECMO require large amounts of potassium (4–5 mEq/kg/day). This requirement is not fully understood but may be related to the effect of decreased pulsatile flow on the kidney and the increased renin production seen in these infants (5,6). Calcium replacements of 30–40 mg/kg/day of elemental calcium are required.

After day 3 of life, hyperalimentation can be started. Because the circuit can be considered as a central line, glucose can be increased to D_{25} if needed. Most infants only require D_{15} to D_{18} to attain adequate serum glucose levels and meet nutritional requirements. Protein can be increased to 2.5 mg/kg/day with intralipids increased to 4 g/kg/day. Some centers avoid use of intralipids in infants with pulmonary failure. They should continue to follow their center's practices. Although there is theoretical concern, there are no data indicating that intralipids interfere with membrane lung function. It is recommended that at least 0.5 gm/kg/day be given to ensure that the infant receives adequate essential fatty acids.

After urine output increases and edema has improved, fluids can be increased to 120–140 mL/kg/day. It must be remembered that after ECMO infants will require less potassium and more sodium in their maintenance fluids.

DAILY HEPARIN MANAGEMENT

Heparin is administered continuously into the ECMO circuit to avoid clotting. Heparin will prolong the clotting time of whole blood by blocking the clot formation at various sites in the normal coagulation system, notably conversion of prothrombin to thrombin and fibrinogen to fibrin. Heparin management will vary depending on pre-ECMO and ECMO events, which will be discussed below. Optimal heparin management will achieve the level of anticoagulation needed to decrease the risk for fibrin and clot formation in the circuit, while minimizing the risk for bleeding complications in the patient. Because anticoagulation must be evaluated rapidly and at the bedside, most centers use the ACT, which is given in seconds (7). This system uses a clotting time value determined from a system that causes activation of the clotting cascade, usually by glass beads or other substances contained in the tube into which the blood is placed. When the tube is inserted in the ACT machine, the specimen is warmed, and clotting occurs at an accelerated rate. This test will give a normal value of 80–120 seconds in a normal infant and 120–160 seconds in an infant who has heparin in his intravenous lines, as opposed to standard nonactivated bleeding time values of over five minutes (8). Platelet levels should be kept above $60,000/mm^3$ in the noncomplicated cases and above $100,000/mm^3$ in cases complicated by bleeding (9).

Fluid management must be considered when initiating the heparin drip. Most infants require 20–70 units/kg/h of heparin. Therefore, to keep the amount of fluid at a minimum, the heparin drip should be mixed with 25 kg/cc in a 5% dextrose solution. The average rate will then be 2 mL/h or 50 units heparin/kg/h.

Death in the ECMO population is most commonly related to bleeding complications. Intracranial hemorrhage (ICH) is the most common of the bleeding complications. The risk factors associated with the development of an ICH include significant hypoxic/ischemic cerebral insult prior to ECMO, sepsis with a coagulopathy, and/or gestational age less than 37 weeks. Initial heparin management should be based on pre-ECMO risk factors. If there is a high risk for ICH, the ACTs should be maintained at 190–210 seconds for at least the first 48 to 72 hours (using the Hemochrome system). Most intracranial bleeds occur during this time period. If the infant is not at risk for ICH, the ACTs should be kept at 220–260 seconds. The range can be narrowed, depending on the number of risk factors present.

It must be remembered that fibrin deposition is related to flow, and when the circuit is at low blood flow rates, the heparin rates will have to be increased to decrease the risk for clot formation. At the beginning of a run, the blood flows will be high, and the ACTs can be lower. At the end of a run, the ACTs will have to be increased, especially at "idling" (60–80 mL/min). Once the flow rate falls below 150 mL/min, the ACTs should be increased to 220–260 seconds. At idling, they should be maintained at 240–260 seconds. New centers should keep ACTs slightly higher until their team has had experience with heparin management, which is definitely an art and not a science. Clinical factors that affect the ACT values are 1) renal function (i.e., if the infant begins to increase urine output, heparin will be excreted and the heparin drip will have to be increased); 2) transfusion of coagulation factors or platelets, which will cause the ACT to drop; 3) a significant patent ductus arteriosus (PDA) with a left-to-right shunt, which may decrease renal blood flow and cause a decrease in renal output and thus heparin excretion, resulting in decreased heparin requirement; and 4) any coagulopathy associated with decreased levels of clotting factors or platelets.

An infant who develops a bleeding complication on ECMO, such as a pulmonary or gastrointestinal hemorrhage, will require special management. These infants should have their ECMO blood flow fixed at 300 mL/min or greater, with their ACTs in the 190–200-second range. Keeping the ECMO blood flow rates high will decrease the risk for fibrin formation in the circuit. When this is done, oxygenation can be altered by varying the Fio_2 into the membrane lung. Fibrinogen levels should be monitored and kept above 150 mg% with transfusion of either fresh frozen plasma or cryoprecipitate. Platelet counts should be kept above 100,000/mm^3.

To evaluate whether bleeding is due to heparin therapy alone or other causes, one must remember that the partial thromboplastin time (PTT) and thrombin time (TT) are both affected by heparin. The reptilase test uses a snake venom that acts on fibrinogen in a manner similar to that of thrombin, but is not inhibited by heparin (8). A prolonged reptilase time would indicate that factors other than heparin should be considered as the cause of bleeding. This test should be interpreted the same way that prolonged thrombin time is interpreted in patients without heparin therapy. It can also be used in cases in which heparin overdose is suspected. If the ACT has increased to levels greater than 500 seconds as the result of a heparin overdose, the reptilase time will be normal.

SEDATION

If the infant is paralyzed prior to ECMO, paralysis is stopped to allow the patient to breathe spontaneously and to awaken and become alert. A complete neurological examination can be done at this time, as well as appropriate bonding of the infant with the parents. It is important to keep the child slightly sedated to protect the ECMO catheters, but not so sedated that respiratory drive is decreased. Most centers use a combination of fentanyl (2–3 mcg/kg every 2–3 hours), chloral hydrate (30 mg/kg every 3–4 hours), or valium (0.1 mg/kg every 3–4 hours). The most important component in keeping the child calm is nursing care. Drugs should not be substituted for good bedside nursing care. Infants can be swaddled if they become too active. Withdrawal from narcotics can be a problem if infants are kept on high-dose fentanyl for prolonged periods. Fentanyl has a central effect, shifting the CO_2 response curve and thus decreasing respiratory drive. The longer an infant is on ECMO, and the greater the total dose of fentanyl, the higher the postmembrane Pco_2 levels must be kept to keep the infant breathing. Because the blood return from the pump enters the aortic arch close to the takeoff of the left carotid artery, the postmembrane Pco_2 level affects the brain's respiratory response more than the patient $Paco_2$. It is not uncommon to have set the postmembrane Pco_2 as high as 50–55 mm Hg at the end of the run to keep the patient breathing. It must also be remembered that fentanyl binds to the membrane lung, and if the circuit is changed, the infant may require larger doses of fentanyl for a few hours (10).

PULMONARY MANAGEMENT ON ECMO

Typically, pulmonary opacification is seen after only a few hours of ECMO (Figures 13.2– 13.4) (3,11). The etiology of this "white-out" lung is unknown, but it may be a combination of several factors. It is known that complement is activated by the initiation of ECMO because of interactions between blood and artificial surface (see Chapter 8). Animal studies have shown that this activation causes a transient capillary leak syndrome. In addition to this phenomenon, ventilation-perfusion relationships are markedly altered. The infant is on high peak pressure and rates prior to ECMO and shortly thereafter is placed on "rest settings." Many think this may result in atelectasis, which can be decreased by using higher peak end-expiratory pressure (PEEP)

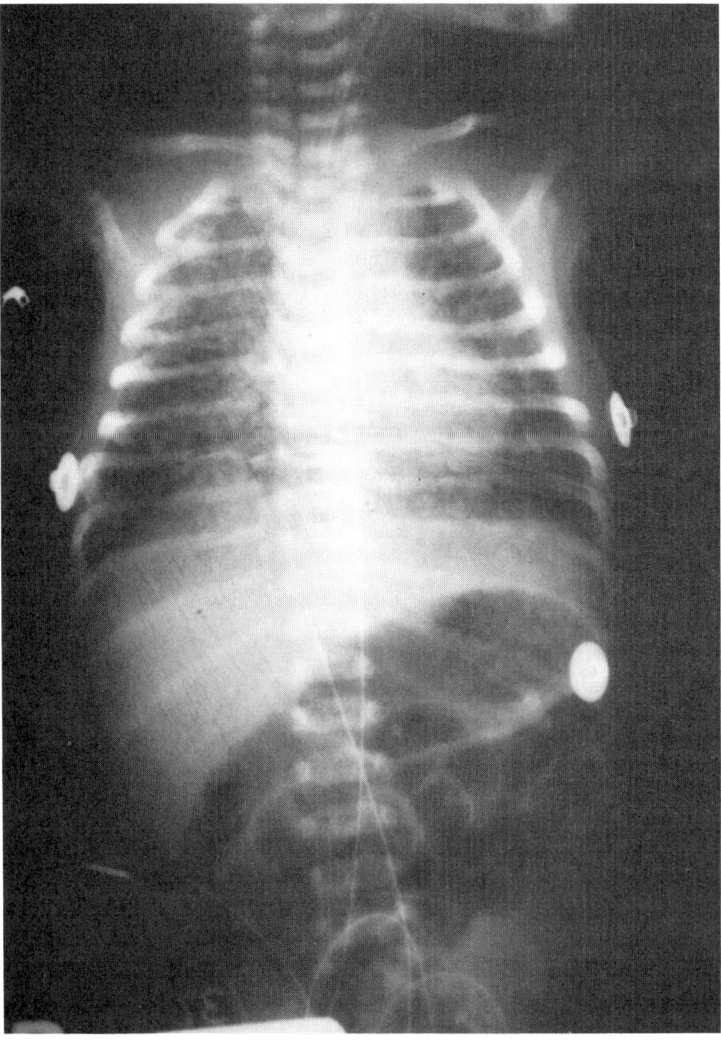

FIGURE 13.2 The typical x-ray findings of an infant with meconium aspiration pre-ECMO.

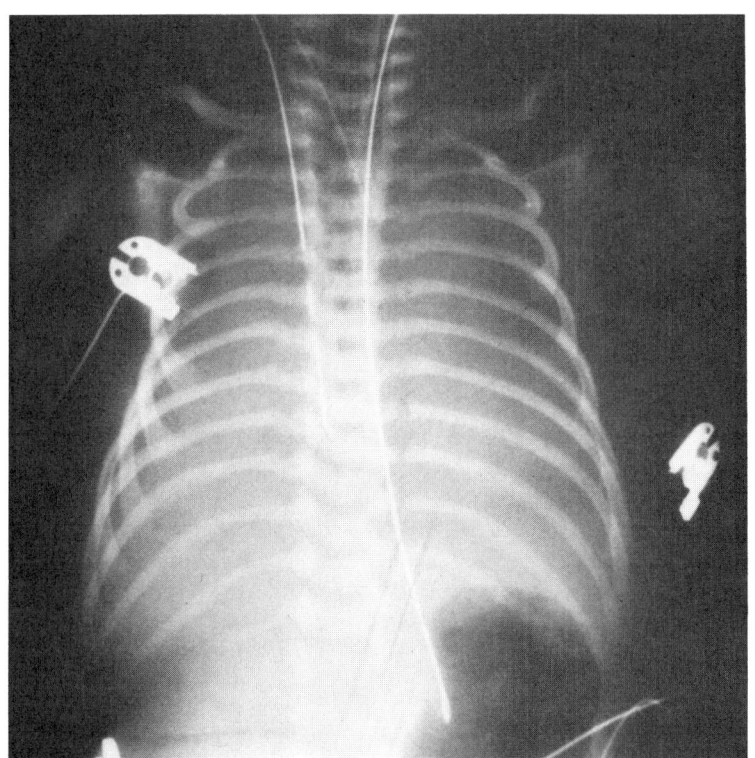

FIGURE 13.3 The same infant 24 hours after being placed on ECMO, showing the typical white-out lung.

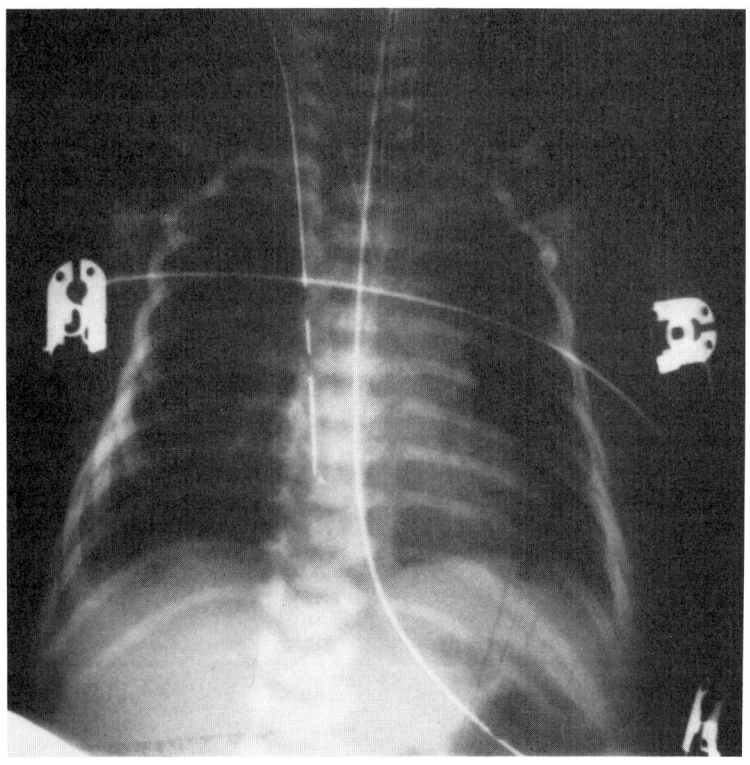

FIGURE 13.4 The same infant on day 5 prior to coming off ECMO, showing total clearing of the lungs.

levels. Keszler et al. (12) have shown that in some infants, the use of PEEP levels of 12–14 cm H_2O will improve lung compliance and decrease time on ECMO. Infants with significant lung damage prior to ECMO or with a significant PDA did not respond as well. Another hypothesis is that these infants have sustained significant lung injury prior to ECMO, resulting in surfactant deficiency (13). Surfactant apoprotein levels from endotracheal aspirates of infants on ECMO are low at the initiation of ECMO, increasing to almost adult levels by the end of the run (Figure 13.5). The other factor that plays a part in this whiteout picture is a left-to-right shunt across a PDA. This occurs in almost all ECMO patients within the first few hours to days on ECMO and is related to the decrease in pulmonary artery pressures (see Chapter 9). It is reasonable to think that all of the factors mentioned are involved in the development of the characteristic radiographic picture and that pulmonary management should be individualized.

Central registry data show that routine ventilator settings on ECMO are Fio_2 0.27 ± 0.11, peak inspiratory pressure (PIP) 21 ± 6 cm H_2O, rate 17 ± 17 breaths per minute (bpm), PEEP 6 ± 4 cm Hg, and mean airway pressure (MAP) 9 ± 3 cm H_2O. Infants can be suctioned as usual, but because of anticoagulation, care should be taken to not suction below the endotracheal tube. Although it is difficult to move the patient for optimal chest physiotherapy, vibrations can be used.

BLOOD GAS MANAGEMENT ON VENOARTERIAL ECMO

Once ECMO is initiated, the primary source of oxygenation and CO_2 removal is the membrane lung. However, an important concept must be understood. Since there are effectively two cardiopulmonary units, it is important to identify which is doing the primary work. The infant's lungs and heart represent one unit, and the ECMO pump and membrane lung represent the other. When an abnormal blood gas value is identified, it is necessary to determine

FIGURE 13.5 The relationship of time on ECMO to SP-A, surfactant protein A (SP-A), lung compliance (C), and the radiographic score. (Reprinted with permission from Lotze A, Whitsett JA, Kammerman LA, et al. Surfactant protein A concentrations in tracheal aspirate fluid from infants requiring extracorporeal membrane oxygenation. J Pediatr 1990;116:435–440.)

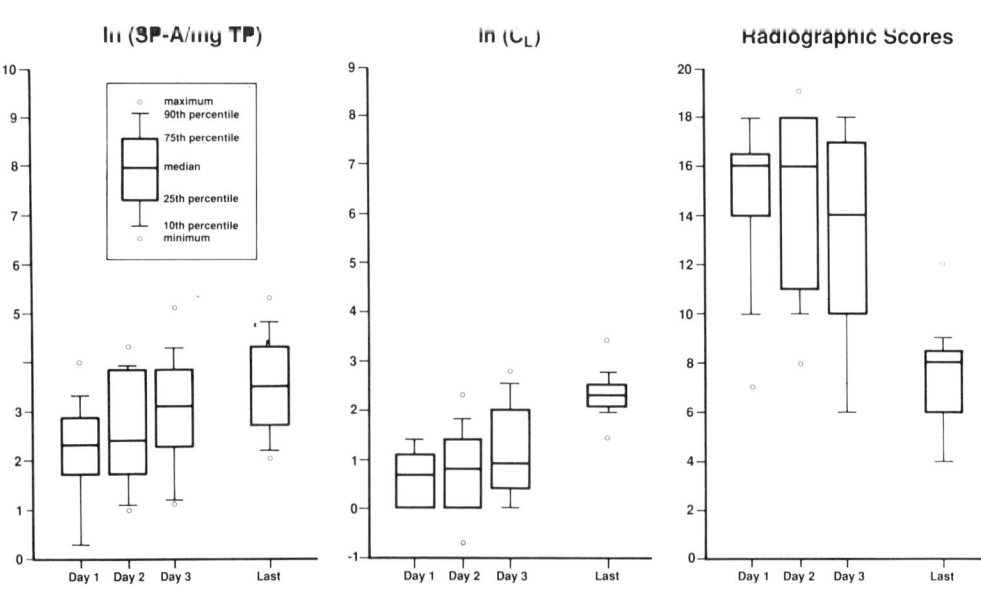

whether the problem lies in the artificial heart/lung or in the patient.

At the beginning of a run, the patient is almost totally dependent on the ECMO circuit for respiratory support. Therefore, when blood gas analysis indicates inadequate oxygen delivery, the pump flow should be turned up. The concept of "percent bypass" is important to understand. Echocardiographic data have shown that, before ECMO, the cardiac output of an infant can range from 150 to 300 mL/kg/min. Our center has chosen to use 200 mL/kg/min as an average cardiac output. The term "percent bypass," then, refers to the percent of the cardiac output going through the ECMO circuit or the amount of "work" being done by the ECMO circuit in relationship to that done by the patient. As an example, in a 3-kg infant, 60% bypass is calculated by the following equation: cardiac output × weight × percent, or 200 mL/kg/min × 3 kg × 0.60, which is 360 mL/min. If the concept of percent bypass is used, it is easy to understand that if the patient is on 30% bypass, abnormal blood gas indicates that the patient must be evaluated as much as the pump system. This is particularly important for the patient who has been on a pump more than three to four days. It is during this period that sedation with such drugs as fentanyl will decrease respiratory drive. If the patient is on 30% bypass, meaning that he/she is doing 70% of the work, and quits breathing, the blood gases will worsen, and a decrease in oxygenation and an increase in $Paco_2$ will result. If the patient no longer supplies most of the "work," only the 30% supplied by the pump occurs. The treatment is to make the patient breathe more by increasing the postmembrane Pco_2 without increasing the ECMO support (see section on CO_2 management below).

During the first 1 to 3 days, most infants require 300–400 mL/min flow or 60% to 70% bypass and are usually dependent primarily on the pump for oxygenation (see Chapter 7). Oxygenation is achieved by diverting more of the cardiac output through the ECMO circuit, thus replacing the patient's nonfunctioning lung with the circuit's functioning lung. This is done very simply by increasing the pump blood flow. Usually only 10–20-mL increases are needed. If the patient develops a significant PDA, oxygenation may decrease and fail to respond to increased pump flow. Increasing the pump flow will increase systemic arterial flow while decreasing pulmonary flow, making the PDA shunt worse. This results in recirculation and flooding of the lungs in a manner similar to that seen in premature infants (see section on PDA below). Another factor in oxygenation, specifically oxygen delivery, is the hemoglobin concentration or hematocrit. The hematocrit should be kept between 40% and 45% to ensure appropriate oxygen-carrying capacity and consequent delivery. In summary, the primary ways to increase oxygenation during ECMO are 1) increasing pump flow, 2) decreasing the left-to-right shunt, and 3) increasing hemoglobin concentration.

A note on using the venous saturation monitor to determine sufficiency of oxygenation: One must understand the concepts of oxygenation, i.e., oxygen content and oxygen delivery, before using these systems independent of an arterial blood gas. The venous blood gas from the ECMO circuit is a right atrial blood gas and not a true "mixed venous" gas. This becomes significant clinically when there are cardiac shunts present. Because most infants on ECMO develop left-to-right shunts, which can occur at the level of the foramen ovale, venous saturations must be considered with other clinical signs. The following concepts must be reviewed:

$$C_vO_2 = C_aO_2 - Vo_2/\text{flow} \quad (1)$$
$$\text{Oxygen content} = Hb \times \%\text{ saturation} \times 1.36 + 0.0031 \times Po_2 \quad (2)$$

where C_vO_2 is venous oxygen content, C_aO_2 is arterial oxygen content, Vo_2 is oxygen consumption, and flow is cardiac output.

As one can see from these equations, for venous saturations to give a true indication of arterial oxygen content, several assumptions must hold true: 1) the cardiac output remains stable and does not change, 2) hemoglobin stays stable, and 3) the metabolic rate of the patient does not change. Any of these factors can cause a change in venous saturation. Therefore, careful evaluation of the patient should take place before this parameter is used solely to wean ECMO flows. Arterial blood gas values are necessary to determine the pH and $Paco_2$ status of the patient, as described in the next section.

Carbon dioxide diffuses across the membrane lung very easily, but because the pressure differential from blood to the membrane gas is small (see Chapter 11), removal of CO_2 is achieved by increasing ventilation to the membrane lung (as with the natural lung) or decreasing the concentration of CO_2 in the membrane gas mixture. Therefore, CO_2 management involves changing the gas flow rates and not the blood flow rates. If the CO_2 is too low, retention of CO_2 can be achieved by decreasing the oxygen flow (decreasing ventilation) or increasing the amount of CO_2 going into the membrane. Again, the concept of percent cardiac bypass is important. If the patient $Paco_2$ is high and the patient is only on 30% bypass, the patient should be evaluated for respiratory rate. If this has dropped significantly due to sedation, the sedation needs to be decreased or the postmembrane Pco_2 increased to stimulate the respiratory drive. Decreasing the postmembrane Pco_2 will only lower the Pco_2 that the brain is "seeing" and cause the patient to breathe less, resulting in a worsening of CO_2 retention. Postmembrane blood gases every 6–8 hours are important because CO_2 flow meters are not accurate and the Pco_2 can drop. The ECMO rule is: If an abnormal patient blood gas is obtained, a postmembrane blood gas must be obtained to allow a proper diagnosis of the problem. If membrane gases are fine, other clinical parameters, such as a chest x-ray for pneumothorax or evaluation for a PDA, must be considered.

WEANING FROM ECMO

In the typical patient, a "white-out" picture on chest x-ray will develop within the first hours of ECMO. This picture correlates with a low measured lung compliance. Over the next three to four days, the lung picture will clear, and lung compliance will markedly improve to a value greater than 0.8 mL/cm H_2O/kg (3). During this period, the arterial blood gas values will improve, permitting a decrease in ECMO blood flow. Very little weaning occurs in the first 24 to 48 hours. There may be a worsening of blood gas values in the first two to three days because of a left-to-right shunt across a PDA. After the PDA closes, weaning will again be possible. As the ECMO specialist obtains an arterial Po_2 that is higher than that specified in the daily parameters, the ECMO blood flow can be decreased. This decrease in flow is gradual (10–20-mL decreases every hour) as the blood gas values allow. Venous saturations can be used with the limitations as stated in the section on blood gas management.

When ECMO blood flow is decreased to approximately 30% of cardiac output (usually 120–150 mL/min), oxygen is added into the ventilator (Fio_2 of 0.30) that will assist weaning. When the flows are decreased to approximately 10% of the cardiac output, or 50–60 mL/min in most cases, this is called "idling." To ensure that the patient will not develop recurrent pulmonary hypertension and hypoxia, idling should be maintained for at least four hours; in most centers this is done for six to eight hours. Some centers have a "trial off" period in which the patient is taken off ECMO by clamping of the catheters. Blood circulates through the bridge while the amount of ventilator support required by the infant is determined. This should not be done for prolonged periods (>20 minutes) because of the risk of clot formation in the catheters. During this trial, the ACTs should be kept >300 seconds, and the heparin drip should be infused into the infant and not the pump. The catheters can be flushed by opening and closing the clamps every five minutes. At CNMC, it is not routine to do a "trial off." If the patient has idled for four to six hours, with Pao_2s in the 70–80-mm Hg range, we have not observed recurrent pulmonary hypertension. If there is a question concerning the patient's ability to come off ECMO, we use lung compliance values, as stated previously. With this weaning technique, ventilator settings after decannulation will usually be Fio_2 0.30 to 0.40, PIP 15 to 20 mm Hg, and 40 to 45 bpm. At CNMC, the average time to extubation after ECMO is 24 hours, and most infants are off oxygen within five days (except for infants with CDH).

The preceding description of weaning is for patients without bleeding complications. In the case of infants with bleeding complications who have ACT levels of 210 seconds or lower, blood flow cannot be weaned, even with good oxygenation. Instead, the oxygen concentration delivered to the membrane lung can be weaned, which will decrease the arterial Pao_2 levels appropriately. When the blender is on an Fio_2 of 0.40 or less, the infant is usually ready to come off ECMO. Lung compliance data are critical in this case. If the lung compliance is 0.8 mL/cm H_2O/kg or greater, heparin should be increased and blood flows should be weaned, with the goal of reaching idling blood flow levels over the next 24 hours.

CARE OF THE PATIENT AFTER ECMO

Decannulation techniques are discussed elsewhere (see Chapter 12). An intermediate-duration neuromuscular blocking agent should be used at decannulation so that the patient cannot aspirate air into the right atrium but can awaken and start breathing within a few hours after decannulation. It is common for the patient on ECMO to require high $Paco_2$ levels (45–55 mm Hg) for respiratory drive by the end of the ECMO run. These levels of $Paco_2$ should be maintained after ECMO to stimulate respiratory drive. Many of these infants have been receiving fentanyl for sedation and will have to be weaned from it slowly for the next two to three days. Pao_2 levels of 60–70 mm Hg should be accepted at this time, and every effort should be made to wean the patient. The patient with CDH is an exception to this rule because this group requires slower weaning to avoid recurrent pulmonary hypertension (see Chapter 17).

Following decannulation, laboratory values, including hemoglobin, hematocrit, calcium, and electrolytes, should be obtained within eight hours. These can then be monitored every 12 to 24 hours thereafter. Of importance, the platelet count should be followed closely (values every eight hours for 24 hours) because there can be a secondary thrombocytopenia which may require platelet transfusion. Fluid administration should be altered to provide sodium at 2–3 mEq/kg/day and potassium at 1–2 mEq/kg/day. If a central line is not in place, the dextrose concentration should be decreased appropriately. Prophylactic antibiotics should be stopped within 24 hours.

The neck wound should be examined daily for any signs of infection or bleeding. A dressing of 4-inch × 4-inch gauze or Opsite can be used for a few days, and then the wound is left open.

After extubation, the infant will usually require oxygen therapy for another five to seven days. But during this period, enteral feedings can be started if the respiratory rate is <60 bpm. Feedings can be advanced as with any term newborn, but most ECMO infants are poor feeders and may require gavage feeding for a few days. This finding is common and does not predict long-term feeding problems.

The infant should have a cranial computed tomography (CT) scan before discharge because of the high incidence of abnormalities missed on ultrasound studies. Basal auditory evoked responses should also be evaluated before discharge or back-transfer to detect any hearing abnormalities. If the infant is stable, he/she should be seen by the follow-up team for a neurologic assessment prior to back-transfer or discharge. All infants must be followed in a neonatal follow-up program (see Chapter 16).

SUMMARY

Care of the ECMO patient is a team effort, requiring the services of nurses, respiratory therapists, ECMO specialists, and ECMO physicians. The team must continually evaluate its areas of responsibility, as with any new therapy, and make changes when appropriate. With this team approach, even the most difficult patients can be managed safely and with minimal complications.

REFERENCES

(1) Butch SH. Technical aspects of transfusion. In: Luban NLC, Keating LJ, eds. Hemotherapy of the infant and premature, 1st ed. Arlington: American Association of Blood Banks, 1983.

(2) Moroff G, Friedman A, Robkin-Kline L, Gaunthier G, Luban N. Reduction of the volume

of stored platelet concentrates for neonatal use. Transfusion 1982;22:125–7.

(3) Lotze A, Short BL, Taylor GA. The use of lung compliance as a parameter for improvement in lung function in newborns with respiratory failure requiring extracorporeal membrane oxygenation. Crit Care Med 1987;15:226–9.

(4) Sas G, ed. The biology of antithrombins, 1st ed. Boca Raton: CRC Press, 1990.

(5) Marinelli KA, Short BL, Martin GR, Goldstein D. Extracorporeal membrane oxygenation: its effect on renin, aldosterone and natriuretic peptide. Pediatr Res 1989;25:241A.

(6) Sell LL, Cullen ML, Lerner GR, et al. Hypertension during extracorporeal membrane oxygenation: cause, effect and management. Surgery 1987;102:724–30.

(7) Hattersley P. Activated coagulation time of whole blood. JAMA 1966;196:436–40.

(8) Kay LA, ed. Essentials of haemostasis and thrombosis, 2nd ed. New York: Churchill Livingstone, 1988.

(9) Anderson JM, Kottke-Marchant K. Platelet interactions with biomaterials and artificial devices. In: Williams DF, ed. Blood compatibility, vol. I, 1st ed. Boca Raton: CRC Press, 1987.

(10) Hickey RR, Hansen DD. Fentanyl and sufentanyl-oxygen-pancuronium anesthesia for cardiac surgery in infants. Anesth Analg 1984;63:117–24.

(11) Taylor GA, Short BL, Kreismer P. Extracorporeal membrane oxygenation: radiographic appearance of the neonatal chest. Am J Radiol 1986;146:1257–60.

(12) Keszler M, Subramanian KN, Smith YA, et al. Pulmonary management during extracorporeal membrane oxygenation. Crit Care Med 1989;17:495–500.

(13) Lotze A, Whitsett JA, Kammerman LA, et al. Surfactant protein A concentrations in tracheal aspirate fluid from infants requiring extracorporeal membrane oxygenation. J Pediatr 1990;116:435–40.

14

Emergencies During Extracorporeal Membrane Oxygenation and Their Management

❖

Joseph B. Zwischenberger, M.D.
Charles S. Cox, Jr., M.D.

An understanding of the physiology relevant to extracorporeal membrane oxygenation (ECMO), familiarity with the ECMO circuit, and the attainment of a certain level of confidence in managing patients on ECMO prepare one to handle most of the problems routinely encountered with this technique. Unfortunately, it is the nature of long-term heart-lung bypass that things occasionally do not go well at all. Potentially catastrophic complications arise unexpectedly and progress rapidly.

There is a fine line between routine management of the ECMO patient and ECMO complications. Complications are defined as difficult factors or issues often appearing unexpectedly and changing existing plans, methods, or attitudes (1). Early in the experience of ECMO, complications were considered management problems (2). With the founding of the National Registry (now called the Extracorporeal Life Support Organization (ELSO) Registry), ECMO centers were able to compile mechanical and patient "complications" so that these "management problems" could be tabulated and reviewed. Release of the National ECMO Registry in July 1990 showed that a total of 3,876 neonates had been treated with ECMO, with an overall survival rate of 83%.

We surveyed 47 of 53 active ECMO centers in the fall of 1989 to document equipment usage and use of safety devices during ECMO. Ninety-six percent of programs used a roller pump, and 2 of 47 used a centrifugal pump. The majority of programs (85%) used Super Tygon S65HL tubing for the raceway, 11% used regular polyvinyl chloride (PVC) tubing, and 2% used polyurethane tubing. Sixty-eight percent used thin-wall PVC tubing, and 15% used thick-wall PVC tubing for the circuit. One hundred percent of programs used a SciMed Kolobow (spiral coil) membrane lung oxygenator (SciMed Life Systems, Inc., Minneapolis, Minnesota) Ninety-one percent used a SciMed Heat Exchanger, and 9% used the Electromedics Heat Exchanger (Electromedics, Inc., Englewood, Colorado). There is currently controversy regarding routine changeout of the SciMed Heat Exchanger during ECMO. The manufacturer recommends routine changeout at five days, but many programs will avoid the difficulties of changeout if there are no apparent problems.

For a heat source, 43% used a Gaymar T-pump (Gaymar Industries, Inc., Orchard Park, N.Y.), 25% used Seabrook Medical Systems, Inc. (Cincinnati, Ohio), and 23% used Cincinnati Sub-zero (Cincinnati Sub Zero, Inc., Cincinnati, Ohio); various other manufacturers supplied the equipment for 8%. Although all programs arrange their heat exchanger to serve as a bubble trap, only 11% use an arterial bubble trap to help prevent air embolism. Six percent use an in-line arterial line filter, most commonly the Healthdyne (Delta) model K-37 (Healthdyne Cardiovascular Inc., Costa Mesa, California). Use of an arterial filter or trap is controversial because of the possibility that clot formation may cause arterial emboli. ECMO utilizes relatively low flows and moderate anticoagulation compared with cardiopulmonary bypass, for which these filters were designed.

A bladder box servoregulated to the roller pump is used by 87% of programs to detect decreases in venous return. The other programs presumably use a pressure-regulated cutoff or a centrifugal pump which does not require a bladder box. Seventy-nine percent monitor circuit pressures between the pump and the patient, with 64% measuring both pre- and postmembrane pressures. An air bubble detector on the arterial side of the circuit is used by 17% with no dominant brand. Gas line pressures are monitored by 32% of programs; 32% use a gas line pop-off valve. A continuous in-line blood gas monitor is used by 68% to measure mixed venous oxygen saturation. Nine percent monitor venous Pco_2, venous Po_2, and arterial Pco_2. None of the programs uses an in-line monitor for blood chemistries.

An oxygen analyzer is used by 51% to monitor the oxygenator sweep gas; 17% use a blood flow meter in the circuit. A blood temperature monitor in the circuit is used by 51%. All programs monitor activated clotting time, but several different products are available for this purpose. The most common is a Hemochron (International Technidyne Corp., Edison, N.J.) (72%), followed by ACTester (Trimed, Inc., Huntington Beach, California (21%) and Hemotec (Hemotec, Inc., Englewood, Colorado) ACT (4%), and one program does hand-held activated clotting times.

Controversy abounds regarding requirements for the background and the level of training of an ECMO technical specialist. The background experience of the person monitoring the patient at the bedside and the ECMO circuit is of vital importance, yet economic realities and local availability influence the trained personnel in each program. Exclusive use of registered nurses (RNs) with intensive care unit experience is reported by 53% of programs. Twenty-six percent use RNs and respiratory therapists (RTs) and 6% use RNs, RTs, and certified clinical perfusionists (CCPs). One program uses CCPs only; one uses RTs only; one uses perfusion assistants only; and one uses RNs, RTs, and resident physicians. Twenty-eight percent of programs use CCPs to prime and troubleshoot the circuit. The average length of didactic instruction for an ECMO technical specialist was 25.3 hours, with 18.5 hours in the animal laboratory and 6.4 hours of water drills. The average length of clinical supervision or preceptorship was 34.2 hours. This survey recognized trends and frequency of use and in no way implies standard of care. However, the variability in personnel, training, equipment, and monitoring all impact upon the frequency, recognition, and management of complications.

MECHANICAL COMPLICATIONS

Mechanical complications are listed in order of frequency in Table 14.1. Complications are related to each major component of the circuit. Revealingly, the most common (11%)

TABLE 14.1 Mechanical complications (Total cases: 3,876)

Complication	Incidence (%)	Survival (%)
Cannula Problem	8	75
Oxygenator failure	5	66
Clots in major parts	5	77
Tubing rupture	2	83
Pump failure	2	86
Heat exchanger malfunction	1	71
Air in circuit	1	73
Mechanical—other	11	81

July 1990 ELSO National Registry.

mechanical complication listed in the Registry is that of "other." This reflects the fact that, in addition to the identifiable components listed above, the entire circuit is subject to failure, including the bladder box, connectors, electrical components, power sources, plugs, oxygen sources, carbogen tanks, blenders, and circuit monitoring equipment. Table 14.2 outlines the management plan for many of the mechanical complications (3).

Cannula problems can relate to both the venous and arterial cannulas. Ideally, the venous cannula is threaded through the right internal jugular vein into the right atrium, and the arterial cannula is inserted into the common carotid so that its tip rests at the entrance or within the aortic arch. The largest catheters that fit comfortably inside the artery and vein are used. Cannulas are inserted with great care to avoid vascular damage during insertion, since loss of control of the internal jugular vein can result in massive mediastinal bleeding, and dissection of the carotid artery intima can progress to a lethal aortic dissection. The venous cannula, however, can be advanced too little or too much, either of which can cause cannula obstruction. Likewise, the venous catheter can enter the subclavian vein. Anatomic variations of the right atrium (aneurysmal atrial septum or redundant eustachian valve) can interfere with venous return. After insertion, venous catheter position can be identified by chest x-ray or echocardiogram. The venous catheter position can be checked for adequate venous drainage at the time of insertion by increasing flow to 120 to 150 cc/kg to insure full supportive flow.

Problems with arterial cannulation include insertion too far into the ascending aorta, insertion too far down the descending aorta, or misdirection into the subclavian artery. Insertion too far into the ascending aorta can cause increased afterload to left ventricular outflow and may contribute to left ventricular failure. In addition, the cannula can cross the aortic valve, causing aortic insufficiency or valvular infection. Insertion too far down the descending aorta can compromise coronary and cerebral oxygenated blood flow as well as "streaming," in which peripheral arterial PaO_2 monitoring will yield an excessively high PaO_2. This is seen when a high umbilical catheter selectively samples oxygenated blood from the ECMO circuit. The distance from the orifice of the innominate artery to the takeoff of the right subclavian artery can be a remarkably short 1 to 1.5 cm. If the arterial cannula is pulled out to the point at which the arterial infusion selectively enters the right subclavian artery, the right upper extremity can be infused with the entire postoxygenator blood flow while the rest of the body is hypoxic and cyanotic.

Oxygenator failure recorded in the ELSO National Registry has decreased in frequency to 5%; however, the ELSO Registry does not record the method of determining oxygenator failure. Controversy exists as to the best method by which oxygenator failure can be demonstrated. Many programs only change an oxygenator when it fails to transfer oxygen or

TABLE 14.2 Management of mechanical complications

Mechanical complications	Rationale and treatment
Tubing rupture	Take patient off bypass.
Air in circuit	Increase ventilator to pre-ECMO parameters.
Oxygenator malfunction	Aspirate air, repair circuit, replace oxygenator. Be prepared to resuscitate infant.
Power failure	Always plug pump into hospital's emergency power supply.
	Hand crank until emergency power is available.
Decannulation	Apply firm pressure. Come off bypass; increase ventilator parameters. Repair vessel; replace blood volume. Be prepared to resuscitate infant.

Reprinted by permission of Neonatal Network. Nugent J. Extracorporeal membrane oxygenation in the neonate. April 1986; Vol. 4(5): 33–6.

carbon dioxide (CO_2). Other programs monitor pre- and postoxygenator pressure gradients, platelet count, plasma free hemoglobin, and fibrin split products to demonstrate when the oxygenator may be causing a consumptive coagulopathy. Early in the ECMO experience, most programs used an oxygenator bypass loop to facilitate exchange of an oxygenator; however, this loop has been associated with frequent thrombosis which requires changeout or permanent clamping of the tubing. The ECMO team at Galveston has implemented a double-diamond tubing arrangement with dual connectors both pre- and postoxygenator, which allows in-line replacement of the oxygenator without interrupting ECMO flow.

Tubing rupture has become much less frequent with the introduction of Super Tygon TM raceway tubing (Norton Performance Plastics, Inc., Akron, Ohio) (4). Previously, PVC tubing required advancement of the raceway every 24 hours to prevent tube fatigue and rupture. Pump failure, likewise, has become more rare as direct and belt-driven pumps have been manufactured specifically with long-term extracorporeal support in mind. Although heat exchanger malfunction occurs in only 1% of cases, it may cause severe hypothermia or hemodilution in the infant. Also, defective heat exchangers have been responsible for aluminum particle emboli; redesign of the oxygenator has eliminated this problem (5).

Occasionally during an ECMO run, the tubing of the circuit must be repaired because a connection has come loose or because the tubing itself is damaged. Tubing may be cut easily with the jaws of a tubing clamp when the tubing is too close to the hinged joint of the clamp; it may be pierced by such tools as penetrating towel clamps (used to secure the neck lines to the patient's bed); or it may occasionally crack from fatigue (usually seen at the main bridge or in the raceway).

The management response to replace malfunctioning equipment, especially if the circuit is squirting blood or pumping air, is shown diagrammatically in Figure 14.1. The bedside technician immediately clamps the venous and arterial lines and opens the bridge to remove the patient from ECMO. The pump is turned off to allow correction of the problem in the circuit. The only exception is massive air embolism, in which the arterial line should be clamped first (discussed later). The patient is now airway dependent, so hand bagging with 100% Fio_2 or replacement on pre-ECMO ventilator settings is necessary to ensure adequate respiratory support. A clamp is placed on either side of the damaged tubing segment, and the damaged segment is sterilized with betadine. Using sterile bandage scissors, the piece of tubing in question is cut out, leaving at least $1\frac{1}{2}$ inches of tubing beyond each clamp. A sterile connector is inserted into one of the free ends, and both ends are filled with fluid. After these are joined together, a careful search for air in the circuit is made. All extraneous clamps are removed from the circuit, and the pump is turned on to recirculate. Once this process is completed, the patient is placed back on ECMO.

If repair necessitates the removal of a large segment of tubing, such as the raceway, then a replacement piece should be inserted where the damaged portion was removed. This is done by making the connection to one of the loose ends while the clamps are still in place. The replacement piece is filled with fluid from its free end, while it is held upright. It is easiest to do this with a large syringe and an 18-gauge needle (especially blunt tipped) placed well into the piece of tubing so that it touches the inside of the tube. Fluids that froth easily, such as albumin or fresh frozen plasma, should be avoided for this purpose. When the insertion segment is filled, the connection is made and the procedure is completed as described above.

The ECMO circuit is designed to pump blood safely and efficiently, but a large bolus of air can develop and circulate rapidly into the infant. This complication, though rare, is commonly fatal. There are several potential sources of such an embolus. When the partial pressure of oxygen in the blood is very high, as seen following oxygenation in the membrane, oxygen can easily be forced out of solution. Hitting the membrane or operating the circuit in a low ambient pressure environment (such as in flight in an up-pressurized airplane cabin) may produce foam in the top of the oxygenator. Operating the pump with a clamp on the venous side of the circuit, with the bladder in the "prime" mode or with the outlet arm of the bladder kinked (as can occur during "walking" of the raceway), can generate a markedly negative pressure in the blood path and pull

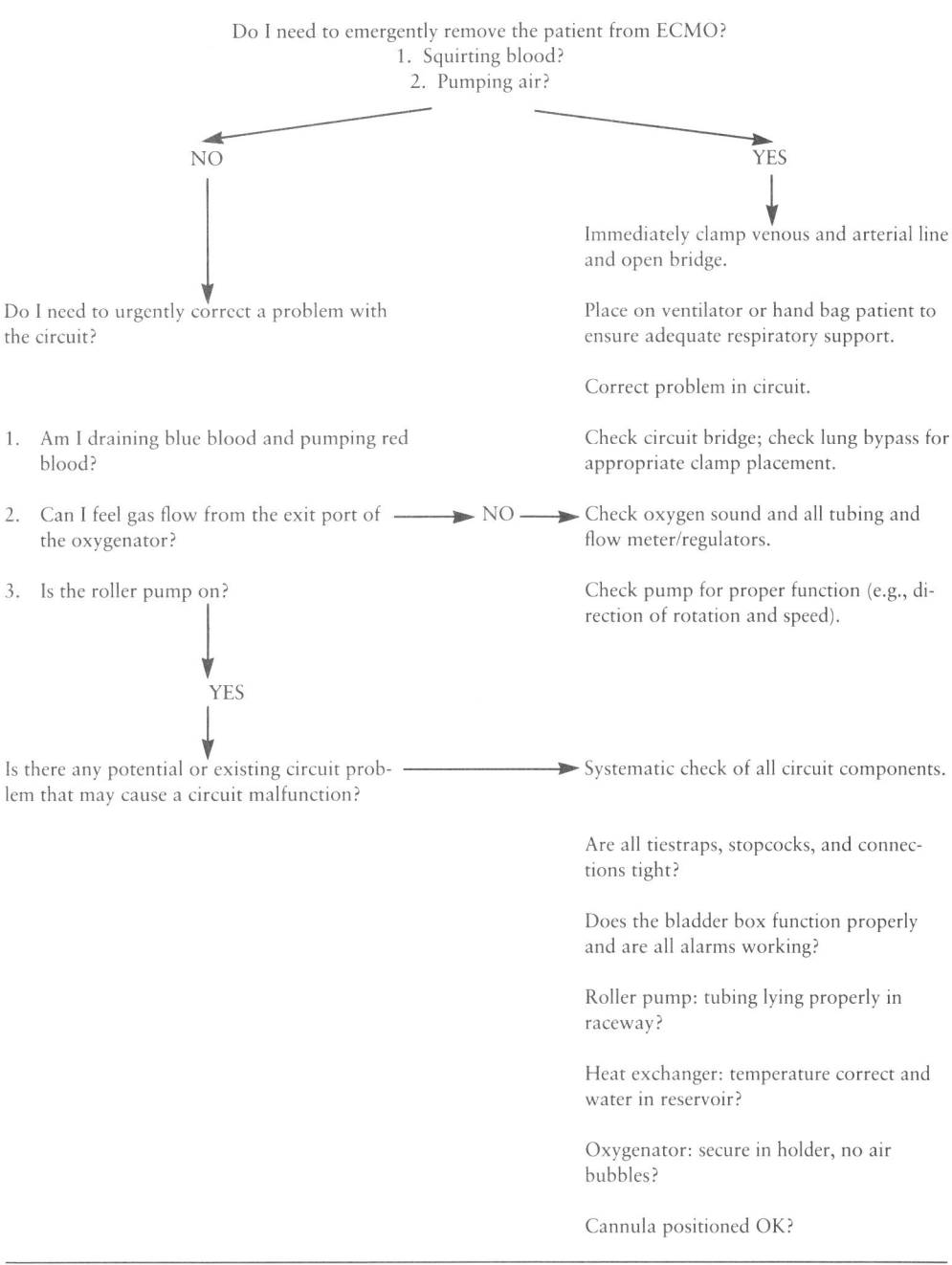

FIGURE 14.1 Management algorithm for replacement of malfunctioning equipment.

large amounts of gas out of solution, called cavitation. This is precisely the problem that the bladder box system is designed to avoid.

Probably the most dramatic air embolus occurs when a small tear develops in the membrane which permits blood to leak into the gas path of the oxygenator. The blood gradually moves down to the gas exhalation port where it may either be blown out in small drops onto the floor or accumulate and form a clot. If this clot obstructs the egress of gas, back pressure will develop inside the gas path of the oxygenator. When the gas pressure exceeds that of the blood, a large bolus of air crosses the membrane and appears in the blood path. As it surges out of the membrane to the heat exchanger (and the arterial line filter, if it is used), the gas-trapping capacity of these two devices (on the order of 45 mL for each) may rapidly be exceeded, and the embolus will push into the arterial line toward the infant's aorta.

Obviously, the solution to these problems rests on prevention and a rapid response when air embolism is recognized. Keeping the Pao_2 in the postmembrane blood at 400 mm Hg or less, carefully monitoring the toggle switches on the bladder box so that the bladder box is always functioning, strictly prohibiting placement of extraneous clamps on the circuit, and adhering to precautions with regard to the procedure for "walking the raceway" will eliminate most problems. Lightly touching the gas exhalation port of the membrane with a finger as part of the hourly circuit check will alert the practitioner when blood rather than water alone is being expelled. However, occluding the gas exhalation port even briefly can cause a precipitous rise in the gas phase pressure across the membrane, risking a membrane rupture and/or air embolus.

Strict adherence to the hourly protocol and general vigilance for problems will permit the fastest possible response time once an air embolus develops. If a bolus of air is sighted but has not yet entered the patient, the responses shown in Figure 14.1 should be followed. *If the air is headed toward the arterial cannula, a clamp is immediately placed on the arterial tubing close to the baby.* Then the pump is immediately turned off, the main bridge is unclamped, and the venous line is clamped. The baby should be hand bagged or the ventilator should be returned to its pre-ECMO settings, and the problem in the circuit should be identified and corrected (with the pump running again, if possible). If, however, air has already entered the patient, additional protective measures should be undertaken. Once the baby is "off bypass," lower the head relative to the body as much as possible in order to move any air pockets away from the cerebral circulation. Using a sterile catheter-tipped syringe, aspirate any accessible air from the arterial cannula. High doses of inotropic drugs may be necessary in the short term if any air has entered the coronaries and caused acute cardiac decompensation. Identify the cause of the air leak and correct it. If a hyperbaric chamber is available and the patient is stable, its immediate use should also be considered.

Occasionally, the pump "cuts out" and quits pumping blood. This is a manifestation of inadequate venous return to the pump for a variety of reasons. Figure 14.2 outlines our management approach to this problem. All causes of inadequate venous return must be considered. This may simply be a response to hypovolemia which can be corrected easily with intravascular volume expansion. The

FIGURE 14.2 Management of inadequate venous return to the pump (pump cutting out).

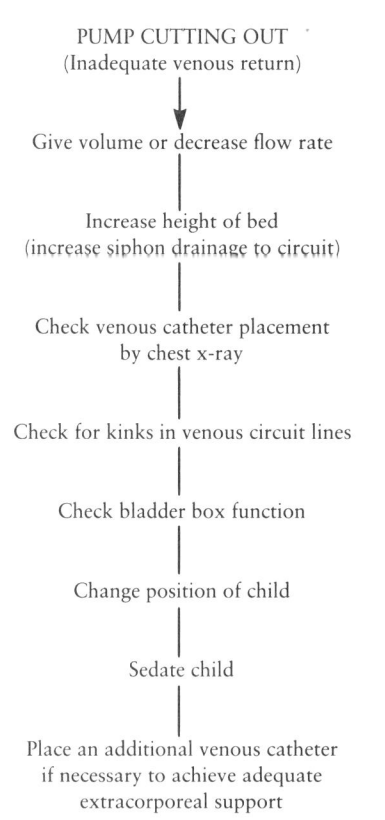

circuit must be checked to rule out any kinks or obstructions to venous return. Likewise, venous catheter placement must be confirmed by chest roentgenogram. Echocardiography may be required to ensure that cardiac tamponade is not causing obstruction to venous return. If these maneuvers do not uncover the etiology of inadequate venous return, placement of an additional venous drainage catheter may be necessary.

PATIENT COMPLICATIONS

Patient complications in descending order of frequency according to the ELSO National Registry include intracranial hemorrhage, seizures, surgical site hemorrhage, cardiac dysfunction, hemofiltration/dialysis, hypertension, abnormal creatinine, electrolyte abnormalities, hemolysis, pneumothorax, positive blood culture (sepsis), gastrointestinal hemorrhage, and arrhythmias (Table 14.3). Table 14.4 briefly outlines management of many patient complications. Because of systemic anticoagulation, bleeding complications are common. Moderate bleeding (<10 cc/h) is frequently seen at the neck cannulation site. This problem is minimized by liberal use of electrocautery at the time of surgical exposure, systemic anticoagulation during cannulation *after* achieving vessel exposure and initial wound hemostasis, repeat surgical hemostasis after anticoagulation, and liberal use of a topical hemostatic agent, such as cryoprecipitate/topical thrombin glue or gelfoam thrombin. At the University of Texas ECMO Center, neck wounds are packed with a topical hemostatic agent prior to closure, which decreases the incidence of bleeding for the duration of the ECMO course and is easily removed at decannulation.

If during the course of ECMO, bleeding (<10 cc/h) from the neck wound is observed, local pressure, topical placement of hemostatic agents (gelfoam thrombin, oxycel, topical thrombin) and injection of cryoprecipitate topical thrombin glue into the wound have all been successful. If the standard practice of securing the ECMO cannulas with two silk ties over a vessel loop is followed, the neck bleeding is usually from a small vessel in the wound, not from the cannula insertion site. If topical treatment methods are unsuccessful, consider decreasing the heparin infusion rate to keep the activated clotting time (ACT) between 180 and 220 s and maintaining the platelet count >100,000. Anytime the neck incision bleeds more than 10 cc/h for 2 h despite the treatment strategies outlined above, the wound should be explored. Once hemostasis is achieved with electrocautery, the wound should be packed with a topical hemostatic agent and reclosed.

Significant bleeding that is not attributable to the neck incision is *not* routine and must be handled aggressively. A decreasing hematocrit (which decreases faster than would be anticipated as a result of routine blood drawing), a rising heart rate, a fall in the blood pressure, or a progressive rise in the Pao_2 disproportionate to observed improvements in the patient's pulmonary status all suggest bleeding. In addition, neurologic changes noted at the development of seizures, intrathoracic tamponade, or abdominal distension would all lead one to suspect the presence of bleeding into these areas. Such findings should be evaluated by cranial, thoracic, or abdominal ultrasound, by x-rays of the chest or abdomen, or by computed tomography (CT) scan, as appropriate to the case.

Bleeding into the site of a previous invasive procedure is surprisingly frequent, so it is incumbent upon the ECMO practitioner to monitor these locations in particular. Previous surgery, for example, to repair a congenital

TABLE 14.3 Patient complications
(Total cases: 3,876)

Intracranial hemorrhage	16%
Seizures	15%
Surgical site hemorrhage	13%
Cardiac dysfunction	11%
Hemofiltration/dialysis	11%
Hypertension	9%
Abnormal creatinine	9%
Electrolyte abnormalities	9%
Hemolysis	8%
Pneumothorax	5%
Positive blood culture	5%
GI hemorrhage	4%
Arrhythmias	3%

July 1990 ELSO National Registry.

TABLE 14.4 Management of patient complications

Physiological complications	Rationale and treatment
Electrolyte/glucose/fluid imbalance	Additional maintenance electrolytes may be required because of increased total blood volume in the ECMO circuit. Anticoagulant calcium replacement may be required if citrate is a component of blood. Hyperglycemia may occur if citrate-phosphate-dextrose (CPD) anticoagulated blood is used. Reduce dextrose concentration of maintenance and heparin infusions. Maintain total fluid intake 100–150 mL/kg/day. Fluid intake should balance output; Lasix may be required if positive fluid balance occurs.
CNS deterioration: cerebral edema, intracranial hemorrhage, seizures	This most significant complication of ECMO is related to pre-ECMO hypoxemia, acidosis, hypercarbia. Drug of choice for seizures is phenobarbital. Serial EEGs and cranial ultrasounds may be required.
Generalized edema	Extracellular space is enlarged by distribution of crystalloid solution in the prime solution and the action of aldosterone and antidiuretic hormone. Lasix may be given if edema causes brain or lung dysfunction.
Renal failure	Acute tubular necrosis results from pre-ECMO hypotension and hypoxia. Monitor output and indicators of renal failure: blood urea nitrogen (BUN), creatinine, electrolytes. Increase renal perfusion by increasing pump flow and use of dopamine (5 μg/kg/h). Continuous hemofiltration may be added to the circuit if necessary.
Bleeding/thrombocytopenia	Large foreign surface of ECMO circuit lowers platelet function and count. Most common in infants requiring surgery or chest tubes. Minimized with good control of ACT and judicious use of platelets and fresh frozen plasma. All surgical procedures must be done with electrocautery. (See Figure 14.2.)
Decreased venous return/hypovolemia	Infants must have adequate circulating volume to obtain adequate flow rates. Manifest by decrease in extracorporeal flow rate, arterial pressure, and arterial pulse amplitude. Blood sampling, wound drainage, peripheral dilatation may account for hypovolemia. Check for pneumothorax or partial venous catheter occlusion, which may decrease venous return. Replace volume with packed cells, fresh frozen plasma. Treat pneumothorax with chest tube placement.
Hypervolemia	Caused by overinfusion of blood products, which causes larger amounts of blood to pass through malfunctioning lungs. Manifest by widening arterial pulse amplitude and decreasing systemic oxygenation at a fixed extracorporeal flow rate. Treat by removing blood from the circuit.
Patent ductus arteriosus	Left-to-right shunting may occur, with blood crossing atrial septum and draining into extracorporeal circuit, necessitating high pump flows without an expected increase in Pao$_2$. Ligation may be indicated.

Reprinted by permission of Neonatal Network. Nugent J. Extracorporeal membrane oxygenation in the neonate. April 1986; Vol. 4(5):33–6.

diaphragmatic hernia, is an obvious site for bleeding risk, but so is a needle puncture site used to aspirate a pneumothorax or pneumomediastinum, to perform a "bladder tap" or lumbar puncture, or for paracentesis.

Intracranial, gastrointestinal, intrathoracic, abdominal, and retroperitoneal bleeding have all been observed in neonates on ECMO. Managment includes decreasing the heparin infusion rate to maintain the ACT between 180 and 220 s, ensuring that the platelet count remains greater than 100,000/mL, and other specific measures relevant to the site of the bleeding. Occasionally, one can justify suspension of the heparin infusion for 1 to 2 h as a desperate measure. These measures, may, of course, lead to clotting in the circuit, particularly in the membrane lung.

With increasing regularity, major surgical procedures, particularly diaphragmatic hernia repair, are performed immediately before or during ECMO (7). The following protocol has been adopted for patient management under such circumstances. Before surgery, stabilize platelet count greater than 100,000, maintain ACT at 180 to 200, and maximize supportive ECMO flow. At the start of surgery, infuse 1 U of platelets and 10 cc/kg of fresh frozen plasma. Have 15 cc/kg of packed red blood cells at the pump for immediate infusion if necessary. Stop the heparin infusion during the actual surgery and restart it upon completion or when ACT is less than 170 s. (Be prepared to replace the circuit following surgery if the circuit should fail.) Cut all tissues, including skin, with electrocautery on coagulation setting. Dissect slowly with meticulous hemostasis to seal even minute bleeding. Ligate all identifiable vessels. When closing a diaphragmatic hernia with a prosthesis, close the defect without tension rather than attempting a primary closure with extensive dissection. Once surgery is complete, use a generous amount of topical hemostatic agent (cryoprecipitate/topical thrombin glue, gelfoam thrombin, etc.). Do not close until the field is absolutely dry. Use running sutures for hemostasis during closure.

Intrathoracic, abdominal, or retroperitoneal hemorrhages may be decompressed by effective drainage of blood. Allowing such bleeding to tamponade is rarely a successful management technique and can lead to profound hemodynamic decompensation. Drainage is dramatically facilitated by the ultrasound-directed placement of a guidewire, over which a drainage catheter may then be introduced (the Seldinger technique). Blood loss should be replaced on a volume-for-volume basis. In the event that bleeding is not controlled by these measures, more aggressive surgical approaches should be considered. One should not hesitate to reexplore any wound or surgical site. Gastrointestinal bleeding may be due to fairly mild gastritis and may respond to the measures outlined, plus iced saline lavage and administration of antacids, and/or cimetidine. In extreme cases, vasopressin may be used. Esophageal bleeding may be treated similarly, or balloon tamponade may be applied. The general strategy for the management of bleeding is summarized in Figure 14.3.

The subject of intracranial hemorrhage in neonates has been reviewed extensively (8–15). As a rule, appearance of a new intracranial hemorrhage or enlargement of a preexisting bleed are indications to discontinue ECMO support if possible. Factors that increase the pressure gradient between the blood vessel lumen in the germinal matrix and the surrounding brain tissue increase the likelihood of small-vessel rupture and hemorrhage. Hypoxia may directly injure brain capillary endothelial cells. Factors contributing to intracranial hemorrhage in all critically ill neonates include hypoxia, hypercapnia, acidosis, ischemia, hypotension, sepsis, coagulopathy, thrombocytopenia, venous hypertension, seizures, birth trauma, and rapid infusions of colloid or hypertonic solution (12). Mechanical ventilation has been associated with increased rates of intracranial hemorrhage in premature infants with respiratory distress syndrome (13).

During ECMO, infants are exposed to a number of conditions that may increase the risk of intracranial hemorrhage. Ligation of the right internal jugular vein is routine in all ECMO patients. Patients in whom venoarterial ECMO is used commonly have ligation of the right common carotid artery. Krummel et al. (16) used Doppler vascular studies to evaluate cerebral blood flow in six surviving patients seen at one to two years of age, who had previously been treated with ECMO. They

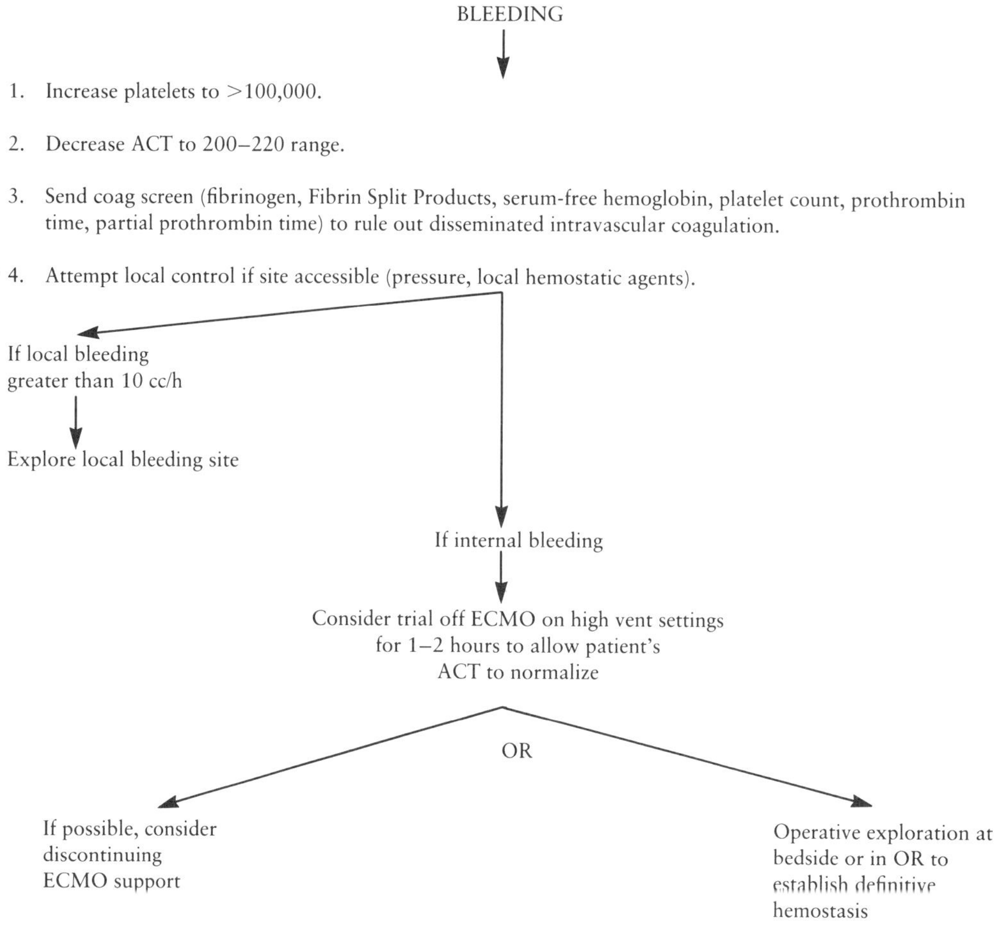

BLEEDING

1. Increase platelets to >100,000.

2. Decrease ACT to 200–220 range.

3. Send coag screen (fibrinogen, Fibrin Split Products, serum-free hemoglobin, platelet count, prothrombin time, partial prothrombin time) to rule out disseminated intravascular coagulation.

4. Attempt local control if site accessible (pressure, local hemostatic agents).

If local bleeding greater than 10 cc/h

Explore local bleeding site

If internal bleeding

Consider trial off ECMO on high vent settings for 1–2 hours to allow patient's ACT to normalize

OR

If possible, consider discontinuing ECMO support

Operative exploration at bedside or in OR to establish definitive hemostasis

FIGURE 14.3 Management of bleeding.

found "adequate" right-sided cerebral blood flow in all patients. Right ophthalmic artery flow was prograde in five and retrograde in one patient. Towne et al. (17) performed noninvasive carotid evaluation on 11 survivors of long-term ECMO aged 4 to 11 years. Prograde internal carotid flow was demonstrated in 10 patients, achieved by retrograde external carotid artery flow. Taylor et al. (18) evaluated intracranial flow patterns with a range-gated, pulsed Doppler imaging system. At the onset of ECMO, the systolic phase broadened, diastolic flow velocities markedly increased, and the mean pulsatility index value decreased. With initiation of ECMO, marked increases were noted in the area under the velocity curve, which tended to decrease during the course of ECMO. These studies suggest that, in neonates, when the common carotid artery is ligated, collateral circulation is readily established. However, the cerebral effects of changes in pulse contour during venoarterial ECMO are unknown.

During ECMO, infants are anticoagulated with heparin infusions of 30 to 60 U/kg/h to maintain activated clotting times two to three times normal. Although anticoagulation *may not cause* intracranial hemorrhage, it may allow rapid progression of hemorrhage with atypical sonographic characteristics of intracranial hemorrhage (19). The extracorporeal circuit also exposes the infant's blood to a large surface area of foreign material, creating the setting for ongoing blood-surface interactions. Thrombocytopenia requiring platelet transfusions, altered platelet function, and activation of complement and white blood cells (WBCs) all occur during extracorporeal circulation (20). This list of potentially detrimental factors that may increase the risk or extent of intracranial hemorrhage must be balanced against the cardiovascular stabilization and reversal of hypoxia, hypercapnia, and acidosis afforded by ECMO.

Many investigators have reported intracranial hemorrhage associated with the use of ECMO. In 1971, White et al. (21) used right internal jugular vein to umbilical vein ECMO in three neonates weighing 1.0, 1.25, and 1.73 kg, respectively. All infants died, and intracranial hemorrhage was found in each at autopsy. Kirkpatrick et al. (22) reported the deaths of two 2.5- and 3.1-kg infants with intraventricular hemorrhage diagnosed by cranial ultrasound. These infants had suffered severe perinatal asphyxia. In their early experience using ECMO in neonates, Bartlett et al. (23) treated 10 patients with respiratory distress syndrome who weighed less than 2 kg. Cranial ultrasound was not available at that time, and decisions were based on the fullness of the fontanel and findings at neurologic examination. Four of the seven who died underwent autopsy. Intracranial hemorrhage was found in three. Towne et al. (17) have reported long-term follow-up results in the three survivors. One neonate (1.84 kg, 35 weeks' gestation) who was developmentally normal at one year of age has since been lost to follow-up. Another infant (1.9 kg, 32 weeks' gestation) has developmental delay and cerebral palsy. A 1.4-kg neonate (35 weeks' gestation) is alive, with normal growth and development at six years of age.

In a retrospective analysis of neonates undergoing ECMO therapy, birthweight and gestational age were the most significant correlates with intracranial hemorrhage occurring during ECMO (14). Eight of eight infants younger than 35 weeks' gestational age (birthweight 1.0 to 2.2 kg) sustained intracranial hemorrhage. Extracorporeal membrane oxygenation was stopped before lung recovery occurred in six (all less than 2.0 kg), and all died. In the other two (2.1 and 2.2 kg), lung function was adequate to sustain life; however, both patients had severe brain damage and died before one year of age. Two of 27 infants older than 34 weeks' gestational age sustained intracranial hemorrhage (birthweight 2.6 and 3.2 kg). Both had lung recovery. One had severe brain damage and died at 18 months; the other is normal at two years of age.

These findings are consistent with the decrease in intracranial hemorrhage seen with advancing gestational age in neonates not treated with ECMO, and they support the hypothesis that intraventricular or periventricular hemorrhage is related to the maturity of the blood vessels in the periventricular germinal matrix. After 34 weeks' gestation, these vessels are better able to withstand the adverse effects of respiratory failure and its treatment, as well as any additional injury that may be caused by ECMO. Of note, the two normal survivors from the early ECMO experience who weighed less than 2 kg were more than 35 weeks' gestational age.

Attention to the details of management during ECMO can minimize the risk of intracranial hemorrhage. Thrombocytopenia must be avoided by platelet transfusion as often as necessary to maintain adequate platelet counts during, as well as after, ECMO when thrombocytopenia may occur. Heparin infusion rates must be carefully adjusted to prevent large variations in the degree of anticoagulation. Measurement of activated clotting time must be done frequently with whole blood. Adequate oxygenation must be maintained and rapid changes in systemic blood pressure avoided. Before ECMO treatment, cranial ultrasound is mandatory in all patients to identify those in whom significant intracranial hemorrhage is already present.

The management of infants who sustain intracranial hemorrhage while on ECMO is never easy. Although no hard-and-fast rules can be established, the following principles, based on our experience, have been adopted to deal with the problem. ECMO is electively discontinued in infants when intracranial hemorrhage is associated with profound clinical deterioration, including flaccidity and fixed pupils. Infants without clinical signs of intracranial hemorrhage (ultrasound diagnosis only) are maintained at the lowest possible activated clotting time (180 to 200 s), with platelet count kept greater than 100,000. Repeat cranial ultrasound examinations are performed. ECMO is discontinued if intracranial hemorrhage progresses or as soon as mechanical ventilatory support can be achieved even if higher ventilator settings are necessary.

Thrombocytopenia is expected during the use of ECMO as platelets are altered and as platelet aggregates form in the extracorporeal circuit and are preferentially sequestered in the lung, liver, and spleen (24). Thrombocytopenia in the neonate is significant in that existing bleeding may be exacerbated or bleeding may occur spontaneously. A platelet count less than 100,000/mm^3 is considered abnormal by most programs. Thrombocytopenia during ECMO may be a result of the following mechanisms: 1) decreased production, 2) increased consumption, 3) sequestration in or removal to extravascular sites, and 4) dilution. Hypoxia has been shown to be a factor in the inhibition of platelet production by blood-forming organs. Thrombocytopenia can occur up to four days after the termination of ECMO for the treatment of neonatal respiratory failure; therefore, platelet counts should be measured frequently during this critical period (8, 18). Neonates with meconium aspiration syndrome or sepsis, those whose ECMO courses are notable for technical complications, and those with rapid rates of platelet loss are at greatest risk for thrombocytopenia. Severe antecedent hypoxia has also been correlated with the development of thrombocytopenia after ECMO.

Ultrasound of the kidneys to exclude major anatomic anomalies is mandatory in the presence of any elevated creatinine or persistently poor response to intravenous furosemide (1 to 2 mg/kg). Oliguria during ECMO is common, especially during the first 24 to 48 h. Sell et al. (25) report the use of continuous hemofiltration (CH) for renal failure during ECMO. CH removes plasma water and dissolved solutes, while retaining proteins and cellular components of the intravascular space. The classic indications for dialysis hold true for continuous hemofiltration on ECMO: hypervolemia, hyperkalemia, and azotemia. Hyperkalemia and hypervolemia are easily managed with CH, but azotemia is more difficult to manage due to chronic hemolysis and occult gastrointestinal bleeding. The CH apparatus is easily added in line to the ECMO circuit and permits removal of up to 10 mL/kg/h.

Systolic hypertension is a dangerous side-effect of ECMO. Sell et al. (26) reported that 38 of 41 newborns treated with ECMO developed systolic blood pressures greater than 90 mm Hg. Forty-four percent developed detectable intracranial hemorrhage, and 27% developed clinically significant intracranial hemorrhage. The development of a medical management protocol using hydralazine, nitroglycerine, and captopril decreased the incidence of clinically significant intracerebral hemorrhage from 50% prior to protocol therapy to 9% after protocol therapy. We currently use hydralazine 0.1 mg/kg IV for systolic hypertension greater than 90 mm Hg. Rarely are more than two doses required to control systolic hypertension.

It is unusual to have catastrophic hemodynamic deterioration while a patient is on venoarterial bypass. The factors that deserve immediate evaluation when this occurs include venous catheter placement, adequacy of systemic volume status, and the possibility of extracorporeal circuit failure (see Table 14.5). Major cardiac dysfunction is usually not appreciated during venoarterial bypass when full supportive flow (120 mL/kg/min) can be provided. In infants, some degree of cardiac depression is fairly common early in the course of ECMO, particularly with severely asphyxiated patients. Dickson et al. (27) reported a group of six neonates who met echocardiographic criteria for "stunned myocardium" after ECMO. This is defined as left ventricular shortening fraction (LVSF) decreasing by ≥25% with initiation of ECMO and returning to normal after 48 hours on ECMO. This syndrome occurs despite relief of hypoxia. They postulate that impaired filling of the coronary arteries and persistent subendocardial ischemia during the early high-flow phases may precipitate the lower LVSF (27). Venoarterial bypass is preferred over venovenous support in these cases. ECMO can provide univentricular or biventricular cardiac support, thus extending the application of ECMO to infants and children who develop refractory

TABLE 14.5 Differential diagnosis of acute cardiorespiratory decompensation ECMO

Cause	Findings	Management
Pericardial tamponade (from blood or air)	Blood pressure (BP) down, pulse pressure narrowed, marked rise in PaO_2 followed by fall in ECMO flow, *poor perfusion.*	Echocardiogram for diagnosis. Must decompress pericardium ("needle the heart") acutely, then place pericardial drain. Control bleeding.
Tension hemothorax or pneumothorax	Chest and abdomen distended, not moving well with ventilator breaths. Marked rise in PaO_2 followed by BP down, pulse pressure narrowed. ECMO flow down and *poor perfusion.*	Chest x-ray or transilluminate for diagnosis. Must decompress chest ("needle the chest") acutely, then place chest tube. Control bleeding (with cautery).
Respiratory failure (acute hypoxia)	Endotracheal tube "out or plugged," ventilator malfunction, oxygenator failure, sweep O_2 disconnected.	Check endotracheal tube ventilator, ECMO circuit.
Electrolyte imbalance, myocardial ischemia, drug effects	Dysrhythmia, heart rate up or down, BP down, perfusion poor, poor contractility on echo.	Support cardiac output with ECMO, inotropes, fluids. Oxygenate, correct electrolytes, treat infection.
Massive hemorrhage (especially intracranial)	Pallor or cyanosis, heart rate up, then down, hematocrit down, BP down, perfusion poor. May see no clinical change if on ECMO.	Cranial ultrasound, echocardiogram, abdominal ultrasound or CXR for diagnosis. Aspirate stomach, stool guaiac, ACT 180–220, platelets >100,000, manage coagulation, decompress or control bleeding.
Overwhelming sepsis	Shock, poor perfusion, disseminated intravascular coagulation (DIC) picture.	Sepsis work-up (*not* LP) Change antibiotics, pressors volume, WBCs, cultures.

postoperative cardiogenic shock after repair of congenital heart defects (28).

If cardiac arrest, dysrhythmia, or a drop in cardiac output secondary to severe myocardial dysfunction occurs, the initial treatment of choice while the patient is on ECMO is simply to turn up the pump flow. This may require the addition of blood volume to the circuit. The cause of the acute event can then be determined and treated. Continued ECMO/circulatory support is likely to be one of the most effective therapeutic measures. Treatment may include the administration of standard "arrest" medications, some adjustments of the electrolyte levels, addition of an antiarrhythmic agent, treatment with sympathomimetics or inotropes, or even countershock. If the pump flow cannot be increased sufficiently to compensate for the fall in intrinsic cardiac output, the episode must be handled much the same as a cardiac arrest in any other patient. Do not forget that the most common cause of cardiac dysfunction in ventilated neonates is hypoxia from respiratory—not cardiac—failure. First, check the ECMO circuit, oxygenator etc. (see Table 14.5 and Figure 14.1). Then check the endotracheal tube, listen for breath sounds, and hand ventilate the patient. Assess the infant for inadvertent extubation or development of a tension pneumothorax. The reason why one cannot achieve the desired ECMO flows may be that venous return to the patient's heart is being impeded by the accumulation of blood or air in the chest or pericardium (29). Assign someone to begin chest compressions, bearing in mind that the infant is still anticoagulated. Administer the routine cardiotonic drugs (epinephrine, atropine, sodium bicarbonate, calcium, etc.).

Extreme acid-base imbalance caused by the addition of too much or too little CO_2 to the sweep gas, hypoxia caused by removal (or absence) of the tubing to the gas inlet port of the oxygenator, or hypovolemia from failure to clamp the main bridge are just a few examples of the numerous ways in which circuit problems can precipitate such an event. In any case, the goal is to restore normal cardiac and respiratory function in the most rapid and least traumatic manner possible. Once the potential problems outlined above have been eliminated, one should consider intrathoracic complications that can cause immediate hemodynamic deterioration on ECMO: pericardial tamponade and tension hemothorax or pneumothorax (30).

Pericardial tamponade and tension hemothorax and/or pneumothorax have the common pathophysiology of increasing intrapericardial pressure and decreasing venous return (see Figure 14.1). Perfusion initially is maintained by the nonpulsatile flow of the ECMO flow and progressive hemodynamic deterioration. With decreased venous return to the heart, pulmonary blood flow is decreased, the native cardiac output is decreased, and the relative contribution of the extracorporeal circuit to peripheral perfusion is increased. Therefore, peripheral perfusion is initially maintained by the nonpulsatile flow of the ECMO circuit (postoxygenator $Po_2 > 300$ mm Hg). The peripheral arterial partial pressure of oxygen (Pao_2) will increase, but the patient will actually have decreased peripheral perfusion with a decreased pulse pressure and decreased Svo_2. Decreased Svo_2 confirms a decrease in oxygen delivery achieved by the ECMO flow and further hemodynamic deterioration of the patient. The triad of increased Pao_2 and decreased peripheral perfusion (as evidenced by decreased pulse pressure and decreased Svo_2), followed by decreased ECMO flow with progressive hemodynamic deterioration, is consistently associated with tension pneumothorax (31) (Figures 14.1 and 14.4).

The diagnosis of tension hemothorax and pneumothorax may be suggested by transillumination of the chest but is best confirmed by chest roentgenogram. ECMO does not affect the classic appearance of tension hemothorax or pneumothorax on chest roentgenogram.

FIGURE 14.4 Management of hemodynamic deterioration possibly associated with tension pneumothorax or hemothorax.

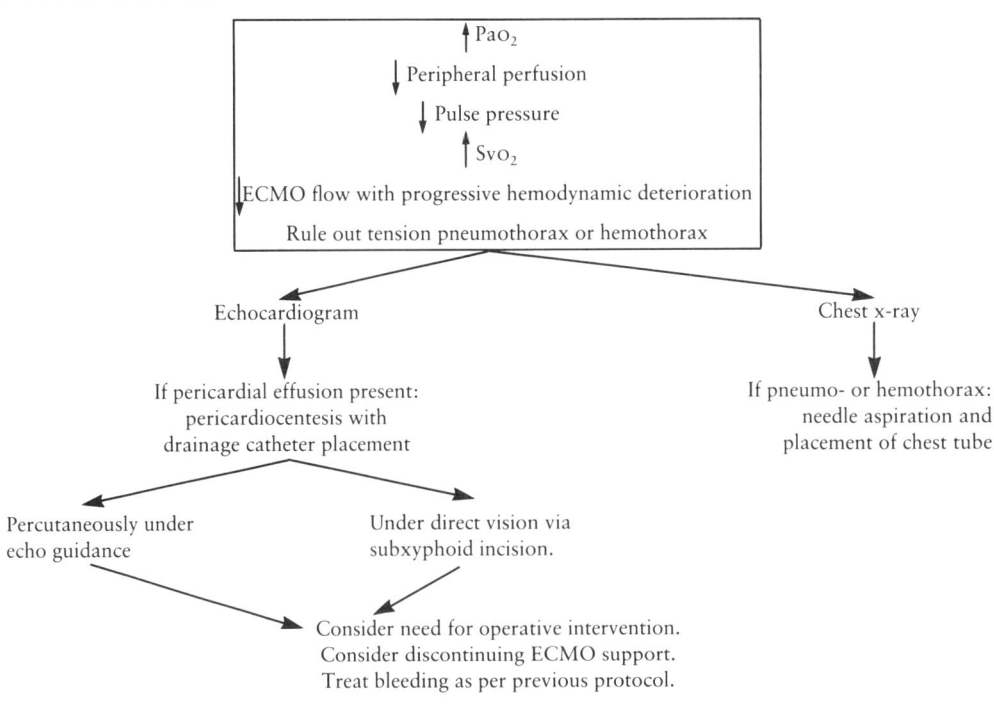

Likewise, pericardial tamponade may be suggested on chest roentgenogram by enlargement of the cardiac silhouette. Most helpful, however, is an echocardiogram, which will demonstrate a pericardial effusion and may also localize a hemothorax.

For emergency treatment of both tension hemothorax and pneumothorax and pericardial tamponade, I recommend placement of a percutaneous drainage catheter or reverse the developing pathophysiology. For pericardial tamponade, placement of an angiocatheter into the pericardium using ultrasound guidance seems most safe and reliable. Once partial drainage using the angiocatheter has relieved the tamponade, a guidewire may be passed using modified Seldinger technique to place a multiholed drainage tube. I have successfully used a No. 5 French pediatric feeding tube for this purpose. A peritoneal dialysis catheter or any of the commercially available multiholed drainage catheters may be used. For tension hemothorax and pneumothorax, a needle, angiocatheter, and chest tube are all options for emergent decompression. If these measures are unsuccessful or if the patient responds initially but later hemodynamically deteriorates, emergency thoracotomy may be necessary for drainage of a hemothorax or a hemopericardium (see Figure 14.4). As noted, anytime a site of abnormal bleeding is identified during ECMO, the immediate strategy is to modify the anticoagulation as outlined in Figure 14.2. Sepsis is both an indication for and a complication of ECMO. However, only 5% of all patients requiring ECMO develop positive blood cultures (2). This is a remarkably low incidence given the duration of cannulation, the large surface area involved, and the frequency of access to the circuit.

The pathophysiology of persistent fetal circulation is a right-to-left shunt and a patent ductus arteriosus (PDA) during severe respiratory failure in the newborn. Therefore, when ECMO is initiated, a PDA is always present. When pulmonary vasospasm relaxes, flow through the ductus reverses (becomes left to right), and the ductus usually closes within 24 h. The ductus may remain patent with major left-to-right shunting. A persistent left-to-right shunt across the ductus arteriosus may lead to pulmonary edema. Decreased systemic oxygenation may result both from pulmonary edema and from decreased systemic blood flow. Both of these effects will require the operator to increase the ECMO flow to maintain adequate gas exchange and perfusion. Likewise, if renal failure occurs and a previous hypoxic or ischemic insult cannot be identified, then the possibility of decreased renal perfusion during ECMO as a result of a PDA must be considered. Therefore, PDA on ECMO may present with any of the following: a decreased Pao_2, an increased $Paco_2$, decreased peripheral perfusion, decreased urine output, acidosis, and rising ECMO flow and volume requirements. The clinical diagnosis may be confirmed, as with other neonatal patients, with Doppler echocardiography or angiography. Some centers have tried using intravenous indomethacin to treat PDA in neonates on ECMO. However, many practitioners strongly discourage this approach because of its effects on platelet function that increase the risks of bleeding in patients on ECMO. Once the diagnosis is established, most programs will "run the patient relatively dry" while maintaining supportive ECMO flow until the PDA closes. While this often means a few additional days on ECMO, surgical ligation is rarely necessary. If this is deemed necessary after three to four days of consecutive treatment, the surgeon should be aware of the potential for bleeding complications. Special measures should include maintaining the ACT between 180 and 220 s, infusing platelets during surgery, keeping the platelet count above 100,000/mL, using electrocautery exclusively during surgery, administering fresh frozen plasma (10 cc/kg) during and every six hours after surgery for 24 hours, maximizing ECMO support, and providing ongoing blood and volume replacement (on a volume-for-volume basis) both during and after the ligation. Liberal use of topical hemostatic agents is also mandatory. Table 14.4 outlines the physiologic/metabolic complications associated with ECMO and the treatment for each complication.

Hemolysis is a complication often related to the ECMO membrane and/or circuit (23). Clots in the circuit or membrane may promote a coagulopathy by activation of complement white blood cells, platelets, or coagulation factors to cause erythrocytes to adhere and lyse on the fibrin strands. These theories are reinforced by data that show a decreased plasma free hemoglobin after membrane and circuit changeout (23). The management response to hemolysis is outlined in Figure 14.5.

Occasionally, after one week of ECMO, a patient cannot be weaned. We routinely return to use of either diuretics and/or a hemofilter to remove excess fluid to birthweight. Ventilator support is increased to the maximal acceptable pressures and inspired oxygen. An echocardiogram is repeated to ensure that a PDA with predominant left-to-right shunt is not present and to once again rule out total anomalous venous return. We then attempt a trial off ECMO with the increased ventilator settings. If the trial off ECMO is unsuccessful, then cardiac catheterization and/or open lung biopsy must be performed to rule out potentially correctable problems. If no correctable lesions are found, a decision must be made to discontinue ECMO support or continue it indefinitely if there are objective signs of improvement with no complications. The management response to failure to wean is outlined in Figure 14.6.

FIGURE 14.5 Management response to hemolysis.

HEMOLYSIS
↓
Check ACT, platelet count, fibrinogen, fibrin split products, and serum-free hemoglobin, prothrombin time, partial prothrombin time to rule out disseminated intravascular coagulation.
↓
Check circuit for clots or circuit kinks, arterial catheter occlusion, temperature of heat exchanger or circuit pressures 300 mm Hg.
↓
Change oxygenator pump head, or entire circuit as indicated.
↓
Alkalinize urine and keep urine flow greater than 3 cc/kg/h with fluids, furosemide, or mannitol.

FAILURE TO WEAN
↓
Diurese to birthweight (Lasix, mannitol, or hemofilter).
↓
Increase ventilator pressures, e.g., 30/4, IT 1.0, BUR 10, FiO_2 40% (attempt to decrease lung atelectasis).
↓
Recheck echocardiogram for congenital heart disease or patent ductus with predominant left-to-right shunt.
↓
Wean with PaO_2 = 60, maintaining venous saturation >60.
↓
Trial off ECMO with increased ventilator settings.
↓
If still unable to wean, must obtain cardiac catheterization on ECMO to rule out congenital heart disease, especially total anomalous pulmonary venous return.
↓
Discontinue ECMO support at high ventilator settings if necessary or continue indefinitely if signs of improvement or no progressive complications (possible irreversible lung disease—bronchopulmonary dysplasia).

FIGURE 14.6 Management algorithm for failure to wean patient from ECMO.

SUMMARY

The complications encountered in ECMO can be classified as mechanical or patient complications (see Table 14.6). Any mechanical component of the ECMO apparatus may fail, and constant system checks and monitoring prevent most complications from becoming management disasters. The incidence of these complications are listed in the text. Patient complications are often related to systemic heparinization; intracranial hemorrhage, gastrointestinal hemorrhage, and cannula site

TABLE 14.6 ECMO emergencies

Coming off ECMO
If something disastrous occurs to the circuit, remove the patient from the circuit.
1. Clamp the venous cannula.
2. Unclamp the bridge.
3. Clamp the arterial cannula.
4. Place patient on emergency ventilator settings.
5. Turn off the sweep gas.
6. Turn off water heater.
7. Stop all infusions, especially heparin, into the circuit if off longer than 10–15 min.
8. Follow the patient's ACT.
9. Provide glucose to the patient.

Air in the circuit
This is one of the most likely, and one of the worst, disasters. Unless air is on the venous side of the circuit and can be easily aspirated from the bladder, remove the patient from ECMO and remove it.

If air is in the preoxygenator circuit, check for cracks or leaks in the circuit, connectors, pigtails, stopcocks, or cannula connectors. Make certain that no bubbles are being infused from the drips or the pressure monitor. Be extremely careful not to introduce air as you flush the stopcocks and pigtails.

If air is in the postoxygenator circuit, remove the patient from ECMO immediately; this is a true emergency. Air has either traveled through the entire circuit or is leaking from the oxygenator. If the oxygenator is leaking air into the circuit the oxygenator must be changed. Aspirate air on the arterial side from either the cooximeter side or from the postoxygenator, platelet infusion site.

If air is widespread throughout the circuit, something disastrous has happened. Take the patient off and reprime an entirely new circuit.

Accidental decannulation
Avoid this by adequately sedating and restraining the infant and by carefully supervising all manipulations of the infant. A decannulated patient is already off ECMO. Your primary goals are to turn off the pump, turn up the ventilator, stop the bleeding with local pressure, and start replacing the blood that has sprayed all over the room. Don't fail to call the surgeons to repair the vessel. If the patient is too sick to remain off ECMO, and only one catheter has been dislodged, keep the patient heparinized so that catheter does not clot off.

Cannula kink
If a kink occurs in the right atrial catheter, the venous reservoir will collapse and the pump will shut off. If it occurs in the aortic catheter, the high-pressure alarm should shut off the pump. However, if the alarm has become disconnected, the circuit will rupture at its weakest point. If this happens, turn up the ventilator and replace the blood that is lost. You will need a new circuit.

One of the most common causes of occlusion of the aortic catheter is inadvertently clamping/unclamping in the wrong order as the patient comes off or goes on ECMO. Never have the aortic catheter and the bridge clamped at the same time.

Tubing rupture, connector separation
Remove the patient from ECMO and repair the circuit. To ensure that the circuit is entirely free of air, circulate it through the bridge before putting the patient back on ECMO.

Loss of power
The battery pack should work. If it does not, crank the pump by hand. Remember that only the relay box and the pump are powered by the battery pack.

Reprinted by permission of Neonatal Network. Nugent, J. Extracorporeal membrane oxygenation in the neonate, Vol. 4(5) April 1986:33–6.

bleeding are all due to anticoagulation. Other metabolic problems are seen, but they are less common. Thrombocytopenia is a result of ECMO but may be exacerbated by sepsis. The management of these complications is discussed in detail, and management algorithms are shown as guides to systematic treatment.

REFERENCES

(1) Webster's Ninth New Collegiate Dictionary. Springfield, MA: Merriam-Webster Inc., 1984: 290.

(2) Extracorporeal Life Support Organization Registry—July 1990. Ann Arbor, MI: University of Michigan, 1990.

(3) Nugent J. Extracorporeal membrane oxygenation in the neonate 1986;4:33–6.

(4) Toomasian JM, Kenby KA, Chapman R, et al. Performance of a rupture-resistant polyvinyl chloride tubing. Proc Am Acad Cardiovasc Perfusion 1987;8:56–9.

(5) Vogler C, Sotelo-Avila C, Lagunoff D, et al. Aluminum containing emboli in infants treated with extracorporeal membrane oxygenation. N Engl J Med 1988;319:75–9.

(6) Allison PL, Kurusz M, Graves DF, Zwischenberger JB. Devices and monitoring during neonatal ECMO: survey results. Perfusion 1990;5: 193–201.

(7) Langham MR, Krummel TM, Greenfield LJ, Drucker DE, et al. Extracorporeal membrane oxygenation following repair of congenital diaphragmatic hernia. Ann Thorac Surg 1987;44:247–52.

(8) Ahmann PA, Lazzara A, Dykes FD, et al. Intraventricular hemorrhage in high-risk preterm infants: incidence and outcome. Ann Neurol 1980;7:118–24.

(9) Harck HT, Naeye RL, Storch A, et al. Perinatal cerebral intraventricular hemorrhage. J Pediatr 1972;80:37–42.

(10) Leech RW, Kohnen P, et al. Subependymal and intraventricular hemorrhages in the newborn. Am J Pathol 1974;77:465–76.

(11) DeCourten GM, Rabinowicz TH. Intraventricular hemorrhage in premature infants. Reappraisal and new hypothesis. Dev Med Child Neurol 1981;23:389–403.

(12) Volpe JJ. Neonatal intraventricular hemorrhage. N Engl J Med 1981;304:886–91.

(13) Tarby TJ, Volpe JJ. Intraventricular hemorrhage in the premature infant. Pediatr Clin North Am 1982;29:1077–1104.

(14) Cilley RE, Zwischenberger JB, Andrews AF, et al. Intracranial hemorrhage during extracorporeal membrane oxygenation in neonates. Pediatrics 1986;78:699–704.

(15) Babcock DS, Bokyung KH, Weiss RG, Ryckman FC. Brain abnormalities in infants on ECMO: sonographic and CT findings. AJR 1989;153:578–6.

(16) Krummel TM, Greenfield LJ, Kirkpatrick BV, Moelle DG, et al. The early evaluation of survivors after extracorporeal membrane oxygenation for pulmonary failure. Pediatr Surg 1984;19:585–90.

(17) Towne BN, Lott IT, Hicks DA, et al. Long-term follow-up of infants and children treated with ECMO: a preliminary report. J Pediatr Surg 1985;20:410–14.

(18) Taylor GA, Fitz CR, Miller MK, Garin DB, et al. Intracranial flow patterns in infants undergoing extracorporeal membrane oxygenation: preliminary observations with Doppler US. Radiology Acc 1987;165:671–4.

(19) Bowerman RA, Zwischenberger JB, Andres AF, et al. Cranial sonography in the evaluation of the infant treated with extracorporeal membrane oxygenation. AJNR 1985;6:377–89.

(20) Anderson HL III, Cilley RE, Zwischenberger JB, et al. Thrombocytopenia in neonates after extracorporeal membrane oxygenation. Trans ASAIO 1986;32:534–7.

(21) White JJ, Andrews HA, Risemberg H, et al. Prolonged respiratory support in newborn infants with a membrane oxygenator. Surgery 1971;7:288–96.

(22) Kirkpatrick BV, Krummel TM, Mueller DA, et al. Use of extracorporeal membrane oxygenation for respiratory failure in term infants. Pediatrics 1983;72:872–6.

(23) Bartlett RH, Andrews AF, Toomasian JM, et al. Extracorporeal membrane oxygenation for newborn respiratory failure: forty-five cases. Surgery 1982;92:425–33.

(24) Steinhorn RN, Isham-Schupt B, Smith C, et al. Hemolysis during long-term extracorporeal membrane oxygenation. J Pediatr 1989;115: 625–30.

(25) Sell LL, Cullen ML, Whittlesey GC, et al. Experience with renal failure during ECMO: treatment with continuous hemofiltration. Pediatr Surg 1987;22:600–2.

(26) Sell LL, Cullen ML, Lerner GR, et al. Hypertension during extracorporeal membrane oxygenation: cause, effect and management. Surgery 1987;102:724–30.

(27) Dickson M, Hirthler M, Simon J, et al. Stunned myocardium during ECMO: a reperfusion injury mediated by oxygen free radicals? Proc ELSO 1989;1:47.

(28) Klein MD, Shaheen KW, Whittlesey GC, Pinsky WW, Arciniegas E. Extracorporeal mem-

brane oxygenation for the circulatory support of children after repair of congenital heart disease. J Thorac Cardiovasc Surg 1990;100:498–505.

(29) Zwischenberger JB, Bartlett RH. Extracorporeal circulation for respiratory or cardiac failure. In: Civetta JM, Taylor RW, Kirby RR, eds. Critical care. Philadelphia: J.B. Lippincott, 1992.

(30) Zwischenberger JB, Cilley RE, Hirschl RB, Heiss KF, Conti VR, Bartlett RH. Life-threatening intrathoracic complications during treatment with extracorporeal membrane oxygenation. J Pediatr Surg 1988;23:599–604.

(31) Zwischenberger JB, Bowers RM, Dickens GJ. Tension pneumothorax during ECMO. Ann Thorac Surg 1989; 47:868–71.

(32) Oeveren M, Kazatchkine A, et al. Deleterious effects of cardiopulmonary bypass. J Thoracic Cardiovasc Surg 1985;89:888–9.

15

Risks of Neonatal ECMO

R.E. Schumacher, M.D.

The delivery of (good) medical care is to do as much of nothing as possible.
—*The Fat Man (1)*

The nearly exponential growth in the number of ECMO centers (and hence ECMO patients) in the past several years is testimony to the lifesaving capabilities of the ECMO procedure. Earlier reports on long-term morbidity are equally gratifying in that the overwhelming majority of neonatal ECMO survivors lead normal to near-normal lives. (2–4). However, when a new technology is introduced, additional and sometimes novel risks are often associated with the procedure. This is the case for newborns who receive extracorporeal membrane oxygenation.

Many of the risks associated with neonatal ECMO are theoretical and/or controversial in nature. The ability to identify ECMO-specific risks is hampered by several factors. One is that individual practices in the pre-ECMO management of infants, selection criteria for patients on ECMO, and specific ECMO techniques themselves can produce great interinstitutional variability in the incidence of adverse sequelae. Another variable that confounds the interpretation of neonatal risks of ECMO is that there exists no comparable group of equally ill newborns to serve as a control and/or comparison group. Only two randomized controlled studies of ECMO have been reported to date, with a total of 11 control infants described (5,6). While these studies have documented the efficacy of ECMO in terms of improved survival rates, they have, by the nature of their design, failed to provide an adequate cohort of control infants from which to ascertain ECMO-specific risks. By reviewing data from the national Extracorporeal Life Support Organization (ELSO) registry, some insight can be gained into the nature and relative frequency of certain complications (7). However, even with these data, one is left in the less-than-desirable position of trying to assign cause-and-effect relationships between ECMO and adverse sequelae where only associations exist.

Risks are incurred when, through the introduction of new technology, medicine intervenes and alters or replaces "natural" physiology (or pathophysiology). In the case of ECMO, this occurs (and hence, risk occurs) via two basic alterations in physiology.

The first deals with blood-surface interactions. ECMO requires that blood (both the patient's and a substantial quantity of transfused blood) come in contact with foreign surfaces, notably the ECMO circuit tubing, the membrane lung, and the heat exchanger. Because of these blood-surface interactions, the risk of thrombus formation and subsequent embolization is high. This fact, in turn, necessitates systemic anticoagulation of the infant, thus introducing the risk of bleeding diathesis.

When blood does come in contact with foreign surfaces, the interaction of some of the formed elements, white cells, or platelets, or both, with these surfaces causes the release of a number of vasoactive substances into the systemic circulation. The release of such substances, notably complement factors and arachidonic acid metabolites, has been documented by many investigators (8–10). Figure 15.1 demonstrates substantial increases in the circulating concentration of thromboxane B_2 in a group of infants on bypass. During the first several hours of bypass, these infants often exhibited substantial increases in plasma thromboxane values (11). The consequences of the release of these vasoactive substances have not been studied well, but there exists theoretical risk from alterations in vasomotor tone, permeability, and blood flow.

The interaction of blood with foreign surfaces can also lead to leaching of potentially toxic substances from the foreign surfaces into the circulation (12,13). Finally, the need for continuous blood sampling, ongoing platelet consumption, and the frequent need for blood transfusion with its inherent risk for acquired infections must all be regarded as significant sources of risk when an infant undergoes ECMO therapy.

The other major way in which ECMO alters the basic physiology is by changing patterns of blood flow throughout the body. When using a nonpulsatile-flow roller head pump, as is common practice in neonatal ECMO, alterations in the pressure wave form presented to the systemic circulations are seen. This can have consequences in that certain organs (e.g., brain, carotid bodies) rely on pulse pressure to provide information concerning intravascular volume.

Patterns of blood flow are also changed by occlusion of the right internal jugular vein and right common carotid artery, both of

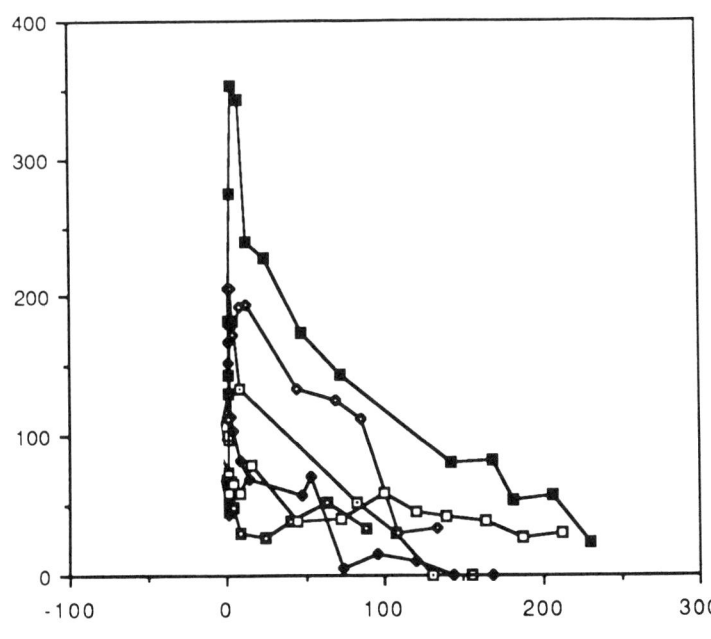

FIGURE 15.1 Percent increase from baseline (pre-ECMO) for values of plasma thromboxane B_2 vs. age in hours for six infants treated with extracorporeal membrane oxygenation.

which can affect the pattern of cerebral blood flow (14).

Additionally, at very high ECMO flows the lung, which normally receives 100% of cardiac output, is bypassed, the consequences of which will be discussed below.

Chiefly as a result of these two factors (blood-surface interactions and changing patterns of blood flow), almost every organ system is at risk for adverse side-effects from the ECMO procedure. The following sections will address both realized and theoretical risks on a system-by-system basis, beginning with the most controversial, the central nervous system.

CENTRAL NERVOUS SYSTEM RISKS

Chief concerns about ECMO and the central nervous system (CNS) include the risk of intracranial hemorrhage and the effects of acute jugular vein and carotid artery blood vessel ligation on CNS perfusion. Hemorrhage is a concern, especially in premature infants. Cilley et al. (15) reported a series in which eight of eight infants younger than 35 weeks' gestational age developed intracranial hemorrhage. This report formed the basis for the current recommendation that premature infants not receive ECMO routinely.

Factors known to predispose to intracranial hemorrhage in newborns include rapid changes in the patterns of blood flow and pressure, rapid changes in the partial pressure of carbon dioxide (CO_2) and perhaps oxygen (which in turn affect blood flow patterns), alterations in the patterns of vasoactive substances and, particularly in low-birthweight infants, systemic heparin therapy (16).

With ECMO, rapid changes in the distribution of CNS blood flow can occur with ligation of either the jugular vein or the carotid artery. In a lamb model of asphyxia, Stolar et al. (17) demonstrated acute changes in intracranial pressure following vessel ligation. In a study using baboons, Kinsella and co-workers (18) found ocular pathologic changes that were presumed to be secondary to venous congestion from jugular vein ligation; the investigators suggested that unilateral jugular ligation alone may contribute to changes in regional intracranial blood flow distribution. Gangitano et al. (19) presented similar concerns over vein ligation.

In a lamb model of central nervous system blood flow, Gleason, Short, and Jones (20) demonstrated that rapid changes in the partial pressure of CO_2 (a phenomenon often seen upon initiation of bypass) can dramatically change cerebral blood flow. These investigators suggested that changes in cerebral blood flow seen with ECMO may be caused by dramatic swings in the partial pressure of CO_2 and that a posthypocapneic hyperemia could contribute to an increased incidence of hemorrhage with ECMO. Alterations in arterial blood flow with ECMO were documented in infants by Raju et al. (14). These investigators reported that within 15 minutes of common carotid artery ligation, blood flow was detected in one infant's middle cerebral artery, but at a velocity 50% of the pre-ECMO value. They also noted that after carotid ligation the vertebrobasilar and the contralateral internal carotid systems appeared to be the main source of reperfusion of the right cerebral hemisphere.

Work by Ment and others (21,22) suggests that endogenous circulating vasoactive arachidonic acid metabolites can contribute to the incidence of intracranial hemorrhage in newborns. As noted above, alterations in circulating concentrations of arachidonic acid metabolites can be caused by ECMO blood-surface interactions and thus place an infant at risk for hemorrhage.

Lesko and co-workers (23) suggest that an excessive amount of heparin delivered to low-birthweight infants (primarily via total parenteral nutrition) places infants at risk for intracranial hemorrhage. ECMO, with its systemic anticoagulation, would seem to contribute to that risk, especially in preterm newborns. In the presence of hemorrhage, heparin therapy may put an infant at risk for expansion of the hemorrhage.

Despite these theoretical risks, reports of infants with intracranial hemorrhage successfully treated with ECMO have been made (7). Moreover, steps can be taken to lower the risk of hemorrhage. Draining of the distal jugular vein with a second catheter may lessen the effects of acute jugular vein ligation (19). Venovenous ECMO, now being used at several centers, may obviate the need for carotid artery ligation (24). The use of ECMO prime without platelets may lessen the change in the vasoactive profile seen with ECMO initiation. The use of heparin-bonded circuits, now under study, may obviate the need for systemic heparinization of the infant (25). These modifications or alterations of the current ECMO procedure should lower the overall risk of hemorrhage and may soon allow successful ECMO runs in even small premature infants.

Much controversy exists over the effects of jugular vein and/or carotid ligation during the use of ECMO in the term infant, and whether or not CNS damage can occur ipsilateral to the side of vessel ligation. In response to early reports that right-sided brain lesions had not been seen with the use of ECMO, Schumacher et al. (26) reported several cases in which infants had evidence of right-sided brain lesions post-ECMO (Figure 15.2). These lesions were manifest on computed tomography (CT) brain scan as right-hemispheric stroke, right parasagital injury, and right-sided infarcts of the basal ganglia. The investigators noted that at their institution, when unilateral central nervous system injury occurred post-ECMO, it was invariably right-sided. No lesions were seen exclusively on the left hemisphere. The study suffered from the fact that, although cranial ultrasound studies were routinely obtained in all infants, brain scans were not done on all ECMO patients; since the report dealt with CT findings, the potential for a Type 1 error existed. However, these investigators also provided electroencephalographic (EEG) findings (which were routinely obtained in all infants receiving ECMO) in the same cohort, which showed an increase in the incidence of slowing and attenuation on the side ipsilateral to the ligation procedure. These types of EEG findings are compatible with ischemia pro-

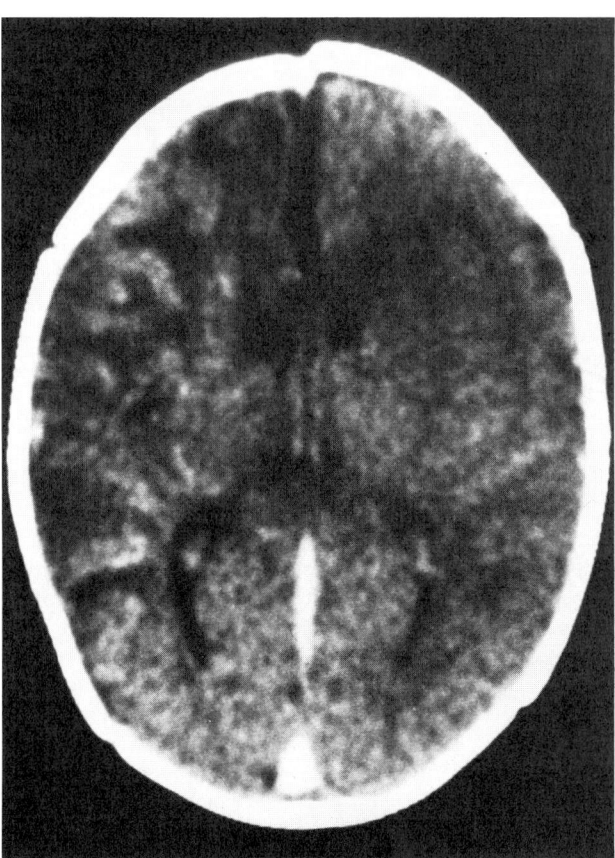

FIGURE 15.2   CT brain scan of a term infant, after venoarterial ECMO, demonstrating findings compatible with a large hemorrhagic infarction in the distribution of the right middle cerebral artery.

duced by either carotid artery or jugular vein ligation. Early follow-up reports from the same institution found evidence of a left hemiparesis in seven of 23 infants, whereas no infants demonstrated a right hemiparesis.

Although some investigators have cited similar findings, others have disagreed, presenting very thorough CT brain scan studies that show no increase in the incidence of right-sided brain lesions. (27,28). Taylor et al. (29) found no evidence of an increased incidence of right-sided CNS damage.

Neither Schumacher nor Taylor et al. have any comparable non-ECMO control with which to compare findings. This seems particularly important in view of the fact that, when one reviews the literature on stroke in the term newborn, there appears to be a tendency to left-brain injury (29,30). If this selective vulnerability of the left brain exists, reports citing no difference in the incidence of right- or left-sided brain injury post-ECMO may actually be supportive of a relative increase in right-sided injury (or, alternatively, an ECMO-induced decrease in the left hemisphere's vulnerability to injury).

More insight on the possible effects of the ECMO procedure on the brain may be gained through the use of animal models. A lamb model of ECMO is being studied by Gleason and Short. In a report from their laboratory, Bender et al. (31) showed that prolonged hypoxemia in lambs produced compensatory increases in cerebral blood flow so as to maintain oxygen delivery to the brain. Additionally, in the absence of antecedent hypoxia/ischemia, the ECMO procedure itself does not seem to effect cerebral oxygen metabolism (32). Subsequent carotid artery ligation was *not* shown to affect cerebral blood flow, oxygen delivery, or cerebral metabolic rate. In contrast, in a rat pup model of CNS hypoxic-ischemic injury, Silverstein et al. (33) found that carotid artery ligation and 15 min of hypoxia produced substantial hemispheric brain injury. These rats also showed characteristic unilateral EEG and motor behavior symptoms, suggesting selective damage to the brain ipsilateral to the ligation. Although the use of animal models in such situations may be helpful, questions regarding species-specific changes and/or study design must be taken into account.

EEG monitoring of the CNS function before and after ligation has been investigated at several institutions. Wiznitzer and co-investigators (34) reported on EEG findings before and during ECMO. They concluded that lateralized abnormalities in their ECMO patient's EEGs were the consequence of pre-ECMO cerebral dysfunction and were unrelated to transient changes in cerebral perfusion after carotid ligation. Studies at the University of Michigan using compressed spectral array EEG have demonstrated EEG changes during carotid artery ligation. An example is shown in Figure 15.3 that demonstrates a loss of electrical power in both hemispheres after carotid artery ligation. Lott et al. (35), using long-latency auditory and somatosensory evoked potentials, showed consistent reduction in the amplitude of right hemispheric evoked potentials in children aged four to nine years post-ECMO. These investigators speculated that the findings reflected redirected cerebral blood flow patterns after ECMO.

The degree of pre-ECMO CNS damage present may determine an infant's susceptibility to major vessel ligation. Except in a few patients with anomalies of the circle of Willis, ligation of the carotid in and of itself should not affect an infant whose cardiac output is sufficient to maintain oxygen delivery to the CNS. But many ECMO patients have elements of hypoxic-ischemic encephalopathy or evidence of very low cardiac output prior to ligation. If an infant's cardiac output in compromised to the point that only marginal or insufficient oxygen delivery exists, it is reasonable to assume that ligation of vessels will further compromise oxygen delivery and damage will follow. Indeed, seven of eight infants with right hemispheric damage reported by Schumacher et al. (26) were extremely hypotensive prior to ECMO cannulation. In a recent report from the institution that reported no right-left differences in brain injury, Taylor et al. (36) correlated brain CT findings with those at autopsy in a group of infants who expired following ECMO (and presumably were among the most compromised before ECMO). In this report, four infants exhibited significant unilateral brain pathology, three had right-sided, ischemic-type lesions, and only one exhibited exclusive left-sided changes. Preventing such injury can be achieved by

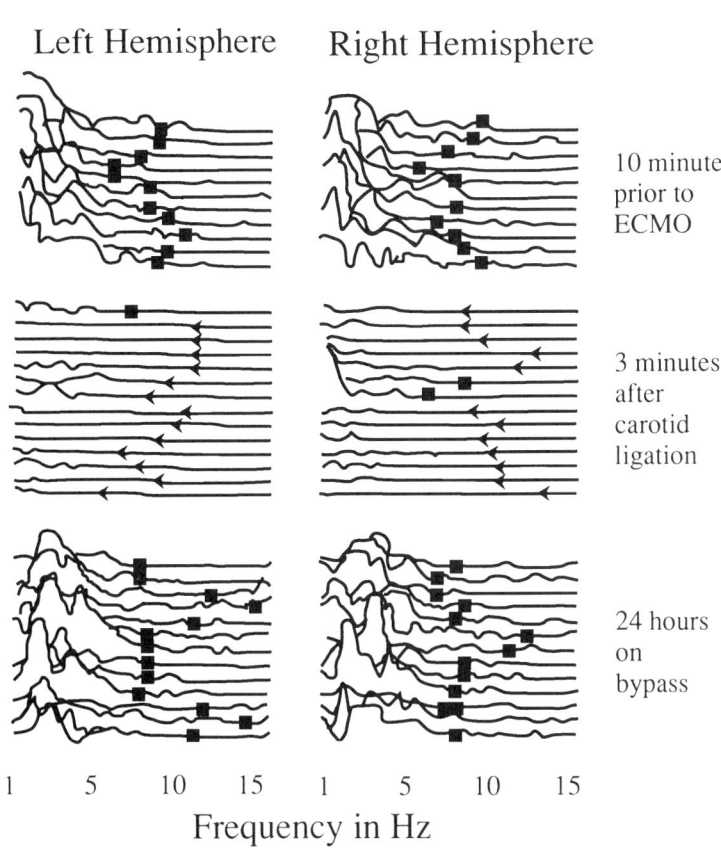

FIGURE 15.3 Compressed spectral array EEG findings of the right and left hemispheres in an infant before, during, and after cannulation for veno-arterial ECMO. Each line represents 16 seconds of electrical activity, with height above baseline being directly proportional to electrical power at that frequency. Three minutes after carotid ligation, the infant demonstrated acute loss of power from both cerebral hemispheres. A return to "baseline" was seen the next day. ■ = two standard deviations (SD) of electrical power lie to the left of this marker. < = not enough signal to calculate 2 SD.

improving selection criteria such that vulnerable patients are recognized early. Additionally, the success of venovenous ECMO can obviate the need for carotid artery ligation.

Taylor et al. (37) have also described a larger-than-expected number of infants with midline or posterior fossa hemorrhage, raising the question as to whether ECMO or jugular vein ligation or both predispose to such injury. A subsequent review of autopsy findings over five years, done by the same investigators, found five infants with posterior fossa hemorrhages. All were identified prospectively by cranial ultrasound examinations (38). An example of such a lesion is shown in Figure 15.4. Unilateral retinal vascular changes have been reported to occur following ECMO (39). Investigators hypothesized that these changes were secondary to vessel ligation. The changes seen were not expected to interfere with vision.

Brain-stem function may also be affected following jugular venous and/or carotid artery ligation. Schumacher et al. (40) reported relative prolongation of brain-stem auditory evoked responses emanating from the right brain stem following ECMO. Figure 15.5 shows prolongation of interpeak latency period I–V during ECMO cannulation.

CARDIAC PROBLEMS

Cardiac stun or a dramatic decrease in apparent cardiac performance has been noted in a subset of infants receiving ECMO (41,42). Martin et al. (41) made the diagnosis of cardiac stun in a group of infants when aortic pulse pressure was less than or equal to 10 mm Hg or arterial Po_2 was greater than 350 mm Hg

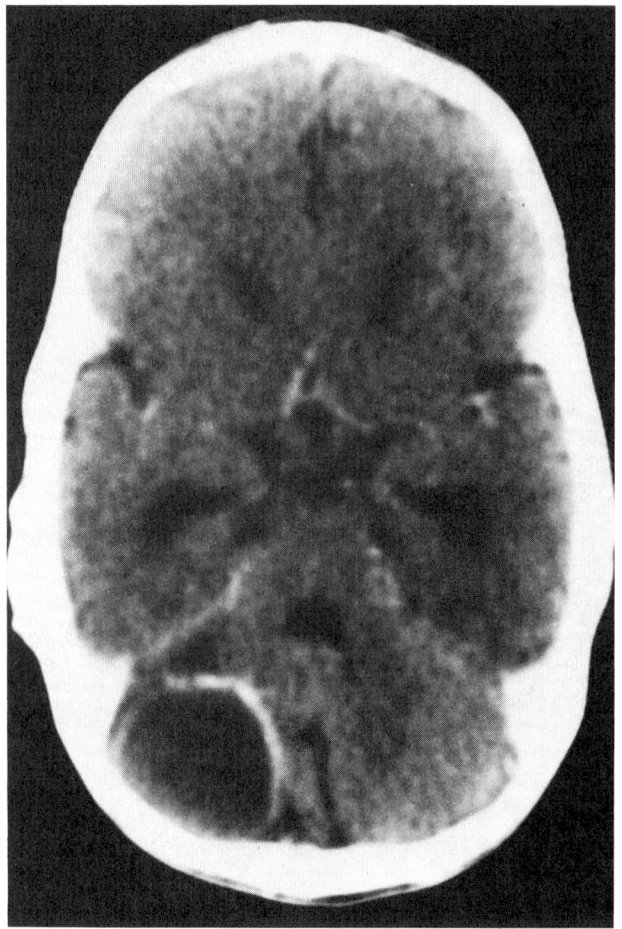

FIGURE 15.4 CT brain scan from an infant one month after ECMO, which shows a posthemorrhagic, right-sided posterior fossa extraaxial cyst. Obstructive hydrocephalus ensued.

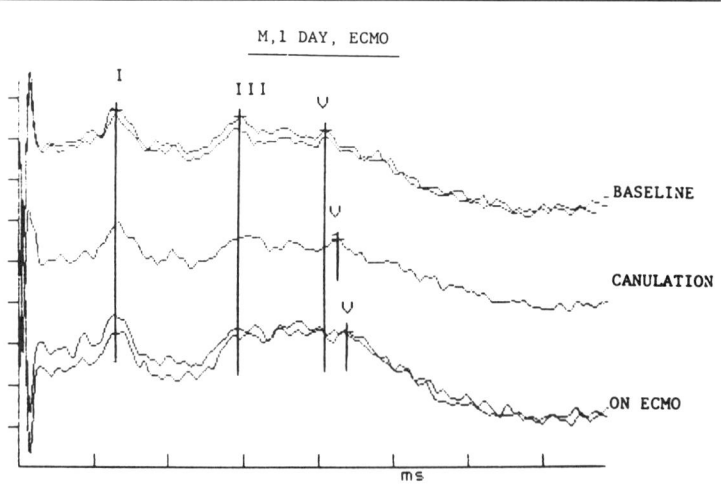

FIGURE 15.5 Brainstem auditory responses during cannulation for ECMO that demonstrate prolongation of interpeak latency periods occurring with ligation of major blood vessels.

(suggesting little contribution to total Po_2 from the native heart and lung). The investigators found that 5% of all infants receiving ECMO at their institution fulfilled the criteria for cardiac stun. Patients with cardiac stun had lower pre-ECMO Po_2 values, and pre-ECMO cardiac arrests were more common. Patients with cardiac stun had higher overall mortality rates after ECMO. However, cardiac stun itself was almost always transient in nature. Some have speculated that these findings represent a free radical mediated reperfusion injury (43). However, there are reasons why ECMO might be implicated as being contributory. First, blood-surface interactions cause the release of vasoactive substances (e.g., serotonin, thromboxane) which can contribute to myocardial ischemic changes. Secondly, Gerstman et al. (44), using microspheres to study coronary artery blood flow, demonstrated during venoarterial ECMO that blood flow to the coronary arteries was derived chiefly from the native heart and lung which, during ECMO, are likely to have low oxygen content. This model suggested that coronary artery oxygen delivery in ECMO patients may sometimes be suboptimal or even contribute to myocardial oxygen deprivation and cardiac dysfunction. The presence of retrograde, ECMO-generated flow in the proximal aorta may actually increase left ventricular afterload in ECMO patients. Support for this theory comes from Martin et al. (41) who, in their study of myocardial stun, documented increased left ventricular afterload in ECMO patients.

Hemopericardium has been seen in several infants following ECMO. At the University of Michigan, this has been seen exclusively in infants who have had previous cardiac arrest and/or pneumopericardium and either received intracardiac injections of epinephrine or had pericardial tubes placed for drainage of air. It is presumed that the systemic anticoagulation necessary for ECMO subsequently permitted bleeding at former puncture sites.

PULMONARY PROBLEMS

Although the principal reason for venoarterial ECMO is to afford an infant's lungs a period of rest, there is reason to suspect that ECMO has some adverse side-effects on the pulmonary system. Most infants undergo total pulmonary opacification and dramatic decreases in pulmonary compliance within a day of being placed on bypass (45). This can be explained on the basis of the "rearrangement" of Starling forces: A decrease in the alveolar distending pressure allows for greater transcapillary fluid escape into and across what, in an infant with respiratory failure, is usually a damaged alveolar wall. Such edema decreases pulmonary compliance and increases the work of breathing. This transcapillary fluid leak can also inhibit surfactant production, delaying lung recovery (46). Keszler et al. (47) have shown that through the use of high positive end-expiratory pressure (PEEP) during ECMO, the incidence of pulmonary opacification is decreased and the overall ECMO run is shortened.

Initial interactions of blood with foreign surfaces in the ECMO circuit can release vasoactive substances, some of which are capable of altering vascular permeability and some of which are capable of exacerbating pulmonary hypertension. Support for this second period of vascular permeability is found in the "re-white-out" of chest x-ray following a membrane lung change during an ECMO run. In this instance, a new foreign surface is made available for interaction with blood.

The lung is normally an area of intense metabolic activity. By virtue of its large vascular surface area and the fact that it receives 100% of the cardiac output, it has the ability to influence circulating concentrations of a large number of substances. Numerous vasoactive agents (such as angiotensin I, 5-hydroxytryptamine, norepinephrine, various prostaglandins, and leukotrienes) are synthesized, removed, stored, or metabolized in the lung (48). ECMO, by altering the percent of cardiac output delivered to the pulmonary vasculature, has potential of dramatically altering the lungs' ability to influence an infant's circulating "vasoactive profile." The consequences of such alterations remain to be studied.

Upper airway obstruction from right vocal cord paresis has been seen in up to 4% of patients following ECMO. This finding, which is thought to be due to vagal or right laryngeal nerve damage secondary to adjacent ECMO catheters, is usually transient in nature (49).

RENAL PROBLEMS

Urine output often decreases dramatically once an infant is placed on bypass. Oliguria or anuria or both are commonly reported complications of ECMO. Similarly, several centers report problems with systemic hypertension in infants receiving ECMO. There are multiple theoretical explanations for both phenomena.

ECMO, by unloading the right atrium is capable of affecting concentrations of circulating atrial naturetic factor. Palermo and co-workers (50) reported elevated blood concentrations of atrial naturetic factor in patients receiving ECMO, suggesting that this finding could explain the increase in extracellular fluid volume, oliguria, and hypertension seen in these patients.

Exceedingly high values of plasma renin activity have been seen in some infants on bypass (51). This may be due to a loss of feedback inhibition from angiotensin II when, at high levels of pulmonary bypass, a substantial percentage of cardiac output is not made available to pulmonary angiotensin-converting enzyme. This may, in part, account for the alterations in fluid status and blood pressure seen in some infants.

At high pump flows, an infant's pulse pressure can be damped, sending a "false message" to the kidney or the carotid baroreceptor. Following carotid artery ligation, the right carotid baroreceptor is not receiving a legitimate flow signal, the consequences of which have not been studied.

Aluminum toxicity to the kidneys is also a potential ECMO risk (12,52). Vogler et al. (12) reported aluminum-containing emboli found in infants who had undergone prolonged bypass. These investigators cited evidence that the aluminum came from the mixing rods of the ECMO circuit heat exchanger. Kelly et al. (52) reported on aluminum toxicity in ECMO infants but demonstrated that the large amount of serum albumin used to prime the ECMO circuit was probably the source of the aluminum.

Oliguria and fluid overload is treated at many institutions by diuretic therapy, hemofiltration, or both. Caution should be used with this approach because the benefits of forced diuresis have not been demonstrated consistently, and overly aggressive hemofiltration may decrease intravascular volume to dangerous levels.

Systemic hypertension on bypass occurs in approximately 12% of patients but has been reported to occur in as many as 93% of infants at some ECMO centers (51). Sell and co-workers (51) suggested that the etiology of hypertension was multifactorial in nature and that increased extracellular fluid volume and elevated circulating values for renin activity, aldosterone, epinephrine, prostaglandin E_2, thromboxane, and antidiuretic hormone were all potentially contributing factors. In sharp contrast to the opinion of Sell et al. are the findings of Boedy and co-workers (53). These latter investigators could not relate the development of hypertension to increased plasma renin activity or sodium or colloid loads. Hypertension, when present, has usually been transient and has been treated successfully with a variety of agents, including diuretics, hydralazine, and angiotensin-converting enzyme inhibitors. Sell et al. (51) speculated that the presence of hypertension could contribute to intracranial hemorrhage. Boedy's work does not support a role for hypertension contributing to intracranial hemorrhage (53). ECMO registry data suggest that the presence of hypertension does not adversely effect survival (7).

GASTROINTESTINAL PROBLEMS

Difficulties with various aspects of the gastrointestinal system have been noted in infants during and following ECMO. Anecdotal reports of swallowing dysfunction and/or gastroesophageal reflux in babies following ECMO are numerous. Although it is reasonable to assume that sick infants per se do not feed well, certain complications of ECMO may be contributory. Taylor and Short (54) demonstrated gastroesophageal reflux and megaesophagus in infants following ECMO. Vocal cord paralysis can interfere with infant feeding ability. Both megaesophagus and vocal cord paresis may occur as a result of ECMO-induced vagal nerve neuropraxis. Although great care is taken during dissection of the neck for placement of ECMO cannulas, and the vagus nerve is always identified during this operation, the ECMO cannulas are stiff and are placed immediately adjacent to the right vagus nerve, which contains the fibers for the esophageal plexus as well as fibers that innervate the right vocal cord.

Direct hyperbilirubinemia has been reported in infants following ECMO (13). Pre-ECMO factors that can contribute to cholestasis in ECMO patients include hypoxia, acidosis, and hypotension. Contributing factors during ECMO could include complement activation, hemolysis (especially when a hemofilter is used with ECMO), and a toxic effect of circuit plasticizing agents. Shneider et al. (13) reported the presence of significant concentrations of di-2-ethylhexyl phthalate, a plasticizer found in ECMO circuit tubing, in the blood of ECMO infants. Shneider speculated that this substance, presumably leached from the plastic tubing in the ECMO circuit, contributed to hepatic canalicular dysfunction in patients with direct hyperbilirubinemia who were receiving ECMO. As noted above, toxic levels of aluminum can be present in ECMO patients, which could also contribute to hepatic dysfunction. Almond and co-workers (55) reported biliary calculi in an infant following ECMO. These investigators hypothesized that the hemolysis associated with ECMO, plus systemic hyperalimentation, predispose to early calculous disease.

Finally, there exists the theoretical risk of gastrointestinal bleeding in a newborn. The risk of hemorrhage from stress and the use of tolazoline before ECMO may be made more significant in the presence of systemic anticoagulation. Morbidity from postoperative bleeding, especially in infants with diaphragmatic hernia, has been notable (56).

RISK OF INFECTION

The risk of infection on bypass is acquired from the threat of transfusion-transmitted infection, alterations in immune (leukocyte) function, and the presence of multiple portals of entry (stopcocks, cannulas, etc.) in the ECMO circuit. A positive blood culture while on bypass is reported by the ELSO neonatal registry to occur in 5% of cases, with the pre-ECMO diagnosis of sepsis being a predictor of a positive culture on ECMO. Leukopenia (white blood count < 1,500) occurred in approximately 1% of cases. Minifee and Zwischenberger (8), using a sheep model of ECMO, demonstrated a significant and acute fall in the white blood cell count within minutes of institution of bypass; however, by 24 hours of bypass, the cell count had returned to above-normal values. In contrast, Zach et al. (57) demonstrated decreases in both absolute neutrophil count and absolute lymphocyte count that persisted for days in infants on bypass. In their study of 16 patients, four (25%) ECMO-treated newborns developed "serious infections." Hocker et al. (58) reported that patients undergoing ECMO experience a transient decrease in absolute neutrophil count, but neutrophil phagocytosis and oxidative burst remained unchanged during the first 48 hours of bypass. They did note activation of the complement system in infants on bypass. DePalma and co-workers (59) performed flow cytometric analysis of eight different lymphocyte populations in neonates on ECMO. Absolute lymphocyte counts decreased on day 1 of ECMO. In contrast to findings in adults, no significant changes in percentages of any of the lymphocyte subpopulations were seen as a result of ECMO. Hirthler and investigators (10) documented "late" (>4 days of bypass) changes in inflammatory mediators in 16 infants on ECMO and speculated that subclinical sepsis as a result of system contamination could account for the changes seen. Concern over the risk of transfusion-acquired infection prompted a study by Luban et al (60). These workers documented an average of 22 donor exposures and a mean volume of 1,348 mL of blood products in 168 infants receiving ECMO. In a subset of this same cohort, one in 37 infants (3%) developed what could be considered a transfusion-related infection (non-A, non-B hepatitis). No incidence of transfusion-acquired infection has been reported to the ELSO international registry.

THE INTERNATIONAL ELSO REGISTRY: COMPLICATIONS IN THE FIRST 3,000 CASES

The international Extracorporeal Life Support Organization (ELSO) maintains a data base that includes patient complications on bypass. The original registry lists 35 different possible complications of neonatal ECMO (Table 15.1). In a report detailing outcome in the first 715 neonatal ECMO cases, Toomasian and co-workers (61) cited an average of 1.77 complications per patient. These investigators noted that the presence of hemorrhage, neurologic abnormalities, renal insufficiency, and certain metabolic abnormalities occurred more frequently in infants who died. A predictive model relating complications to survival found that the most significant complications were intracranial hemorrhage, need for dialysis, "severe neurologic impairment," need for surgery on ECMO, elevated creatinine, low pH, and the presence of seizures. Toomasian et al. (61) also demonstrated the presence of a learning curve with experience, noting that the number of complications per patient for a center's first 10 cases averaged 2.29, while the average for all subsequent patients decreased to 1.60 ($p = 0.001$ by Student's t test).

The ELSO registry now holds data on more than 3,000 neonatal ECMO cases. Data from the first 3,000 cases list one or more complications occurring in 63% of all patients. Complications occurred >1% of the time in 25 of 35 of the categories listed in Table 15.1. The presence of one or more complications was associated with a decreased survival rate. Survival rate for patients with ≥1 complication was 75% vs. a survival rate of 95% for patients with no complications ($p < 0.0001$, chi square). By individual chi square analysis, most complications were by themselves associated with decreased survival. Of the complications occurring in >1% of cases, only the presence of "ECMO jitters," serum potassium <2.5 mEq/dL, systemic hypertension, and intracranial hemorrhage diagnosed by CT brain scan were *not* associated with decreased survival. The more commonly occurring complications (>5% incidence), along with survival rates given each complication, are presented in Figure 15.6.

Simple observation of registry data suggests that some patients are more prone to certain

TABLE 15.1 Physiologic complications during ECMO

1. ICH US*†	19. Other cardiovascular factors*
2. ICH CT scan*	20. Pneumothorax*
3. GI hemorrhage*‡	21. Other pulmonary factors*
4. Surgery site hematoma*	22. Positive culture*
5. >5 units platelet/day*	23. Low WBC <1,500
6. Hemolysis*	24. Other infection
7. Other hematology*	25. Potassium <2.5*
8. Severe neuroimpairment*	26. Potassium >7.5
9. Seizures*	27. Sodium <120
10. Jitteriness*	28. Sodium >160
11. Other neurologic factors*	29. Calcium <6.0
12. Creatinine >1.5,<3.0*	30. Calcium >14
13. Creatinine >3.0*	31. Glucose <20
14. Dialysis/hemofiltration*	32. Glucose >350
15. Other renal factors*	33. pH <7.05
16. CPR*§	34. pH >7.75
17. Arrhythmia*	35. Hypertension*
18. Vasodilator used*	36. Other*

* = occurring in >1% of reported cases.
†ICH = intracranial hemorrhage; US = ultrasound.
‡GI = gastrointestinal.
§CPR = cardiopulmonary resuscitation.

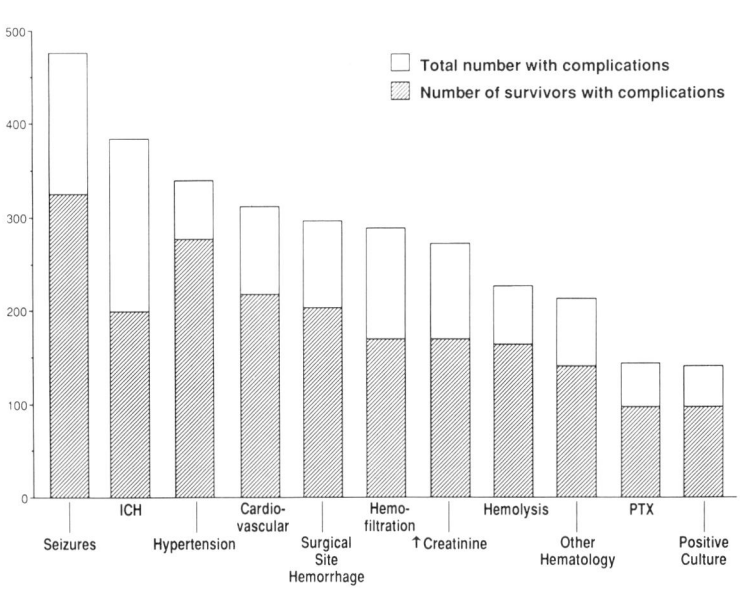

FIGURE 15.6 Complications while on ECMO occurring with an incidence of >5%, $n = 2,934$ patients in the registry.

complications than others. To find a model predicting the presence or absence of several serious complications, we performed stepwise logistic regression analyses using data from the first 3,000 neonatal cases. Complications on ECMO that were looked at included intracranial hemorrhage diagnosed by ultrasound, seizures, a positive blood culture on ECMO, an elevated serum creatinine (>1.5 mg/mL), and the need for hemodialysis or hemofiltration. Independent variables examined included respiratory diagnosis and pre-ECMO complications (seizures, renal failure, pH < 7.20, or $Paco_2$ > 60 mm Hg), and criteria for ECMO (oxygenation index > 40, $AaDO_2$ > 620, cardiac arrest, acute respiratory deterioration, or failure to respond to conventional medical management).

Factors associated with an increased probability of intracranial hemorrhage included the diagnoses of respiratory distress syndrome (RDS) or sepsis and the pre-ECMO complications of seizures, renal failure, pH < 7.20, or $Paco_2$ > 60 mm Hg. The diagnosis of meconium aspiration syndrome was associated with an increased probability of no intracranial hemorrhage. It is likely that the diagnosis of RDS serves as a marker for prematurity and its inherent risk for hemorrhage.

An increased probability of seizures during ECMO was associated with the diagnosis of sepsis, the pre-ECMO conditions of seizures, renal failure, pH < 7.20, or $Paco_2$ > 60 mm Hg, and the indications for ECMO of cardiac arrest or oxygenation index > 40. If criteria for ECMO was "failure to respond to conventional medical management," the probability of seizures during ECMO was decreased.

The probability of a positive culture on ECMO was increased by association with the pre-ECMO diagnoses of sepsis, meconium aspiration syndrome, or congenital diaphragmatic hernia. The criteria for ECMO "failure to respond to convention medical management" or an oxygenation index >40 was associated with decreased probability of a positive culture.

An increased probability of renal insufficiency (serum creatinine ≥1.5 mg/dL) occurred in infants with the pre-ECMO complication of renal failure or pH <7.20. The diagnosis of meconium aspiration syndrome or the indication for ECMO being "failure to respond" or oxygenation index >40 decreased the probability of an elevated creatinine level during ECMO.

Interestingly, and in contrast to the previous model, the model for "need for dialysis or hemofiltration" found that the indications for

ECMO of "failure to respond" or oxygenation index >40 increased the probability of this complication. In addition, the indication for ECMO of cardiac arrest, the diagnoses of sepsis, RDS, or diaphragmatic hernia, combined with pre-ECMO renal failure, increased the probability that dialysis or hemofiltration would be necessary. The fact that the predictive models for elevated creatinine level and the need for dialysis or hemofiltration have different "predictors" allows one to speculate that, in the absence of renal insufficiency, hemofiltration is used by some to treat fluid overload.

SUMMARY

The risks of neonatal ECMO are many and involve every organ system. What is most remarkable is that, despite these multiple risks, the overwhelming majority of neonatal survivors of ECMO will lead normal lives. We are still in a period when complications and their specific incidence are being defined. Continued input to the international registry will help tremendously in identifying the risk of certain complications. Once the risks are defined, many can be lessened by modifications of existing procedures. To deny the existence of ECMO-specific complications is short-sighted and does a disservice to future patients and to those who have worked so hard to bring this exciting new treatment to the place where it is today.

REFERENCES

(1) Shem S. House of God. New York: Richard Marek Publishers, 1978.

(2) Glass P, Miller M, Short B. Morbidity for survivors of extracorporeal membrane oxygenation: neurodevelopmental outcome at 1 year of age. Pediatrics 1989;83:72–8.

(3) Towne BH, Lott IT, Hicks DA, Healey T. Long-term follow-up of infants and children treated with extracorporeal membrane oxygenation (ECMO): a preliminary report. J Pediatr Surg 1985;20:410–14.

(4) Andrews AF, Nixon CA, Roloff DW, Bartlett RH. One to three year outcome of fourteen neonatal ECMO survivors. Pediatrics 1986;78:692–8.

(5) Bartlett RH, Roloff DW, Cornell RG, et al. Extracorporeal circulation in neonatal respiratory failure: a prospective randomized study. Pediatrics 1985;76:479–87.

(6) O'Rourke PP, Crone RK, Vacanti JP, et al. Extracorporeal membrane oxygenation and conventional medical therapy in neonates with persistent pulmonary hypertension of the newborn: a prospective randomized study. Pediatrics 1989;84:957–63.

(7) International Extracorporeal Life Support Organization Registry, Ann Arbor, MI.

(8) Minifee PK, Zwischenberger JB, Flick GR, Nevelle N, Herndon DN. Leukopenia and eicosanoid release parallel hypoxemia during extracorporeal membrane oxygenation. J Pediatr Surg (in press)

(9) Darling EM, Harris WE, Cooper S, Hatchell J, Macphee AA. Complement activation during long-term extracorporeal membrane oxygenation in neonates. Gothenburg, Sweden: Scandinavian Association for ECMO Conference, 1989.

(10) Hirthler MA, Simoni J, Dickson M, Goldthorn J. Late changes in inflammatory mediators during ECMO: consistent with subclinical sepsis. Ann Arbor, MI: National Extracorporeal Life Support Organization Charter Meeting, 1989.

(11) Bui KC, Hammerman C, Hirschl RB, et al. Plasma prostanoids in neonates with pulmonary hypertension treated with conventional therapy and with extracorporeal membrane oxygenation. J Thorac Cardiovasc Surg 1991;101:973–83.

(12) Vogler C, Sotelo-Avila C, Lagunoff D, Braun P, Schreifels JA, Weber T. Aluminum-containing emboli in infants treated with extracorporeal membrane oxygenation. N Engl J Med 1988;319:75–9.

(13) Shneider B, Maller E, VanMarter L, O'Rourke PP. Cholestasis in infants supported with extracorporeal membrane oxygenation. J Pediatr 1989;115:462–5.

(14) Raju TN, Kim SY, Meller JL, Srinivasan G, Ghai V, Reyes H. Circle of Willis blood velocity and flow direction after common carotid artery ligation for neonatal extracorporeal membrane oxygenation. Pediatrics 1989;83:343–7.

(15) Cilley RE, Zwischenberger JB, Andrews AF, et al. Intracranial hemorrhage during extracor-

poreal membrane oxygenation in neonates. Pediatrics 1986;78:699–704.

(16) Volpe JJ. Neurology of the newborn, 2nd ed. Philadelphia: W.B. Saunders Company, 1987.

(17) Stolar CJ, Reyes C. Extracorporeal membrane oxygenation causes significant changes in intracranial pressure and carotid artery blood flow in newborn lambs. J Pediatr Surg 1988;23:1163–8.

(18) Kinsella JP, Gerstmann DR, deLemos RA. Ocular blood flow following unilateral carotid ligation. Ann Arbor, MI: National Extracorporeal Life Support Organization Charter Meeting, 1989.

(19) Gangitano ES, Vogt JF, Muenchow SK, et al. Proposal for a multicenter controlled trial to study the effects of cannulation of the cephalad segment of the internal jugular vein during extracorporeal membrane oxygenation in the neonate. Ann Arbor, MI: National Extracorporeal Life Support Organization Charter Meeting, 1989.

(20) Gleason CA, Short BL, Jones D. Cerebral blood flow and metabolism during and after prolonged hypocapnia in newborn lambs. J Pediatr 1989;115:309–14.

(21) Ment LR, Duncan CC, Ehrenkranz RA, et al. Randomized low-dose indomethacin trial for prevention of intraventricular hemorrhage in very low birth weight neonates. J Pediatr 1988;112:948–55.

(22) Rennie JM, Doyle J, Cooke RWI. Elevated levels of immunoreactive prostacyclin metabolite in babies who develop IVH. Acta Pediatr Scand 1987;76:19–23.

(23) Lesko SM, Mitchell AA, Epstein MF, Louik C, Ciacoia GP, Shapiro S. Heparin use as a risk factor for intraventricular hemorrhage in low-birth-weight infants. N Engl J Med 1986;314:1156–60.

(24) Anderson HL III, Otsuro T, Chapman RA, Bartlett RH. Venovenous extracorporeal life support in neonates using a double lumen catheter. Trans ASAIO 1989;35:650–3.

(25) Toomasian JM, Hsu LC, Hirschl RB, Heiss KF, Hultquist KA, Bartlett RH. Evaluation of Duraflo II heparin coating in prolonged extracorporeal membrane oxygenation. Trans ASAIO 1989;34:410–14.

(26) Schumacher RE, Barks JDE, Johnston MV, et al. Right-sided brain lesions in infants following extracorporeal membrane oxygenation. Pediatrics 1988;92:155–61.

(27) Campbell LR, Bunyapen C, Holmes GL, et al. Right common carotid artery ligation in extracorporeal membrane oxygenation. J Pediatr 1988;113:110–13.

(28) Zak LK, Donn SM. Functional brain injury associated with neonatal ECMO. Pediatr Res 1989;25:127A.

(29) Taylor GA, Short BL, Fitz CR. Imaging of cerebrovascular injury in infants treated with extracorporeal membrane oxygenation. J Pediatr 1989;114:635–9.

(30) Schumacher RE, Donn SM. Cerebrovascular injury during extracorporeal membrane oxygenation. J Pediatr 1989;115:505–6.

(31) Bender KS, Short BL, Walker KL, et al. Effects of prolonged hypoxemia, carotid artery ligation and jugular vein ligation on cerebral blood flow (CBF) and cerebral oxygen consumption ($CMRO_2$) in the newborn lamb. Gothenburg, Sweden: Scandinavian Association for ECMO Conference, 1989.

(32) Short BL, Walker LK, Gleason CA, Jones MD Jr, Traystman RJ. Effect of extracorporeal membrane oxygenation on cerebral blood flow and cerebral oxygen metabolism in newborn lambs. Pediatr Res 1990;28:50–3.

(33) Silverstein F, Buchanan K, Johnston MV. Pathogenesis of hypoxic-ischemic brain injury in a perinatal rodent model. Neurosci Lett 1984;49:271–7.

(34) Wiznitzer M, Horwitz SJ, Stork EK, Walsh M. Electroencephalographic findings before and during extracorporeal membrane oxygenation. Ann Arbor, MI: National Extracorporeal Life Support Organization Charter Meeting, 1989.

(35) Lott IT, McPherson D, Towne B, Johnson D. Starr A. Long-term neurophysiologic outcome after neonatal extracorporeal membrane oxygenation. J Pediatr 1990;116:343–9.

(36) Taylor GA, Fitz CR, Kapur S, Short BL. Cerebrovascular accidents in neonates treated with extracorporeal membrane oxygenation: sonographic-pathologic correlation. Am J Roentgenol 1989;153:355–61.

(37) Taylor GA, Fitz CR, Miller MK, Garin DB, Catena LM, Short BL. Intracranial abnormalities in infants treated with extracorporeal membrane oxygenation: imaging with US and CT. Radiology 1987;165:675–8.

(38) Bulas DI, Taylor GA, Revenis ME, Glass P, Ingram JD. Posterior fossa intracranial hemorrhage in infants treated with extracorporeal membrane oxygenation. AJR 1991;156:571–5.

(39) Patrias MC, Rabinowicz IM, Klein MD. Ocular findings in infants treated with extracorporeal membrane oxygenation support. Pediatrics 1988;82:560–4.

(40) Schumacher RE, Spak C, Standish C, Kileny P. Asymmetric brainstem evoked responses in infants treated with extracorporeal membrane oxygenation. Ear Hear 1990;11:359–62.

(41) Martin GR, Short BL, Abbott C, O'Brien AM. Cardiac stun in infants undergoing extracorporeal membrane oxygenation. J Thorac Cardiovasc Surg 1991;101:607–11.

(42) Cater G, Lotze A, Miller M. Short B. Stunned myocardium in an infant treated with extracorporeal membrane oxygenation. J Pediatr Surg 1988;23:1011–13.

(43) Dickson M, Hirthler M, Simoni J, Bradley C, Goldthorn J. Stunned myocardium during extracorporeal membrane oxygenation: reperfusion injury mediated by oxygen free radicals? Am J Surg 1990;160:644–6.

(44) Gerstman BM, Nose K, Kinsella JP, Cornish JD. Left carotid artery (LCA) and coronary (CA) arterial flow partitioning during neonatal ECMO (abstract). Pediatr Res 1989;25:37A.

(45) Lotze A, Short BL, Taylor GA. Lung compliance as a measure of lung function in newborns with respiratory failure requiring extracorporeal membrane oxygenation. Crit Care Med 1987;15:226–9.

(46) Bloom BT, Merritt TA. Inhibition of human surfactant by human plasma proteins (abstract). Pediatr Res 1987;21:111A.

(47) Keszler M, Subramanian KN, Smith YA, et al. Pulmonary management during extracorporeal membrane oxygenation. Crit Care Med 1989;17:495–500.

(48) Said SI. Metabolic functions of the pulmonary circulation. Circ Res 1982;50:325–33.

(49) Schumacher RE, Weinfeld, IJ, Bartlett RH. Neonatal vocal cord paralysis following extracorporeal membrane oxygenation. Pediatrics 1989;84:793–6.

(50) Palermo ML, Outwater KM, O'Rourke PP. Effect of extracorporeal membrane oxygenation on arterial natriuretic factor. Pediatr Res 1989;25:42A.

(51) Sell, Cullen ML, Lerner GR, et al. Hypertension during extracorporeal membrane oxygenation: cause, effect, and management. Surgery 1987;102:724–30.

(52) Kelly AT, Short BL, Rains TC, Kapur S, Mullick F. Aluminum contamination in extracorporeal membrane oxygenation: new findings. Pediatr Res 1989;25:101A.

(53) Boedy RF, Goldbergh AK, Howell CG Jr, Hulse E, Edwards EG, Kanto WP Jr. Incidence of hypertension in infants on extracorporeal membrane oxygenation. J Pediatr Surg 1990;25:258–61.

(54) Taylor GA, Short BL. Esophageal dilatation and reflux in neonates on extracorporeal membrane oxygenation after diaphragmatic hernia repair (letter). AJR 1988;151:1055.

(55) Almond S, Adolph V, Steiner R, Hill C, Falterman K, Arensman R. Calculous disease of the biliary tract in infants: a complication of neonatal ECMO. Gothenburg, Sweden: Scandinavian Association for ECMO Conference, 1989.

(56) Redmond C, Heaton J, Calix J, et al. A correlation of pulmonary hypoplasia, mean airway pressure, and survival in congenital diaphragmatic hernia treated with extracorporeal membrane oxygenation. J Pediatr Surg 1987;22:1143–9.

(57) Zach TL, Steinhorn RH, Georgieff MK, Mills MM, Green TP. Leukopenia associated with extracorporeal membrane oxygenation in newborn infants. J Pediatr 1990;116:440–4.

(58) Hocker J, Wellhausen S, Ward R, Cook L. Effect of extracorporeal membrane oxygenation on leukocyte function in neonates. Artif Organs 1991;15:23–8.

(59) DePalma L, Short BL, Van Meurs K, Luban NL. A flow cytometric analysis of lymphocyte subpopulations in neonates undergoing extracorporeal membrane oxygenation. J Pediatr 1991;118:117–20.

(60) Luban N, MacDonald M, Przygocki R, Bors S, Kammerman L. Blood use and transfusion transmitted infection in extracorporeal membrane oxygenation (ECMO). Snowmass, CO: 5th Annual Children's Hospital National Medical Center ECMO Symposium, 1989.

(61) Toomasian JM, Snedecor SM, Cornell RG, Cilley RE, Bartlett RH. National experience with extracorporeal membrane oxygenation for newborn respiratory failure: data from 715 cases. Trans ASAIO 1989;34:140–7.

16

Patient Neurodevelopmental Outcomes after Neonatal ECMO

Penny Glass, PH.D.

ECMO survivors represent a unique group of infants and children, most of whom would have died previously. Pre-ECMO events and the risks associated with the ECMO procedure itself place the patient receiving ECMO at risk for injury to the developing brain. The fact that as many as half of the survivors of ECMO may have some hemorrhagic or nonhemorrhagic brain lesion documented by routine cranial ultrasound and computed tomography (CT) in the neonatal period suggests that a significant number have sustained a degree of neurologic injury. Yet overall outcome is surprisingly good.

To date, neurodevelopmental outcome has been published from six institutions employing ECMO (1–6), with significant handicap ranging from 10% to 15%. However, the studies are limited in scope and emphasize major morbidity, and currently only 11 survivors are reported at school age. It is well established that major handicap alone is insufficient to describe morbidity among risk groups (7). Even transient dysfunction may be a marker of problems at school age (8). Therefore, although only a 10% to 15% significant morbidity exists, the remaining ECMO survivors are at risk for learning impairment at school age and should be followed closely.

Concerning the pre-ECMO risk, only a limited number of outcome studies involve either full-term children who sustained neonatal brain damage or who had respiratory failure (e.g., persistent pulmonary hypertension) not treated by ECMO. Even data regarding this latter group annul the fact that most survivors of ECMO would have died prior to the availability of ECMO. All ECMO centers conducting follow-up studies have the sense that they are approaching an undefined entity.

The purpose of this chapter is to present what is known about the neurodevelopmental outcome of neonates treated with ECMO. To provide a framework, the outcome of infants with perinatal asphyxia and of neonates not treated with ECMO who have sustained a documented insult to the brain will be reviewed, followed by the outcome of non-ECMO infants with persistent pulmonary hypertension of the neonate (PPHN). The description of neurodevelopmental outcome of ECMO-treated neonates commences at the time of hospital discharge. Center-specific data and data from recent survey responses of a broad representation of

ECMO centers are used. Finally, specific sequelae are detailed.

CNS INSULT IN NEONATES

Before the initiation of ECMO, potential candidates have all experienced significant hypoxia and acidosis which can affect the developing brain. In addition, most infants receiving ECMO have some degree of perinatal asphyxia. A clear marker of asphyxial insult in the neonate is clinically apparent hypoxic/ischemic encephalopathy (HIE), which has been classified into three stages of severity by Sarnat and Sarnat (9): Stage I = hyperalert; Stage II = lethargic with suppressed primitive reflexes; Stage III = comatose with absent primitive reflexes. Infants with intractable seizures may be either Stage II or Stage III. The outcome of infants who have HIE in the first week of life is related to the degree of HIE present and the rate of recovery. Neurologic handicap has been reported as virtually 100% for infants with Stage III HIE (9). More recently, however, using a slightly modified determination of severe HIE, Low et al. (10) reported that 50% of infants with Stage III HIE were normal at one year of age. Moderate HIE portends a handicap rate of approximately 20%, with the remaining 80% at increased risk for learning problems at school age (11). Clearly, HIE is a marker of central nervous system (CNS) insult, with consequences for neurodevelopmental outcome. The potential for recovery is also apparent.

After failure of conventional respiratory management, potential ECMO candidates are typically paralyzed with pavulon and treated with hyperventilation and systemic alkalosis in an attempt to reduce pulmonary hypertension (12). This form of therapeutic management is recognized as having the potential to alter the flow of blood to the brain (13,14). A number of studies have suggested that asphyxia, severe respiratory disease, and other disorders of the newborn are accompanied by abnormal cerebral blood flow regulation. This may lead to ischemic and (or) hemorrhagic damage in the developing brain (15). Cerebral infarction has been reported in critically ill neonates not treated with ECMO (16). Neonatal ischemia, as defined by a reduction in cerebral blood flow, is associated wtih cerebral atrophy and neuropsychological deficits at preschool age (17).

Major hemorrhagic and nonhemorrhagic brain lesions are also identified with significant handicap, but not consistently so. Most of the literature regarding severe intraventricular hemorrhage (IVH) concerns premature infants. The effect of hemorrhage on the developing brain is likely to depend on the maturity of the brain at the time of insult (18). Unfortunately, little attention has been given to outcome among *full-term* neonates following hemorrhagic or nonhemorrhagic brain lesions, or to more subtle manifestations of brain injury other than major neurologic handicap. Mannino and Trauner (19) reported four cases of full-term neonates with large cerebral infarcts. Two were normal on follow-up. Nanba et al. (20) studied 13 full-term neonates with intracranial hemorrhage. Three died; of the remaining 10, only three were normal at follow-up (ages 8 to 18 months). Menezes et al. (21) presented three cases of term neonates with posterior fossa hemorrhages. The neurological status of all three was subsequently normal. In contrast, Cheek et al. (22) reported poor outcome in all five term infants who had cerebellar hemorrhages. In the latest study to date, Bergman et al. (23) followed 17 full-term survivors of intracranial hemorrhage (ICH) at one to seven years of age. They reported normal outcome in nine; two had severe mental and motor handicaps; and three were profoundly impaired (untestable). Given the small sample and the short-term follow-up conducted, conclusions regarding outcome of full-term infants who have sustained an intracranial hemorrhage or a stroke are limited, but the consequences range from severely impaired to potentially normal. Again, the potential for recovery is apparent.

Neurodevelopmental follow-up of neonates in severe respiratory failure managed with hyperventilation is limited, and the diagnosis of PPHN varies in the literature. However, evidence suggests that significant sequelae occur in up to 30% of survivors. For example, Bernbaum et al. (24) reported significant sequelae in 22% ($N = 10$) of survivors of

PPHN. Likewise, Bifano and Pfannenstiel (25) and Ferarra et al. (26) reported significant developmental delay in 19% ($N = 21$) and 18% ($N = 11$), respectively. On the other hand, Sell et al. (27) evaluated 40 infants at one to four years of age and found severe handicap in only 7%. More recently, John et al. (28) evaluated 23 survivors of severe PPHN at 12 to 36 months and reported significant motor handicap in seven (30%); two of the seven also had significant mental handicaps. Despite the fact that hyperventilation may affect cerebral blood flow, the consensus has been that the sequelae reported among survivors of PPHN are related to the severity of illness per se and not to the method of treatment (29). Neuroimaging was not routine in these studies. It would be more prudent to suggest that the sequelae typical of critically ill infants not treated with ECMO also require a more comprehensive evaluation.

ECMO and the Developing Brain

ECMO therapy may also compromise the developing brain. The initiation of bypass disrupts the normal flow of blood in the brain and may theoretically even "steal" blood from the contralateral hemisphere. Changes in cerebral blood flow have been documented in infants undergoing ECMO (30). Alteration of cerebral blood flow, in addition to the use of systemic anticoagulant, may increase the risk for intracranial hemorrhage. The rate of either hemorrhagic or nonhemorrhagic intracranial lesions among ECMO-treated infants is high (31,32). Although there is no concurrent comparison group, the type and locus of lesions are unusual. In addition, venoarterial bypass requires permanent ligation of the right internal jugular vein and right common carotid artery, which has raised specific concerns regarding possible right-sided brain lesions and subsequent left hemiparesis (see Chapter 15). Finally, some centers have begun to reanatomose the ligated vessels. The consequences of any one of the above factors imposed on a sick newborn are unknown. In fact, the effect of the ECMO procedure itself cannot be differentiated from the background disease without a randomized study in the neonatal period. Randomization for the purpose of evaluating morbidity is not ethical if one outcome is death. Morbidity among ECMO survivors is being evaluated in the majority of ECMO centers.

Neurodevelopmental Outcome of ECMO-Treated Neonates

Neurobehavioral alterations are apparent in neonates who have received ECMO even after the acute disease process is passed and the infant nears discharge (approximately one month of age). Virtually all of these infants exhibit signs of general CNS depression, including lethargy, hypotonia (which is particularly evident in poor head control), and weak or absent primitive reflexes. In other words, moderate HIE may persist for up to one month in the majority of ECMO-treated survivors. Parents are taught techniques of positioning and handling the infant at discharge. The overriding concern is more often feeding.

Difficulty in establishing full oral feeding is routine in neonates discharged after receiving ECMO. The cause varies and should be assessed carefully in each individual infant. Most feeding problems appear to have no significant mechanical or respiratory component. These infants have normal ability to suck and can coordinate sucking, swallowing, and breathing appropriately within a few days after extubation. However, when they feed, they will suck initially, then stop. Thus, their oral intake may not be adequate for their current weight (although monitoring actual weight gain rather than total calories consumed may be a more prudent criterion given the low activity level of these infants). Delaying hospital discharge until full oral feeding is established is probably unnecessary for this group if there are no other medical problems (e.g., congenital diaphragmatic hernia). Parents are taught gavage feeding, and weight gain is closely monitored after discharge. Routinely, parents give up on the gavage within a few days, and the problem returns. Consistent feeding style and patience yield success.

A number of hypotheses regarding this type of feeding problem have been generated, but not tested: 1) Poor feeding is known to be a sign of general CNS depression and is reported in non-ECMO infants as well, 2) poor feeding may be related more specifically to manipulation of the vagus nerve during cannulation.

A minority of infants who have received ECMO have difficulty with the oral motor component of feeding. Again, the problem is typically transient and responds to therapeutic intervention. There is always the possibility that respiratory compromise may be contributing to the feeding difficulty. Careful assessment of all physiologic responses to feeding, not just oxygen saturation, is essential. Supplemental oxygen by nasal cannula may be useful during feeding as a temporary bridge. Competent nursing and education of parents help to pace the infant so (s)he is not overstressed.

At the far end of the continuum are infants with chronic lung disease or congenital diaphragmatic hernia who may require prolonged nasogastric feeding or even a gastrostomy in order to maintain adequate growth. Specialized follow-up within two weeks of discharge is prudent. Reestablishment of oral feeding in the latter group is typically problematic and requires sustained medical attention and therapeutic intervention.

Remarkably, by four months of age, the typical infant discharged from ECMO is functioning in the normal range as defined by both mental and motor scales of the Bayley (90 or above). Residual hypotonia or mild asymmetry persists in approximately 25%. Mild motor delay typically accompanies the hypotonia. These infants often function reasonably well in the supine position but lack precursors for rolling and sitting. They cannot respond appropriately to test items requiring activity at the table. Head control is usually at the three-month level. We believe that referrals for physical therapy or occupational therapy for abnormalities of tone are appropriate at this time and are generally supportive for parents. At the least, parents can be instructed in ways to encourage development. The prognosis is generally good. The remaining 10% to 15% of infants exhibit significant neurologic abnormality and (or) have motor function more than 2 standard deviations (SD) below the norm (DQ < 70). They should be evaluated carefully and managed by a neurologist or psychiatrist with appropriate therapeutic prescriptions.

In ECMO survivors at one year of age, the

TABLE 16.1 ECMO survivors at age one year (33)

Survivors at one year	814
Centers reporting	29
Infants with known outcome	563
Significant neurologic impairment	57

Information in ELSO National Registry.

rate of significant handicap among reporting ECMO centers currently ranges from 0% to 20% (Table 16.1). The most commonly reported handicap, although it is rare, is neuromotor abnormality in the form of cerebral palsy of the spastic quadraparesis type. Spastic diplegia occurs among ECMO-treated neonates who were preterm. Motor handicap occurs without mental handicap. Mental handicap is most often accompanied by motor delay at this age.

Published reports of one-year outcome are consistent with the national survey. Early studies by Andrews et al. in Michigan (2) evaluated 14 ECMO survivors at one to three years of age and found significant deficits (IQ < 60) in 29%; the remaining children functioned normally. Krummel et al. (4) reported normal outcome in five of six ECMO infants at 18 months of age, with one infant (17%) having a significant neurologic deficit. Redmond et al. (5) identified neurologic complications among three of 42 survivors at six to 27 months of age.

Among 17 Bayley exams, the mean mental and motor scores were in the normal range. The number of individuals identified as delayed was not specified. Using a standard neurologic examination and the Bayley scales (3), we also found normal growth and development in the majority of survivors at one year, with Bayley Mental and Motor Scales both >90 for 60% of infants. Mild neuromotor lag (DQ 70–90), typically accompanied by slightly decreased tone, occurred in 20%. Subtle fine motor lags are not uncommon. Significant delay (index <70) occurred in 10% of the sample; 5% had a significant neuromotor abnormality. Only one infant in this group of 100 infants was profoundly impaired (index <50). A second child was determined to be positive for human immunodeficiency virus (HIV) at four months

TABLE 16.2 ECMO survivors at age two years (33)

Survivors at two years	386
Centers reporting	16
Infants with known outcome	283
Significant neurologic impairment	26

Information in ELSO National Registry.

of age as a result of a transfusion while on bypass. She spent the first year of her life chronically infected, in a room in the intensive care unit, and was not testable.

According to the 1989 national survey (33), developmental outcome in survivors of ECMO at two years of age is fairly consistent for rate of significant abnormality (10% to 15%) (Table 16.2), but more subtle problems that may be related to later learning disabilities in school begin to emerge (3,34). For example, at this age, although 60% have normal cognitive functioning, 25% to 30% are considered suspect and have a specific lag of four to nine months in either language or perceptual skills. It is unclear whether this is a precursor of learning problems at school age or a normal variant. The language lag is dominated by males; the perceptual lag is dominated by females. The HIV-infected infant mentioned above was discharged home at 13 months of age and was ambulatory. By age two, she was delayed and deviant, as would be expected from prolonged hospitalization, but she remained free from infection and progressed to the point of walking and beginning to talk (and laugh) around her tracheotomy.

The results of preschool testing have been similar. Wilkerson et al. (35) evaluated 19 three-year-olds, two of whom (11%) were abnormal. One of the two had marked language delays and behavioral problems. The other had a chromosomal anomaly with absence of the corpus callosum and profound mental retardation. We have found problems in visual/motor integration even among normal three-year-olds. Figure 16.1 depicts performance on the Beery Test of Visual Motor Integration for a representative sample of five of 20 ECMO survivors who otherwise had normal cognitive skills. The task requires *copying* of simple geometric forms. All of the

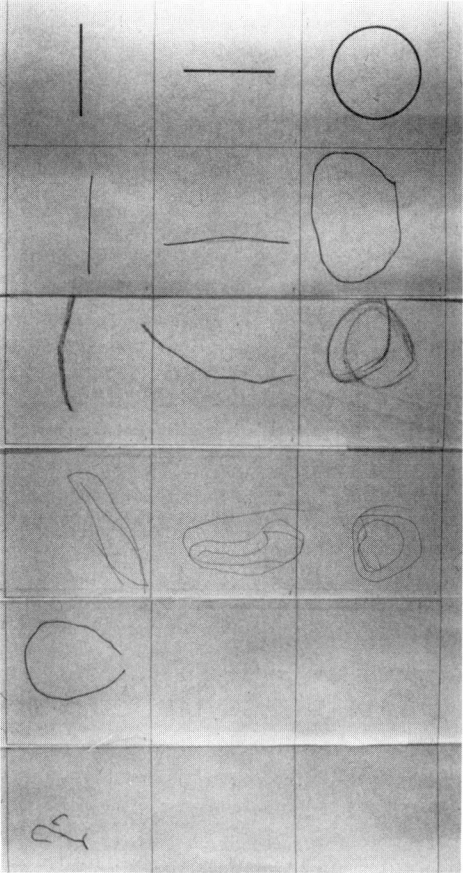

FIGURE 16.1 Developmental Test of Visual Motor Integration: Variation in performance among five normal three-year-old children treated with ECMO as neonates. The first two rows are considered appropriate responses for three-year-old children.

children whose performance is depicted in Figure 16.1 were able to *imitate* the forms following the Beery, indicating that failures were not due to simple fine motor coordination. *None* of the three-year-old ECMO survivors who were classified as suspect or delayed passed the Beery. Deficits in language, perceptual skills, or visual/motor integration are hallmarks of learning disabilities at school age. Comprehensive neuropsychological and neuromotor evaluations at age five are currently under way.

The reports of ECMO survivors beyond

early childhood are generally limited to small samples; however, these are also consistent for major handicap. Towne et al. (6) evaluated 16 children between the ages of four and 11 who were among the first survivors of neonatal ECMO. Neuromotor, cognitive, and speech and language functions were assessed, revealing moderate-to-severe problems in 21%. Schumacher et al. (personal communication) found that two of 11 (18%) children evaluated at age five or older were handicapped. They reported that, more recently, ECMO-treated children appear to be faring better. Overall, the studies indicate that the rate of significant morbidity is probably comparable to that reported for similarly ill infants who are not treated with ECMO at other institutions (0 to 29%). However, more subtle problems have not been evaluated adequately and may be much more pervasive.

PREDICTORS OF NEURODEVELOPMENTAL OUTCOME

Our outcome study at one year of age was of sufficient size to permit initial evaluation of potential predictors of short-term neurodevelopmental status. We were able to identify factors associated with developmental delay at one year: chronic lung disease, major intracranial hemorrhage, a diagnosis of sepsis, a gestational age <37 weeks at birth, and visual attention (3,36).

Chronic lung disease among ECMO survivors is uncommon (<15%), but the course is typical of other infants with lung disease. Neurodevelopmental status is generally dependent on lung recovery, with motor skills being more frequently compromised. This profile is consistent with that of infants not treated with ECMO who have chronic lung disease (37). Infants expend energy resources on breathing. Recovery is often complicated by poor somatic growth.

We previously reported the relationship of neonatal neuroimaging abnormalities to short-term developmental outcome (Bayley scales) in one-year-old ECMO survivors (3,32). Hemorrhagic and nonhemorrhagic abnormalities detected on routine cranial ultrasound and CT were given a score of severity for bleeding, ventricular dilatation, and other parenchymal lesions. Degree of abnormality was associated with outcome at one year of age. Pilot data of neuroimaging and outcome at age two are consistent with these findings. Infants with normal or minor abnormality on neuroimaging had a 70% chance of normal function at age two and only a 10% chance of delay. Conversely, only 25% of infants with moderate-to-severe neuroimaging abnormality were normal at age two, and 40% were delayed. The relationship between neonatal brain lesions in ECMO survivors and outcome at age five is currently being evaluated.

Given the increased mortality among infants treated with ECMO who are younger than 37 weeks' gestation and their higher incidence of ICH, if a candidate is less than 37 weeks' gestation, our explanation of risk given to the parents is somewhat different from explanations given to parents of more mature neonates (38). The developmental delay encountered among ECMO infants of <37 weeks' gestation may be partially accounted for by a higher rate of severe ICH. New ECMO centers are generally advised to set the lower birthweight limit at 2.5 kg rather than 2 kg until they have gained experience.

Finally, performance on a visual attention task (P-VAT) in the neonatal period is related to developmental outcome at one year of age. Forty-five infants were evaluated at one month of age if they were medically stable. Of the 27 who "passed" the P-VAT, 20 (78%) tested normal at one year on the Bayley. Conversely, of the 18 who "failed" the P-VAT, only 7 (39%) tested normal at one year (33). This would suggest that evaluation of visual attention provides a useful adjunct to the discharge examination and alerts professionals to infants who need closer follow-up.

Lateral Asymmetry

Asymmetry as a result of the ECMO procedure has been a concern from the beginning, both in terms of possible right-sided brain lesions and deficits in lateralized function. Schumacher et al. (39) reported an increased incidence in right-sided brain lesions evidenced by asymmetric CTs and electroencephalograms (EEGs) in a subsample of their ECMO population. Perhaps even more interesting is a recent report of lateralized lesions that were dependent on whether the lesions were hemorrhagic or nonhemorrhagic. Mendoza et al. (40) found more right-sided hemorrhagic lesions and more left-sided nonhemorrhagic lesions, which was consistent with their predicted alterations in cerebral blood flow. In contrast to these reports, we found no increase in right-sided brain lesions on neuroimaging (32), since most were bilateral. It is possible that differences in technique and management contribute to variable distributions of lesions. A multicentered study to evaluate this issue is warranted.

With regard to functional asymmetry, one problem has been the presence of normal postural asymmetry in the newborn period, followed by the emergence of a normal lateral preference in the first year of age. Subtle postural asymmetry in the newborn is difficult to evaluate. Preferential head position off midline is characteristic of the normal newborn. The ECMO infant may "prefer" a head posture to the left because of prolonged position during the ECMO run or "prefer" a head posture to the right due to the healing wound dressing on the ECMO incision site. If the examiner is careful to maintain the infant's head in midline, then subtle asymmetries may be revealed. For example, differences in passive tone in the upper extremities have been reported (Schumacher, personal communication). However, it is difficult to determine which side is deviant. A further caution is that asymmetric responses also occur at a higher rate among preterm infants and thus may reflect a general disturbance of CNS integration rather than a focal lateralized lesion.

What may be evident in follow-up is not so often asymmetry as it is a lack of appropriate bimanual integration. Lateral preference among infants is difficult to evaluate and may vary depending on the task (just as in adults) and the age. Lateral preference also shifts during the first year (41). To further complicate interpretation, some infants are noted to have greater dexterity with their left hand and yet preferentially use the right. Indeed, reach and grasp are not even controlled identically by the contralateral hemisphere. It is not surprising that functional asymmetry in ECMO survivors has been an inconsistent finding.

Towne et al. (6) found one child in a sample of 16 who had a motor deficit indicative of unilateral right hemisphere damage. Krummel et al. (4) reported right-handedness in all six infants in their study. However, right lateral preference occurs in approximately 80% of normal one- to 2-year-old infants (42). We reported a decreased incidence of right lateral preference in our two-year-old group of ECMO survivors (67%) (43). A *lower* frequency of right-handedness is consistent with reports of other high-risk populations (44) and warrants further investigation. Additionally, we found an interesting association between lateral preference and developmental status. Normal two-year-old toddlers were more likely to demonstrate a right lateral preference (87%) than those classified as suspect or delayed (30%). As a caveat, none of the studies have differentiated between normal lateral preference and abnormal asymmetry. No long-term assessment is currently available. The most reasonable conclusions to draw from all of the above evidence are that lateralized lesions do occur that may or may not be related to carotid and jugular ligation. However, functional asymmetry need not be indicative of focal lesions to the contralateral hemisphere.

It is tempting to speculate that lateralized brain lesions in ECMO survivors would have consequences in childhood with respect to the lateralization of cognitive functions such as language (left hemisphere) and visual spatial skills (right hemisphere). In one respect, there is strong evidence in studies of adult brain damage but little evidence in the literature on neonatal brain damage to support such findings (45). However, the sample sizes have been small and the lesions difficult to document (46). Furthermore, there has never been a cohort like the ECMO survivors.

Hearing Loss

A number of studies of infants with histories of PPHN have reported a 20% to 50% incidence of progressive sensorineural hearing loss in this population, which suggests that ECMO-treated neonates (who predominantly have had PPHN) are at similar risk for hearing loss. Schumacher et al. (personal communication) reported sensorineural hearing loss in 16% of 81 survivors. We found no predilection for *progressive* sensorineural hearing loss. All significant hearing loss in this sample of 50 at age two was detected prior to discharge, using the basal auditory evoked response (BAER) (47). None of the children with a hearing loss performed in the normal range cognitively when tested at age two. Thus, a routine BAER near the time of discharge or in the early months is important, with close follow-up of any abnormal examination. Hearing evaluations after one year of age can probably be limited to infants who have recurrent otitis or any signs of mild developmental delay.

Vision

Retinopathy of prematurity has not been reported as a consequence of ECMO, despite the hyperoxic conditions during bypass. Among our first 100 eye examinations made at the time of discharge, retinopathy of prematurity (ROP) was detected in two infants, both of whom were younger than 37 weeks' gestation. These cases involved minor changes in the temporal periphery with no sequelae. It has been well established that the primary cause of ROP is immaturity of the retina. Hyperoxia to a mature retina, while it may not be harmless, does not result in ROP. Routine eye examinations on all ECMO survivors to rule out ROP are probably unnecessary, given current published recommendations. Examination of the retina of any infant receiving ECMO who is younger than 38 weeks' gestation is probably still prudent. With the advent of new technology leading to the use of ECMO in even younger infants, ROP may surface as a complication.

A few rare cases of vision loss have been reported by individual centers. Cortical blindness occurs as part of the clinical picture in cases of severe cerebral palsy, but that is not unique to ECMO. One center reported blindness of unknown etiology in an otherwise normal infant. The patient had bilateral retinal detachments but not as a consequence of ROP.

We have a unique case of progressive blindness that was first diagnosed in a one-year-old patient. Both optic nerves appeared pale, although magnetic resonance imaging (MRI) at the time was negative. A year later, the patient had complete loss of vision in his right eye, and a repeat MRI revealed a blood clot in the right ophthalmic artery. This patient had bilateral hypoplastic kidneys at birth and prune belly syndrome, requiring chronic peritoneal dialysis. He failed two attempts at kidney transplants due to clotting and was placed on daily heparin and aspirin. He was reported to have normal vision in his left eye. Growth was impaired. Cognitively, he was normal at age $2\frac{1}{2}$. He died recently at age three, following recurrent medical complications.

Psychosocial Issues

The birth of an infant who immediately becomes critically ill can potentially affect the manner in which the family relates to the child and can contribute to behavior problems manifested by the child (48). Issues of family stress are just beginning to be explored. Some researchers question whether the findings are really unique to ECMO. Similar issues have been addressed among families with premature infants. A comparison of these groups would be interesting. Parents of infants receiving ECMO often have other children later. When a number of those parents were asked after the subsequent birth what they were most concerned about during labor and delivery, it was the knowledge that something could potentially go wrong with the baby. This same awareness is also held by most health professionals.

Social/emotional problems may also have an organic basis and thus should receive clinical attention at any visit. Returning to the concern regarding carotid ligation, the right hemisphere is theoretically understood to be preprogrammed to serve a special role in affective regulation (49). An adaptively debilitating "social learning disability" profile has been well documented in children with neuropsychological evidence of severe right hemisphere deficits. Thus, ECMO survivors may show higher elevations than control subjects on measures of hyperactivity, maladaptive behavior, and immature socialization.

SUMMARY

Early brain damage can have devastating effects on overall cognitive or motor development, or both, although specific functions may be spared entirely or selectively (50). Most children who have experienced early brain trauma may appear globally intact, both cognitively and neurologically, but are likely to show specific neuropsychological deficits in the areas of language, memory, or sensory/motor integration, particularly vulnerability regarding complex tasks. Neurological "soft" signs or minor neuromotor dysfunction are found among children with learning disabilities. "Sparing" may be at the expense of other functions, and thus the pattern of brain organization may differ from that of the normal population. Finally, a major consequence of early brain damage may also appear as psychosocial maladjustment, including hyperactivity, social/emotional immaturity, or behavioral disturbance. Thus, the literature on early brain injury suggests that it is vital to evaluate ECMO survivors in depth over the course of their development.

This chapter represents a delineation of the neurodevelopmental consequences of a new, but increasingly utilized drastic care modality (ECMO) which has implications for the health care system. Systematic and long-term evaluation of these children provides parental support and guidance for delayed or handicapped infants and children, an internal audit of each ECMO center, and a unique opportunity for learning about the plasticity and organization of the developing brain.

REFERENCES

(1) Adolph V, Ekelund C, Smith C, Starrett A, Falterman K, Arensman R. Developmental outcome of neonates treated with extracorporeal membrane oxygenation. Pediatr Surg 1990;25:43–6.

(2) Andrews AF, Nixon CA, Cilley RE, Roloff DW, Bartlett RH. One-to-three year outcome for 14 neonatal survivors of extracorporeal membrane oxygenation. Pediatrics 1986;78:692–8.

(3) Glass P, Miller M, Short B. Morbidity for survivors of extracorporeal membrane oxygenation: neurodevelopmental outcome at 1 year of age. Pediatrics 1989;83:72–8.

(4) Krummel TM, Greenfield LJ, Kirkpatrick BV, et al. The early evolution of survivors after extracorporeal membrane oxygenation for neonatal pulmonary failure. Pediatr Surg 1984;19:585–90.

(5) Redmond CR, Graves ED, Falterman KW, Ochsner JL, Arensman RM. Extracorporeal membrane oxygenation for respiratory and cardiac failure in infants and children. Thorac Cardiovasc Surg 1987;93:199–204.

(6) Towne BH, Lott IT, Hicks DA, Healey T. Long-term follow-up of infants and children treated with extracorporeal membrane oxygenation (ECMO): preliminary report. Pediatr Surg 1985;20:410–14.

(7) Seigel L. The prediction of possible learning disabilities in pre-term and full-term children. In: Fields T, Sostek A, eds. Infants born at risk: physiological, perceptual, and cognitive processes. New York: Grune & Stratton, 1983.

(8) Amiel-Tison C, Grenier A. Neurological assessment during the first year of life. Oxford: Oxford University Press, 1986.

(9) Sarnat HB, Sarnat MS. Neonatal encephalography following fetal distress: a clinical and electroencephalographic study. Arch Neurol 1976;33:696–705.

(10) Low JA, Galbraith RS, Muir DW, Killen HL, Pater EA, Karchmar BA. The relationship between perinatal hypoxia and newborn encephalopathy. Am J Obstet Gynecol 1985;152:256–60.

(11) Robertson CMT, Finer NN. Educational readiness of survivors of neonatal encephalopathy associated with birth asphyxia at term. Dev Behav Pediatr 1988;9:298–306.

(12) Duara S, Gewitz MH, Fox WW. Use of mechanical ventilation for clinical management of persistent pulmonary hypertension of the newborn. Clin Perinatol 1984;11:641–52.

(13) Reuter JH, Disney TA. Regional cerebral blood flow and cerebral metabolic rate of oxygen during hyperventilation in the newborn dog. Pediatr Res 1986;20:1102–6.

(14) Gleason CA, Short BL, Jones MD. Cerebral blood flow and metabolism during and after prolonged hypocarbia in newborn lambs. Pediatrics 1989;115:309–14.

(15) Perlman JM. Neonatal cerebral blood flow velocity measurement. Clin Perinatol 1985;12:179–93.

(16) Scher MS, Klesh KW, Murphy TF, Guthrie R. Seizures and infarction in neonates with persistent pulmonary hypertension. Pediatr Neurol 1986;2:332–9.

(17) Skov H, Lou H, Pederson H. Perinatal brain ischaemia: impact at four years of age. Dev Med Child Neurol 1984;28:353–7.

(18) Pape KE, Wigglesworth JS. Haemorrhage, ischaemia and the perinatal brain. Philadelphia: J.B. Lippincott, 1979.

(19) Mannino FL, Trauner DA. Stroke in neonates. Pediatrics 1983;102:605–10.

(20) Nanba E, Eda I, Takashima S, Ohta S, Ohtani K, Takeshita K. Intracranial hemorrhage in the full-term neonate and young infant: correlation of the location and outcome. Brain Dev 1984;6:435–43.

(21) Menezes AH, Smith DE, Bell WE. Posterior fossa hemorrhage in the term neonate. Neurosurgery 1983;13:452–6.

(22) Cheek WR, Fishman MA, Speer MA, Williamson WD, Laurent JR. Cerebellar hemorrhage in the term neonate. Concepts Pediatr Neurosurgery 1985;5:48–56.

(23) Bergman I, Bauer RE, Barmada MA, et al. Intracerebral hemorrhage in the full-term neonatal infant. Pediatrics 1985;75:488–96.

(24) Bernbaum JC, Russell P, Sheridan PH, Gewitz MH, Fox WM, Peckman GJ. Long-term follow-up of newborns with persistent pulmonary hypertension. Crit Care Med 1984;12:579–83.

(25) Bifano EM, Pfannenstiel A. Duration of hyperventilation and outcome in infants with persistent pulmonary hypertension. Pediatrics 1988;81:657–61.

(26) Ferrara B, Johnson DE, Chang PN, Thompson TR. Efficacy of neurologic outcome of profound hypocapneic alkalosis for the treatment of persistent pulmonary hypertension in infancy. Pediatrics 1984;105:457–61.

(27) Sell EJ, Gaines JA, Gluckman C, Williams E. Persistent fetal circulation: neurodevelopmental outcome. Am J Dis Child 1985;139:25–8.

(28) John E, Roberts V, Burnard ED. Persistent pulmonary hypertension of the newborn treated with hyperventilation: clinical features and outcome. Aust Paediatr J 1988;24:357–61.

(29) Ballard RA, Leonard CH. Developmental follow-up of infants with persistent pulmonary hypertension of the newborn. Clin Perinatol 1984;11:737–45.

(30) Taylor GA, Short BL, Glass P, Ichord R. Cerebral hemodynamics in infants undergoing extracorporeal membrane oxygenation: further observations. Radiology 1988;168:163–7.

(31) Miller MM, Short BL, Glass P, Lotze A, Anderson KD. Outcome of 100 infants treated with extracorporeal membrane oxygenation (ECMO) (abstract). Pediatr Res 1987;21(4):369A.

(32) Taylor GA, Fitz CR, Glass P, Short BL. CT of cerebrovascular injury after neonatal extracorporeal membrane oxygenation: further observations. Radiology 1988;168:163–7.

(33) Ann Arbor, MI: Extracorporeal Life Support Organization (ELSO) National Registry. National Survey of ECMO Centers. University of Michigan, 1989.

(34) Glass P, Short BL. Neuro-developmental outcome at age 2. Pediatr Res 1989;25:253A.

(35) Wilkerson SA, Stewart DL, Cook LN. Developmental outcome of ECMO patients over a four year span. Snowmass, CO: 6th Annual ECMO Symposium, 1990.

(36) Glass P. Assessment of visual attention in high risk neonates (PVAT): association with intracranial hemorrhage and Bayley outcome at 1 year of age. Washington, D.C.: International Conference of Infant Studies, 1988.

(37) Grobstein J, Ballard RA. Outcome after neonatal intensive care. In: Ballard RA, ed. Pediatric care of the ICN graduate. Philadelphia: W.B. Saunders, 1988.

(38) Revenis ME, Glass P, Sanchez L, Short BL. Outcome of low birth weight (LBW) babies on extracorporeal membrane oxygenation (ECMO). Pediatr Res 1990;27(4):254A.

(39) Schumacher RE, Barks JDE, Johnston MV, Scher MS, Bartlett RH. Right-sided brain lesions in infants following unilateral carotid ligation for extracorporeal membrane oxygenation. Pediatr Res 1987;21(4):375A.

(40) Mendoza JC, Shearer LT, Cook LN. Lateralization of brain lesions following ECMO. Snowmass, CO: 6th Annual ECMO Symposium, 1990.

(41) Young G, Segalowitz S, Misek P, Alp I, Boulet R. Is early reaching left-handed? Review of manual specialization research. In: Young G, Segalowitz S, Corter C, Trehub S, eds. Manual specialization and the developing brain. New York: Academic Press, 1983.

(42) Ramsay DS. Onset of unimanual handedness in infants. Infant Behav Dev 1980;3:377–85.

(43) Glass P, Short B. Right lateral preference in 2 year old infants treated with ECMO. Pediatr Res 1988;23(4):447A.

(44) Henry RR, Satz P, Saslow E. Early brain damage and the ontogenesis of functional asymmetry. In: Robertson CR, Finger S, eds. Early brain damage: research orientations and clinical orientations, vol. 1. Orlando: Academic Press, 1984.

(45) Witelson SF. On hemisphere specialization and cerebral plasticity: Mark II. In: Best CT, ed. Hemispheric function and collaboration in the child. Orlando: Academic Press, 1985.

(46) Dennis M, Whitaker HA. Hemisphere equipotentiality and language acquisition. In: Segalowitz SJ, Gruber FA, eds. Language development and neurological theory. New York: Academic Press, 1977.

(47) Lipsi K, Glass P, Short BL. Presence of hearing loss in children following ECMO therapy: a follow-up study at 2 years of age. Pediatr Res 1990;27(4):247A.

(48) Macey TJ, Harmon RJ, Easterbrouks MA. Impact of premature birth on the development of the infant in the family. Consult Clin Psychol 1987;55:846–52.

(49) Ross E. Disturbances of emotional language with right hemisphere lesions. In: Ardila A, Ostrosky-Solis F, eds. The right hemisphere: neurology and neuropsychology. New York: Gordon & Breach, 1984.

(50) Taylor HG. Early brain injury and cognitive development. In: Robertson CR, Finger S, eds. Early brain damage: research orientations and clinical observations, vol. 1. Orlando: Academic Press, 1984.

17

Management of Infants with Congenital Diaphragmatic Hernia Using ECMO

❖

Charles J.H. Stolar, M.D.
Mitchell E. Price, M.D.
Marilyn W. Butler, M.D.
Eric L. Lazar, M.D.

One of the earliest autopsy reports of the gross anatomy associated with congenital diaphragmatic hernia was by Dr. George McCauley, an associate of Dr. John Hunter and was reported in the Proceedings of the Royal College of Physicians, London, in 1754(1):

This child was born in the lying-in-hospital, in Brownlow Street, on the 24th of August, 1752; and was a fully grown boy, remarkably fat and fleshy. He was the fifth child of a healthy young woman, who was well during her pregnancy. The child, when first born, started and shuddered; so that the nurse apprehended his going into fits. He breathed also with difficulty, and it was some time before he could cry; which when he did, there was something particular in the note. He seemed to revive a little in about half an hour, and breathed more freely: but soon relapsed, and died before he was quite an hour and a half old. Being informed of these particulars by the mother, the matron, and the nurse, I was desirous of examining the body.... I laid open the abdomen ... ; and found none of the intestines were contained in that cavity, except part of the colon which was distended with meconium. Before I proceeded further in the dissection, I sent to acquaint my ingenious friend, Dr. Hunter. We together dissected and examined this curious subject; and, at the same time, committed to writing the most remarkable appearances.

When the sternum was raised, the stomach with the greatest part of the intestines, with the spleen, and part of the pancreas were found in the left cavity of the thorax; having been protruded through a discontinuation, or rather an aperture of the diaphragm, about an inch from the natural passage of the esophagus.

From the extraordinary bulk of the parts contained in the left side of the thorax, the mediastinum, the heart, the esophagus, and the descending aorta, were forced a considerable way to the right side of the thorax; because there was not the least mark of rupture or inflammation about the edges of this chasm: and because it is probable that the diminished size of the left lobes of the lungs, and the heart and mediastinum being pushed to the right side, were gradually affected by the bulk and increase of the viscera.

As the esophagus was pushed to the right side by the stomach and the bowels, in the cavity of the thorax, it kept the same course and pierced the diaphragm, not at the usual place, but considerable further to the right side: and the aperture through which it passed, was backwards and to the right side, with respect to that for the vena cava.

I have preserved the heart and lungs, to show the disproportioned sizes of the lobes. And I have dried and prepared the diaphragm, with its connections to the vertebrae and sternum, to show the preternatural aperture through which the bowels passed into the thorax; as also the passage of the esophagus in the right side of the diaphragm. These preparations were at the same time shown to the Society.

The first understanding of pulmonary hypoplasia was reported by Morgagni (2) in 1769 in his treatise describing all manner of congenital diaphragmatic defects. In that treatise, he reported the small size of the ipsilateral lung. Cooper in 1827 (3) and Laennec in 1834 (4) not only reported the earliest clinical descriptions and gross pathology, but also suggested that a laparotomy might be the proper approach for reduction and correction of the hernia. Bowditch in 1847 (5) was the first to make the bedside diagnosis and further emphasized the clinical criteria for diagnosis. Although Bochdalek's (6) understanding of the embryology in 1848 was wrong, the congenital defect continues to carry his name. He speculated that the hernia resulted from a posterolateral rupture of the membrane, separating the pleuroperitoneal canal into two cavities. He also speculated incorrectly that the best way to repair the defect was through the bed of the twelfth rib. The record is not clear as to whether this was actually attempted. The earliest, although unsuccessful, attempts to repair congenital diaphragmatic hernia (CDH) were by Nauman in 1888 (7), and O'Dwyer in 1890 (8), but the first successful operation for this problem in a child was reported by Heidenhain in 1905 (9). The groundwork for treating this problem in the newborn period was laid by Hedblom (10) whose review of the reported cases showed that 75% of 44 congenital cases died in the newborn period. He suggested that earlier intervention might improve survival. Successful repair of congenital diaphragmatic hernia remained rare until 1940 when Ladd and Gross (11) reported nine of 16 patients surviving, the youngest being 40 hours old. It was not until 1946 (12) that Gross reported the first infant less than 24 hours old surviving after operative repair of the defect.

Although alluded to by Morgagni, the histopathology of pulmonary hypoplasia was first detailed by Campanale and Rowland (1953) (13) and Reid (1963) (14). Our current understanding of the pulmonary hypoplasia associated with congenital diaphragmatic hernia features a spectrum of abnormalities that are related to the point in lung development that the defect occurs. The usual understanding of the etiology of diaphragmatic hernia is based on the concept advocated by Wells (15) and Bremmer (16). A persistent defect in the diaphragm separating the pleuroperitoneal canal into the chest and abdomen allows the abdominal viscera to migrate into the thorax. This may result from an intrinsic developmental abnormality of the diaphragm or an incoordination of the developmental timing between the development of the diaphragm and the return of the midgut from the umbilicus into the abdomen. Other embryologic concepts are worth mentioning. Gattone and Morse (17) and Iritani (18) suggested that an intrinsic abnormality of the lung rather than the diaphragm resulted in pulmonary hypoplasia which in turn allowed abdominal viscera to herniate into the chest. Discussions by these authors as to the origin of the myoblasts that come to populate the diaphragm suggest that a pleuroperitoneal membrane with faulty or inadequate myoblasts could be vulnerable to herniation.

The consequence of these events is to create a space-occupying lesion in the chest at a time when the developing lungs are in a very vulnerable glandular stage. De Lorimer et al. (19) showed that many of the cardinal features of diaphragmatic hernia can be mimicked by placing a prosthetic space-occupying mass in the thorax of the fetal lamb at appropriate times in development. He also emphasized that although the ipsilateral lung is more severely affected than the contralateral, both lungs are affected by congenital diaphragmatic hernia. The volume of intestinal herniation, its timing with respect to gestation and lung development, and the persistence/intermittence of the hernia all combine to yield a spectrum of both histopathologic observations and clinical courses.

Acknowledging this spectrum, the microscopic description of diaphragmatic hernia is generally characterized as grossly abnormal. The abnormality is not uniformly distributed throughout the lungs and affects the various lung components—airways, blood vessels, gas exchange surfaces, and surfactant systems—differently. In all cases, the lung wet and dry weights are reduced, the ipsilateral lung more than the contralateral. In addition, detailed work by Price et al. (20) in animal models suggests that the lobe closest to the ipsilateral diaphragm is more severely affected than all others. This is confirmed by total protein and RNA/DNA determinations.

Reid's studies showed (21) that no further bronchial division occurs after the sixteenth week of gestation. It should be no surprise, since congenital diaphragmatic hernia usually occurs at 10–12 weeks, that there is a profound reduction of bronchial divisions in all lobes of affected infants. Although there are suggestions that diaphragmatic hernia is a dynamic process (22), information from those severe enough to result in autopsy suggests that pathology is relatively fixed in the tenth to twelfth week of gestation.

Alveoli are present in the lungs of infants dying with diaphragmatic hernia, and, although the number of alveoli per acinus is probably normal, the total number of alveoli is reduced because of the reduced number of bronchial divisions. The arterial abnormalities have been best described by Geggel et al. (23). Morphometric analysis of the lungs, when related to clinical course, showed that infants who died immediately or after a brief period of adequate gas exchange have smaller preacinar arterioles than usual, as well as excessive precocious medial muscular hypertrophy. These findings were more pronounced in the group that never had a period of adequate gas exchange. The status of the surfactant system in diaphragmatic hernia is largely unknown, although animal work by Pringle (24) suggests an abundance and hypermaturity of the type II pneumocytes in ovine models. Reports by Glick et al. (25) suggest a paucity of surfactant in studied human infants, while reports by Gandy et al. (26) demonstrate normal surfactant levels in both diaphragmatic hernia and renal agenesis.

Although the histopathologic appearance of diaphragmatic hernia would appear static, the clinical reality is dynamic. Despite the varying degrees of pulmonary hypoplasia, it is the minority of infants that cannot be ventilated to physiologic levels of CO_2. The variable difficulty in maintaining oxygen delivery, as well as the varying degree of right-to-left shunting with resultant pre- and postductal oxygen gradients, is a reflection of the waxing and waning of pulmonary vasomotor tone. Work from our laboratory (27) and others (28) has suggested that the site of the pulmonary hypertensive response to hypoxia is in the alveolar precapillary arterioles. If, as is the case with congenital diaphragmatic hernia, this bed features excessive and precocious amounts of vascular smooth muscle, and if this muscle has difficulty accomplishing the remodeling that ordinarily accompanies the time of birth changes in pulmonary vasomotor tone, then it comes as no surprise that these histopathologic findings and pathophysiologic responses result in a clinical spectrum that characterizes congenital diaphragmatic hernia. The decreased size of the pulmonary vascular bed burdened with excessive muscularization combine and conspire to yield an exaggerated response to hypoxemia that in turn accelerates the diversion of blood from an opportunity for meaningful gas exchange. Other factors known to exacerbate and contribute to increased pulmonary vasomotor tone—alveolar hypoxia, arterial hypoxemia, hypercapnia, acidosis, hypothermia, and disturbances of vasoactive mediator homeostasis—become superimposed on this vulnerable situation and contribute to a vicious cycle of increased pulmonary hypertension and hypoxia.

CLINICAL MANAGEMENT

The diagnosis is usually made in a newborn infant with respiratory distress who has a scaphoid abdomen and absent or diminished breath sounds in one hemithorax. A chest radiograph confirms the diagnosis, although upper gastrointestinal series or position of nasogastric tube may be needed to remove obfuscation caused by cystic adenomatoid malformation. The infant is promptly intubated and ventilated to maximize gas exchange. Mask ventilation is dangerous because it will increase distension of the thoracic viscera. A nasogastric tube will minimize this distension and vent swallowed air.

Venous access can be established through the umbilical vein and passed, on occasion, to the level of the right atrium for monitoring of mixed venous oxygen saturation and administration of vasoactive drugs directly into the pulmonary circulation. Arterial access is easily accomplished through the umbilical artery for blood pressure and blood gas monitoring in the postductal position. We feel strongly that a preductal arterial site should also be accomplished in either the right radial or superficial temporal arteries. Significant right-to-left shunting consequent to pulmonary hypertension can be reflected as postductal hypoxemia and masquerade the gas exchange abilities of the lungs. A preductal measurement can more accurately reflect the gas exchange abilities and adequate pulmonary parenchyma, while postductal assessment may lead the clinician to act precipitously. The preductal assessment of oxygen content will also more accurately reflect oxygen delivery to the brain and can allow the clinician to be comfortable spending more time in preoperative resuscitation. If arterial access is not possible in a pre- and postductal location, oxygen saturation can be reasonably monitored noninvasively by transcutaneous pulse oximetry. Noninvasive measurement of Po_2 can be obtained from transcutaneous Po_2 electrodes in both positions.

These noninvasive measures have the advantages of being continuous, allowing the clinician the opportunity to appreciate trends, and generating useful information without disturbing the infant. Although physical examination and chest radiograph are usually the only diagnostic studies needed in the preoperative period, the frequent association of congenital diaphragmatic hernia with structural abnormalities of the heart require cardiac evaluation with two-dimensional color cardiac ultrasound and duplex Doppler scanning. The air-filled viscera in the chest may make this difficult until the hernia is reduced and repaired. Antibiotic prophylaxis is administered and blood samples are obtained for complete blood count, electrolytes, and blood banking samples sufficient for ECMO needs.

The amount of time spent in the preoperative resuscitation is variable and in evolution. The work of Bohn et al. (29,30) reflects one extreme. They hypothesize that, if an infant with congenital diaphragmatic hernia has sufficient lung parenchyma for potential survival, it should be possible to ventilate him or her adequately preoperatively. They also hypothesize that, if there is adequate lung parenchyma and if the baby can be adequately ventilated, then there is no need for surgery to be done on an emergency basis. Accordingly, they manage the congenital diaphragmatic hernia infant with a conventional pressure-cycled ventilator, complemented by muscle paralysis-induced alkalosis and some pharmacologic manipulation. If this does not achieve adequate gas exchange and hemodynamic stability, the infant is converted to a high-frequency oscillating ventilator. If stability is achieved with either management, the infant is operated on electively one to four days after birth. Infants who are not stabilized with either approach are deemed to have pulmonary hypoplasia incompatible with life and expire without an operation.

The other extreme, advocated by Connors et al. (31) and Wilson et al. (32), employs ECMO as an additional preoperative resuscitative tool. In their practice, if an infant cannot be stabilized preoperatively by conventional means, they report using ECMO to achieve adequate gas exchange and hemodynamic stability. While their experience demonstrates that this can be done with acceptable morbidity, identifying an appropriate infant for preoperative ECMO remains problematic, poorly defined, and a matter of opinion. Certainly, an infant transferred from an outlying hospital to an ECMO center who was doing acceptably well but deteriorated before surgery would be a better operative risk after a period of ECMO resuscitation. However, using ECMO to stabilize all infants who are doing poorly prior to surgery, particularly if there has never been any indication of adequate lung parenchyma, exposes the clinician and the infant to the untenable situation of an infant who is alive only because of ECMO life support with pulmonary hypoplasia to a degree incompatible with life.

RESULTS

It is difficult to quote a survival and death statistic for congenital diaphragmatic hernia because its therapy and referral patterns are in rapid evolution. Many clinicians are in awe of Dr. Gross's 68% survival reported in 1946; yet, to be included in his statistics, an infant had to make it to the operating room at the Boston Children's Hospital. In today's world of helicopter, fixed wing, and ambulance transport of the most critically ill newborns to ECMO centers, not to mention prenatal diagnosis, the patient population is very different. In addition, our ability to stabilize, for at least a short while, the majority of infants with new ventilator and pharmacologic techniques increases the number of infants making it to the operating room. This becomes even more telling when ECMO centers consider whether or not ECMO has made an impact on CDH survival because the infants referred are often outborn infants who are failing conventional therapy at another Level III neonatal intensive care unit. More than 66% of CDH infants in the Extracorporeal Life Support Organization (ELSO) Registry are outborn (33). The point is that ECMO centers are being asked to treat only the sickest of the sick patients and can report on only a seriously skewed population when discussing morbidity and mortality. An ECMO center reporting, for example, 75% survival is reporting 75% survival of the very worst cases of congenital diaphragmatic hernia, not 75% of the entire clinical spectrum.

These kinds of considerations make it impossible to compare congenital diaphragmatic hernia survival with ECMO to any historical control. As difficult as it has been to accomplish any kind of ECMO-versus-conventional-therapy trial for all ECMO diagnoses, none has even been published to date for congenital diaphragmatic hernia. Nevertheless, if one can accept that ECMO centers are treating the most desperately sick infants with congenital diaphragmatic hernia and are reporting 65%–85% (33) survival of infants thought to have at least 80% mortality likelihood, then it is hard to deny that some increased portion of these infants are surviving who would otherwise die. Individual ECMO centers have reported small series of congenital diaphragmatic hernia treated with ECMO who enjoyed 60%–90% survival (34–37). More telling is the much larger group of infants in the Extracorporeal Life Support Organization Registry. The best survival was reported in 1987 with 57/81 (70% survival). In 1989, there were 50/93 (54%) survivors. The cumulative experience since 1980 is 608/996 (61%) survivors (as of October, 1991).

The ECMO survival rate for CDH continues to be significantly worse than all other diagnoses for which ECMO is used. In addition to the considerations already discussed, this may also reflect the general tendency to use ECMO for all congenital diaphragmatic hernia infants who are dying from hypoxemia despite maximal conventional therapy. Infants who die despite ECMO do so as a result of either pulmonary hypoplasia, pulmonary hypertension, brain death, bronchopulmonary dysplasia, or hemorrhage (38). The immediate morbidity is similar to other ECMO entry diagnoses although the proximate surgical correction of the hernia has made hemorrhagic complications more prominent (32,38). The frequency of brain death suggests that earlier ECMO referral, transport, and intervention might decrease the frequency of this cause of death. The frequency of bronchopulmonary dysplasia suggests that alternate respiratory care techniques might decrease this as a cause of death. A similar outcome may be obtained as we gain a better understanding of the etiology of neonatal pulmonary hypertension. Specifically, a cautionary lesson has been learned from a small group of our apparent ECMO survivors who died four to eight weeks later of recurrent pulmonary hypertension. At autopsy, this subset of infants ($n = 3$) had adequate lung parenchyma and alveolar units but with severe pulmonary hypertensive angiopathy which caused their deaths despite prior normalization of pulmonary vascular tone while being treated with ECMO.

Long-term follow-up of the survivors is

limited because of the newness of the therapy. This subject is discussed in detail elsewhere. In our institution, 36 survivors have been followed for up to eight years. Seven of eight children of school age are functioning at age-appropriate levels for both motor and cognitive skills. One child is significantly delayed. Two of the remaining 24 infants have significant neurologic handicaps. Pulmonary function testing is not possible on the youngest survivors and only marginally on the oldest. The children tested ($n = 6$) have normal exercise tolerance and lung volumes and no oxygen requirement. The dynamic compliance has been normal, although there has been slight evidence of restrictive lung disease.

PATIENT SELECTION CONSIDERATIONS

Selection of infants with congenital diaphragmatic hernia who are candidates for ECMO therapy remains confusing and controversial. This is due in part to the previous comments about changing patient population, but also to a diversity of opinions as to what constitutes conventional therapy, what constitutes failure of that therapy, and what degree of failure is associated with which mortality likelihood. Although entry criteria are discussed elsewhere in this book, of all the diagnoses for which ECMO may be a therapy, congenital diaphragmatic hernia is the only one that involves less than two lungs. Consequently, entry criteria for congenital diaphragmatic hernia must be unique for that diagnosis.

In addition, it is extremely difficult to test reasonable entry criteria when the ethical dilemmas of testing a treatment for which the control group is expected to have a very high mortality is compounded by the relatively small numbers of appropriate congenital diaphragmatic hernia patients in any one ECMO center and compared to the heterogenous population of a multicenter study. Entry criteria developed at a single institution, which may be appropriate for that institution, continue to be confounded by at least anecdotal reports of exceptions and contradictions of those criteria from another institution (39).

Although selection of patients with severe pulmonary hypoplasia incompatible with meaningful gas exchange despite prolonged ECMO support is a desirable goal, a common response to this dilemma has been to use ECMO for all infants with intractable respiratory failure despite maximal conventional therapy. Many parameters have been developed to predict mortality risk prenatally, preoperatively, and postoperatively and to classify infants according to severity of pulmonary hypoplasia. Adzick et al. (22), in a series of prenatally diagnosed congenital diaphragmatic hernias, reported that a prenatal diagnosis was associated with 60% mortality, and associated polyhydramnios yielded 85% mortality. These data were collected before ECMO was widely available. In our institution, 13/15 prenatally diagnosed congenital diaphragmatic hernias have survived, seven with ECMO support. Further, 14/18 with polyhydramnios (not all prenatally diagnosed) survived, 11 with ECMO support. Other centers report similar experience (39).

The first postnatal attempts at mortality prediction were by Boix-Ochoa (40) who studied the infant's initial arterial blood gas values and response to therapy prior to and after surgery. Improvement in pH, Po_2, and Pco_2 were more likely to be related to survival than no response with continued acidosis and hypoxemia. Bohn et al. (29,30), as discussed earlier, used this approach and combined it with consideration of the amount of mechanical ventilation required to generate a specific response. When studied preoperatively, they use a ventilatory index (mean airway pressure × respirator rate) plotted against the arterial Pco_2. Infants whose oxygen requirements require a ventilatory index over 1,000 and who yield a Pco_2 no less than 40 mm Hg are considered to have overwhelming pulmonary hypoplasia and are not selected for operation.

Our institution and others (33,41), however, have demonstrated survival in several infants using ECMO who would have met Bohn's criteria for 100% mortality. A role for $AaDo_2$ gradients and oxygenation index (42) on at least an institutional basis has been established for nondiaphragmatic hernia ECMO indications (43). They should be used only by extrapolation for diaphragmatic hernia, yet a sustained $AaDo_2$ gradient over 600 mm Hg and an oxygenation index over 40 for 8–12 hours are clearly associated with significant mortality. A problem with multifactorial indices and gradients is that they are summary statistics, and many of the factors can be manipulated by respiratory care techniques to skew their interpretation. This again emphasizes the importance of each ECMO center developing institutional entry guidelines based on their own concept of maximal "conventional" therapy.

We have favored assessment of the infant after an appropriately timed operation, recognizing that there will be an occasional carefully selected infant with congenital diaphragmatic hernia who will benefit from preoperative ECMO resuscitation. We have also emphasized a physiological assessment of the lungs' potential for gas exchange by paying specific attention to the preductal arterial blood gas measurements. Arterial blood that is studied from a postductal site is a variable mixture of blood that has bypassed the pulmonary capillary bed via a right-to-left shunt and some blood that has been through the lungs. Blood from a preductal site is more representative of the lungs' abilities, although there may be some fraction from right-to-left shunts across the foramen ovale or consequent to ventilation-perfusion mismatching.

If no pre- or postductal Po_2 gradient exists, then these concerns are not an issue. However, as is frequently the case, a measured postductal Po_2 will be much lower than a preductal measurement. If the postductal Po_2 is less than 100 mm Hg, we favor measurement of the preductal Po_2. We have felt that an infant with congenital diaphragmatic hernia who is unable to generate a preductal Po_2 of at least 100 mm Hg at some point in the pre- or postoperative period has pulmonary hypoplasia to a degree incompatible with life despite ECMO. Five such infants with a mean best preductal Po_2 of 33 ± 14 mm Hg despite maximal conventional therapy were not treated with ECMO. All died of intractable hypoxemia and acidosis. At autopsy, all had less than the fifth percentile for lung weight and radial/alveolar counts consistent with the severest pulmonary hypoplasia.

A preductal Po_2 of 100 mm Hg is not entirely arbitrary and was extrapolated from the work of Boix-Ochoa (40) and Bohn (29,30). It has the advantage of being a directly measured physiologic value. It is important to note that it is a guideline, not an absolute number. It should be used to complement other entry criteria already discussed and must be modified as additional experience accrues. Unfortunately, other published reports continue to emphasize only the postductal Po_2 (32,42).

ECMO CONSIDERATIONS SPECIFIC TO CONGENITAL DIAPHRAGMATIC HERNIA

The general management of the infant with congenital diaphragmatic hernia who is being treated with ECMO has already been discussed. There are, however, some specific considerations with respect to congenital diaphragmatic hernia in the ECMO era. The pediatric surgeon responsible for the surgical management should keep in mind the possibility that the infant may need ECMO. If a decision has been made to treat the infant with ECMO prior to repair of the hernia, the repair should be delayed until oxygen delivery has been normalized, along with myocardial contractility, renal function, neurologic recovery, and all other biochemical and physiologic parameters. When the general condition of the infant is optimum, the operation can be commenced. We recommend repairing the infant while on ECMO but weaning the flow as much as is reasonable first. This should obviate concern for recurrent pulmonary hypertension precipitated by the operative procedure, and hopefully minimize postoperative ECMO support of the heparinized patient. Connors et al. (31) maintain that this can be done without additional morbidity despite systemic heparinization, particularly if a prosthetic patch is used liberally. The activated clotting time should be 180–200 seconds and the platelet count 80–100,000/mm^3. Liberal use of fibrin glue may be a useful adjunct. If ECMO is anticipated after the repair rather than before, potential bleeding from surgical sites should be anticipated. This can be minimized by limiting dissection only to that which is absolutely needed. An uncomplicated primary closure of the diaphragm without undue tension using a nonabsorbable suture material is desirable. Extensive attempts to mobilize the abdominal and chest walls along with the endothoracic muscle layers should be avoided. Instead, only sufficient tissue should be identified so as to allow secure placement of a prosthetic material such as Gortex. Loss of abdominal domain is a variable but constant feature of congenital diaphragmatic hernia. In infants where the abdomen can be closed only with tension and pressure that compromises respiratory excursion and venous return, we have made liberal use of Teflon-reinforced silicone sheeting sutured to the abdominal wall fascia to augment the abdominal wall. In four such cases, we have had no additional morbidity, and the prostheses were removed 48 hours after decannulation from ECMO. The use of tube thoracostomies has been controversial. Although a traditional approach has been to place them in both hemithoraces and subject them to 5–10 cm of negative pressure, if there is no contralateral pneumothorax, we favor using the tube only on the ipsilateral side attached to 2 cm of water seal only. We use this as a passive drain and remove it when drainage has stopped and is no longer needed. Serous drainage will usually continue until the ipsilateral lung fills its pleural space. If, after an extended trial, the lung does not fill the space, the tube can be removed, and pleural fluid will occupy space not taken by lung.

Bleeding and hemorrhage are a constant concern in these recent operative infants who are systemically heparinized while on ECMO. In addition, the ECMO circuit consumes platelets. The resultant thrombocytopenia requires periodic platelet transfusions to keep the platelet count greater than 75,000/mL. The heparin infusion is monitored by keeping the activated clotting time between 180 and 200 seconds. Delaying ECMO as long as is reasonably possible after surgery will maximize clot formation at surgical sites. Surgical dressings should be weighed, and chest tube and abdominal drain losses must be quantitated to monitor bleeding. Serious bleeding, manifest as loss of greater than 20% of the circulating blood volume in 8 h, or progressive abdominal distension will mandate surgical reexploration. The reexploration may not be satisfying, as a focal bleeding site is seldom located.

Monitoring of oxygen delivery is best done by complementing measurements in the dorsal aorta with continuous monitoring of mixed venous oxygen saturation. If the hemoglobin concentration and cardiac output are adequate, then the SVo_2 is extraordinarily useful. If there is continued difficulty with oxygen delivery despite high extracorporeal support, consideration should also be given to using vasoactive drugs such as priscoline, prostacycline, and nifedipine to dilate the pulmonary arterial bed in an attempt to ameliorate the increased pulmonary vascular tone. The clinician should also be aware of the spectrum of endocardial cushion defects that are associated with about 15% of congenital diaphragmatic hernias.

SUMMARY

This chapter discusses how the embryologic development of congenital diaphragmatic hernia results in neonatal lungs that reflect an extraordinarily complex interface between pulmonary hypoplasia and pulmonary hypertension. The morphologic and physiologic manifestations of this interface result in a broad spectrum of clinical conditions, some of which clearly benefit from resuscitation with extracorporeal membrane oxygenation. We continue to be confused as to how best to identify a reasonable infant who will benefit from the therapy. As more thoughtful experience develops, the place of ECMO in the therapeutic armamentarium for congenital diaphragmatic hernia will become clearer.

REFERENCES

(1) Macaulay G. An account of viscera herniation. Phil Trans Roy Coll Phys 1754;6:25–35.

(2) Morgagni GB. Seats and causes of disease investigated by anatomy, vol. 3. Alexander B, translator. London: Miller and Caldwell, 1769:205–6.

(3) Cooper AP. The anatomy and surgical treatment of abdominal hernia. London: Longman, Rees, Orme, Brown, and Green, 1827.

(4) Laennec RTH. 1834, cited by Ravitch MM. Congenital diaphragmatic hernia. In : Nyhus LM, Harkins H, eds. Hernia. Philadelphia: JP Lippincott, 1964.

(5) Bowditch HI. Peculiar case of diaphragmatic hernia. Buffalo Med J 1853;9:65–95.

(6) Bochdalek VA. Einige Betrachtungen uber die Enstehung des angeborenen Zwerchfellbruches. Als Bietrag Zur pathologischen Anatomie der Hernien vjschr Prakt Heilk 1848;18:89–99.

(7) Nauman G. Hernia diaphragmatica; Laparotomi, dod. Hygiea 1888;50:524–8.

(8) O'Dwyer J. Operation for relief of congenital diaphragmatic hernia. Ann Surg 1890;11:124–9.

(9) Heidenhain L. Gesichte eines Falles von chronisher Incarceration des Mageus in einer angehorenen Zwerchfellhernie welcher durcher Laparotomie geheilt wurde, mitansheissenden Bermerkungen uber die Moglichkeit, das Kardiacarcinom der Speiserihre zu reseciren. Dt Z Chir 1905;76:394–407.

(10) Hedblom CA. Diaphragmatic hernia: a study of 378 cases in which operation was performed. JAMA 1925;85:947–53.

(11) Ladd WE, Gross RE. Congenital diaphragmatic hernia. Engl J Med 1940;223:917–25.

(12) Gross RE. Congenital hernia of the diaphragm. Am J Dis Child 1946;71:579–92.

(13) Campanale RP, Rowland RH. Hypoplasia of the lung associated with congenital diaphragmatic hernia. Ann Surg 1955;142:176–89.

(14) Areechon W, Reid L. Hypoplasia of the lung associated with congenital diaphragmatic hernia. Br Med J 1963;1:230–3.

(15) Wells LJ. Development of the human diaphragm and pleural sacs. Contr Embryol Carneg Inst 1954;35:107–37.

(16) Bremer JL. The diaphragm and diaphragmatic hernia. Arch Pathol 1943;36:539–49.

(17) Gattone VH, Morse DE. A scanning electron miscroscopic study of congenital diaphragmatic hernia. J Submicrosc Cytol 1982;14:483–90.

(18) Iritani I. Experimental study on the embryogenesis of congenital diaphragmatic hernia. Anat Embryol 1984;169:133–9.

(19) de Lorimer AA, Tierney DF, Parker HR. Hypoplastic lungs in fetal lambs with surgically produced diaphragmatic hernias. Surgery 1967;62:12–17.

(20) Price MR, Galantowicz ME, Stolar CJH. Mechanical forces contribute to neonatal lung growth: the influence of altered diaphragm function piglets. J Pediatr Surg 1992 (in press).

(21) Reid L. The embryology of the lung. In: de Reuck AVS, Porter R, eds. Development of the lung. London: Churchill, 1967;109–30.

(22) Adzick NS, Harrison MR, Glick PL, Nakayama D, Manning F, de Lorimier A. Diaphragmatic hernia in the fetus. Prenatal diagnosis and outcome in 94 cases. J Pediatr Surg 1985;20:357–61.

(23) Geggel RL, Murphy JD, Langleben D, Crone RK, Vacanti JP, Reid LM. Congenital diaphragmatic hernia: arterial structural changes and persistent pulmonary hypertension after surgical repair. J Pediatr 1985;107:457–64.

(24) Turner JW, Pringle KC. Frequency of mature type II cells in normal and abnormal fetal lamb lung and 110 days gestation. Anat Rec 1984;208:3099–112.

(25) Glick P. Congenital diaphragmatic hernia in humans is a surfactant deficient state. J Pediatr Surg 1992 (in press).

(26) Gandy G. Bradsbrooke JG, Naidoo BT, Gardiner D. Comparison of methods for evaluating surface properties of lung in the perinatal period. Arch Dis Child 1968:43:8–16.

(27) Galantowicz ME, Price MR, Stolar CJH. Differential effect of alveolar and arterial oxygen tension on pulmonary vasomotor tone in ECMO perfused, isolated piglet lungs. J Pediatr Surg (in press).

(28) Marshall C, Marshall BE. Influence of perfusate P_{O_2} on hypoxic pulmonary vasoconstriction in rats. Circ Res 1983;52:691–6.

(29) Bohn DJ, James I, Filler RM, Ein SH, Wesson DE, Shandling B, et al. The relationship of $PaCO_2$ and ventilation parameters in predicting survival in congenital diaphragmatic hernia. J Pediatr Surg 1984;19:666–70.

(30) Bohn D, Masanori T, Perrin D, Barker G, Rabinovitch M. Ventilatory predictors of pulmonary hypoplasia in congenital diaphragmatic hernia, confirmed by morphologic assessment. J Pediatr 1987;111:423–31.

(31) Connors RH, Tracy T Jr, Bailey POV, Weber T. Congenital diaphragmatic hernia repair on ECMO. J Pediatr Surg (in press).

(32) Wilson JM, Lund DP, Lillehei CW, O'Rourke P, Vacanti J. Delayed surgery and preoperative ECMO does not improve survival in high risk congenital diaphragmatic hernia. J Pediatr Surg (in press).

(33) Stolar CJH, Snedecor S, Bartlett RH. Ex-

tracorporeal membrane oxygenation and neonatal respiratory failure: experience from the Extracorporeal Life Support Organization. J Pediatr Surg 1991;26(5):563–71.

(34) Weber TR, Connors RH, Pennington DG, Westfall S, Keenan W, Kotagal S, et al. Neonatal diaphragmatic hernia: an improving outlook with extracorporeal membrane oxygenation. Arch Surg 1987;122:615–8.

(35) Stolar CJH, Dillon PW, Reyes C. Selective use of extracorporeal membrane oxygenation in the management of congenital diaphragmatic hernia. J Pediatr Surg 1988;23:207–11.

(36) Sawyer SF, Falterman KW, Goldsmith JP, Arensman RM. Improving survival in the treatment of congenital diaphragmatic hernia. Ann Thorac Surg 1986;41:75–8.

(37) Langham MR, Krummel TM, Greenfield LJ, Drucker DE, Tracy TF, Mueller DG, et al. Extracorporeal membrane oxygenation after repair of congenital diaphragmatic hernia. Ann Thorac Surg 1987;44:247–52.

(38) Price MR, Galantowicz ME, Stolar CJH. Congenital diaphragmatic hernia, ECMO, and death: a spectrum of etiologies. J Pediatr Surg 1991;26(7):1023–8

(39) Newman KD, Anderson K, Van Muers K, Short BL. Extracorporeal membrane oxygenation and congenital diaphragmatic hernia—should any infant be excluded? J Pediatr Surg (in press).

(40) Boix-Ochoa J, Peguero G, Seijo G, Natal A, Canals J. Acid-base balance and blood gases in prognosis and therapy of congenital diaphragmatic hernia. J Pediatr Surg 1974;9:49–54.

(41) Bailey PV, Connors RH, Tracey T Jr. A critical analysis of extracorporeal membrane oxygenation for congenital diaphragmatic hernia. Surgery 1990;106:611–6.

(42) Beck R., Anderson KD, Pearson GSD. Criteria for extracorporeal membrane oxygenation in a population of infants with persistent pulmonary hypertension of the newborn. J Pediatr Surg 1974;9:49–54.

(43) Wilson, JM, Lund DP, Lillehei CW, Vacanti JP. Congenital diaphragmatic hernia: predictors of severity in the ECMO era. J Pediatr Surg 1991;26(9):1028–33.

18

Venovenous ECMO

Martin Keszler, M.D.
Theodor Kolobow, M.D.

The need to sacrifice the right common carotid artery in the course of standard venoarterial (VA) ECMO has always been a major impediment to wider acceptance of this lifesaving procedure. During the early days of extracorporeal life support, a number of different approaches to vascular access were explored. Arteriovenous via the umbilical (1), femoral (2,3), and neck (4) vessels, jugular to femoral venous (3,5), and jugular to umbilical venous (6,7) routes were all tried with varying degrees of success. However, VA bypass emerged as the dominant approach in clinical practice, primarily because of its great effectiveness in terms of O_2 delivery and the ability to provide cardiac support (8). Nonetheless, when respiratory support is the sole goal of therapy, venovenous (VV) perfusion remains an attractive alternative to traditional VA bypass.

In addition to the obvious benefit of sparing the carotid artery, VV perfusion may have other advantages. Two of the most obvious are infusion of possible emboli into the pulmonary rather than systemic (i.e., cerebral) circulation, and perfusion of the pulmonary vascular bed with oxygenated blood, possibly resulting in a more rapid fall in pulmonary vascular resistance. Other important benefits are the preservation of normal pulsatile flow, maintenance of pulmonary blood flow, and improved myocardial oxygen delivery. Lack of cardiac support, partial recirculation of oxygenated blood, and lower systemic Pao_2 are among the important disadvantages of this approach (Table 18.1).

In this chapter, we shall discuss the theoretical benefits and limitations of VV ECMO, describe various techniques of VV perfusion, and review available experimental and clinical data.

PHYSIOLOGIC CONSIDERATIONS

The reinfusion of oxygenated blood on the venous side of the circulation results in some admixture with desaturated blood. Consequently, systemic Pao_2 during VV ECMO tends to be lower than with VA perfusion. However, this is likely to be tolerated well by the patient since, with adequate cardiac output and oxygen carrying capacity, tissue oxygen delivery is not impaired even with Pao_2 in the 40–50-mm Hg range. This limitation could be

TABLE 18.1 Comparison of venovenous and venoarterial ECMO

Venovenous	Venoarterial
Advantages	
Sparing of the carotid artery	Direct cardiac support
Preservation of pulsatile flow	Excellent gas exchange
Avoidance of hyperoxia	Rapid stabilization
Perfusion of lungs with oxygenated blood	Extensive clinical experience
Perfusion of myocardium with oxygenated blood	
Avoidance of infusion of possible emboli directly into systemic arterial circulation	
Normal pulmonary blood flow	
Disadvantages	
No cardiac support	Carotid artery ligation
Partial recirculation	Nonpulsatile flow
Lower systemic Po_2	Reduced pulmonary blood flow
Limited clinical experience	Potential for cerebral/retinal hyperoxia
Fluctuating central venous pressure and blood pressure (tidal flow system)	Lower myocardial O_2 delivery
Possible unforeseen adverse effects	

eliminated if it were possible to safely and reliably direct the return catheter into the right ventricle. However, the danger of damage to the tricuspid valve and its chordae limits the usefulness of this approach.

As with VA ECMO, the O_2 delivery with VV perfusion is largely a function of bypass flow and hemoglobin level. The return of oxygenated blood into the venous rather than systemic arterial circulation results in partial recirculation. Some of the oxygenated blood just reinfused from the circuit will be immediately drained out again without reaching the patient. This is wasted flow. Depending on technique, recirculation flow may amount to as much as 50% of the total flow. Thus, higher bypass flow is needed to maintain equivalent O_2 delivery. In other words, the admixture of highly oxygenated blood increases the O_2 saturation of the venous blood reaching the oxygenator. Therefore, less oxygen can be added to any given volume of blood.

Another significant limitation of VV ECMO is its inability to provide direct cardiac support. Babies with persistent pulmonary hypertension of the newborn (PPHN) frequently have myocardial dysfunction. This may be the consequence of perinatal asphyxia, or it may reflect the increased afterload, greater wall tension secondary to ventricular dilatation, and relative hypoxemia that are the hallmarks of this disorder. Furthermore, with suprasystemic right-sided pressures and short duration of diastole, coronary blood flow may be impaired, leading to ischemia. Indeed, papillary muscle necrosis has been described in a large percentage of newborns who die of persistent pulmonary hypertension (9). With the current strict ECMO entry criteria, many babies demonstrate significant cardiac decompensation before ECMO and thus may not be candidates for VV ECMO. These considerations may become less important when ECMO is employed earlier in the course of the disease process.

Under normal conditions of VA ECMO, the coronary arteries are perfused predominantly by relatively desaturated blood from the left ventricle (10). With more highly saturated blood directly perfusing the coronary arteries during VV ECMO, rather than depending on uncertain retrograde flow from the aortic arch, myocardial oxygen delivery may be improved, which may in turn lead to improved myocardial contractility. Severe, transient depression of myocardial contractility during VA bypass is found in some infants whose myocardial function appeared to be adequate prior to ECMO (11). The nature of this phenomenon, known as "myocardial stun," is not well understood but may be related to suboptimal myocardial O_2 delivery during and/or before VA ECMO. Depending on its etiology, the incidence of myocardial stun may be reduced by VV perfusion. However, should myocardial stun develop during VV ECMO, rapid conversion to VA bypass would be required to provide cardiac support.

The normal pulsatile flow pattern in the arterial circulation is preserved during VV perfusion, and this may be of major physiologic significance. An extensive body of literature suggests that nonpulsatile flow adversely affects renal function. Decreased urine output, decreased sodium excretion, redistribution of renal blood flow away from the outer cortex, ischemic changes, and increased renin release have all been reported. On the other hand, pulsatile cardiopulmonary bypass techniques appear to promote normal renal function. Pulsatile flow may also be necessary for optimal regulation of circulating blood volume and blood pressure. Animal and adult human studies have demonstrated increased peripheral vascular resistance and alterations in a variety of reflex and humoral factors involved in the regulation of blood volume. Hickey et al. (12) have prepared an exhaustive review of this subject. These issues, which may have important implications for ECMO as well as the effect of pulsatile versus nonpulsatile perfusion on other organs such as the brain, have not been adequately studied in the newborn population.

Another issue in need of further study is the possible advantage of maintaining pulmonary blood flow at a normal or near-normal level. During VA bypass, lungs are usually ventilated, but pulmonary blood flow is greatly reduced. The resulting very high V/Q ratio may lead to alkalosis at the tissue level, possibly severe enough to cause tissue necrosis. Kolobow et al. (13) have reported massive hemorrhagic infarction of the lungs in spontaneously breathing lambs on total VA bypass when the animals were breathing room air. The degree of lung damage could be decreased by the addition of 1% CO_2 to the inspired gas and abolished completely by breathing air with 5% CO_2. The experimental conditions may have exaggerated somewhat the risk associated with clinical ECMO, since induced ventricular fibrillation resulted in virtually total cessation of pulmonary blood flow.

A major advantage of VV ECMO, made possible by the maintenance of normal pulmonary blood flow, is the potential for supplemental oxygen uptake through the natural lungs by a variant of "apneic oxygenation." This is because VV ECMO takes advantage of the rarely appreciated fact that the two gas exchange functions of the lung, oxygen uptake and CO_2 elimination, can occur independently of each other. Thus, oxygen can enter the blood through the lungs even if relatively little ventilation is accomplished.

It is generally accepted that the major contributor to pulmonary barotrauma is mechanical tissue stress due to large fluctuations in airway pressure necessary for tidal volume ventilation. With healthy lungs, apneic oxygenation can maintain normal PaO_2 for extended periods when oxygen taken up by the lungs is continuously replaced by a low flow of O_2 through a catheter at the level of the carina. However, CO_2 will rapidly accumulate, leading to intolerable respiratory acidosis. When metabolically produced CO_2 is continuously removed by an extracorporeal membrane lung, normal arterial gas composition can be maintained virtually indefinitely (14). This important concept has led to the development of a technique known as low-frequency, positive-pressure ventilation with extracorporeal CO_2 removal (LFPPV-$ECCO_2R$) (15). In this system, the low-frequency "sigh" breaths are used not to generate effective minute ventilation but to maintain functional residual capacity. The natural lungs supply the bulk of O_2 uptake, and the membrane lung is utilized almost exclusively to remove CO_2. This is accomplished at flows of as little as 20% of cardiac output, making possible a variety of peripheral cannulation routes. Oxygen toxicity appears not to be a problem, since alveolar gas is in equilibrium with pulmonary capillary gases which, in turn, are largely determined by the composition of the ventilating gas of the membrane oxygenator (14). Oxygen molecules diffuse down to the alveolar level only as fast as is necessary to replace O_2 taken up by the lungs.

Pulmonary O_2 uptake in newborns with PPHN is often limited by decreased pulmonary blood flow, rather than by parenchymal lung disease. Inadequate pulmonary blood flow may prove to be the limiting factor for extracorporeal techniques that rely substantially on the natural lungs for O_2 uptake. It remains to be seen whether perfusion of the pulmonary circulation with oxygenated blood is capable of lowering pulmonary vascular resistance rapidly enough to provide adequate pulmonary blood flow during the critical early stages of VV ECMO. In addition, unless entry criteria become less stringent, the severity of lung disease in babies presently qualifying for ECMO may preclude major reliance on pulmonary O_2 uptake. This would be particularly true with the traditional approach to lung rest. Most ECMO patients treated with "rest" settings of positive inspiratory pressure (PIP) 18–20 cm H_2O and positive end-expiratory pressure (PEEP) 3–5 cm H_2O experience near-total loss of pulmonary function once they are on bypass. We have demonstrated that the use of PEEP at 12–15 cm H_2O can safely prevent this deterioration in a majority of patients and accelerate lung recovery (16,17). This approach to lung management, because of its ability to maintain inflation and the gas transfer capability of the lungs, will most likely become an essential component of VV ECMO.

VV TECHNIQUES

VV perfusion can be accomplished using either single- or double-cannula systems (Figure 18.1). In the following paragraphs, each technique will be examined in detail.

Two-Cannula System

This is the simplest form of VV perfusion. The ECMO circuit is virtually identical to that used for VA bypass. The only difference is that the return cannula is inserted into the femoral vein rather than the carotid artery (Figure 18.2).

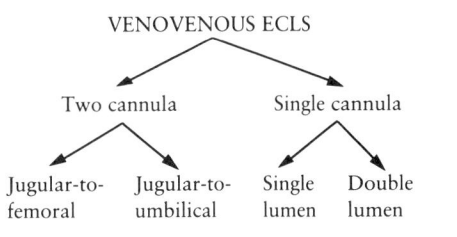

FIGURE 18.1 Possible vascular access sites for venovenous ECLS.

Andrews et al. (18) studied the ability of this system to provide respiratory support in adult sheep. Full respiratory support was achieved, but blood flow 20% higher than with VA ECMO was needed because of recirculation.

Klein et al. (19) reported success in eight of 11 newborns treated with this technique at the University of Michigan between 1981 and 1984. Patients on VV ECMO had somewhat lower, but adequate, PaO_2 and required mean bypass flow of 138 ± 30 mL/kg/min, compared to 94 ± 42 mL/kg/min for VA patients. More time was required to stabilize these babies after initiation of bypass, but, once this was accomplished, bypass proceeded smoothly in most patients. There were no adverse effects on renal or hepatic function. Three patients required conversion from VV to VA perfusion because of low cardiac output (two cases) or insufficient respiratory support (one case). The need for two separate cutdowns led to longer cannulation time and increased bleeding during ECMO. In addition, there was significant morbidity related to the femoral venous catheter, including severe venous insufficiency of the leg with persistent swelling, frequent wound infection, and leg length discrepancy. As a result of these difficulties, VV ECMO in this form has largely been abandoned. By contrast, the two-cannula system using the femoral or saphenous veins has been used successfully in adult patients (20). Venous insufficiency is avoided because cannulation and drainage of both the distal and proximal segments of the femoral vein are technically much more feasible in larger patients. Most recently, percutaneous cannulation of the saphenous vein, which is simple, rapid, and also avoids venous insufficiency, has become widely used (see Chapter 20).

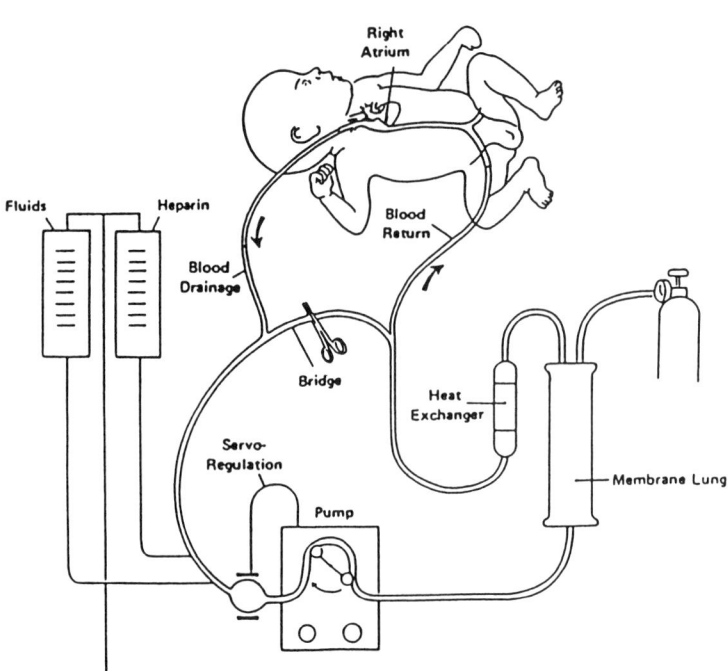

FIGURE 18.2 Two-cannula VV ECMO approach using the jugular and femoral veins. (Reprinted with permission from Bartlett RH. ECMO technical specialist manual, 7 ed. University of Michigan Hospitals, 1984.)

A variant of the two-cannula approach, using the umbilical vein as the return cannula, has recently enjoyed renewed interest sparked by improved catheter technology. Jugular venous-to-umbilical veins bypass was used in the initial clinical experience of White et al. (6). In these cases and in subsequent laboratory work (7), the return catheter was inserted only a short distance into the proximal umbilical vein. However, it appears that reinfusion of bypass flow proximal to the liver may be injurious to the liver and intestines. With newer thin-walled, flexible catheters, passage of a sufficiently large cannula through the ductus venosus into the inferior vena cava and right atrium is now feasible. While this approach has recently been used successfully in two patients, it is not without risk: perforation of the atrium occurred in a third case (Cornish JD, 1988, unpublished observation).

Single-Cannula Systems

The future of VV ECMO in neonates most likely lies with the single-cannula techniques. The attractiveness of this approach rests in the use of a single cannula to drain and reinfuse blood via the jugular vein, thus eliminating the problems associated with a second venous cannula. This can be accomplished in two ways. In one method, a double-lumen cannula drains blood through one lumen, while reinfusing oxygenated blood through the other. With the second method, blood is alternately drained and reinfused through a single-lumen cannula (tidal flow system).

Single-Lumen Tidal Flow System

The VV single-lumen tidal flow system was developed and used extensively in the laboratory by Kolobow et al. (21–23). In addition to standard ECMO circuit components, it includes a venous drainage reservoir and an externally pressurized reinfusion reservoir (Figure 18.3). The pressure within the reinfusion reservoir is adjustable so that the force driving the reinfusion of blood can be directly controlled. A pair of pneumatically-driven tubing occluders directs the flow of blood. When the return occluder is activated and the drainage occluder opens, desaturated blood drains from

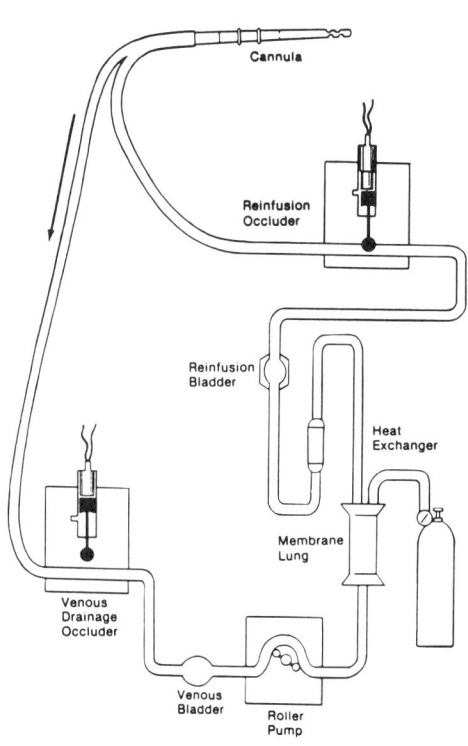

FIGURE 18.3 Components of the tidal flow single-cannula system.

the patient, filling the drainage reservoir; after passing through the membrane lung, it accumulates in the return reservoir. When the drainage occluder is closed and the return occluder opens, accumulated blood driven by pressure in the infusion reservoir is returned to the patient. The roller pump operates continuously, primed by the blood stored in the drainage reservoir.

Two main variables determine the performance of tidal flow VV ECMO. The first is the ratio of drainage to infusion time (the *D:I* ratio). Because drainage occurs passively by gravity, it requires more time than reinfusion. As the proportion of time dedicated to drainage during each cycle increases, maximum attainable ECMO flow will increase. Eventually, however, insufficient time remains to reinfuse each tidal volume without excessive reinfusion pressure. The second variable is the total length of each cycle, which determines the number of cycles/minute and, consequently, at any given pump flow, the "tidal volume" (TV). Within limits of hemodynamic tolerance, the longer the cycle (i.e., the larger the TV), the greater the efficiency of the tidal flow system. This is because: 1) each change in direction of flow recirculates the "dead space" of the cannula (approximately 2 mL), and 2) some of the oxygenated blood that has just been infused into the right atrium is withdrawn at the beginning of the next drainage cycle. Thus, with longer cycles, the bulk of each drainage cycle contains uncontaminated venous blood.

Previous work with this system in the laboratory has employed relatively low blood flow, relying on the natural lungs for much of the O_2 delivery. Because we were concerned that, with present ECMO entry criteria, the infants' lungs may have limited potential for O_2 uptake, we wished to test the limits of the system's O_2 delivery. As with traditional VA ECMO systems, to provide adequate systemic oxygenation, a critical proportion of venous return must be diverted through the artificial lung.

Preliminary studies in our laboratory have demonstrated that the progressive increase in attainable ECMO flow with increasing *D:I* ratios plateaus at a *D:I* ratio of approximately 3.5:1. Furthermore, at ratios of more than 3:1, the pressure required to reinfuse each tidal volume over a very short period of time became very high (>350 mm Hg). High reinfusion pressures can increase the risk of tubing rupture, hemolysis, and injury to the right atrium. Consequently, we prefer to limit reinfusion pressure to ≤250 mm Hg. With reinfusion pressures of 250 mm Hg, maximal flow is attained at a *D:I* ratio of 2:1 and is independent of cycle length.

We then studied the efficiency of oxygen delivery with the VV system at varying cycle lengths in newborn lambs, using a 2:1 ratio of drainage to infusion time. Total length of the drainage/infusion cycle varied from 2 to 6 s (30 cycles/min to 10 cycles/min), resulting in tidal volume of 17 to 50 mL. With longer cycles, recirculation progressively fell from 35.4% ± 5.3% with a 2-s cycle to 10.6 ± 5.2% with a 6-s cycle ($p < 0.001$). Effective bypass flow (total flow − recirculated flow) rose from 102 ± 19 mL/kg/min at 2 s to 132 ± 24 mL/kg/min at 6 s ($p < 0.001$); O_2 delivery increased from 3.7 ± 0.6 mL/kg/min at 2 s to 4.8 ± 0.5 mL/kg/min at 6 s ($p < 0.001$). Oxygen delivery was limited by low O_2 carrying capacity (mean hemoglobin = 8.1). These studies confirmed that longer cycles minimize recirculation, achieving sufficient effective bypass flow to assure adequate O_2 delivery with normal hemoglobin levels (24).

We have also studied right and left ventricular pressures, dimensions, and outputs during tidal flow VV ECMO in five healthy newborn lambs. We explored the effects of increasing tidal volume, first under baseline conditions and then during simulated pulmonary artery hypertension. Ventricular function was not compromised as cycle length progressively increased from 2 s to 6 s. The progressively larger tidal volumes led to increasing excursions in pressures and volumes between minimal values at the end of the drainage period and maximal values at the end of the reinfusion period. However, mean end-diastolic pressures, end-diastolic dimensions, aortic and pulmonary flows, and stroke work remained stable across the full range of cycle lengths (25).

Finally, we studied six newborn lambs instrumented for measurement of systemic, right ventricular, left ventricular, right atrial, and intracranial pressure (ICP) during 24 to 48 hours of tidal flow perfusion at maximal attainable pump flows. Cardiac output was measured with microspheres. Severe respiratory failure was induced by insufflating meconium into the trachea until sustained $AaDo_2$ of ≥600 mm Hg on Fio_2 1.0, PIP ≥ 36 cm H_2O was achieved. After four hours of ventilator support, bypass was initiated, and ventilator settings were reduced to PIP of 24 cm H_2O, PEEP of 14 cm H_2O, and intermittent mandatory ventilation (IMV) of 10. Fio_2 was reduced to <0.40 once adequate ECMO flow was established. The system provided adequate gas exchange in all animals. Calculated ECMO O_2 delivery ranged from 5.0 to 9.6 mL/kg/min. Hemodynamic variables remained stable throughout the experiment. No adverse effects on intracranial pressure were observed. Gross pathology revealed only mild bruising in the right atrial wall (26).

This study confirmed that long-term full respiratory support with the tidal flow system is possible without adverse effects. It also demonstrated the reliability of a prototype tidal flow system using solenoid-driven occluders from a modified Cobe Sentry II single-needle dialysis system (Cobe Laboratories, Lakewood, Colorado). This module can be attached to a standard VA ECMO system, allowing for interchangeability of equipment. If necessary, conversion from VV to VA ECMO can rapidly be accomplished by cannulating the carotid artery, removing the Y connector from the jugular cannula, and reconnecting the circuit in the standard VA ECMO mode. Both occluders must be maintained open; the pressure in the reinfusion reservoir is released. To facilitate conversion, it is preferable to dissect the carotid artery free during the initial cannulation procedure.

Another variant of this technique uses a similar occluder mechanism but eliminates the reinfusion reservoir, relying instead on intermittent pump operation directed by a pair of sensors capable of detecting volume in the drainage reservoir (27). This approach, however, appears to offer no significant advantage over the standard single-lumen technique. A different approach to tidal flow VV technology was described by Saito et al. (28). A microprocessor-driven two-pump system is used to generate a tidal flow pattern without occluders. The device is intended for low-flow ECO_2R use, with reported flows of 20–30 mL/kg/min. No hemodynamic data were reported.

Chevalier et al. (29) recently reported successful clinical use of tidal flow VV ECMO in 20 newborn infants using the Hospal Collin Cardio nonoccusive roller pump (Collin Cardio, Inc., Arcueil, France) with a Gambro single-needle dialysis alternating clamp device (Gambro Inc., Lincolnshire, Illinois) (29). The pump has a distensible, compliant segment of tubing stretched around its rollers. The tubing is not compressed against a raceway; occlusion is created by the tension of the tubing against the rollers. This feature allows the header tubing to function as a capacitance reservoir, eliminating the need for both the drainage and reinfusion bladders of the standard tidal flow system. Because the volume of blood in the header tubing varies according to available venous return, the pump is self-regulating and remarkably safe. When outflow obstruction occurs (such as when the return occluder is closed), blood accumulates in the header tubing segment. As the tubing distends, it becomes progressively less occlusive, so that overpressure is avoided. When the return occluder is released, blood is rapidly infused, driven first by the elastic recoil of the tubing and then by the large stroke volume of the distended header tubing. As the tubing empties, forward flow decreases and ceases completely if venous drainage is obstructed. The tubing is never totally occlusive, so that negative pressure and "degassing" do not occur (Figure 18.4). The only disadvantage is that flow is somewhat variable and must be measured independently.

Despite extensive favorable laboratory experience and the clinical success of Chevalier et al., the introduction of the tidal flow system into clinical practice in the United States has been delayed by lack of an FDA-approved, commercially available model. Other considerations are the need for reliable battery backup to power the occluder system in case of electrical failure. Lingering concerns about possible adverse effects of fluctuations in central venous and systemic arterial pressure may also be dampening enthusiasm for this approach.

Double-Lumen Cannula System

The double-lumen catheter system has been used for some time in VV perfusion in adults. The major attraction of this system is its simplicity. The circuit components are identical to those used in VA bypass, allowing for easy and rapid conversion from VV to VA ECMO. More importantly, no new equipment is needed, reducing the need for retraining of personnel and eliminating concerns about product liability with homemade equipment. The continuous flow pattern generated by simultaneous drainage and reinfusion may also be more physiologic than the tidal flow system. On the other hand, the double-lumen system is inherently less efficient than the single-lumen device. This is because, while the latter gives up a proportion of drainage time, it maintains maximal diameter of the drainage lumen, whereas that diameter is reduced in the double-lumen system. Since resistance to flow is inversely related to the fourth power of the radius, it follows that a reduction in catheter lumen will limit drainage considerably more than a reduction in drainage time in the tidal flow system. In addition, because of simultaneous drainage and reinfusion, recirculation is relatively high: 20% to 50% of total flow.

Attempts at reducing recirculation by varying catheter configuration have met with limited success. Zwischenberger et al. (3) compared the characteristics of both methods of single-cannula VV ECMO in a short-term animal study. A 13 Fr outer diameter (OD) spring wire-reinforced polyurethane single-lumen catheter developed by Kolobow and Zapol (31) was used with the tidal flow system. The wall thickness of this prototype manually fabricated device was 0.3 mm. The double-lumen cannula was made of two ultrathin-walled stainless steel tubes (wall thickness 0.08 mm) in a concentric configuration. The inner reinfusion cannula had an OD of 2.1 mm, and the outer drainage cannula was 4.6 mm OD (14 Fr). The tidal flow system was used with a *D:I* ratio of 3:1 and a short cycle length of 1.8 s to 2.5 s. Both techniques maintained adequate systemic oxygenation (O_2 saturation of 80% and 77% for the tidal flow and continuous flow systems, respectively). Preoxygenator O_2 saturation was higher in the double-lumen cannula than in the single-lumen cannula (79.3 ± 8.1% versus 72.1 ± 7.4%, $p < 0.01$), signifying greater recirculation. Consequently, significantly higher flows were necessary with the double-lumen system in order to maintain similar extracorporeal O_2 delivery. Mechanical trauma to the right atrium, attributed to the rigid double-lumen metal cannula, was observed in all animals after only six hours. Flexible cannulas that were previously available had thicker walls and did not provide adequate flow in the double-lumen configuration.

In 1989, an improved double-lumen catheter was developed and tested by Otsu et al. (32). The catheter is made from thin-walled polyurethane. This material is relatively rigid when cold, allowing easy cannulation, but becomes softer when warmed to body temperature. The drainage lumen of this 14 Fr catheter is approximately five times larger than the return channel. Maximizing drainage lumen size permitted flows as high as 1,000 mL/min at 100 cm H_2O

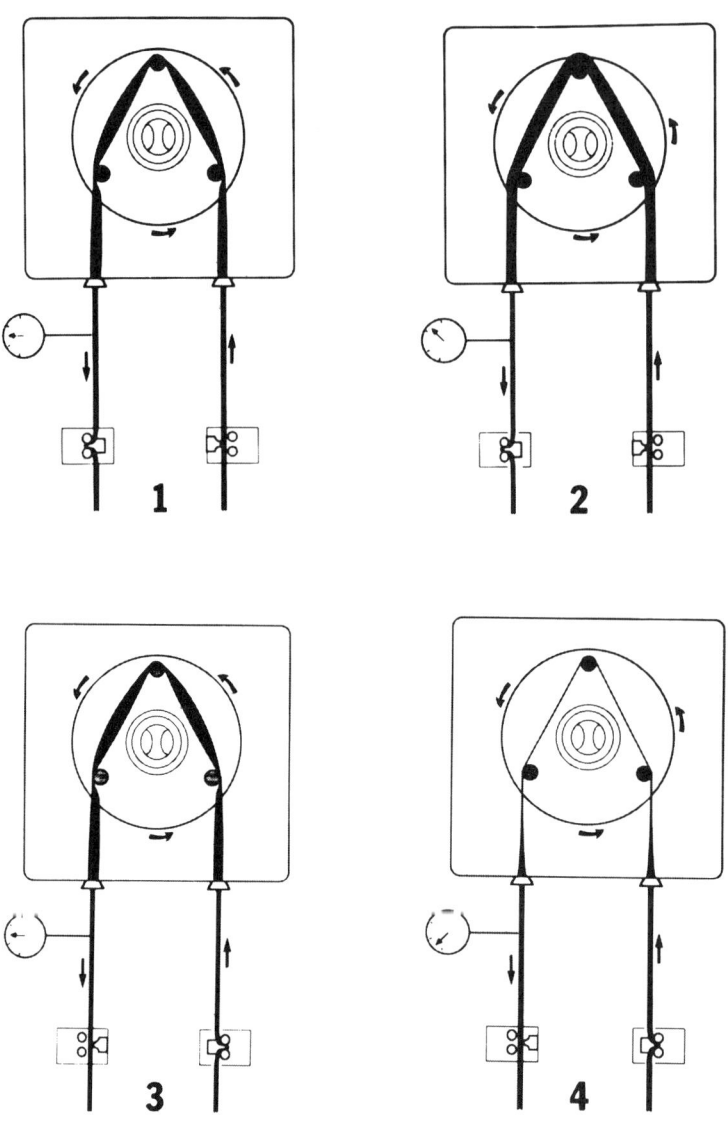

FIGURE 18.4 Principles of operation of the Collin Cardio pump. Step 1 shows the pump midway through the drainage phase. The drainage occluder is open, and the return occluder is closed. The capacitance tubing is partly distended with blood, and the pressure is at a moderate level. In Step 2, the tubing is distended and becoming less occlusive. The system pressure is approaching the point where it will trigger the opening of the return occluder. Step 3 shows the pump midway through the reinfusion phase. The return occluder is open, and the drainage occluder is closed. Blood stored in the header tubing segment is infusing into the patient, and the system pressure is falling. Step 4 shows the pump at the end of the return cycle. The header tubing segment has collapsed, forward flow of blood has ceased, and the system pressure has fallen to the point at which opening of the drainage occluder occurs and the next cycle begins. (Reprinted with permission from Durandy Y, et al. Single-cannula venovenous bypass for respiratory membrane lung support. J Thorac Cardiovasc Surg 1990;99:404–9.)

siphon, *using water*. In vivo, the maximum flow was reached because of the greater viscosity of blood, but was still in excess of 500 mL/min. Despite the high reinfusion pressures (300 mm Hg at 500 mL flow) resulting from the resistance of the small return lumen, hemolysis was not a significant problem. Recirculation rose in a linear fashion with increasing extracorporeal flow and ranged from 5% to 40%. The authors estimated that, under circumstances of clinical ECMO, recirculation would be approximately 20%, and they concluded that the device appeared to be suitable for full respiratory support in the clinical setting.

Clinical experience with this approach was recently reported from the University of Michigan (33). Between November 1988 and May 1989, 21 patients were selected for VV ECMO on the basis of good hemodynamic function and relatively stable clinical status. Double-lumen catheter cannulation was successful in 17 patients. Two patients subsequently required conversion to VA ECMO due to hemodynamic instability or inadequate oxygenation. The mean duration of ECMO was 111 ± 7.7 h in the remaining patients, and all 15 survived. Extracorporeal flow was 100 to 150 mL/kg/min. No significant elevation of serum free hemoglobin was noted despite reinfusion pressures of 300 mm Hg at full support. Respiratory support was adequate despite recirculation of 35% at 300 mL/min and 53% at 400 mL of ECMO flow. No unexpected adverse effects were reported. Currently, a collaborative data collection effort on the first 100 VV ECMO patients is in progress. This study was organized by ELSO to rapidly acquire data on the clinical application of this technique "in the field." Preliminary data suggest that this approach is effective in the majority of patients >3 kg, but that more time is required to stabilize the patients, inotropic support must be continued, and ventilator settings must be weaned much more slowly than with VA ECMO. The smaller 12 Fr catheter that has just become available has not yet been evaluated in the clinical setting.

The double-lumen catheters now have FDA approval and are available for general use. At this time, the double-lumen system, despite some limitations, appears to be more ready for clinical use than the currently available tidal flow systems. When improved tidal flow technology becomes available in the United States, it may become an attractive alternative, particularly for smaller infants in whom catheter lumen size is limited.

IMPLICATIONS FOR THE FUTURE

The introduction of VV single-cannula techniques into clinical practice makes possible the use of extracorporeal lung assist earlier in the course of the disease process. Avoiding ligation of the carotid artery is likely to encourage earlier referral of patients from outlying hospitals. This, in turn, may decrease the number of potential ECMO candidates who are in extremis by the time of referral and who subsequently die at the referring center, during transport, or shortly after arrival at the ECMO center while preparations for cannulation are in progress.

More importantly, we believe that the less invasive VV techniques will lead to an important conceptual change in our use of extracorporeal support technology. The current practice of waiting until the natural lungs become severely dysfunctional and then having to almost completely support cardiopulmonary function will give way to the concept of early lung assist. In cases in which ECMO is offered to prevent immediate demise, the patient becomes totally dependent on the extracorporeal system and is at risk if technical problems develop or if discontinuation of support is necessitated by hemorrhagic complications prior to significant recovery of the lungs. In addition, infants' lungs have been exposed to extremes of ventilator pressures and FiO_2, and, as a result, prolonged hypoxia, hypotension, or both may have ensued. As a consequence, residual chronic lung disease occurs in 10% to 25% of ECMO patients. The extent to which neurologic sequelae following ECMO are related to perinatal complications, pre-ECMO events, or the procedure itself is unknown. However, earlier application of the procedure would offer the promise of improved neurologic outcome as well.

With the emerging concept of lung assist, the emphasis will be on CO_2 removal, which is safer and technically simpler since it requires relatively low bypass flow. The major benefit will be avoidance of large tidal volume ventilation and mechanical tissue distortion, which are believed to be responsible for most cases of acute and chronic barotrauma. Without the need for large tidal breaths, lungs can be safely maintained in moderate inflation by PEEP of 12 to 15 cm H_2O and thus provide effective O_2 uptake without exposure to excessively high Fio_2.

Acceptance of this approach will be increased by recognition of the central role that positive pressure ventilation plays in causing and perpetuating lung injury. Recent studies (34) have demonstrated that positive pressure ventilation alone, without increased Fio_2 or hypocarbia, is capable of causing fatal lung injury in sheep with previously normal lungs. The injury occurred over two to four days when PIP of 30 cm H_2O was used, but emerged after only 12 to 36 h when PIP of 50 cm was employed. Hyperventilation can accelerate the degree of injury, particularly if pulmonary blood flow is reduced, resulting in a V/Q ratio much greater than 1. While lacking concurrent controls, the recent reports of Wung et al. (35) and Dworetz et al. (36) are consistent with these concepts.

It is likely that, in the near future, "heparinless" perfusion circuits will further reduce the risks associated with extracorporeal life support (see Chapter 8). This type of low-flow, single-cannula, heparinless VV lung assist will then justify early application of this "third lung," preempting the rise of ventilator settings to dangerous levels. Indeed, with improved technical design, increased automation, and miniaturization, the system may require less personnel, making its use almost as routine as mechanical ventilation. It may then be appropriate to manage most neonates in respiratory failure with continuous positive airway pressure (CPAP), utilizing $ECCO_2R$ to control $Paco_2$, and avoiding the adverse effects of intubation and mechanical ventilation altogether. Because minute ventilation is unimportant under these circumstances, CPAP could be tailored purely to optimize oxygenation. Substantial decreases in respiratory and neurologic morbidity may then be realized.

REFERENCES

(1) Dorson WJ, Baker E, Cohen ML, et al. A perfusion system for infants. Trans Am Soc Artif Intern Organs 1969;15:155–60.

(2) Rashkind WJ, Freeman A, Klein D, Toft RW. Evaluation of a disposable plastic low volume, pumpless oxygenator as a lung substitute. J Pediatr 1965;66:94–102.

(3) Pierce EC, Thebaut AL, Kent BB, et al. Techniques of extended perfusion using a membrane lung. Ann Thorac Surg 1971;12:451–70.

(4) Kolobow T, Zapol W, Pierce JE, et al. Partial extracorporeal gas exchange in alert newborn lambs with a membrane artificial lung perfused via an A-V shunt for periods up to 96 hours. Trans Am Soc Artif Intern Organs 1968;14:328–34.

(5) Sarin CL, SenGupta A, Taylor HP, Kolff WJ. Further development of an artificial placenta with the use of membrane oxygenator and venovenous perfusion. Surgery 1966;60:754–60.

(6) White JJ, Andrews HG, Risemberg H, et al. Prolonged respiratory support in newborn infants with a membrane oxygenator. Surgery 1971;70:288–96.

(7) Pesenti A, Kolobow T, Buckhold K, et al. Prevention of hyaline membrane disease in premature lambs by apneic oxygenation and extracorporeal carbon dioxide removal. Intens Care Med 1982;8:11–17.

(8) Bartlett RH, Gazzaniga AB, Fong SW, Jefferies MR, Haiduc N. Extracorporeal membrane oxygenator support for cardiopulmonary failure: experience in 28 cases. J Thorac Cardiovasc Surg 1977;73:375–86.

(9) Donnelly WH, Bucciarelli RL, Nelson RM. Ischemic papillary muscle necrosis in stressed newborn infants. J Pediatr 1980;96:295–300.

(10) Gerstmann DR, Koichiro N, Kinsella JP, et al. Left carotid artery (LCA) and coronary (CA) arterial flow partitioning during neonatal ECMO. Pediatr Res 1989;25:37A.

(11) Carter G, Lotze A, Miller M, Short B. Stunned myocardium in an infant treated with extracorporeal membrane oxygenation. J Pediatr Surg 1988;23:1011–8.

(12) Hickey PR, Buckley MJ, Philbin DM. Pulsatile and nonpulsatile cardiopulmonary bypass: review of a counterproductive controversy. Ann Thorac Surg 1983;36:720–37.

(13) Kolobow T, Spragg RG, Pierce JE. Massive pulmonary infarction during total cardiopulmonary bypass in unanesthetized spontaneously breathing lambs. Intern J Artif Org 1981;4:76–81.

(14) Kolobow T, Gattinoni L, Tomlinson T, Pierce JE. An alternative to breathing. J Thorac Cardiovasc Surg 1978;261–6.

(15) Gattinoni L, Kolobow T, Tomlinson T, et al. Low-frequency positive pressure ventilation with extracorporeal carbon dioxide removal (LFPPV-ECCO$_2$R): an experimental study. Anesth Analg 1978;57:470–7.

(16) Keszler M, Siva Subramanian KN, Smith YA, et al. Pulmonary management during extracorporeal membrane oxygenation. An alternate approach. Crit Care Med 1989;17:495–500.

(17) Keszler M, Ryckman F, McDonald JV Jr, et al. A prospective multicenter randomized study of high vs. low positive end-expiratory pressure during extracorporeal membrane oxygenation. J Pediatr 1991 (in press).

(18) Andrews AF, Toomasian J, Oram A, Barlett RH. Total respiratory support with veno-venous (VV) ECMO. Trans Am Soc Artif Intern Organs 1982;28:350–3.

(19) Klein MD, Andrews AF, Wesley JR, et al. Veno venous perfusion in ECMO for newborn respiratory insufficiency. A clinical comparison with venoarterial perfusion. Ann Surg 1985;201:520–6.

(20) Gattinoni L, Pesenti A, Mascheroni D, et al. Low-frequency positive-pressure ventilation with extracorporeal CO_2 removal in severe acute respiratory failure. JAMA 1986;256:881–6.

(21) Kolobow T, Fumagalli R, Arosio P, et al. The use of extracorporeal membrane lung in the successful resuscitation of severely hypoxic and hypercapnic fetal lambs. Trans Am Soc Artif Intern Organs 1982;28:365–8.

(22) Kolobow T, Moretti MP, Mascheroni D, et al. Experimental meconium aspiration syndrome in the preterm fetal lamb: successful treatment using the extracorporeal artificial lung. Trans Am Soc Artif Intern Organs 1983;29:221–5.

(23) Kolobow T, Borelli M, Spatola R, et al. Single catheter veno-venous membrane lung bypass in the treatment of experimental ARDS. Trans Am Soc Artif Intern Organs 1988;34:35–8.

(24) Keszler M, Moront MG, Cox C, et al. Oxygen delivery with a tidal flow veno-venous system for extracorporeal membrane oxygenation. Clin Res 1988;36:49A.

(25) Moront MG, Keszler M, Cox CB, et al. The effect of variable preload on left ventricular function in a single cannula system for extracorporeal membrane oxygenation. Surg Forum 1988;38:238–41.

(26) Keszler M, Cox C, Miller D, et al. Longterm support with tidal flow veno-venous extracorporeal membrane oxygenation (ECMO). Pediatr Res 1989;25:241A.

(27) Funakubo A, Fukui Y, Kawamura T. A compact neonatal extracorporeal oxygenator (ECMO) system using a single lumen catheter. Trans Am Soc Artif Intern Organs 1987;33:429–32.

(28) Saito Y, Terasaki H, Otsu T, et al. Extracorporeal lung assist with a single catheter in puppies. Crit Care Med 1985;13:501–3.

(29) Chevalier JY, Durandy Y, Batisse A, et al. Preliminary report: extracorporeal lung support for neonatal acute respiratory failure. Lancet 1990;335:1364–6.

(30) Zwischenberger JB, Toomasian JM, Drake K, et al. Total respiratory support with single cannula veno-venous ECMO: double lumen continuous flow vs. single lumen tidal flow. Trans Am Soc Artif Intern Organs 1985;31:610–15.

(31) Kolobow T, Zapol W. A new thin-walled nonkinking catheter for peripheral vascular cannulation. Surgery 1970;68:625–9.

(32) Otsu T, Merz SI, Hultquist KA. Laboratory evaluation of a double lumen catheter for venovenous neonatal ECMO. Trans Am Soc Artif Intern Organs 1989;35:647–50.

(33) Anderson HL, Otsu T, Chapman RA, Bartlett RH. Veno-venous extracorporeal life support in neonates using a double lumen catheter. Trans Am Soc Artif Intern Organs 1989;35:650–3.

(34) Kolobow T. Acute respiratory failure. On how to injure healthy lungs (and prevent sick lungs from recovering). Trans Am Soc Artif Intern Organs 1988;34:31–4.

(35) Wung JT, James LS, Kilchevski E, et al. Management of infants with severe respiratory failure and persistence of the fetal circulation, without hyperventilation. Pediatrics 1985;76:488–94.

(36) Dworetz AR, Moya FR, Sabo B, et al. Survival of infants with persistent pulmonary hypertension without extracorporeal membrane oxygenation. Pediatrics 1989;84:1–6.

19

Extracorporeal Life Support in Children

❖

Robert M. Arensman, M.D.
Vincent R. Adolph, M.D.

Extracorporeal life support (ECLS) was originally attempted in adults and older children (1). Success in these groups was relatively infrequent and led to a near abandonment of the technique (2). However, neonates have done well on ECLS circuits (3), and extracorporeal life support has been used for almost 20 years in an attempt to improve the survival of neonates with reversible cardiorespiratory failure (4). Familiarity with ECLS use for neonates has fostered confidence with the technique and an understanding of problems and complications sufficient to lead us back to its use in older children and adults once again. In Chapter 20, Dr. Müller discusses the use of long-term perfusion in adults. This chapter focuses on ECLS in children who have suffered severe pulmonary failure.

INDICATIONS

Whenever any therapeutic intervention is undertaken, there should be a valid indication for its use. ECLS is no exception, but, as with any new procedure or device, a single indication may initiate its use. Further use and study may lead to the addition of other indications or the disappearance of the original or early indications that fail to be favorably influenced by the therapy.

In the case of neonates, early indications were meconium aspiration, persistent pulmonary hypertension of the neonate, and congenital diaphragmatic hernia (5–8). Either the high mortality of these conditions or their frequency made them easily identifiable diagnoses that might be benefited by ECLS. In contrast, the diagnosis of beta-hemolytic streptococcal sepsis (or indeed any type of major infection) was at first thought to preclude the use of ECLS. It was thought that the introduction of large cannulas into the circulation of an infected baby would result in continued sepsis and ultimate demise. Ultimately, children with this diagnosis were placed on ECLS with the idea that the sepsis was secondary to a bacteria usually quite sensitive to antibiotics (9). In addition, it was surmised that ECLS should provide good support for the hypotension and shock present in many of these children when the sepsis was severe. This proved to be the case. Survival in these children was good, and

77% of those who meet criteria and undergo ECLS survive at present (10). Viral pneumonias, air leak syndrome, and hyaline membrane disease in the larger neonate have all been added as diagnoses that may benefit from ECLS when conventional therapies fail (11–16). Stated most broadly, it is reasonable today to say that any neonate with fulminant respiratory failure should be considered for ECLS if demise is imminent. Many of these babies will be rejected because of contraindications, but all should be seriously evaluated.

When one considers the indications for ECLS in older children, it is reasonable once again to first consider the more common and lethal causes of respiratory failure. Certainly, this list would include bacterial and viral pneumonias, plus all the reasons for which children develop adult respiratory distress syndrome (ARDS). Some of the more common problems that lead to ARDS in children are near-drowning, aspirations of a large number of noxious substances, and trauma with intraparenchymal lung damage.

In addition, there are rarer diseases that may result in respiratory failure, such as the collagen vascular diseases or the immunodeficiency syndromes. Many children with relative immunodeficiency are the patients who have undergone some form of tissue or organ transplantation. The need for drugs that reduce the rejection reaction render these children highly susceptible to opportunistic infections which often infect the lungs, create pneumonias that are difficult to treat, and ultimately result in respiratory failure. Pneumonias secondary to cytomegalovirus, a host of rarer viruses, and *pneumocystis carinii* are all examples that have been evaluated for ECMO support by the University of Chicago ECMO team during the past two years. The list of diagnoses for which children have received ECMO support beyond the neonatal period as found in the Extracorporeal Life Support Organization (ELSO) Registry are listed in Table 19.1.

Once again, it becomes impossible to list all the possible indications for ECMO in older children. Rather, the same approach should be taken as indicated previously for neonates. If a child has developed fulminant respiratory failure and maximal, conventional therapy is failing to result in improvement, the care providers should ask the question: "Should ECMO therapy be considered as a possible therapeutic modality for this individual?" Most of the patients under consideration will be rejected because other therapeutic choices are available that are less invasive, less dangerous, and less costly. Still other patients will be rejected because of clear-cut contraindications to undertaking vascular cannulation or systemic anticoagulation, but no child should die from isolated respiratory failure in the last decade of the twentieth century without at least a brief consideration of using ECMO therapy.

CRITERIA

It is a bit surprising that so few prospective ventilatory management trials have been done,

TABLE 19.1 Indications for pediatric ECMO

		Survivors	
	Total	Number	%
Bacterial pneumonia	23	9	39
Viral pneumonia	92	44	48
Intrapulmonary hemorrhage	3	3	100
Aspiration	31	19	61
Pneumocystis carinii pneumonia	5	2	40
ARDS*	79	33	42
Others	52	25	48

*ARDS = adult respiratory distress syndrome.

since mechanical ventilators have been in use in the United States since the 1950s. General principles have slowly evolved, but the exact techniques of safe and efficacious ventilation are still imperfectly known. The result is that there is no agreement as to what parameters indicate a failure of mechanical ventilation and a probable fatal outcome.

Retrospective analysis of deaths associated with ventilation in neonates have indicated that $AaDo_2$ gradients and oxygenation index (OI) have some predictive value over time. Variation from center to center has been as great as 20%–25% in the predictive value of either of these parameters; however, mortality of 70%–90% was demonstrated in each of four reports from University of Michigan, Medical College of Virginia, Children's National Medical Center, and the Ochsner Medical Institutions. It appears that the retrospective data are sufficiently valid to predict when death is more likely than survival. This allows a consideration of ECMO therapy before a fatal outcome, even if ECMO therapy is subsequently rejected.

In children beyond the neonatal period, even data as meager as those available for neonates are not found. As recently as 1979, when the results of the adult ECMO trial were published, patients who required an Fio_2 of 0.5 or greater and remained on mechanical ventilation more than 24 hours had a mortality rate of 67%. If multiple organ failure occurred (respiratory failure plus the failure of any one additional organ system), mortality rose to 90%. The resilience of youth, greater ability to repair pulmonary parenchymal damage, and probably greater ability to manage mechanical ventilation with less pulmonary damage make it extremely unlikely that mortality rates would be so high if a similar group of pediatric patients were studied today. However, affected patients have a high mortality, ranging from 30%–74% (17–19). Survival in patients with ARDS is not improving significantly despite advances in ventilatory support (20).

Nevertheless, there must be some set of predictive parameters that indicate that the usefulness of mechanical ventilation is exhausted. At that point, continued use of high oxygen concentrations and high pressure settings with attendant oxygen toxicity and barotrauma make an unfavorable outcome more likely than a favorable one. At that point, consideration of ECMO therapy should begin. Until recently, there have been little predictive data in pediatric respiratory failure. Zobel and his colleagues have proposed a Respiratory Severity Index (RSI) that predicts 100% mortality if greater than 0.75 after 48 hours of mechanical ventilation (21). Butt and McDougall found that a peak inspiratory pressure greater than 40 mm Hg and an alveolar-arterial gradient of greater than 580 predicts an 80% mortality (22). Tamburro et al. reported that an alveolar-arterial gradient of greater than 450 mm Hg for 16 hours predicts mortality with a 90% sensitivity and a 100% specificity (23). This group also reported a 90% sensitivity and 92% specificity with a gradient of 450 mm Hg for greater than 12 hours.

ELSO has designed a national, prospective data acquisition study to obtain information on what constitutes failure of mechanical ventilation and indicates the need to consider ECMO. Until that study is approved and completed, each ECMO center will have to individualize treatment. Generally, the ECMO team at the University of Chicago has relied on a consensus of the physicians caring for a patient. The group must collectively feel that mechanical ventilation has failed and will likely result in progressive damage if continued. There must be a reasonable expectation that the underlying disease process is reversible with time, and, in almost all cases, there should be the possibility of continuing some form of therapeutic intervention in addition to the lung rest achieved by ECMO. Children for ECMO should meet the criteria for the diagnosis of ARDS listed in Table 19.2.

TABLE 19.2 Criteria for the diagnosis of ARDS

1. Pao_2 <75 on Fio_2 >50% and Pao_2/Fio_2 <200
2. Diffuse bilateral radiographic changes
3. Noncardiogenic pulmonary infiltrates
4. Initiating event or ventilator support >7 days

TABLE 19.3 Equipment choices according to patient size

Weight (kg)	Oxygenator (m²)	Heater	Tubing (in.)	
			Arterial	Venous
>6	0.8	P=714	¼	¼
6–10	1.5	P=714	¼	⅜
11–15	2.5	Integrated	⅜	⅜
16–20	3.5	Integrated	⅜	⅜
>20	4.5	Integrated	⅜	⅜
>20	4.5	Series arrangement for greater CO_2 removal		
>20	4.5	Parallel arrangement for greater O_2 addition		

CIRCUIT DESIGN

The circuit used for older ECMO patients is very similar to the standard neonatal ECMO circuit. However, modifications must be made in several areas to avoid major technical problems. Modifications are necessary in the following components of the circuit: membrane, heat exchanger, tubing size, raceway tubing, and bladder.

Membrane

Our experience to date has been exclusively with the Kolobow/SciMed silicone membrane oxygenator. A membrane for the circuit is always chosen so that its rated flow is at least twice the flow that the patient is expected to require (Table 19.3). The larger membrane can be used in conjunction with a second membrane. When two membranes are used within the same circuit, they can be inserted in series or in parallel to increase the adequacy of oxygenation or ventilation. The larger membrane size is necessary to ensure adequate ventilation in older children; it also provides "respiratory" reserve since older patients frequently require longer ECMO runs (two to four weeks). This reserve decreases the need to change oxygenators while on bypass.

Heat Exchanger

For children with weights up to 11 kg, the SciMed P-714 heat exchanger can be used. This is the same heat exchanger commonly used in neonatal circuits. For children whose weight exceeds 11 kg, it is necessary to use a 2.5 m² oxygenator or one of the larger sizes up to 4.5 m². These oxygenators have an integrated heat exchanger that simplifies the construction of the circuit.

Tubing Size

For patients who require the 0.8-m² or 1.5-m² oxygenator, ¼-inch tubing can be used throughout the circuit. Oxygenators in the series from 2.5 m² and above have ⅜-inch blood ports. Consequently, it is easier to use ⅜-inch tubing throughout the entire circuit.

Raceway Tubing

Super-Tygon tubing has extremely long-lasting properties and is generally recommended for use within the raceway. Personally, we continue to advance this portion of the tubing every 100–110 hours or earlier if it shows signs of wear.

Bladder Bridge

Historically, most neonatal circuits have incorporated a bladder box to servoregulate the circuit by detecting low venous outflow. As the circuit is enlarged to accommodate the amount of venous outflow from a larger child, the bladder box becomes a site of resistance to flow. If there is reluctance to switch to a pressure-controlled system, the bladder box can be continued in the circuit with a bladder bridge constructed around the bladder box.

This bridge will divert the majority of the flow around the bladder but allow sufficient flow through the bladder box so that it continues its servoregulation function. In our experience, patients whose anticipated ECMO flow requires a 2.5-m^2 oxygenator and ⅜-inch tubing will also require a bladder bridge.

CANNULATION TECHNIQUES

The majority of older children who have undergone ECMO have had cannulation in a manner very similar to neonates. The approach is through the right neck to the internal jugular vein and the common carotid artery. Cannulas of the appropriate size are inserted through a small arteriotomy or venotomy and advanced downward into the chest. The artery and vein above the insertions sites are ligated. Chest x-ray confirms the correct position of the cannulas, and ECMO is initiated.

In older children, all the concerns about carotid artery ligation are present. In fact, these concerns are heightened since we know that carotid artery ligation carries an increasing chance of causing stroke as individuals grow older. As present, it appears that this increase occurs at middle age, but one approaches the possibility of carotid artery ligation in a teenager with considerable concern. Our experience is limited in this area, but carotid artery ligation and insertion have been our standard approach in children up to teenage years. Beyond the beginning of teenage years, we have chosen to insert the cannulas through the groin, utilizing the femoral artery. This technique is not without its own complications since the femoral artery is the only major inflow artery in children. They generally do not have a large amount of collateral flow since they do not have advancing arteriosclerosis. When we have used the femoral artery for ECMO return flow, it has been necessary to place a small side cannula into the distal femoral artery to maintain good arterial inflow to the lower leg. The femoral artery cannot be permanently ligated without serious consequence for the lower leg, so arterial reconstruction must be planned at the time of decannulation.

Similarly, in older children it may be necessary to use the femoral vein as the ECMO venous outflow site. In some of the larger children, both the internal jugular vein and the femoral vein have required cannulation to obtain sufficient venous drainage. Once again, a small side cannula to drain the leg may be needed to prevent venous congestion and edema of the lower extremity. When the ECMO run is complete, serious consideration must be given to venous reconstruction to prevent long-term lower leg edema. The use of the venovenous ECMO cannula may eliminate some of these problems in candidates suitable for this form of ECMO.

During the past five years, two or three ECMO centers, including our own, have seriously considered arterial and, more rarely, venous reconstruction at the conclusion of ECMO (24). Several small series have been reported with good initial success rates, i.e., successful reconstruction, Doppler-proven patency, and antegrade blood flow. Children deemed suitable for reconstruction are generally those who have short runs, clean cervical wounds at the end of the ECMO run, and are stable enough to withstand a local procedure that generally takes 45 minutes to one and a half hours. No long-term results are available to date.

Arguments in favor of reconstruction include the following: 1) it restores normal anatomy, 2) it is generally easily achieved, and 3) it restores blood flow to the brain via its normal circulatory pattern. There is concern that the high rate of arteriosclerosis in our population will result in a fairly high rate of carotid occlusion. Theoretically, it is advantageous to have both carotid arteries, particularly with advancing age.

Conversely, it has been argued that carotid artery ligation has been done in several thousand children with a very low rate of complications and no evidence of sequelae from developmental follow-up (25). Reconstruction may restore blood flow, but the clinical situation already indicates whether the child has had any adverse result from the ligation. Later reconstruction will not reverse an ischemic infarct, may result in thrombosis or embolism, and may create a stenotic lesion that will more easily develop an atherosclerotic plaque in the future. At the moment, a recommendation for or against carotid artery and possibly jugular vein reconstruction can be made. If centers are willing to undertake this surgery, it should be with a firm commitment to study these patients in the future in an attempt to provide further information on the benefits or potential dangers of reconstruction.

TECHNIQUES OF MANAGEMENT

Generally, the techniques of patient management do not differ greatly between the neonatal and pediatric ECMO patients. Most centers have perfected their techniques by first doing neonatal ECMO and then extending their services to older children. Slight modifications of the existing protocols allow this to be done quite successfully and point out how similar management for the two sets of children are.

Anticoagulation

Systemic heparin is administered to maintain the activated clotting time (ACT) between 200 and 220 s. With increasing experience, the ACT at our center has been slowly decreased and is often maintained now between 180–200 s. If active bleeding is present and not easily handled with wound reexploration, the ACT would be decreased to 160–180 s. Platelet counts are checked every eight hours and kept above 75,000 with platelet transfusion. Again, if risks are high or bleeding present, the platelet counts are maintained at higher levels, usually 100,000–125,000.

Antibiotics

Two broad-spectrum antibiotics are given with the initiation of ECMO. Initial choices are usually an aminoglycoside and ampicillin. In the older children, suspicion of infection complicating the respiratory failure often results in several antibiotics being given before the consultation with the ECMO team. In those cases, the same antibiotics are generally continued for the indications present before the ECMO therapy. Changes are made according to surveillance culture results obtained daily from the blood stream, lungs, or other sites as indicated.

Sedation

Children on ECMO will generally require both pain medication and sedation. The presence of a host of tubes (endotracheal, urinary, nasogastric, arterial, intravenous, ECMO cannulas) subject most children to some degree of pain. Judicious use of opiates intravenously via the pump is indicated to relieve this pain. In addition, anxiety associated with a strange place, strange people, and many strange procedures and manipulations is severe in most of these children. The older child is more capable of grasping tubes and dislodging them. Consequently, most of them require restraints that also increase anxiety. For all these reasons, the use of sedation is recommended. Paralysis is avoided if at all possible to allow the child to be awake and alert and to interact with his family, nurses, and doctors. However, if intravenous sedatives and pain medication fail to quiet a child, continuous drip paralysis and sedation should be instituted.

Nutrition

Nutritional support is begun shortly after the initiation of ECMO. Standard formulations of amino acids, fats, and glucose are given to achieve full replacement calories. Vitamins and minerals are added daily to prevent deficiency states. Most children, as well as neonates, are overhydrated at the start of ECMO, so formula concentrations are purposely kept high to avoid free water administration. The ability to administer the hyperalimentation via the ECMO circuit eliminates many problems of administration, hypertonicity, and access.

Pulmonary Therapy

Chest physiotherapy treatments are given throughout the run but may vary according to the underlying disease. If a pulmonary function computer is available, static and dynamic compliance, as well as inspiratory and expiratory resistance, should be measured on a daily or every-other-day schedule. Ventilator management and respiratory therapy can be frequently altered and tailored to the individual based on the computer's results. Changes in compliance may reflect improvement in patients who are undergoing ECMO and may also help identify those patients who develop progressive fibrosis.

Psychology

Older children have a wider world experience than neonates and most experience far greater fears and separation anxiety. It appears valuable to involve the child life program personnel with these children as much as possible. The use of toys, television, radio, tapes, videos, and books is important therapy for these children. Visitation with family members, even those who would not normally be admitted to the intensive care unit, should be encouraged and arranged whenever possible.

PATIENT DESCRIPTION AND RESULTS

The combined experience of the ECMO teams of the Ochsner Medical Institutions and the University of Chicago now reaches over nine years. Neonates were first treated with ECMO at each institution, and, with mastery of those cases, both teams initiated the use of ECMO for older children with respiratory failure. The following data represent the pediatric ECMO cases from these two institutions over this nine-year period (Table 19.4).

Twenty-nine patients with pulmonary failure were treated with ECMO. These patients ranged in age from 2–180 months (mean 29 months); weight ranged from 3–70 kg (mean 14 kg). Twenty-one patients had ARDS, as defined in Table 19.2, and 10 of those patients survived (48%). Two children had respiratory failure due to respiratory syncytial virus infection; both of these children survived with a combination of standard therapy and ECMO. Four children developed respiratory failure after orthotopic liver transplantation (OLT). In three of these children, an opportunistic pulmonary infection with *pneumocystis carinii*, cytomegalovirus, or influenza B virus was documented. In the fourth patient, the exact etiology of the pulmonary disease has never been delineated by cultures or lung biopsy. Three of these children survived ECMO therapy (75%), but one died immediately upon cessation of ECMO support. Finally, one patient had severe barotrauma complicating the management of reactive airway disease and survived with ECMO, while one patient with desquamative interstitial pneumonitis died despite ECMO support. Overall, 16 of 29 patients survived (55%). It is interesting to note that only two of the first 10 patients survived, but 14 of the last 19 patients are survivors (74%).

The average time of mechanical ventilation prior to ECMO was 11 days (range 2–42). For

TABLE 19.4 ECMO for patients with pulmonary failure

Number	Age (months)	Weight (kg)	Diagnosis*	Barotrauma†	Days on ventilator	Hours	Survival	Extubated
1	60	20	ARDS Valproic acid toxicity	Y	28	32	N	—
2	1	10	ARDS Aspiration	N	2	112	Y	36
3	76	18	DIP Desquamative interstitial pneumonitis	Y	10	197	N	—
4	16	11	ARDS Hydrocarbon ingestion	Y	6	312	N	—
5	15	20	ARDS Reye's syndrome	Y	42	140	N	—
6	17	10	ARDS Hydrocarbon aspiration	N	2	450	N	—
7	11	9	ARDS Near drowning	Y	4	68	N	—

TABLE 19.4 Continued

Number	Age (months)	Weight (kg)	Diagnosis*	Barotrauma†	Days on ventilator	Hours	Survival	Extubated
8	18	10	ARDS Stevens-Johnson syndrome	Y	15	61	N	—
9	32	14	ARDS Near drowning	Y	9	261	N	—
10	13	20	ARDS Hydrocarbon aspiration	Y	14	595	N	—
11	8	5	Pneumonia Respiratory syncytial virus	N	6	450	Y	‡
12	45	15	ARDS Trauma	Y	9	176	Y	72
13	20	9	ARDS Near drowning	Y	5	249	Y	55
14	55	19	ARDS Near drowning	Y	5	337	N	—
15	10	8	ARDS Near drowning	Y	8	138	Y	64
16	100	35	ARDS Trauma	Y	14	516	N	—
17	17	12	RAD Reactive airway disease	Y	4	89	Y	72
18	14	8	Pneumonia Respiratory syncytial virus	N	#	112	Y	72§
19	2	3	ARDS ? Viral pneumonia	Y	4	107	N	—
20	2	4	ARDS S/P lobectomy	Y	7	475	Y	‖
21	47	17	ARDS Trauma	Y	5	91	Y	28
22	105	35	ARDS ? Aspiration/barotrauma	Y	2	68	Y	72
23	13	13	OLT/Pneu Cytomegalovirus and *pneumocystis carinii*	Y	7	406	Y	288 (12 d)
24	180	70	ARDS Trauma	Y	9	39	N	—
25	16	7	OLT/Pneu Cytomegalovirus	N	14	306	Y	552 (23 d)
26	18	8	OLT/Pneu Influenza B virus	N	3	434	N	—
27	26	12	ARDS Aspiration	N	11	165	Y	120 (5 d)
28	3	3	ARDS Aspiration	—	7	266	Y	—
29	6	5	OLT/Pneu Opportunistic infection undetermined	N	28	338	Y	¶

Note: ARDS = adult respiratory distress syndrome; RAD = reactive airway disease; OLT = orthotopic liver transplantation; Pneu = pneumonia.
*Diagnosis with description or initiating event.
†Indicates if patient met standard neonatal barotrauma criteria for ECMO. Y = yes, N = no.
‡Prolonged ventilator support required after ECMO, but survived and extubated.
§Returned to prior ventilator settings.
‖Required ventilator support beyond three months after ECMO decannulation.
¶Required tracheostomy and prolonged ventilator support.

survivors, the average was seven days (range 2–28), and, for nonsurvivors, the average was 14 days (range 2–42). Only one patient on mechanical ventilation for 10 days or longer prior to ECMO survived. Results are consistently better when extracorporeal life support is instituted early. This fact emphasizes the need for predictive criteria that can be used early after the onset of respiratory failure.

The average time on ECMO was 242 hours (range 32–595). Survivors were on ECMO for an average of 219 hours (range 68–475) compared to an average of 271 hours for patients who died (range 32–595). Nine of the 16 survivors were extubated shortly after decannulation, with the average time to extubation being 72 hours. (range 28–72). Three patients required mechanical ventilation for more than two weeks after ECMO but survived to extubation. Two patients are still on mechanical ventilation more than three months after ECMO. One patient with respiratory syncytial virus infection required ventilator support prior to infection and ECMO because of bronchopulmonary dysplasia. That child was able to return to the same level of respirator support within 72 hours of decannulation from ECMO.

Statistical analysis of pre-ECMO ventilator settings, $Paco_2$, Pao_2, pulmonary compliance, $AaDo_2$, oxygenation index, and the limited published predictive criteria for pediatric ARDS have not helped identify patients who will or will not survive with the addition of extracorporeal life support.

COMPLICATIONS

Ten of the 29 patients (35%) had uncomplicated courses on ECMO that range from 39–338 hours. All of these children survived to extubation except for one child who has required a tracheostomy and continued low-level ventilator support. Nineteen of the 29 patients had at least one complication on ECMO (66%). The most significant complications have been hemorrhagic. Earlier in the series, platelets were given when thrombocytopenia was associated with bleeding, and the ACTs were generally kept between 250–350 s. Using the 200–250-s ACT range and maintaining platelet counts above 75,000 have lowered the incidence and severity of hemorrhagic complications. Further familiarity with the entire process of ECMO in older children has led us to further reduce the ACT times. Currently, the target range is 180–220 s.

Seven of the first ten patients had significant hemorrhagic complications, while only six of the last 19 children had significant bleeding. In addition, in only two of the last 12 patients was a hemorrhagic complication the direct cause of death. By contrast, in four of the first 10 patients, bleeding either directly led to the patient's death or was significant and required discontinuation of ECMO, shortly after which the patient died. There have been no thrombotic complications in these patients.

Intracranial hemorrhage (ICH), confirmed by computed tomography (CT) scan, or acute neurologic deterioration attributed to ICH occurred in four patients, and two patients developed severe intrapulmonary hemorrhage that prompted decannulation. One patient died after ECMO was discontinued due to a rapidly expanding retroperitoneal hematoma that developed at the same time as an acute neurologic change. Seven other patients had significant blood loss from the gastrointestinal tract or from surgical sites, but the bleeding was not sufficiently severe to prompt decannulation. Overall, 12 of the 29 patients (41%) had a hemorrhagic complication on ECMO.

Mechanical complications were secondary only to hemorrhagic complications in frequency and severity. In the first 14 circuits, Tygon tubing was used for the circuit and raceway tubing. In four cases, raceway rupture complicated the ECMO run; in two cases, raceway rupture occurred twice despite periodic advancing of the raceway tubing. In all subsequent cases, Super-Tygon tubing has been used and advanced through the raceway every 100–110 hours. No further raceway ruptures have occurred, even in runs as long as 516 hours.

Oxygenator deterioration requiring replacement or addition of a second oxygenator occurred for seven patients. In one patient, the membrane failed within minutes of initiating bypass; because of the suspicion of clot in the oxygenator, it was immediately changed. The membrane was found to contain several large clots occupying almost the entire surface area. The cause of this widespread clot could not be determined, and the subsequent oxygenator functioned without problems.

Pump failure mandated change in one patient. Fortunately, the patient tolerated exclusion from the circuit, and another pump was substituted without difficulty. Two patients required repositioning of cannulas after the original placement because of later migration. This was tolerated without problems. During the ECMO run in one child, air was found in the venous cannula. No source of entry was identified, the air was aspirated from the bladder, and the run was completed satisfactorily. In all, mechanical complications occurred in 10 of the 29 children (45%).

Four patients developed renal insufficiency or failure during the course of the ECMO therapy to the extent that hemofiltration or dialysis was required. All four of these children died. Mild renal insufficiency (elevated creatinine; no dialysis or hemofiltration) occurred in two patients, both of whom did well.

Six patients had culture-proven infections during the course of ECMO. Mortality was high in this group. Four died and two survived.

FOLLOW-UP

Very little data are available on the long-term follow-up of these patients. Thirteen of the 16 survivors were extubated during the original hospital stay. Three of the patients required prolonged ventilator support, and two remain on some form of ventilator support months after the completion of ECMO. One of these patients had chronic ventilator dependence prior to ECMO and still requires ventilator support at night. However, his requirements continue to decrease.

Developmental follow-up is extremely anecdotal since so many of these children were brought long distances for ECMO therapy and cannot easily return for complete neurologic, psychologic, and intellectual testing. None

TABLE 19.5 Results of pediatric ECMO in ELSO International Registry

Year on ECMO	Survivors		Total	Cumulative total
	Number	%		
1982	0	0	1	1
1984	1	50	2	3
1985	3	60	5	8
1986	0	0	6	14
1987	5	42	12	26
1988	13	37	35	61
1989	26	52	50	111
1990	50	45	111	222
1991	37	59	63	285

require supplemental oxygen at this time. None have readily discernible right hemispheric deficits.

REGISTRY RESULTS

ELSO centers have reported pediatric ECMO cases since 1982. Through the third quarter of 1991, a total of 285 cases have been reported, with an overall survival rate of 47%. Considering the severity of illness in these children and the recourse to ECMO as a last-ditch therapeutic intervention, these results are encouraging. In addition, individual centers have reported improving survival with experience, and the general trend of survival as reported in the Registry indicates improving survival. In Table 19.5, the results of the international pediatric ECMO Registry are summarized by diagnosis, year of ECMO initiation, and outcome.

CONCLUSION

ECMO therapy in children other than neonates is in its infancy. Cautious use of this modality for children with fulminant respiratory failure who have exhausted all means of conventional ventilatory support is reasonable and humane. Ideally, centers that have considerable experience in neonatal ECMO should expand their programs to incorporate these patients. Prior to the use of this therapy, centers should make sure that their ECMO team members are appropriately trained, that they are prepared to provide a long-range follow-up program, that they will participate in the ELSO Registry, and that they will contribute to the continued collection of information and experience concerning the uses, benefits, and complications of ECMO. Finally, this chapter concludes with the hope that any child who is dying from pulmonary failure will be fully evaluated for the role that ECMO therapy might play in his or her treatment.

REFERENCES

(1) Hill J, O'Brien T, Murray J. Prolonged extracorporeal membrane oxygenation for acute post-traumatic respiratory failure (shock-lung syndrome). N Engl J Med 1972;286:629–34.

(2) Zapol W, Snider M, Hill J, et al. Extracorporeal membrane oxygenation in severe acute respiratory failure. JAMA 1979;242:2193–6.

(3) Bartlett R, Gazzaniga A, Jeffries M, et al. Extracorporeal membrane oxygenation (ECMO): cardio-pulmonary support in infancy. Trans ASAIO 1976;22:80–8.

(4) Gille J, Bagniewski A. Ten years of use of extracorporeal membrane oxygenation (ECMO) in the treatment of acute respiratory insufficiency (ARI). Trans ASAIO 1976;22:102–8.

(5) Bartlett R, Andrews A, Toomasian J, Haiduc N, Gazzaniga A. Extracorporeal membrane oxygenation (ECMO) for newborn respiratory failure: forty-five cases. Surgery 1982;92:425–33.

(6) Short B, Miller M, Anderson K. Extracorporeal membrane oxygenation in the management of respiratory failure in the newborn. Clin Perinatol 1987;14:737–48.

(7) O'Rourke P, Crone R, Vacanti J, et al. Extracorporeal membrane oxygenation and conventional medical therapy in neonates with persistent pulmonary hypertension of the newborn: a prospective randomized study. Pediatrics 1989;84:957–63.

(8) Loe W, Graves E, Ochsner J, Falterman K, Arensman, R. Extracorporeal membrane oxygenation (ECMO) for newborn respiratory failure. J Pediatr Surg 1985;20:684–8.

(9) Redmond C, Goldsmith J, Sharp M, Falterman K, Arensman R. Extracorporeal membrane oxygenation for neonates. J La State Med Soc 1986;138:40–5.

(10) Extracorporeal Life Support Registry Data, University of Michigan.

(11) Bartlett R, Gazzaniga A. Extracorporeal circulation for cardiopulmonary insufficiency. Curr Probl Surg 1978;15:1–96.

(12) Gattinoni L, Pesenti A, Mascheroni D, et al. Low-frequency positive-pressure ventilation with extracorporeal CO_2 removal in severe acute respiratory failure. JAMA 1986;256:881–6.

(13) Snider M, Campbell D, Kofke W, et al. Venovenous perfusion of adults and children with severe acute respiratory distress syndrome. Trans ASAIO 1988;34:1014–20.

(14) Redmond C, Graves E, Falterman K, Ochsner J, Arensman R. Extracorporeal membrane oxygenation for respiratory and cardiac failure in infants and children. J Thorac Cardiovasc Surg 1987;93:199–204.

(15) Steiner R, Adolph V, Heaton B, et al. Pediatric extracorporeal membrane oxygenation in posttraumatic respiratory failure. J Pediatr Surg 1991;26:1011–15.

(16) Egan R, Duffin J, Glynn M, et al. Ten-year experience with extracorporeal membrane oxygenation for severe respiratory failure. Chest 1988;94:681–7.

(17) Holbrook R, Taylor G, Pollack M, Field A. Adult respiratory distress syndrome in children. Pediatr Clin North Am 1980;27:677–85.

(18) Katz R. Adult respiratory distress syndrome in children. Clin Chest Med 1987;8:635–9.

(19) DeBruin W, Notterman D, Greenwald B. Mortality of ARDS in infants and children (Abstract). Crit Care Med 1989;17:S111.

(20) Hudson L. Survival data in patients with acute and chronic lung disease requiring mechanical ventilation. Am Rev Respir Dis 1989;140:S19–S24.

(21) Zobel G, Kuttnig M, Trop H. A respiratory severity index (RSI) for children with ARDS (Abstract). Crit Care Med 1989;17:S110.

(22) Butt W, McDougall P. What is the role of pediatric ECMO in Australia? Aust Paediatr J 1989;25:189–91.

(23) Tamburro R, Chyka D, Bugnitz M. The use of alveolar-arterial oxygen gradient to predict mortality from severe respiratory failure in pediatrics. Breckenridge, CO: Proceedings of the Sixth

Annual ECMO Symposium of Children's Hospital National Medical Center, 1990.

(24) Adolph V, Bonis S, Falterman K, Arensman R. Carotid artery repair after pediatric extracorporeal membrane oxygenation. J Pediatr Surg 1990;25:867–70.

(25) Adolph V, Ekelund C, Smith A, Falterman K, Arensman R. Developmental outcome of neonates treated with extracorporeal membrane oxygenation. J Pediatr Surg 1990;25:43–6.

20

Extracorporeal Respiratory Support in Patients with Adult Respiratory Distress Syndrome

❖

Eckhard Müller, M.D.

Acute respiratory failure (ARF) is characterized by noncardiogenic pulmonary edema as the marker of acute lung injury (1). Moon in 1948 (2) described the natural history of pulmonary histology in patients who died of respiratory failure minutes to one week following shock. The lungs were heavy, and they showed marked capillary engorgement, congestion, severe edema and proteinaceous fluid, gross basilar atelectasis, leukocyte infiltration, capillary hemorrhage, petechiae, pleural effusion, and pneumonia. ARF received greatest attention during the Vietnam War as the major cause of death. It was thereafter also called "Da Nang lung" (1–3).

The histopathological pictures of the Da Nang lung era in the late 1960s reflected changes not seen before. Pathologists observed diffuse hyaline membranes, focal intraalveolar hemorrhage with necrosis of the alveolar walls, cuboidal lining cells (granular pneumocytes), hyperplasia, fibroplasia, fibrosis, and collagen deposition. Gross basilar atelectasis was no longer detectable (1). Those newly observed changes in the histopathology were in tandem with the introduction of mechanical ventilators.

Ashbaugh et al. coined the term "adult respiratory distress syndrome" (ARDS) in 1967 (4) to describe the emergence of a new disease entity. As Teplitz (1), an Army pathologist during the Vietnam era, pointed out:

> There can be no doubt that the pathology of acute respiratory insufficiency (ARI), with diffuse hyaline membrane formation as the modern pathologist now knows it, had its advent at precisely the same time that blood gases became routinely available for monitoring, and Pulmonary Intensive Care Units were first established. This era specifically dates back to around 1963.

and:

> Thus, this end-stage pathologic picture which is indistinguishable from severe, well advanced interstitial pneumonitis with hyaline membranes is not a new disease process discovered during the Vietnam War and given clinical appellations of adult respiratory distress syndrome, post traumatic pulmonary insufficiency, shock lung, and congestive atelectasis, but a result of iatrogenic modification of the pathology of noncardiogenic pulmonary oedema.

This altered histopathologic and clinical picture of ARF, now under the appellation of ARDS, is common in the intensive care units. In the United States, ARDS affects about 150,000 patients per year and complicates the course of one out of 100 hospital admissions (5).

ARDS possesses the following characteristics: refractory hypoxemia due to increased right-to-left shunting, diffuse interstitial and alveolar infiltrates, markedly reduced functional residual capacity (FRC) and lung compliance and, at times, multiorgan system failure (MOSF).

UNDERLYING DISEASES AND STIMULI

ARF/ARDS is essentially not a primary disease. It can occur as a sequel to a broad variety of pulmonary and nonpulmonary disease processes and stimuli (Table 20.1). The evidence is strong that mechanical ventilation at elevated peak airway pressures may contribute to the severity of pulmonary malfunction and may even be the prime reason why mild ARF progresses to ARDS and MOSF (6).

PATHOPHYSIOLOGY OF ARF/ARDS

The natural history of ARF was no doubt altered by the introduction of mechanical ventilation; at present, the natural history of noncardiogenic pulmonary edema can be encountered only in countries and institutions with a level of medical technology similar to what existed in the 1960s. The clinical picture of ARDS has changed to such a degree that it is often impossible to state whether certain clinical and biochemical markers are related to the natural history of the disease process alone or are marked by iatrogenic processes like mechanical ventilation.

It has now been shown repeatedly that the clinical course and the evolving histopathologic picture of ARDS are readily duplicated in animal models at ventilator settings commonly seen in patients with ARDS (7) (Kolobow T, unpublished data). The evolving clinical picture encompasses severe hypoxemia, pulmonary interstitial and alveolar edema, pulmonary hypertension, bilateral diffuse infiltrates on chest roentgenographic films, and MOSF involving the renal, hepatic, and circulatory systems. The histopathologic changes were typical of those found in clinical ARDS. There is strong evidence that overinflating healthy lungs or healthy parts of sick lungs, rather than high airway pressures alone, is the prime factor responsible for the injury process (8,9). The mechanisms of this injury process are not fully understood (9).

Current research is mainly directed at plasma-derived and/or -transmitted factors. There is evidence that, in ARDS, blood coagula-

TABLE 20.1 Underlying diseases and stimuli for adult respiratory distress syndrome

Pulmonary predispositions	Nonrespiratory predispositions
Pneumonia (bacterial/viral)	Hemorrhagic shock
Aspiration of gastrointestinal contents	Massive trauma
Inhalation of toxic fumes	Sepsis from any cause
Chest trauma with pulmonary contusion	Massive burns
High inspiratory oxygen concentrations	Multiple transfusions
Mechanical ventilation with elevated airway pressures	DIC*
	Pancreatitis
	Preeclampsia
	Amniotic fluid embolism
	Severe head trauma
	Cardiopulmonary bypass
	Drugs (e.g., ASA, bleomycin)†

*DIC = disseminated intravascular coagulation.
†ASA = acetosalicylic acid.

tion, fibrinolytic, and complement systems are activated (10). It is thought that complement-induced aggregation of neutrophils and their degranulation, with subsequent release of leukotrienes, prostaglandins, thromboxane, platelet-activating factors, oxygen free radicals, and metabolites of the arachidonic acid cycle, may affect the pulmonary vascular endothelial cell (3). However, the overall roles of the neutrophils, of the degranulation processes and of the release products, of oxygen free radicals, of the endothelial cell, and of cytokines and tumor necrosis factor α are still not completely understood (3,5,10,11).

Pathology

The histopathologic picture of ARF today differs greatly from that seen prior to the introduction of mechanical ventilation (1–3). ARDS presents a predictable evolution in pulmonary histopathology.

Early exudative phase The early exudative phase lasts for 24 to 96 hours after the initial injury. It is characterized by increased microvascular permeability, protein-rich interstitial edema, congestion, interstitial cell infiltration with leukocyte and platelet aggregates, early fibroplasia, vascular macrothrombi, hyaline membrane formation, necrosis mainly of type I alveolar epithelial cells and alveolar walls.

Proliferative phase The proliferative phase (three to 10 days after the initial injury) is characterized by widespread inflammatory infiltrates, thickened epithelium, and rapid proliferation of type II pneumocytes. The interstitium is thickened by edema, leukocytes, and fibroblasts.

Fibrotic phase During the fibrotic phase (commencing seven to 10 days after injury), there is deposition of collagen in the alveolar septa and the hyaline membranes that finally progresses to diffuse fibrosis with dark red, indurated lungs that have diffuse hemorrhagic lobar consolidation and a liverlike consistency. This is the relatively uniform result of treating any of a variety of underlying disease processes with aggressive mechanical ventilation.

The histopathologic features of lung involvement are not uniform. Areas of edema, consolidation, and/or atelectasis are interspersed with regions that appear to be normal. The time course is also variable.

MORTALITY AND MORBIDITY UNDER CONVENTIONAL TREATMENT

Intermittent positive pressure ventilation (IPPV) has been the mainstay of mechanical pulmonary ventilation since the introduction of mechanical ventilation. During the last 20 years, positive end-expiratory pressure (PEEP), super-PEEP, continuous positive airway pressure (CPAP), continuous positive pressure ventilation (CPPV), intermittent mechanical ventilation (IMV), pressure release ventilation (PRV), inverse ratio ventilation (IRV), and different forms of high-frequency ventilation (high-frequency ventilation [HFV], high-frequency jet ventilation [HFJV], and high-frequency oscillatory ventilation [HFO]) have been added to IPPV; new and more sophisticated mechanical ventilators are coming to market every year (6). In spite of all this, mortality from ARDS has not changed during the last 20 years and remains between 60% and 70% (4,12,13), approaching 95%–100% in patients with MOSF.

There are major adverse effects from mechanical ventilation. Some adverse effects, such as barotrauma consisting of extraalveolar air, are well known. The overall incidence of barotrauma in patients with severe ARDS had been reported to be 74% (14). Other adverse effects, such as iatrogenic lung injury and MOSF, have been demonstrated only recently (Kolobow T, unpublished data). Impairment in the hemodynamic, renal, coagulation, and gastrointestinal systems is common. Patients with ARDS die from either their underlying disease process, MOSF, or sepsis (15). Survival has been shown to be related to age and underlying disease (16). Patients without a clear site of infection are often shown at autopsy to have pneumonia, predominantly with gram-negative bacteria (16).

Major insight comes from the Additional Data Collection (ADC) study, conducted as part of the National Institutes of Health

(NIH)-sponsored ECMO study (17) on some 700 patients (18). It was demonstrated that patients who required an Fio_2 of 0.5 or greater while on mechanical ventilation for 24 hours had an expected mortality of 67%, and the presence of just one additional organ system failure raised the mortality to near that of the ECMO patients (about 90%) (18,19).

Montgomery et al. (20) demonstrated that only 16% of patients they studied died of pulmonary failure, with death during the first three days attributed to underlying disease or injury process. Sepsis and MOSF accounted for most of the later deaths (20). MOSF occurs in 93% of infected patients but also in 47% of the noninfected patients (15).

LONG-TERM PROGNOSIS IN SURVIVORS

Lakshminarayan et al. (21) showed that recovery of lung function can be total following ARDS. These results have been confirmed in Marburg (14) and in Milan (22). Near-total recovery in lung function can be expected within the first year following even the most severe forms of ARDS. It is surprising that even extensive fibrosis is reversible.

HISTORY OF EXTRACORPOREAL RESPIRATORY SUPPORT IN PATIENTS WITH ARDS

In 1972, Hill et al. (23) were the first to report survival following extracorporeal membrane oxygenation (ECMO) in an adult patient with acute posttraumatic respiratory failure. Soon thereafter, reports of other successful cases followed (24–26).

Based on these reports, in 1974, the Lung Division of the National Heart and Lung Institute proposed a multicenter, prospective randomized study of ECMO in ARF. The study started in 1975 and lasted two years (17). Patients with respiratory failure were randomly assigned to either conventional mechanical ventilation or conventional mechanical ventilation plus venoarterial ECMO whenever they fulfilled either slow-entry or rapid-entry ECMO criteria (Tables 20.2 and 20.3). The study was initially designed to include 300 patients but was terminated after entry of only 92 patients because survival in both the control and the ECMO group was less than 10% (17). There were major technical complications: bleeding averaged greater than 2 L/day and was the cause of death in a significant number of patients. Extensive and apparently irreversible fibrosis was uniformly found at autopsy (27). It was concluded that mortality from severe ARDS was not altered by extracorporeal gas exchange. As a result, clinical research on ECMO in adults virtually stopped.

Kolobow and associates (19,28) have suggested that the main reasons for the failure of the ECMO study were 1) a lack of concern for continued use of mechanical ventilation with high volumes and pressures, and 2) reduced perfusion of the lungs during ECMO.

While the ECMO study was still in progress, Kolobow et al. (29) showed that pulmonary ventilation was primarily beneficial for the removal of CO_2 rather than for providing a supply of oxygen. In studies conducted in awake sheep, they demonstrated that, when 30% to 50% of metabolically produced CO_2 was continuously removed by means of an extracorporeal membrane lung perfusion system, alveolar ventilation decreased by 30% to

TABLE 20.2 Slow-entry criteria

After 48 hours of maximal respiratory therapy while on Fio_2 0.6

PEEP* 5 cm H_2O or more

$Paco_2$ 30–45 mm Hg

Pao_2 50 mm Hg or less on three occasions 6 hours apart over a 12-hour period

QVA/Q shunt of 30% or more while on Fio_2 1.0 at 5 cm H_2O PEEP for at least 15 min

*PEEP = positive end-expiratory pressure.

TABLE 20.3 Rapid-entry criteria

Continuous Fio_2 1.0

PEEP 5 cm H_2O or more

$Paco_2$ 30–45 mm Hg

Pao_2 50 mm Hg or less on three determinations one hour apart over a two-hour period

50%. When all metabolically produced CO_2 was removed continuously by the membrane lung, virtually all spontaneous breathing stopped. Using the venovenous approach and low flow rates, pulmonary O_2 uptake was provided by apneic oxygenation, first described by Frumin et al. in 1959 (30). They concluded that pulmonary motion was not essential for blood oxygenation during prolonged extracorporeal bypass (31).

Further studies by Gattinoni et al. (32) demonstrated that mechanical ventilation had a beneficial effect in maintaining a normal functional residual capacity (FRC) and total static lung compliance (TSLC) at respiratory rates from less than one breath/min to four breaths/min. Extracorporeal CO_2 removal ($ECco_2R$) and apneic oxygenation were therefore combined with low-frequency positive pressure ventilation (LFPPV-$ECco_2R$) (32). These studies emphasized the overriding importance of mechanical ventilation in CO_2 elimination, while oxygenation was achieved almost entirely by the natural lungs in apnea.

In Milan, Italy, Gattinoni applied LFPPV-$ECco_2R$ to patients with severe ARDS in order to "rest the lung." In 1980, Gattinoni et al. (33) reported the first success in three patients with severe respiratory failure, all of whom had failed mechanical ventilation. These investigators also observed that LFPPV-$ECco_2R$ was greatly beneficial in recovery of cardiac and renal functions (34). The Milan group has continued to apply LFPPV-$ECco_2R$ and has contributed to further improvement of this technique (35). The most active group beside the Gattinoni group is the group in Marburg, Germany, who have treated more than 100 patients with this method. At present, the total number of patients supported with LFPPV-$ECco_2R$ exceeds 250.

PATIENT MANAGEMENT

Patient Management and Selection for $ECco_2R$

Management before $ECco_2R$ Patient management protocols, indications, and contraindications differ somewhat from each center. I will therefore refer to the current practice in Marburg, Germany.

All patients are transferred from the referring hospital by helicopter or ambulance by our own specially designed transportation unit.

Computed tomography (CT) scans and x-rays of the chest are taken immediately after the patient's arrival to document the degree of "barotrauma" and the position of chest drains. If indicated, CT scans and diagnostic tests of other organ systems (e.g., brain) are performed at the same time. Monitoring and infusion devices, including the Swan-Ganz catheter, a catheter for extravascular lung water measurement, and, if necessary, chest drains, are placed. A tracheostomy is then performed. The patient is placed on pressure-controlled IRV, PEEP, and a peak airway pressure limit of 45 cm H_2O with an Fio_2 of 1.0. Data on hemodynamics, gas exchange, and lung function, including TSLC, are recorded. The severity of respiratory failure is then classified according to the score from Morel et al. (36) (Table 20.4).

Indications and Contraindications for ECMO

The indications for and contraindications to extracorporeal respiratory support at our institution are as follows in Tables 20.5 and 20.6. In case there are no contraindications, patients with life-threatening hypoxemia ($Po_2 < 50$ mm Hg, Fio_2 1.0, PEEP ≥ 5 cm H_2O = fast-entry ECMO criteria) are placed on bypass immediately. All other patients are treated in a conventional manner for another 24 hours. Thereafter, patients who fulfilled the criteria of Morel 4 (slow-entry ECMO criteria) are placed on bypass. In patients who do not qualify, the same tests are performed on a daily basis, with the option for bypass at any time that there is no improvement on conventional mechanical ventilation.

Technique and Patient Management during $ECco_2R$

The Technique of LFPPV-$ECco_2R$ The technique of extracorporeal CO_2 removal ($ECco_2R$) with low-frequency positive pres-

TABLE 20.4 Geneva pulmonary failure scoring system

Score	Chest x-ray	AaDo$_2$*/Fio$_2$ (mm Hg)	C$_t$† (mL/cm H$_2$O)	MPAP‡ (mm Hg)
1	Moderately increased interstitial markings	300–375	70–80	20–25
2	Markedly increased interstitial markings	375–450	50–70	25–30
3	Patchy air-space consolidation	450–525	30–50	30–35
4	Extensive air-space consolidation	>525	<30	>35

AaDo$_2$ = alveolar-arterial oxygen gradient.
†C$_t$ = dynamic compliance
‡MPAP = mean pulmonary artery pressure.

sure ventilation (LFPPV) and apneic oxygenation has been described extensively elsewhere (14,22,33,37). Figure 20.1 is a diagram of the bypass circuit showing basic principles of patient management during LFPPV-ECco$_2$R. The purpose of ECco$_2$R is to remove CO$_2$ by extracorporeal means, rest the lungs, and prevent further injury by mechanical ventilation at elevated airway pressures.

As it is readily possible to hyperventilate the membrane lung, metabolically produced CO$_2$ (250–300 mL/min) can be removed at a venovenous bypass flow to 20 to 40 cc/kg/min (approximately 30% of cardiac output) with two membrane lungs in series (or in parallel), using a roller pump, all placed into a temperature-controlled chamber with integrated monitoring and servocontrol devices for blood flow, reservoir, roller pump, pre- and postmembrane pressure monitoring, and continuous oxygen-saturation measurement.

Currently, we use either two Kolobow silicone SciMed membrane lungs with 7- to 9-m^2 surface area, together with a 100-cc silicone rubber reservoir and polyurethane tubing (Contron); or two polypropylene heparin-bonded hollow fiber oxygenators (Carmeda/Maxima) with gas flowing inside the capillaries and blood on the outside and a total surface area of 4 m^2, together with heparin-bonded polyvinyl chloride tubing and catheter system. The membrane lungs are ventilated with an air-oxygen mixture at an initial gas flow of up to 10 L/min for each membrane lung, vacuumed or, in case of the Carmeda lungs, blown through the artificial lung so as to avoid possible air embolism.

When the SciMed membrane lung is used, the gas is well humidified to body temperature; the hollow fiber oxygenators are ventilated

TABLE 20.5 Indications for ECco$_2$R*

Slow-entry ECMO† criteria
Q$_{sp}$/Q$_t$‡ >30%
Peak airway pressure >45 cm H$_2$O
TSLC§ <30 mL/cm H$_2$O
ARDS∥ typical x-ray and/or CT scan
No improvement after 24 h on conventional mechanical ventilation with PC-IRV,¶ PEEP#
Therapy-resistant status asthmaticus

*ECco$_2$R = extracorporeal CO$_2$ removal.
†ECMO = extracorporeal membrane oxygenation.
‡Q$_{sp}$/Q$_t$ = intrapulmonary R to L shunt
§TSLC = total static lung compliance.
∥ARDS = adult respiratory distress syndrome.
¶PC-IRV = pressure controlled inverse ratio ventilation
#PEEP = positive-end expiratory pressure.

TABLE 20.6 Contraindications for ECco$_2$R*

<24 h after major surgery or trauma
<72 h after severe head injury with intracerebral bleeding
Age >65 years
Body weight <10 kg
Hypoxic brain damage
Cancer patients
ARDS† and severe COPD‡

*ECco$_2$R = extracorporeal CO$_2$ removal.
†ARDS = adult respiratory distress syndrome.
‡COPD = chronic obstructive pulmonary disease.

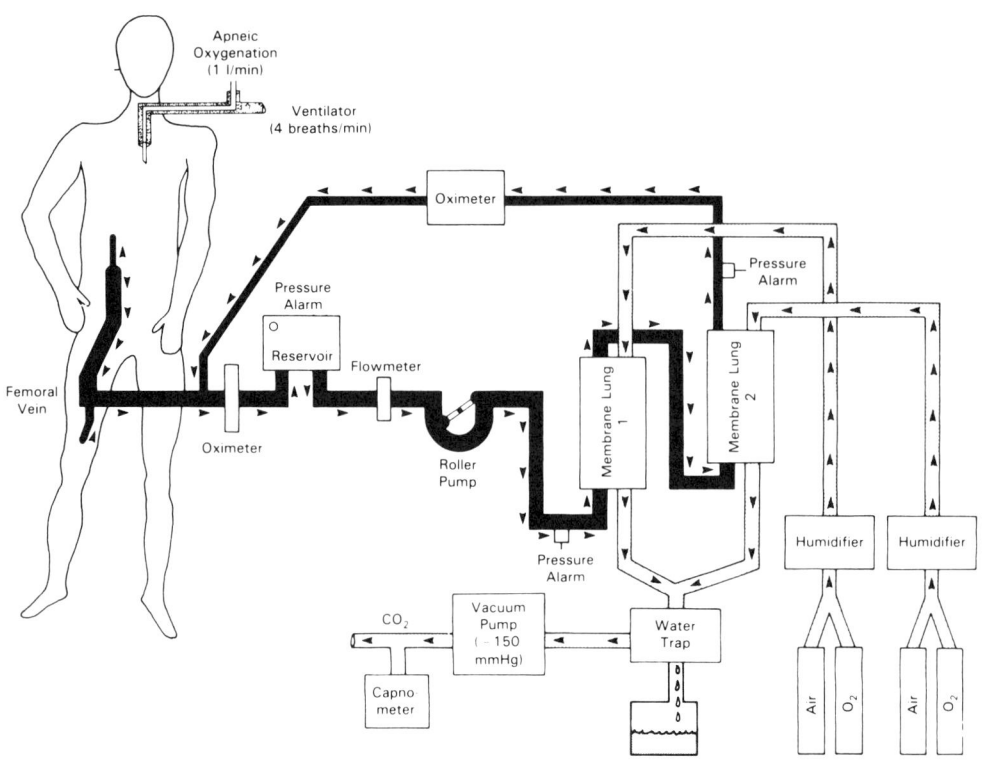

FIGURE 20.1 Flow diagram showing major components in the circuit used to accomplish extracorporeal carbon dioxide removal.

with a dry gas mixture at an inlet temperature approximately 2°C above blood temperature.

The pre- and postmembrane circuit pressures, blood gases, and CO_2 concentration in the ventilation gas are monitored. We make note of clotting in the extracorporeal circuit. When the hollow fiber oxygenators are used, plasma leakage occurs at some point between 8 and 240 hours of use, and the membrane lung must be considered for replacement.

The technique of blood drainage and return has recently undergone important changes. After successful use of the Pesenti double-lumen catheter, we now use the percutaneous approach as the access of choice because of decreased bleeding and avoidance of major surgical procedures for catheter implantation. Blood drainage and return currently in use vary depending on specific needs and are shown in Table 20.7.

TABLE 20.7 Methods of blood drainage and return

Blood drainage	Blood return
Double-lumen catheter	Inferior vena cava
Saphenous vein	Saphenous vein
Right saphenous and left saphenous	Superior vena cava
or	
Inferior vena cava	Right ventricle (through internal jugular vein)
Right atrium	Right ventricle

Patient management

Lung management As mechanical ventilation is greatly reduced, healing of the injured lung is possible. With a bypass flow of approximately 20 to 40 cc/kg/min, the total metabolic CO_2 load can be removed by the extracoporeal system. Only a small part of total oxygen needs, however, can be met through the bypass system. The rest of the O_2 supply is met through apneic oxygenation by the sick lung. A small intratracheal catheter is advanced so that it rests with its tip at the level of the carina to provide the means for apneic oxygenation. The flow of well-humidifed oxygen is set at about 500 cc/min or higher in the presence of a large bronchopleural fistula.

Apneic oxygenation through diseased lungs is feasible in the vast majority of patients. To maintain FRC, initial PEEP levels are currently adjusted by use of an external water seal to between 20 and 35 cm H_2O. This "lung rest" is interrupted by one to four breaths/min (LFPPV) (pressure limited to 35 to 45 cm H_2O). We are presently using a Servo ventilator model 900 C (Siemens Elema, Sweden).

As gas exchange improves, the PEEP level is reduced in gradual steps of 2 to 3 cm H_2O. Once PEEP is reduced to 10 to 15 cm H_2O, all sedation and paralysis are discontinued, and the patient is allowed to breathe spontaneously, either in the pressure support mode or on CPAP. The extracorporeal blood flow is slowly reduced over time.

Bypass is discontinued when the patient is able to maintain adequate blood gases with minimal extracorporeal blood flow, at an FiO_2 of 0.4 and a PEEP of 8 to 14 cm H_2O. Removal of the percutaneous catheters does not require reanastomosis to reconstruct the vessels. Further weaning from respiratory support proceeds in a conventional manner.

Anticoagulation and related problems Anticoagulation is achieved by continuous heparin infusion. The heparin dose depends on the patient's weight as well as on the type of extracorporeal system used. When the Kolobow SciMed membrane lung is used, heparin is administered to achieve an activated clotting time (ACT) of 180 to 220 s and a partial thromboplastin time (PTT) between 55 and 75 s (two to three times normal value). When heparin-bonded perfusion systems are used, the amount of heparin administered is reduced to 10 to 20 units/kg/h. The PTT is maintained between 45 to 55 s, and the ACT is kept between 140 to 160 s. Antithrombin III (AT III) levels are kept at 90% of normal or greater, either by transfusion of fresh frozen plasma (FFP) or commercial AT III.

Platelet levels are remarkably stable following an initial fall at the start of bypass or membrane lung changing. Platelets are transfused at levels less than 30,000/mL. In the presence of bleeding, platelets are transfused to raise the count above 60,000/mL.

Fresh frozen plasma is administered whenever there is a clinical indication (e.g., a coagulation disorder) or after membrane lung exchange because of leakage of plasma. Hematocrit is maintained between 35% and 45% for optimum oxygen transport capacity.

Bleeding complications involving blood losses greater than 500 cc/day are rare (the total incidence is approximately 10%). Bleeding can occur from catheter insertion sites, surgical wounds, and chest drains. In addition, intracerebral, gastrointestinal, and intrapulmonary bleeding are fairly common. Great care must be taken during any interventional procedure. All necessary chest drains should be introduced via a minithoracotomy under direct vision and without trocar by the most experienced staff member. Even with heparin-bonded systems, temporary disconnection from bypass may still be necessary if all attempts to stop bleeding by surgical means or through further reduction in the amount of administered heparin have failed.

Monitoring All patients are continuously monitored with a fiberoptic 7.5 Fr Swan-Ganz catheter to record mixed venous oxygen saturation. A percutaneous O_2 sensor is continuously in place. Blood gases, all ventilation and hemodynamic parameters, pressures and flow rates in the extracorporeal unit, the amount of heparin, and the ACT are recorded hourly. Samples for red blood cells, platelets, white blood cells, electrolytes, renal function parameters, and partial thromboplastin time are taken three times a day. Daily hemodynamic and respiratory function tests at FiO_2 of 1.0 with the measurement of $AaDo_2$, shunt, cardiac index, total static lung compliance, and extravascular lung water are performed. Bedside chest roentgenographic films are made. Other laboratory tests are performed as needed. Blood cultures are taken from the circuit every second day or whenever indicated. A complete microbiologic check is performed every third day. Thus, 106 variables are recorded for each patient during a single day on bypass. A note is made of all minor/major complications and problems.

With increased experience, the need to staff one patient on $ECco_2R$ has been reduced from one experienced physician and one nurse to one experienced nurse per patient.

Hemodynamics during bypass With the venovenous approach, hemodynamic problems are rare even at increased PEEP levels. There is a significant decline in the need for pharmacologic agents to sustain cardiocirculatory function following start of $ECco_2R$ (34).

Septic problems The possibility of septic complications increases with time on bypass. Sepsis is encountered in some 10% of patients. All attempts are made to identify the source of sepsis. Occasionally, the whole bypass circuit is exchanged, even if the circuit is not the likely origin of sepsis. The prophylactic application of antimicrobial drugs is not routine in the Marburg center.

Renal problems In patients with renal failure, hemofiltration is readily included in the extracorporeal perfusion circuit. Blood flows from the membrane lung through the hemofilter into the venous reservoir, using existing pressure gradients. Every attempt is made to keep the fluid balance negative or in balance.

Nutrition during bypass In the vast majority of patients, nutrition can be achieved via the nasogastric tube. In patients with additional needs, parenteral nutrition is instituted either instead of or in addition to enteral feeding.

Recent additions to patient management In addition to the introduction of percutaneous techniques for catheter implantation, there has been a preliminary report on the successful use of high-flow venovenous (VV) bypass (flow ≥75% of cardiac output) and intracardiac return of flow to ensure that no venous admixture occurs. This case involved a patient with respiratory failure, severe right heart failure (cardiac index = 1.2 L/min/m^2) from multiple pulmonary emboli, and severe pulmonary hypertension (38).

Meanwhile, there are initial promising experiences in some patients managed during bypass with mechanical ventilation at low peak inspiratory pressures and respiratory rates without apneic oxygenation, using much lower PEEP levels in combination with a markedly increased extracorporeal blood flow.

RESULTS

Mortality and Morbidity

By August 1990, more than 250 adults and children (excluding neonates) with severe forms of ARDS had been supported worldwide with $ECco_2R$ and LFPPV with apneic oxygenation. Because patient population, indications, contraindications, technique, and experience with extracorporeal support may vary from center to center, the results may be difficult to compare.

In centers with the most experience, all patients were supported with "maximal" conventional mechanical ventilation during the first hours or days after transfer from the referring hospital. They were connected to extracorporeal bypass if available conventional therapy did not lead to improved gas exchange.

Ninety-seven percent to 100% of the patients were transferred from other institutions. The average pretreatment time before transfer was 15.5 days for the Marburg group; the vast majority fulfilled either rapid- or slow-entry ECMO criteria (14,39).

In the Marburg experience, 39% of patients had posttraumatic respiratory failure, 23% had pneumonia, 13% had surgical and postsurgical complications (e.g., sepsis), 17% had complications during pregnancy and birth, and the rest had other underlying diseases such as asthma attack, bleeding, or inhalation of toxic

TABLE 20.8 Long-term survival

Group	Investigator/Country	Number of patients	Survival (%)
Monza/Milano	Gattinoni/Italy	73	48
Stockholm	Bindslev/Sweden	16	50
Salt Lake City	Morris/USA	40	38
Berlin	Falke/Germany	15	47
Paris	Brunet/France	14	43
Marburg	Lennartz/Germany	92	52

fumes (14,37). The average age in this group was 31 years (range 5 to 59). The peak inspiratory pressure (PIP) averaged 53 cm H_2O, $AaDo_2$ with an Fio_2 1.0 was 565 mm Hg, right-left shunt 41% at a average PEEP of 13 cm H_2O just before transfer to Marburg. Ninety-five percent of the patients were on dopamine, MOSF was present in 40%, and 25% had renal failure (Knoch M, unpublished data). Table 20.8 shows the total number of patients and the survival rates from some active centers (40).

The average bypass time was eight days for the Milan group and 15 days for the Marburg group. Recently, the Stockholm group reported one successful case following 54 days on bypass (Olsson E, personal communication. Washington, D.C.: ASAIO meeting, 1991).

The following parameters all appear to be reliable for assessing the clinical course of a patient on $ECco_2R$: changes in $AaDo_2$ at Fio_2 1.0, shunt, chest roentgenographic film, pulmonary artery pressures, TSLC, and extravascular lung water as measured by the double indicator technique.

Lung function improved sufficiently in more than 70% of all patients treated, and those patients were eventually weaned off bypass to CPAP or minimal ventilatory support (14). Some patients succumbed to the underlying disease processes and/or to complications from therapy either during bypass or during weaning following bypass.

Bleeding was the cause of death in 10% of all patients; the average daily transfusion of packed red blood cells was 500 to 1,370 cc/day (range 0–12.25 L), using the SciMed membrane lung (14,39). Platelet levels commonly remained stable; after an initial drop to about 55% at the start of bypass, the level remained between 140,000 and 160,000 throughout the bypass period in the absence of sepsis or bleeding.

Using the Carmeda system, the target anticoagulation level could be achieved with 10 to 20 units heparin/kg/h (Knoch M, unpublished data).

The overall incidence of barotrauma in all patients supported with $ECco_2R$ was 74%; 44% of all pneumothoraces occurred on $ECco_2R$ (14). As reported by Wagner et al. (41), thoracotomy was indicated in 32% of all patients with ARDS while on $ECco_2R$ for large bronchopleural fistula, bullas, pneumothoraces, segmental resection for necrosis, or other complications such as hemothorax. Overall survival rate in this group was 62%.

Hemodynamics remained stable during venovenous extracorporeal respiratory support. There was a general decrease in cardiocirculatory pharmacologic support. Following the start of $ECco_2R$, there was a general improvement in renal function which often occurred within hours after connection to the extracorporeal perfusion system (14,34).

Long-Term Follow-up

The long-term outlook for patients recovering from ARDS is excellent. Following $ECco_2R$, patients were transferred to a rehabilitation clinic. Static and dynamic lung function and spiroergometric tests performed just prior to transfer yielded readings 30% to 40% of normal. Three months later, all measurements had improved to 80% of normal. One year later, more than 90% of the patients showed full recovery in gas exchange, ventilation, and cardiocirculatory variables, and all were fully rehabilitated and had resumed their former activities (14).

Statistical Analysis

To improve selection criteria, we have attempted to predict responders from nonresponders among candidates for bypass at the time of bypass initiation. Gattinoni et al. (40) have shown that patients with ARDS and a TSLC ≤25 mL/cm H_2O have a poor chance of recovery on mechanical ventilation alone and are, therefore, good candidates for LFPPV-$ECco_2R$. Pesenti et al. (39) reported that the duration of preceding mechanical ventilation and elevated $Paco_2$ levels correlated negatively with ultimate outcome. Knoch et al. (14,37) have suggested that gas exchange and hemodynamic parameters before $ECco_2R$ correlate with outcome. In the presence of right heart failure, the outlook is uniformly poor, but this need not be so if, instead of VV bypass, these patients were to be placed on high-flow venoarterial (VA) bypass used for adult ECMO (42).

Regardless of these predictive indices, the decision to attempt VV/VA bypass still has to be made on an individual basis. Reports of greatly delayed response to bypass should not cause the exclusion of anyone who has even a remote chance of recovery.

Heparin-bonded systems: The Carmeda heparin-bonded system has been used on occasion by all major groups, either routinely or when indicated, in more than 50 patients worldwide.

Preliminary data show that the incidence of bleeding complications and daily blood loss are significantly reduced with use of the Carmeda systems (Knoch M, unpublished data). The amount of heparin used is also significantly reduced compared to conventional methods.

As stated earlier, the problem with the Carmeda system is plasma leakage. Hyperbilirubinemia, fat infusions, and drugs such as propofol seem to shorten the life span of these heparin-bonded lungs. Use time may also be influenced by temperature, humidity of the gases, flow rates, and transmembrane pressures. Despite the need to change the mechanical lung, survival rates seem unaffected and are reported to be 67% and better (Knoch M, Falke K, unpublished data). It is not clear whether these rates represent a general trend or are related to the use of the heparin-bonded systems or increased experience with $ECco_2R$ itself.

Nonetheless, the heparin-bonded systems may influence overall survival by reducing bleeding complications. Initial reports of successful major surgery in patients still on extracorporeal bypass are encouraging (43). Reduced risks from bleeding contraindications may permit support of patients with $ECco_2R$ earlier after trauma and/or surgical procedures.

DISCUSSION

The approach to ARDS remains supportive and hence symptomatic; our goal is to create an environment for optimal healing of the injured lungs. The question is posed whether mechanical ventilation at substantially elevated peak airway pressures can provide such an environment.

A review of the literature shows that mortality has been unchanged in ARDS over the last 20 years despite improvements in knowledge, techniques, and care. The reason remains to be elucidated (9,42).

Kolobow et al. (29) have shown that the main purpose of ventilation in patients breathing air enriched with oxygen is the removal of CO_2. Oxygenation can be achieved in apnea with an intratracheal oxygen flow alone (no breathing necessary). These results were confirmed by all active $ECco_2R$ centers, since even the sickest lungs were able to support the major part of oxygen demand via apneic oxygenation when FRC was maintained by PEEP. Hence, the need for mechanical ventilation in ARDS is reduced primarily to control of $Paco_2$ through alveolar ventilation. In patients with severe lung injury and reduced lung compliance, peak airway pressures by necessity become highly elevated, but at what price?

Greenfield et al. (44) reported as early as 1964 that severe pulmonary atelectasis occurred in dogs after two hours of mechanical ventilation at peak airway pressures of "only" 26 to 32 cm H_2O. Yet during the same period, mechanical ventilation was widely introduced for the clinical treatment of patients with acute respiratory failure, at airway pressures sometimes much greater than 30 cm H$_2$O. Also during the same time, Teplitz (1) described the changes in the appearance of the histopathologic picture of ARF.

Tsuno et al. (45) explored lung injury from mechanical ventilation at airway pressures of 30 cm H$_2$O. They observed a progressive deterioration in TSLC, FRC, and arterial blood gases; invariably, they found abnormal chest radiographic changes. At autopsy, there was severe pulmonary atelectasis, increased wet lung weight, and increased minimum surface tension of saline lung lavage fluid.

Borelli et al. (7) induced severe respiratory failure with MOSF and death within days of ventilating healthy laboratory animals at peak airway pressures of 50 cm H$_2$O. These studies provide us with new understanding of the adverse effects of mechanical ventilation. It is not "barotrauma" alone in the context of extraalveolar air that one has to contend with. Mechanical ventilation itself can contribute to the severity of pulmonary dysfunction and may be the prime reason to transform mild ARF into ARDS and MOSF, affecting ultimate survival.

Perhaps this is why mortality from ARDS has not changed during the last 20 years. This may be the main reason why results with ECCO$_2$R are so much better than with mechanical ventilation. Does this information not provide the laboratory proof of Teplitz's research and also explain the failure of the ECMO study? The real question is, what is the mechanism of this type of ventilator-induced lung injury?

As stated earlier, Dreyfuss et al. (8) have shown onset of permeability edema following the start of mechanical ventilation at high PIP, implicating changes in volume rather than in pressure as the likely mechanism of injury. Of course, in the normal course of ventilation, volume changes follow pressure changes.

Spontaneous hyperventilation alone of healthy lungs can also lead to severe respiratory failure and death in the absence of mechanical ventilation (46). It is therefore very likely that healthy lungs (or healthy parts of sick lungs) can, in fact, be destroyed by repeated ventilation.

Computed tomographic studies by Gattinoni et al. (47) have documented distribution of the disease process in ARDS. It is well accepted that, at the beginning of respiratory failure, not all of the lung is involved. As Pesenti et al. (48) pointed out:

> ... the lungs are patchy and dishomogeneous in ARDS. Areas of consolidation, edema, and/or atelectasis are interspersed with what appears to be normal parenchyma

and:

> The normal appearing lung is often reduced to 10%–20% of its usual amount, and this small residual healthy lung has to provide for the gas exchange of the whole adult body.

Thus, mechanical ventilation cannot provide homogeneous ventilation to all regions of the lung. Instead, mechanical ventilation greatly overinflates and, very possibly, injures healthy areas—the likely cause of progression from mild ARF to ARDS and MOSF.

The improvement in arterial blood gases as PIP increases has its price. The price we have to pay for this may be delayed by hours or days, but in the end it leads to further impairment in lung function and the appearance of MOSF (49).

Until now, results from the major ECCO$_2$R groups have shown that survival from severe ARDS can be improved to about 50% to 60% in a patient population with a risk for dying of at least 90%. The question is, why not do better?

The availability of percutaneous techniques and heparin-bonded systems seems to have improved the survival rate in the adult patient population (Knoch M, Falke K, unpublished data). The key to further improvement may be lung management comparable to that currently in practice in neonatal ECMO. The question remains: Can we improve our current method of lung management and create the necessary environment for optimal healing of the lungs?

The way out of this dilemma may be much higher extracorporeal flow rates, thereby eliminating the need for high PEEP levels and inspiratory pressures during ECCO$_2$R; this approach may enable us to keep patients on a more physiologic CPAP and thereby avoid the possibility of further lung injury from mechanical ventilation while on bypass.

There still remain some patients in whom damage to the lungs, failure of the cardiocirculatory system, and MOSF are so advanced that venovenous bypass techniques are insufficient; these patients are likely to benefit from a hybrid VV/VA bypass with flow rates of up to 150 cc/kg/min (46), just as in neonatal ECMO.

A more elegant approach to the problem is prevention of the progression of ARF into ARDS and MOSF. The evidence about ventilator-induced lung injury can no longer be denied. Other possibilities of respiratory support, like controlled hypoventilation (50–52), should be considered early in the course of ARF to avoid lung injury from ventilation at high peak airway pressures. The place of high-frequency ventilation in ARDS has not yet been defined (53).

Recently, we have explored in the laboratory setting a technique that greatly reduces anatomical dead space during mechanical ventilation (54). A continuous intratracheal flow of fresh humidified air/oxygen is introduced through a small catheter with a diffuser at its distal end placed at the level of the carina (Figure 20.2). The catheter can be placed through an endotracheal (tracheostomy) tube or possibly can be passed percutaneously. With a continuous gas flow of four times dead space per respiratory cycle (in adults, 4 × 120 cc = 48 cc), the anatomical dead space can be greatly reduced.

This new technique, intratracheal ventilation (ITV) or intratracheal pulmonary ventilation (ITPV), can be used for respiratory support either alone or in combination with other conventional forms of respiratory support (55). We have first applied this technique to studies in lungs in which the bulk of the lung was excised by surgical means in an attempt to develop effective techniques to ventilate very small lungs (54). We have used ITPV combined with mechanical ventilation in a pressure-controlled mode, with respiratory rate adjusted to between 60 and 120 breaths/min, to effect adequate alveolar ventilation. We could sustain gas exchange on room air in lungs as small as 12% of normal volume without any lung injury; the same lungs subsequently ventilated with mechanical ventilation so as to sustain adequate blood gases resulted, after a short "honeymoon" period, in severe lung injury with progressive hypoxemia, hypercapnia, and acidosis from which the animals died within 12 hours.

In spontaneously breathing patients, receiving either CPAP or no other form of respiratory support, ITV can reduce the work of breathing by greatly reducing anatomical dead space. It is possible that some patients now managed with mechanical ventilation can also be weaned to CPAP while on ITV. Similarly, patients with chronic obstructive lung disease (COPD) might also benefit from ITV alone or in combination. In adults and children, spontaneous breathing or mechanical ventilation with respiratory rates in excess of 60 breaths/min are often not cost-effective; with the new techniques of ITV/ITPV, this constraint no longer applies, and effective ventilation can be extended to respiratory rates between 60 and 120 breaths/min or higher. Higher respiratory rates allow lower tidal volumes, and hence lower PIP, greatly reducing or eliminating the risk of mechanical ventilation-induced lung injury.

However, there will still be patients with progressive respiratory failure in whom gas

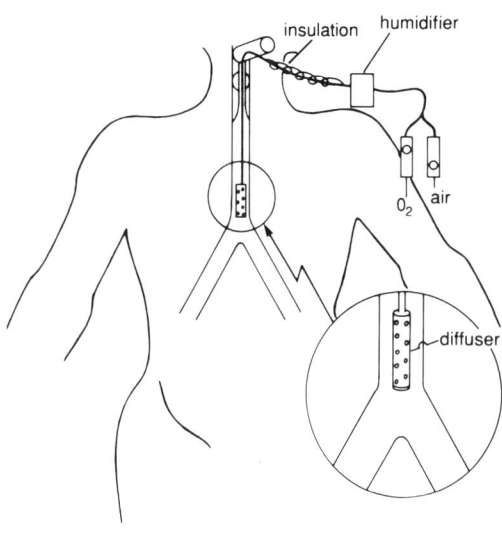

FIGURE 20.2 Diagrammatic representation of the apparatus used to accomplish oxygenation during apneic ventilation.

exchange on mechanical ventilation and ITV/ITPV can no longer be achieved at airway pressures within safe limits, based on studies discussed earlier. These patients may then be placed on partial extracorporeal bypass (ECco$_2$R) using heparinized perfusion systems. This type of support, when employed using the emerging techniques as described earlier, is safe in the hands of experienced personnel.

Physicians are now at a point at which indications for ECco$_2$R can be considered much earlier, for example, when MOSF is first recognized (e.g., when we start to give furosemide and dopamine). At that point, extracorporeal support should be considered when the patient fulfills entry criteria. One is remiss to wait until extracorporeal life support becomes the last resort, and ultimate outcome for the patient will be affected by the appearance of MOSF.

REFERENCES

(1) Teplitz CC. The core pathobiology and integrated medical science of adult respiratory insufficiency. Surg Clin North Am 1976;56:1091–133.

(2) Moon VH. The pathology of secondary shock. Am J Pathol 1948;24:235–73.

(3) Puttermann C. Adult respiratory distress syndrome: current concepts. Resuscitation 1988;16:91–105.

(4) Ashbaugh DG, Bigelow DB, Petty TL, Levine BE. Acute respiratory distress in adults. Lancet 1967;2:319–23.

(5) Langlois PF, Gawryl MS, Zeller J, Lint T. Accentuated complement activated in patient plasma during the adult respiratory distress syndrome: a potential mechanism for pulmonary inflammation. Heart Lung 1989;18:71–84.

(6) Kolobow T, Gattinoni L, Solca M, Pesenti A. A new approach to the prevention and the treatment of acute respiratory failure in the adult and the neonate. Appl Cardiopulmonary Pathophysiol 1989;3:135–46.

(7) Borelli M, Kolobow T, Spatola R, Prato P, Tsuno K. Severe acute respiratory failure managed with continuous positive airway pressure and partial extracorporeal carbon dioxide removal by an artificial membrane lung. Am Rev Respir Dis 1988;138:1480–7.

(8) Dreyfuss D, Soler P, Basset G, Saumon G. High inflation pressure pulmonary edema. Respective effects of high airway pressure, high tidal volume and positive end-expiratory pressure. Am Rev Respir Dis 1988;137:1159–64.

(9) Hickling KG. Ventilatory management of ARDS: can it effect the outcome? Intens Care Med 1990; 16:219–26.

(10) Müller E. Adult respiratory distress syndrome. Activation of complement, coagulation and fibrinolytic systems. Biomedical Progress 1991;1 (in press).

(11) Rinaldo JE. Mediation of ARDS by leukocytes. Clinical evidence and implication for therapy. Chest 1986;89:590–3.

(12) Artigas A. Adult respiratory distress syndrome: changing concepts of clinical evolution and recovery. In: Vincent JL, ed. Update in intensive care and emergency medicine 5. Berlin: Springer Verlag, 1988.

(13) Rollins RJ, Morris AH, Mortensen CJ. Arterial hypoxemia in 1976 predicts a mortality identical to that in 1985 (Abstract). Clin Res 1986;34:79A.

(14) Knoch M. Treatment of severe ARDS with extracorporeal CO$_2$ removal. In: Gille JP, ed. Neonatal and adult respiratory failure. Mechanisms and treatment. Paris: Editions Scientifiques Elsevier, 1989.

(15) Bell RC, Coalson JJ, Smith JD, Johanson WG. Multiple organ system failure and infection in adult respiratory distress syndrome. Ann Intern Med 1983;99:293–8.

(16) Maunder RJ, Kubilis PS, Anardi DM, Hudson LD. Determinants of survival in the adult respiratory distress syndrome (ARDS) (Abstract). Am Rev Respir Dis 1989;140:A220.

(17) Zapol WM, Snider MT, Hill JD, et al. Extracorporeal membrane oxygenation in severe acute respiratory failure. JAMA 1979;242:2193–6.

(18) Bartlett RH, Morris AH, Fairley HB, Hirsch R, O'Connor N, Pontopiddan H. A prospective study of acute hypoxic respiratory failure. Chest 1986;89:684–9.

(19) Kolobow T, Gattinoni L, Pesenti A, et al. ECMO revisited. Int J Artif Organs 1987;10:1–2.

(20) Montgomery AB, Stager MA, Corrico CJ, Hudson LD. Causes of mortality in patients with the ARDS. Am Rev Respir Dis 1985;132:485–9.

(21) Lakshminarayan S, Stanford RE, Petty TL. Prognosis after recovery of adult respiratory

(22) Gattinoni L, Pesenti A, Mascheroni D, et al. Low-frequency positive-pressure ventilation with extracorporeal CO_2 removal in severe acute respiratory failure. JAMA 1986;256:881–6.

(23) Hill JD, O'Brien TG, Murray JJ, et al. Extracorporeal oxygenation for acute post-traumatic respiratory failure (shock-lung syndrome): use of the Bramson Membrane Lung. N Engl J Med 1972;286:629–34.

(24) Schulte HD. Membrane oxygenators in prolonged assisted extracorporeal circulation. Deutsche Medizinische Wochenschrift 1973;98:508.

(25) Geelhoed GW, Adkins PC, Corso PJ, Joseph WL. Clinical effects of membrane lung support for acute respiratory failure. Ann Thorac Surg 1975;20:177–86.

(26) Gille JP, Bagniewski AM. Ten years of use of extracorporeal membrane oxygenation (ECMO) in the treatment of acute respiratory insufficiency (ARI). Trans ASAIO 1976;22:102.

(27) Pratt PC, Vollmer RT, Shelburn JD, et al. Pulmonary morphology in a multihospital collaborative extracorporeal membrane oxygenation project. Am J Pathol 1979;95:191–212.

(28) Kolobow T. An update on adult extracorporeal membrane oxygenation—extracorporeal CO_2 removal. Trans ASAIO 1988;34:1004–5.

(29) Kolobow T, Gattinoni L, Tomlinson TA, Pierce JE. Control of breathing using an extracorporeal membrane lung. Anesthesiology 1977;46:138–41.

(30) Frumin MJ, Epstein RM, Cohen G. Apneic oxygenation in man. Anesthesiology 1959;20:789–98.

(31) Kolobow T, Gattinoni L, Tomlinson T. An alternative to breathing. J Thorac Cardiovasc Surg 1978;75:261–6.

(32) Gattinoni L, Kolobow T, Tomlinson T, et al. Low frequency positive pressure ventilation and extracorporeal carbon dioxide removal (LFPPV-$ECCO_2R$): an experimental study. Anaesth Analg 1978;55:470–7.

(33) Gattinoni L, Agostoni A, Pesenti A, et al. Treatment of acute respiratory failure with low-frequency positive pressure ventilation and extracorporeal removal of CO_2. Lancet 1980;2:292–4.

(34) Gattinoni L, Agostoni A, Damia G, et al. Hemodynamics and renal function during low frequency positive pressure ventilation with extracorporeal CO_2 removal. Intens Care Med 1980;6:155–61.

(35) Pesenti A, Kolobow T, Riboni A, et al. Single vein cannulation for extracorporeal respiratory support. Life Support Systems 1982;1:165–7.

(36) Morel DR, Dargent F, Bachmann M, Suter PM, Junod AF. Pulmonary extraction of serotonin and propanolol in patients with adult respiratory distress syndrome. Am Rev Respir Dis 1985;132:479–82.

(37) Knoch M, Müller E, Höltermann W, Wagner PK, Lennartz H. Extracorporale CO_2-Elimination. Deutsche Medizinische Wochenschrift 1989;114:796–9.

(38) Knoch M, Iverson S, Härtel B, Kussmann J, Sangmeister C. Behandlung einer protrahierten Hypoxie mit dem "high flow" veno-venösen Langzeitbypass und anschließender Thrombendarteriektomie (TEA) der Pulmonalgefäße bei einer jungen Patientin mit chronisch-rezidivierenden Lungenembolien. Thorac Cardiovasc Surg I 1990;38:49–50.

(39) Pesenti A, Gattinoni L, Kolobow T, Damia G. Extracorporeal circulation in adult respiratory failure. Trans ASAIO 1988;11:43–7.

(40) Gattinoni L, Pesenti A, Caspani ML, et al. The role of total static lung compliance in the management of severe ARDS unresponsive to conventional treatment. Intens Care Med 1984;10:121–6.

(41) Wagner PK, Knoch M, Sangmeister C, Müller E, Lennartz H, Rothmund M. Extracorporeal gas exchange in adult respiratory distress syndrome (ARDS). New associated morbidity and its surgical treatment. Br J Surg 1990;77;1395–8.

(42) Kolobow T. Acute respiratory failure. On how to injure healthy lungs (and prevent sick lungs from recovering). Trans ASAIO 1988;11:31–4.

(43) Weidemann H, Fray D, Kaiser D, et al. Major thoracic surgical procedures during $ECCO_2$ removal with heparin coated extracorporeal systems. Thorac Cardiovasc Surg I 1990;38 (Suppl):129.

(44) Greenfield LJ, Ebert PA, Benson DW. Effect of positive pressure ventilation on surface tension properties of lung extracts. Anesthesiology 1964;25:312–16.

(45) Tsuno K, Prato P, Kolobow T. Acute lung injury from mechanical ventilation at moderately high airway pressures. J Appl Physiol 1990;69:956–61.

(46) Mascheroni D, Kolobow T, Fumagalli R, Moretti MP, Chen V, Buckhold D. Acute respiratory failure following pharmacologically induced hyperventilation: an experimental animal study. Intens Care Med 1988;15:8–14.

(47) Gattinoni L, Pesenti A, Bombino M, et al. Relationships between lung computed tomography density, gas exchange, and PEEP in acute respiratory failure. Anesthesiology 1988;69:824–32.

(48) Pesenti A, Kolobow T, Gattinoni L. Extracorporeal respiratory support in the adult. Trans ASAIO 1988;24:1006–8.

(49) Kolobow T. The (ir)relevance of short term studies. Int J Artif Organs 1990;13:1–2.

(50) Lee PC, Helsmoortel CM, Cohn SM, Fink MP. Are low tidal volumes safe? Chest 1990;97:425–9.

(51) Hickling KG, Henderson SJ, Jackson R. Low mortality associated with low volume pressure limited ventilation with permissive hypercapnia in severe adult respiratory distress syndrome. Intens Care Med 1990;16:372–7.

(52) Wung JT, James LS, Kilchevsky E, James E. Management of severe respiratory failure with persistence of the fetal circulation without hyperventilation. Pediatrics 1985;76:488–94.

(53) Carlon GC, Howland SW, Ray C, et al. High frequency jet ventilation. A prospective randomized evaluation. Chest 1983;84:551–9.

(54) Müller E, Kolobow T, Mandava S, et al. On how to ventilate lungs as small as 12% of normal. Intratracheal pulmonary ventilation (ITPV). A new mode of pulmonary ventilation. Ann Arbor, Mi: Extracorporeal Life Support Organization (ELSO), Annual Meeting, November 1990.

(55) Kolobow T, Müller E, Mandava S, et al. Intratracheal ventilation (ITV), and intratracheal pulmonary ventilation (ITPV). A technique whose time has come. Ann Arbor, MI: Extracorporeal Life Support Organization (ELSO), Annual Meeting, November 1990.

21

Extracorporeal Membrane Oxygenation Therapy for Cardiac Disease

❖

Michael D. Klein, M.D.
Grant C. Whittlesey

HISTORY

Heart-Lung Machines for Open Heart Surgery

Heart-lung machines for temporary support during open heart surgery trace their development back to the early work of Alexis Carrel and Charles Lindbergh (1) at the Rockefeller Institute in New York. They were able to maintain a cat thyroid gland for 18 days.

The work of many investigators culminated in the first open heart procedure performed with extracorporeal circulation by John Gibbon in 1954 (2). Much of the work in developing these devices was made possible by Gordon Murray's 1938 (3) introduction of heparin as a clinical drug to provide anticoagulation. Using the direct blood-gas interface of a bubble oxygenator, perfusion times much longer than a few hours resulted in damage to the cellular elements of the blood, as well as denaturation and conversion of plasma proteins to toxic peptides (4,5). Long-term pulmonary support was made possible by the development of membrane oxygenators used by Clowes et al. (6) and Kolobow and Bowman (7). It is this avoidance of a direct blood-gas interface that permits long-term extracorporeal gas exchange, as well as circulation.

Extracorporeal Circulatory Support

In 1956, Dennis (8) reported results of studies using extracorporeal support for the failing heart which could be expected to recover following either surgery or a period of medical treatment (8). The most commonly applied form of this support is the intraaortic balloon pump (IABP), utilizing a counterpulsation technique first suggested by Harken (unpublished presentation at the International College of Cardiology meeting in Brussels, Belgium, 1958) and introduced clinically by Kantrowicz (9). This device improves coronary blood flow during ventricular diastole by rapid balloon inflation, which augments aortic root pressure. Balloon deflation during systole reduces afterload, assisting ventricular ejection, and decreases ventricular end-diastolic pressure. It is particularly appropriate for left heart failure with ischemic myocardial disease. Most children, however, do not have this form of cardiac disease. Moreover, in children, there is increased risk of local arterial injury to the small femoral artery. The IABP is generally ineffective for right heart failure, and it offers limited circulatory assistance at the rapid heart rate of a child. A group at the University of Utah (10) has had some success with specially designed balloons. A pulmonary artery balloon for support of the right heart has been proposed for use either alone or in combination with IABP, but this has not been tested clinically (11).

Left-sided extracorporeal assist devices have demonstrated success in adults, but they do not address right heart failure (12). This is usually done by cannulating the left atrium and perfusing the aorta (Figure 21.1). Incorporating a centrifugal pump will avoid the necessity of controlling the flow rate based on the venous return. These devices are frequently, although not always, used with systemic heparin and offer no control over oxygenation and ventilation. Right-sided extracorporeal pump assist devices are theoretically attractive (13), but access to the pulmonary artery for perfusion is difficult, and direct perfusion of the pulmonary artery can have a deleterious effect on the lung (Figure 21.2) (14).

Ventricular assist devices that are attached directly to the heart offer the advantage of requiring little or no anticoagulation, but they require major operative procedures in the chest and could interfere with the anatomic repair of congenital heart disease. We have previously demonstrated that venovenous ECMO (15,16), in which oxygenated blood is returned to the systemic venous system (Figure 21.3), can salvage newborns dying of respiratory failure (17). This approach may correct acidosis and hypertension enough to treat pulmonary vascular reactive crisis and may have some applications for cardiac support in children who frequently begin with right-sided failure.

In 1988, the Hemopump axial flow pump (Nimbus Inc., Rancho Cordova, California) was introduced for the support of arterial perfusion (18). This device is essentially a 12-French rotor and inlet cannula which is passed, on its 9-French flexible drive shaft, through the

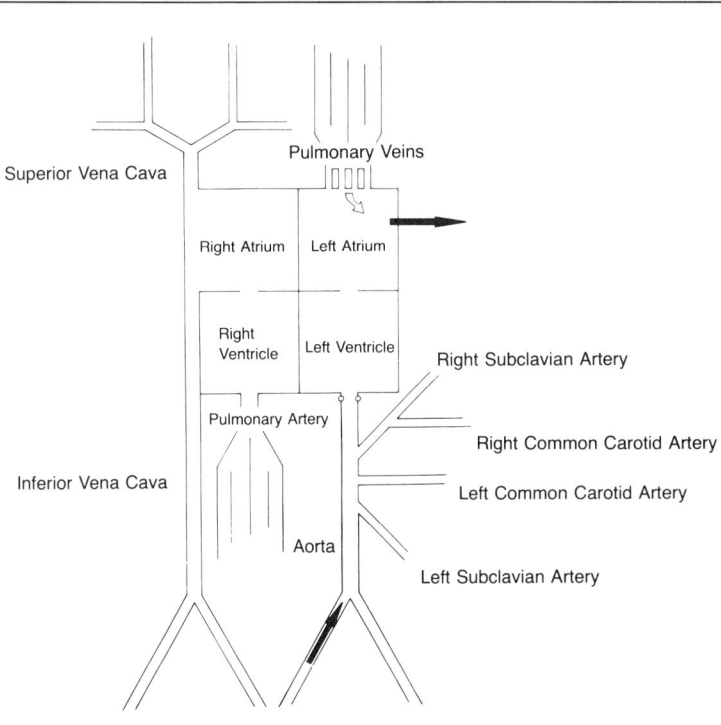

FIGURE 21.1 Schematic presentation of left heart assist cannulation. Solid arrows indicate cannula position. Outlined arrows indicate flow patterns.

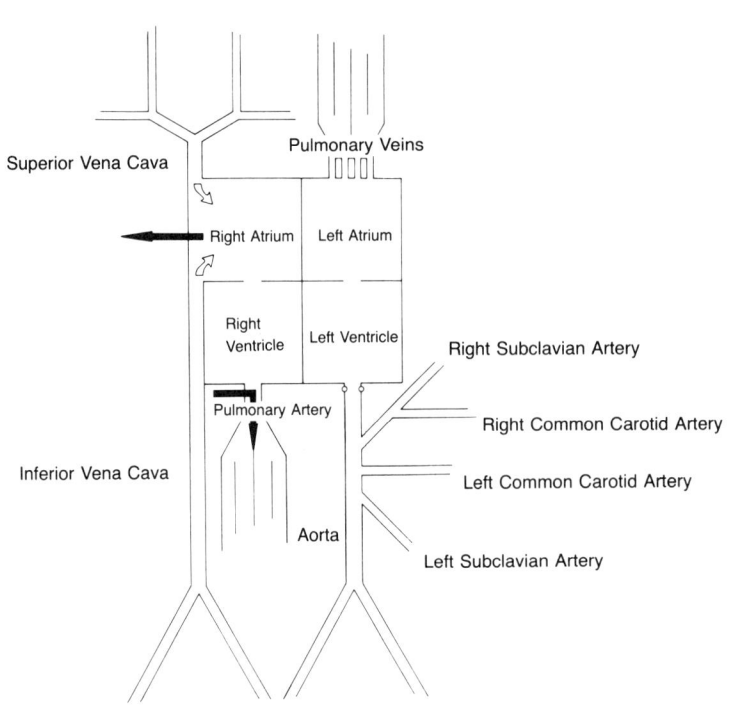

FIGURE 21.2 Schematic presentation of right heart assist cannulation. Solid arrows indicate cannula position. Outlined arrows indicate flow patterns.

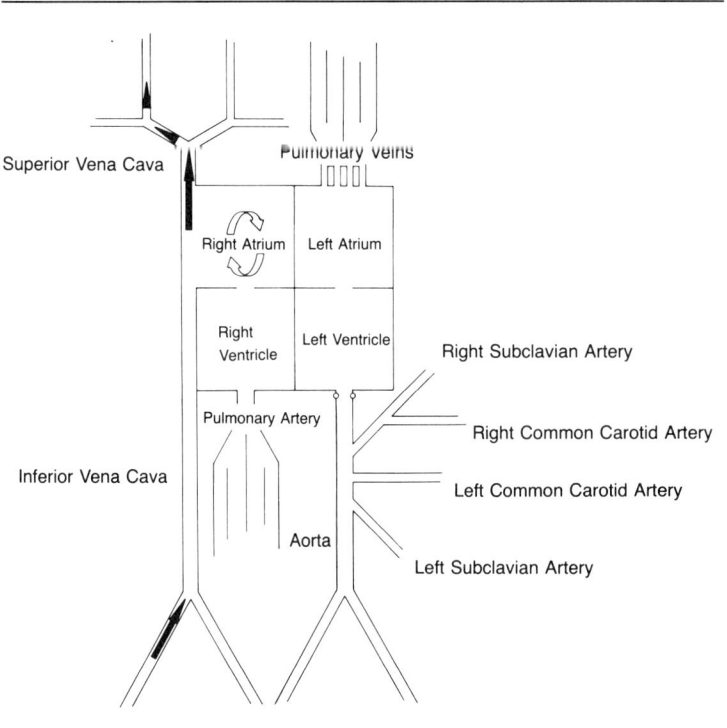

FIGURE 21.3 Schematic presentation of venovenous ECMO cannulation. Solid arrows indicate cannula position. Outlined arrows indicate flow patterns.

aortic valve into the left ventricle from the femoral artery. Blood from the left ventricle is pumped down the aorta to assist arterial perfusion. Its disadvantages in children are similar to those of the IABP.

ECMO

Why consider ECMO for cardiac support? The standard ECMO circuit used for pulmonary support in newborns was not developed specifically with cardiac support in mind. Draining venous blood from the right side of the heart will unload the right ventricle; however, no support for the right ventricle in terms of perfusion of the pulmonary artery is provided. Blood is pumped into the aortic arch supporting the peripheral circulation, but coronary artery perfusion is not provided, and no provision whatsoever is made for decompressing the left heart (Figure 21.4). The left heart is unloaded by decreasing the pulmonary venous return. As blood is removed from the right heart, less flow goes through the lungs.

Two factors have attracted interest in ECMO for cardiac support, especially in children. The first is its convenience of application in the intensive care unit; the second is the availability at many medical centers of a skilled team able to apply this technology at a moment's notice and to care for a patient continuously during its application. In addition, other methods of mechanical support, such as the left ventricular assist device or the intraaortic balloon pump, are often not applicable after the repair of congenital heart disease.

Early use of ECMO for cardiac support Baffes et al. (19) in 1970 were the first to report long-term extracorporeal circulation for the support of children with congenital heart disease. They used this mainly as an adjunct to palliative surgery. In 1972, Hill et al. (20) first reported a survivor who was treated with ECMO in Dusseldorf following repair of tetralogy of Fallot. Soeter et al. (21) reported a similar success in 1973. In 1975, Pyle et al. (22) included two patients treated for cardiac failure in his ECMO

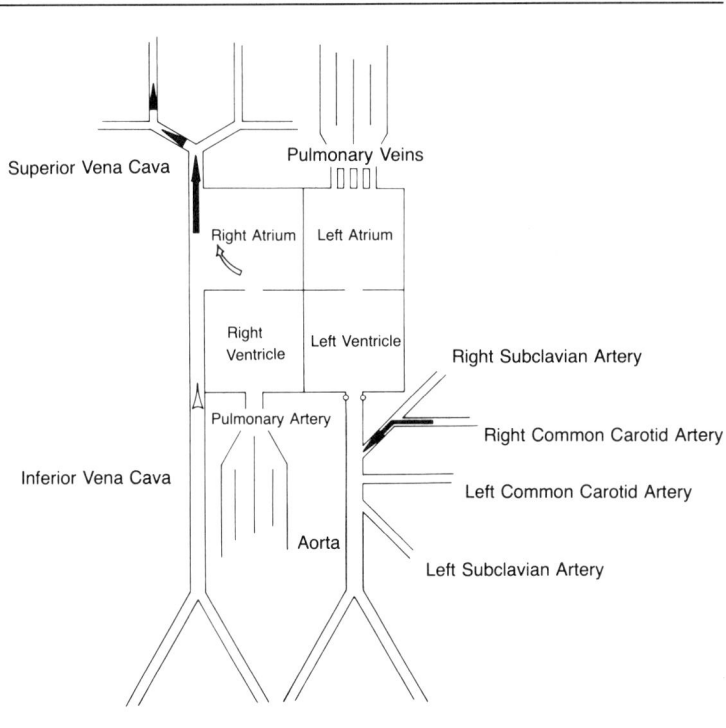

FIGURE 21.4 Schematic presentation of standard venoarterial ECMO cannulation. Solid arrows indicate cannula position. Outlined arrows indicate flow patterns.

series of nine patients. Neither survived. In 1977, Bartlett et al. (23) reported four patients with postcardiotomy cardiogenic shock who were treated with ECMO. One two-year-old treated for 36 hours immediately following a Mustard procedure survived. Since the other patients treated were on ECMO for 15 hours or less, one suspects that they had irreversible organ damage at the time that ECMO was initiated.

INDICATIONS FOR ECMO FOR CARDIAC SUPPORT

General Indications

ECMO has been used for temporary cardiac support in both adults and children. Indications have included low cardiac output from uni- or biventricular failure following the repair of congenital heart defects. In most children, biventricular failure appears to follow from right heart failure. In addition to low cardiac output, children can develop a pulmonary vasoreactive crisis following repair of congenital heart disease, which leads to severe hypoxemia and cardiac arrest (24). This reversible pulmonary artery hypertension is treated on ECMO by both decreasing pulmonary circulation with drainage of the right atrium and by providing oxygen to increase pulmonary arteriolar dilatation.

ECMO has also been used as a bridge to surgery in patients with life-threatening cardiac failure. Most patients requiring extracorporeal support as a bridge to surgery have undergone sudden decompensation, making the applicability of ECMO dependent on its instant availability. However, some patients who have undergone slow decompensation can be placed on ECMO to stabilize them prior to operation. Other patients, especially those with total anomalous pulmonary venous return, may not tolerate induction of anesthesia, thoracotomy, and cannulation for open heart surgery. These patients can be stabilized on ECMO to permit unhurried repair (25). ECMO has been suggested for temporary emergency room support of adults in cardiogenic shock, to stabilize them for further evaluation and treatment (26). This can be instituted using percutaneous inserted femoral arterial and venous cannulas, a centrifugal pump, and membrane oxygenator. This type of urgent application would require that equipment be constantly ready with a crystalloid prime and that experienced personnel be available.

ECMO as a bridge to transplantation requires the availability of an experienced transplant team or a team experienced in the transport of patients on ECMO, as well as the availability of a donor heart (27). ECMO has also been used to treat the cardiac failure accompanying rejection following cardiac transplantation, and survival is reported (Behrendt, D, personal communication).

Of a more speculative nature is the use of ECMO to treat temporary cardiomyopathies which are usually secondary to some other life-threatening disease such as renal failure, severe burns, or myocarditis. ECMO can also be used to treat pulmonary complications following cardiac disease and cardiac surgery.

Practical and Specific Indications

With any form of extracorporeal life support, perhaps the most difficult problem is knowing when to apply the technique. Given the novelty of such therapy and the twin hazards of anticoagulation and major vessel cannulation, there is currently fair agreement that such techniques should be applied only in situations where other forms of therapy are unsuccessful. In cardiac support, alternate forms of therapy that should be utilized first include mechanical ventilation and pharmacologic support with inotropes (dopamine, dobutamine, amrinone lactate, isoproterenol, and epinephrine) and afterload-reducing agents (nitroprusside and nitroglycerin). In patients with pulmonary vasoreactive crisis, agents that dilate the pulmonary arterial tree such as tolazoline, nitroglycerin, and prostaglandin E_1 are also used. Optimal cardiac rhythm must be achieved by normalizing serum electrolytes, use of appropriate drugs, or electrical pacing. In addition, some mechanical devices, such as intermittent abdominal compression (28) and IABP, have been useful. Monitoring of fluid, drug, and ventilator management is critically important. In children, this includes right atrial, left atrial, pulmonary arterial, and systemic arterial pressures, and, in some cases, cardiac output. It is also important to evaluate the anatomic result in postoperative patients carefully to be sure that reoperation is not the treatment of choice.

The Children's Hospital of Michigan Predictor Study

In order to develop some objective criteria to determine who might need extracorporeal life support following surgery for congenital heart disease, we reviewed 312 children at the Children's Hospital of Michigan undergoing open heart surgery between January 1984 and June 1985 (29). Twenty-seven patients (8.7%) died during the early postoperative period. Of these, three patients could not come off bypass and died in the operating room. Twelve of the remaining 24 patients died by eight hours postoperatively, and only five were alive 16 hours following operation. Between patients who lived and patients who died, we found statistically significant differences for age, weight, circulatory arrest time, aortic cross-clamp time, heart rate, systolic blood pressure, right atrial pressure, left atrial pressure, urine output, isoproterenol dose, dopamine dose, volume of colloid administered, volume of crystalloid administered, volume of blood administered, FiO_2, PaO_2, pH, and ventilator rate (Table 21.1).

Translating these differences into rules for predicting mortality was more difficult. Our best guidelines combined two indicators of cardiac output: dopamine dose and urine output. Of the nonsurvivors, 91% had both a urine output <1.2 mL/h and a dopamine infusion >5 µg/kg/min at one hour postoperatively, compared with only 3.1% of all the survivors. Eight hours postoperatively, 82% of those who died had a urine output <2 mL/kg/h and required >10 µg/kg/min of dopamine, compared to only 2.8% of the survivors.

The elegant studies of Kirklin et al. (30) add support to the necessity of evaluating children early in the postoperative course for predictors of mortality. As in our group, they noted that mortality increased significantly in patients with complex cardiac disease. They found that mortality for ventricular septal defect (VSD) repair had decreased and become unrelated to age at operation. However, when VSD was associated with another major lesion, the overall mortality remained high (24%) and was increased further at younger ages (31). They noted that, of a total of 174 patients younger than three months of age who underwent open heart procedures, 142 left the operating room alive (82%). Of these, 43 died postoperatively (30%), for a total mortality of 43%. Among all variables measured, only the nurses' subjective evaluations of the pedal pulses and pedal skin temperature and the measured cardiac index in the first five hours after operation were significantly related to mortality. While our predictors are different, we agree that there is a subgroup of patients operated on for congenital heart disease who have a high mortality and who might benefit from extraordinary means of support.

As time passes, new drugs are introduced, new methods of ventilation are developed, and new techniques of assessing cardiopulmonary function become available. We feel that the message of both the Detroit and Alabama predictor studies is the same: Children with postoperative cardiac failure are often more ill than we suspect. Extraordinary means of support should be considered when *moderate* (not maximal) levels of "conventional" management have been employed, and cardiac output is still inadequate.

CANNULATION TECHNIQUES

Neck

Most children placed on ECMO for cardiac support, including those cannulated in the operating room because they cannot come off bypass postoperatively, have had standard neck cannulation as used in newborns. This involves cannulation of the right atrium via the right internal jugular vein and the aortic arch via the right common carotid artery (Figure 21.4). In most cases, this does not prevent flow to the right subclavian artery. There is controversy as to whether this deleteriously affects cerebral circulation and whether the coronary arteries are adequately perfused. A steal effect may occur by jetting blood flow down the

TABLE 21.1 Differences in patients living and dying following open heart surgery for congenital heart disease (29)

	Hour 1			Hour 8		
Parameter	Lived	P<	Died	Lived	P<	Died
Age (mo)	45.2 ± 59	0.01	13.7 ± 26.7	NA*	NA	NA
Weight (kg)	14.4 ± 13.9	0.01	6.4 ± 5.3	NA	NA	NA
Circulatory arrest time (min)	44.8 ± 18.8	0.01	69.1 ± 31.9	NA	NA	NA
Aortic cross-clamp time (min)	80.2 ± 32.3	0.05	107 ± 49.1	NA	NA	NA
Heart rate	125 ± 33	0.01	149 ± 21	126 ± 22	0.05	144 ± 41
Systolic blood pressure (mm Hg)	112 ± 23	0.01	86 ± 23	86 ± 23	0.001	83 ± 24
Left atrial pressure (mm Hg)	14 ± 5	NS†	17 ± 5	16 ± 5	0.05	21 ± 5
Right atrial pressure (mm Hg)	15 ± 5	0.01	24 ± 7	17 ± 4	0.05	21 ± 9
Urine output (mL/kg/min)	3.35 ± 4.27	0.01	1.12 ± 0.90	2.4 ± 1.5	0.01	1.51 ± 0.92
Isoproterenol (μg/kg/min)	0.11 ± 0.18	NS	0.13 ± 0.09	0.06 ± 0.07	0.05	0.34 ± 0.38
Dopamine (μg/kg/min)	2.29 ± 3.76	0.01	14.13 ± 8.38	7.2 ± 3.5	0.001	19.4 ± 10.1
Colloid administered (mL/kg/h)	9.6 ± 5.9	NS	12.9 ± 3.2	3.2 ± 2.2	0.01	5.7 ± 3.4
Crystalloid administered (mL/kg/h)	2.0 ± 1.0	0.001	3.7 ± 2.8	1.8 ± 0.7	NS	2.2 ± 1.0
Blood administered (mL/kg/h)	9.6 ± 6.9	NS	11.9 ± 5.9	3.2 ± 2.4	0.05	5.2 ± 3.8
Fio_2	0.79 ± 0.08	0.01	0.9 ± 0.1	0.50 ± 0.13	0.001	0.77 ± 0.27
Pao_2	237 ± 106	0.05	168 ± 134	130 ± 40	0.01	75 ± 33
Ventilator rate	21 ± 2.8	0.01	25 ± 6	19.8 ± 5.4	0.01	26.1 ± 8.8
pH	7.39 ± 0.08	0.01	7.26 ± 0.11	7.45 ± 0.06	0.05	7.33 ± 0.18

*NA = not applicable.
†NS = not significant.

aortic arch away from the coronaries. In our own experience at the Children's Hospital of Michigan, there have been very few complications with this technique, and all occurred in newborns being treated for respiratory failure. One arterial cannula entered the right subclavian artery and perfused only the arm. One patient's arterial cannula had gone through the aortic valve into the left ventricle. Both of these problems were easily managed by repositioning the cannula. We have had only one dissection of the carotid intima, treated by removal of the cannula and cannulation of the femoral vein for venovenous ECMO. Neck cannulation has the advantage of speed and easy availability in the intensive care unit. The cannulas are stable, and operative site bleeding is minimal.

Weinhaus et al. (32) in 1989 reported several patients who had both the carotid artery and internal jugular vein repaired following decannulation of the neck. The groups in New Orleans, Cleveland, and San Francisco are also selectively repairing the carotid artery (although not necessarily the internal jugular vein). We have three concerns with carotid reconstruction: 1) there is no evidence that there is a deficit that carotid reconstruction might avoid, 2) embolic phenomena, later turbulent flow, and plaque formation at a stenotic area are possibilities, and 3) whatever damage might be done by ligation of the carotid artery has already been done unless proximal cannulation during ECMO is performed, and one might conceivably induce a reperfusion injury.

Chest

Certain patients are not anatomically suitable for neck cannulation. In our group, this included a patient with a prior left carotid artery ligation for repair of coarctation of the aorta, as well as several patients with Mustard-type repairs in whom it was felt the cannulas might obstruct systemic venous return. We cannulated these patients through the chest in the standard fashion of bypass for cardiac surgery with catheters in the right atrial appendage and the aortic arch. When using chest cannulation, we used Gortex pericardial patch material to cover the chest wall defect. There have been no accidental decannulations of the arch or the atrium. The St. Louis University group (33) reported mediastinitis in three of eight patients using chest cannulation, but neither our group nor others (34) have found this a significant problem. This technique allows for easy decompression of mediastinal tamponade but requires transport to the operating room for both cannulation and decannulation.

Cannulation via the chest allows separate left heart decompression, which we have accomplished by cannulation of the left atrium (Figure 21.5). We have found this especially

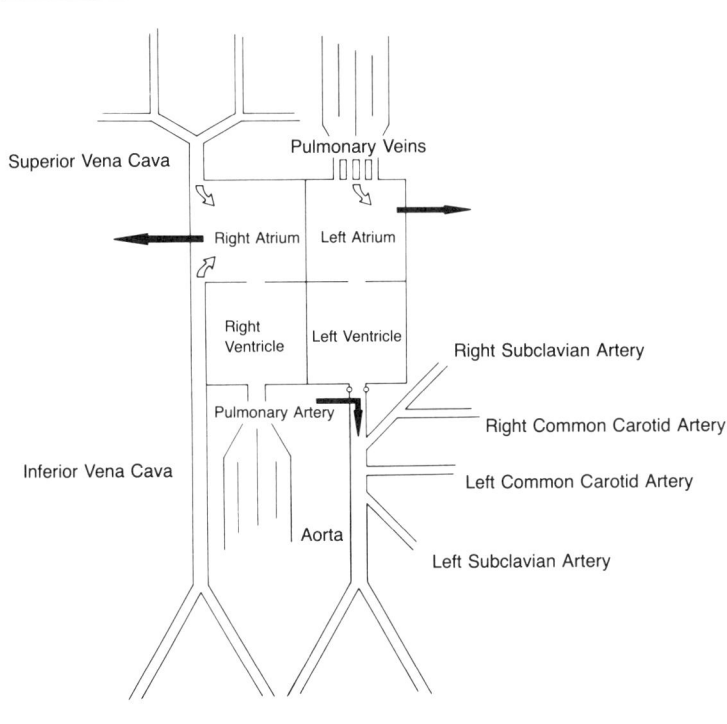

FIGURE 21.5 Schematic presentation of transthoracic cannulation, including left heart decompression. Solid arrows indicate cannula position. Outlined arrows indicate flow patterns.

useful when, after cannulation of the right atrium, there is still significant left heart distension. This probably occurs in patients with primary left heart failure. By using this biatrial cannulation technique, we have obtained our only two survivors among children cannulated in the operating room because they could not come off bypass. We originally believed that our patients who survived directly from the operating room did so because of separate left heart drainage, but it may be because of better coronary profusion with an aortic arch cannula.

Bavaria et al. (35) have noted that ECMO causes progressive increased left ventricular systolic wall stress in the failing heart. Animal studies by Eugene et al. (36) also indicate that for ECMO to be successful in the ischemic heart, left ventricular venting is necessary. Our microsphere flow studies both in rabbits (37) and sheep (38) show a decrease in the percent of cannula flow going to the myocardium. Coronary perfusion consists mainly of the small amount of relatively unoxygenated blood ejected from the left ventricle. This correlates with the anatomic finding of subendocardial ischemia in our animals. Further elucidation of blood flow patterns in patients on ECMO with various forms of cannulation will be necessary before we can fully understand the effect of ECMO on the myocardium.

Kolobow et al. (39) have reported an ingenious technique for decompressing the left side of the heart without direct chest access. This is done by using a percutaneous catheter which floats through the right atrium and right ventricle into the pulmonary artery (Figure 21.6). A special spring coiled on the catheter renders the pulmonary valve partially incompetent. Retrograde pulmonary blood flow then decompresses the left side of the heart as the venous blood drains into the ECMO circuit.

Axillary

Other cannulation techniques have been described but are not in routine use. Wickline et al. (40) investigated axillary artery cannulation

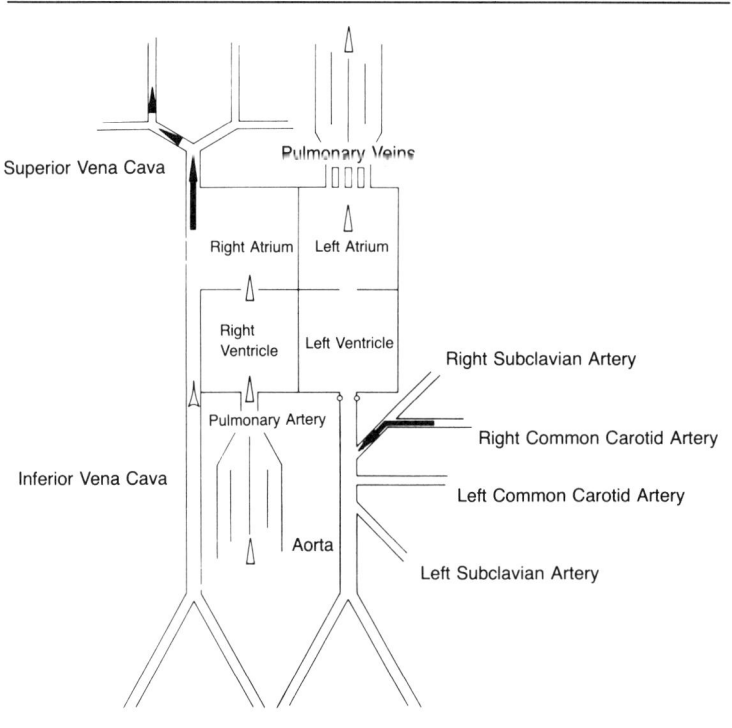

FIGURE 21.6 Schematic presentation of venoarterial ECMO, with pulmonary artery spring catheter for left heart decompression. Solid arrows indicate cannula position. Outlined arrows indicate flow patterns.

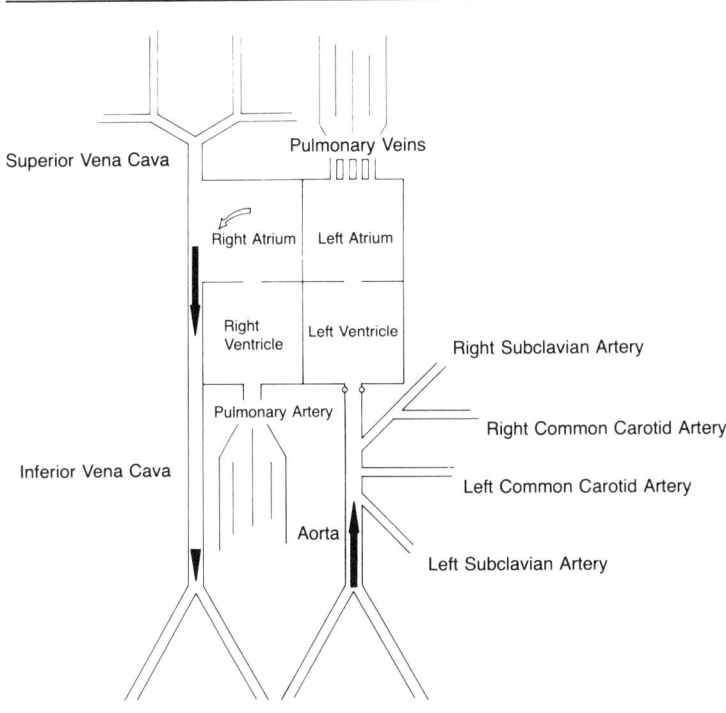

FIGURE 21.7 Schematic presentation of femoral artery and vein ECMO cannulation. Solid arrows indicate cannula position. Outlined arrows indicate flow patterns.

in baboons and found that cerebral circulation was protected but that the myocardium still only received blood ejected from the left ventricle and not blood from the perfusion cannula. This approach does risk ischemia to the arm and can be a difficult operation. Soeter et al. (21) reported a successful 48-hour ECMO case in a 14.5-kg girl with severe pulmonary insufficiency following correction of tetralogy of Fallot and atrial secundrum defect (ASD). They used catheters in the axillary artery and in the femoral vein and right internal jugular veins.

Femoral

At St. Louis University (41), older pediatric patients who have required ECMO for cardiac failure following open heart surgery have been cannulated from the groin using the femoral artery and vein. Early in their experience, these investigators found that proximal cannulation from the groin resulted in vascular insufficiency to the leg (42). This problem may be alleviated by distal femoral artery cannulation.

Femoral artery cannulation (Figure 21.7) may require passage of the perfusion cannula to the level of the aortic arch in order to perfuse the arch branches against the remaining left ventricular output (43).

CIRCUIT

Any number of mechanical circuits can be used. We use gravity drainage to a collapsible venous return monitor (bladder), a roller pump, a silicone membrane oxygenator, and a heat exchanger (Figure 21.8). We have not used arterial filtration or arterial pressure monitoring. A centrifugal pump allows elimination of the bladder but may cause more hemolysis. Until recently, bladders were not available for 3/8-in. tubing, so, for larger patients, we have used the centrifugal pump (Figure 21.9). We also use an Amicon Minifilter (Amicon Division, W. R. Grace & Co., Danvers, Massachusetts) for ultrafiltration, which receives blood from the oxy-

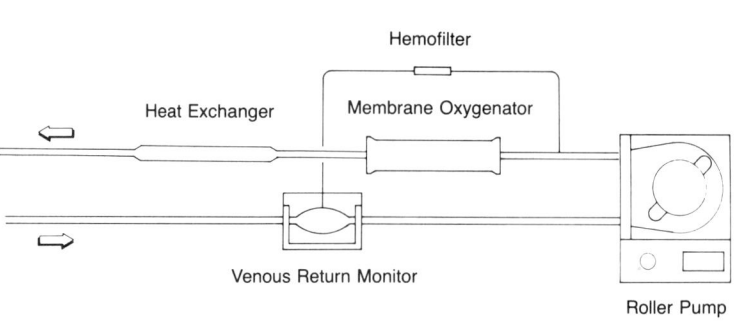

FIGURE 21.8 Schematic presentation of ECMO circuit, including venous return monitor and roller pump. Outlined arrows indicate flow patterns.

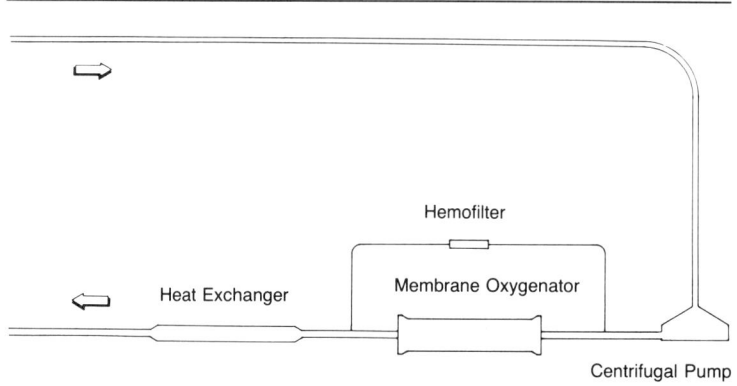

FIGURE 21.9 Schematic presentation of ECMO circuit, including centrifugal pump. Outlined arrows indicate flow patterns.

genator inlet line and drains back into the bladder.

While many cannulas are available, we have had excellent success in neck cannulation using the Elecath (Electro-Catheter Co., Rahway, N.J.) catheters (with side holes and an end hole) when the internal jugular vein will accommodate a 10- to 16-Fr cannula. For larger children, we use 20- and 24-Fr Argyle chest tubes (Sherwood Medical, St. Louis, Missouri). Arterial cannulas have included chest tubes from 8 to 16 Fr, with the distal portion of the catheter, including the side holes, cut off. The growth in ECMO for older patients has stimulated the production of specially designed larger cannulas. We currently use Biomedicus (Eden Prairie, Minnesota) cannulas for both neck and groin cannulation and find we can get much more flow for a given outside diameter than previously. When chest cannulation is employed, we use William Harvey (C. F. Bard, Inc., Santa Anna, California) and Pacifico (DLP, Grand Rapids, Michigan) venous cannulas and angled THI aortic perfusion cannulas (Sherwood Medical, St. Louis, Missouri).

MANAGEMENT

Pump

The goal of ECMO support in the patient after cardiac surgery differs from that in a neonate with hypoxemia secondary to pulmonary hypertension. In the neonate, pump flows are adjusted to achieve satisfactory arterial oxygenation. In patients with low caridac output after cardiac surgery, the goal is to maintain adequate tissue perfusion. This requires nearly complete cardiac bypass to prevent cardiac distension, minimize myocardial energy expenditure, and maximize potential functional cardiac recovery. Flows of 150 mL/kg/min and greater are frequently needed to reduce both right atrial pressure and left atrial pressure. High pump flows are maintained for at least 72 h before attempting to wean from bypass. Since the patient's lungs are usually not significantly impaired, membrane gas exchange can further reduce the $PaCO_2$ and increase the PaO_2. Ventilating the membrane lung with a mixture of air, oxygen, and perhaps CO_2 may be helpful in preventing excessive alkalosis or harmful hyperoxia.

Coagulation

While it is easy to give blood to a patient on ECMO, massive transfusion leads to pulmonary impairment which may not be recoverable. Hemorrhage is not usually a problem for the first 72 hours, even in patients cannulated immediately after cardiopulmonary bypass. Our protocol includes a continuous heparin infusion to maintain an activated clotting time (ACT) at 200 seconds. When bleeding is a problem, the ACT is maintained at an even lower level. Other systemic measures to control bleeding include maintenance of the prothrombin time at or near normal with vitamin K. We administer fresh frozen plasma 10 mL/kg every six hours and administer more if the prothrombin time is abnormal. We maintain the platelet count over 100,000/mm^3 with platelet transfusions.

Local control of bleeding is also important. Operative sites, especially the cannulation site, are treated with fibrin glue made on the surgical field from single-donor cryoprecipitate and thrombin reconstituted with 10% calcium gluconate. Significant bleeding from the cannula insertion site should lead to exploration, although a specific bleeding point may not be found.

Reoperation is mandatory when bleeding has led to pericardial or mediastinal tamponade. This can result, not only in evidence of poor cardiac function, but also in poor venous return to the pump.

Most candidates for cardiac ECMO are beyond the age when intracranial hemorrhage is common. We have, however, seen this in some of our younger patients on cardiac ECMO and therefore perform daily cranial ultrasounds when the fontanelle is open. We also vigorously control hypertension with hydralazine, captopril, and nitroglycerin.

Fluids

Our patients routinely receive antibiotics and, if renal function is good, parenteral nutrition. Fluid management during cardiac ECMO may require ultrafiltration. Most patients going on cardiac ECMO have had prior volume expansion in order to improve cardiac filling and, consequently, cardiac function. Usually this is done at a time when the kidneys are functioning poorly due to low cardiac output. Once the goal becomes decompression of the heart, it is important to remove excess vascular volume. We frequently lower atrial filling pressures after instituting bypass by manually removing blood from the circuit until the desired pressure is obtained. In addition, our bleeding control protocol requires the transfusion of large amounts of fresh frozen plasma and platelets, and the bleeding requires the transfusion of large volumes of blood. Managing this volume overload may require the ability to remove fluids mechanically. Ultrafiltration can also be used to treat patients who have developed renal failure. It must be remembered that, while ultrafiltration is very efficient at removing fluid volume, it is less efficient than dialysis at removing urea and correcting electrolyte abnormalities. Thus, high-volume ultrafiltration must be used in coordination with suitable replacement fluid, such as 0.45% normal saline without potassium.

Weaning

Weaning cardiac patients from ECMO is also different from the technique used in newborns with respiratory failure. In cardiac patients, before weaning can be attempted, the filling volume and atrial pressures must be increased so that maximal cardiac function can be obtained. In addition, we use a moderate inotropic infusion such as 5 μg/kg/min of dopamine. While volume is being restored, the pump flow can be turned down slowly over six to eight hours. If the pulse contour of the arterial tracing, as well as other signs of adequate perfusion (such as urine output), are present, a full trial off ECMO can be attempted.

Evaluating Cardiac Function

Objective assessment of cardiac function during ECMO is difficult to obtain. With the heart empty, normal function cannot be expected. Standard dilution techniques to measure cardiac output are not applicable in patients on partial bypass. The multiple gated acquisition (MUGA) nuclear scan requires temporary discontinuation of ECMO for at least three minutes; even so, the cardiac output displayed is based on a poorly filled heart. Our most useful tools have been the two-dimensional echocardiography and the color flow Doppler ultrasound. With these, as pump flows decrease, myocardial contractility and ventricular ejection in relationship to systolic blood pressure can be assessed subjectively.

RESULTS

The Children's Hospital of Michigan Series

Preoperative cardiac ECMO At the Children's Hospital of Michigan, we treated four children prior to repair of a congenital heart defect. One patient was placed on ECMO for a mistaken diagnosis of primary pulmonary hypertension of the newborn (44). Angiography on ECMO demonstrated the correct diagnosis of obstructed total anomalous pulmonary venous return, and he underwent successful repair. Another patient with cor triatriatum had profound cardiac failure during catheterization and was placed on ECMO. He underwent surgical repair and remained on ECMO for 42 hours postoperatively but died because of irreversible myocardial failure. The third patient had had repair of total anomalous pulmonary venous return at one week of age. Severe pulmonary venous obstruction proximal to the anastomosis associated with right heart failure was evident eight weeks later; as a result, he was placed on ECMO for 24 hours prior to unsuccessful reoperation. A fourth patient had repair of congenital diaphragmatic hernia as a newborn. When hypoxemia was persistent, she underwent echocardiography in preparation for ECMO to treat pulmonary artery hypertension which accompanies congenital diaphragmatic hernia. This study revealed the possibility of total anomalous pulmonary venous return which was confirmed at cardiac catheterization. The patient was placed on ECMO to stabilize her and was taken to the operating room where a total repair was performed. Postoperatively, she remained on ECMO for five days. She was decannulated and did well for three days until progressive pulmonary failure led to death.

Postoperative cardiac ECMO Between August 1984 and October 1989, we used ECMO to treat a total of 46 patients with low cardiac output or severe pulmonary vasoreactive crisis following open repair of congenital heart lesions. Twenty-six of these patients improved sufficiently to permit discontinuation of ECMO support, decannulation, and eventual hospital discharge. One patient died after discharge from the intensive care unit, presumably because of pulmonary vasoreactive crisis. This is a survival of 56% overall.

The mean age of our postoperative patients is 13.1 months (range one day to seven years). Twelve patients had Down syndrome and six of these survived. One also had imperforate anus and duodenal atresia. Other congenital anomalies were rare. One patient had a cleft palate, and one had hypoparathyroidism.

Of the 39 patients treated in our published postoperative ECMO series (29), 13 had biventricular failure, 12 had primarily left ventricular failure, five had primarily right ventricular failure, and six had pulmonary vasoreactive crisis. More patients in the nonsurvivor group had biventricular failure (9/14), and more patients in the survivor group had primarily left ventricular failure (9/22). Cardiac diagnoses included complicated tetralogy of Fallot, complete atrioventricular septal defect, complicated transposition of the great arteries, anomalous left coronary artery from the pulmonary artery, complicated total anomalous pulmonary venous return, complicated ventricular septal defect, and complicated double-outlet right ventricle. Twenty of the 27 patients cannulated four hours or more after operation survived (74%). Of the nine patients cannulated in the operating room because they could not come off bypass, seven died. The two who survived had open chest cannulation with separate decompression of the left atrium.

Once ECMO support was initiated, the patients usually improved dramatically. Arterial pressure rose, atrial pressures fell, and urine output increased (Table 21.2). Most patients required approximately 150 mL/kg/min of pump flow, permitting right atrial pressures to decrease by a mean of 9 mm Hg and left atrial pressures by a mean of 6 mm Hg. The survivors were cannulated for ECMO a mean of 34.5 ± 37.0 hours after operation, and the nonsurvivors 19.2 ± 27.7 hours after surgery. The mean time on ECMO for all patients was 105.4 ± 45.7 hours (109.9 ± 27.8 hours for survivors and 97.9 ± 66.8 hours for nonsurvivors). The nonsurvivors died 26.6 ± 59.2 hours after coming off ECMO. Those who survived spent a mean of 27.6 ± 10.6 days in the hospital.

In any discussion of mechanical support for patients following cardiac surgery, there is one unanswerable question: Would the patient have survived without such support? In Table 21.2, we have demonstrated how similar our survivors and nonsurvivors were before going on ECMO. We do not believe the survivors would have lived without ECMO, because they were just as sick to start with as the nonsurvivors. We also compared our ECMO patients to patients dying in our predictor study (Table 21.3). Our ECMO patients are not very different from the patients who died before ECMO was available. There was no difference in age or weight, and, while the predictor study had longer circulatory arrest times, there was no difference in aortic cross-clamp time. If there was a significant difference in the other variables tested at one hour postoperative, there was no difference in those same variables tested at eight hours postoperative and vice versa. The only consistent difference between the patients placed on ECMO and those who died in the predictor study is that the predictor study patients received larger amounts of dopamine before they died.

Complications Bleeding on ECMO was a common complication in our series (17 patients). Transfusion requirement during ECMO was 3.24 ± 5.14 mL/kg/h. Nonsurvivors and patients requiring cannulation because they could not come off bypass clearly had more bleeding (Table 21.4). Intracranial hemorrhage occurred in four patients, two of whom died.

Mechanical or circuit complications occurred in only three patients. An early model centrifugal pump head failed in a patient who was being weaned from ECMO. The patient was decannulated and lived. Two oxygenators

TABLE 21.2 Data pre-ECMO and on ECMO*

Group	MAP† (mm Hg)		RAP‡ (mm Hg)		LAP§ (mm Hg)		Urine Output (mL/kg/h)	
	Pre-ECMO	On ECMO	Pre-ECMO	On ECMO	Pre-ECMO	On ECMO	Pre-ECMO	On ECMO
All	61 ± 4	76 ± 12	21 ± 6	12 ± 3	18 ± 6	12 ± 4	0.61 ± 0.74	3.5 ± 4.3
Survivors	62 ± 4	82 ± 7	20 ± 4	12 ± 2	18 ± 3	11 ± 2	1.7 ± 2.3	4.3 ± 5.1
Nonsurvivors	55 ± 4	69 ± 13	22 ± 4	12 ± 3	19 ± 6	13 ± 4	0.69 ± 0.5	2.2 ± 2.2

*Average of six hours prior to cannulation. (No pre-ECMO data are available for patients cannulated in the operating room because they could not come off bypass.)
†MAP = mean arterial pressure.
‡RAP = right atrial pressure.
§LAP = left atrial pressure.
Reprinted with permission from Klein MD, Whittlesey GC, Pinsky W, Arciniegas E. Extracorporeal membrane oxygenation (ECMO) for the circulatory support of children after repair of congenital heart disease. J Thorac Cardiovasc Surg 1990;100:498–505.

TABLE 21.3 Comparison of all ECMO patients, with predictor review patients used to prepare predictors

	Hour 1			Hour 8		
Parameter	ECMO patients all	P<	Predictor review patients who died	ECMO patients all	P<	Predictor review patients who died
Age (mo)	13.7 ± 6.2	NS*	13.7 ± 26.7	NA†		NA
Weight (kg)	7.15 ± 2.41	NS	6.4 ± 5.3	NA		NA
Circulatory arrest time (min)	46.0 ± 4.3	0.01	69.1 ± 31.9	NA		NA
Aortic cross-clamp time (min)	97.9 ± 12.2	NS	106.6 ± 49.1	NA		NA
Heart rate	161 ± 7	0.05	149 ± 21	145 ± 27	NS	144 ± 41
Systolic blood pressure (mm Hg)	108 ± 17	0.01	86 ± 23	92 ± 12	NS	83 ± 24
Left atrial pressure (mm Hg)	15 ± 2	NS	17 ± 5	16 ± 2	0.01	21 ± 5
Right atrial pressure (mm Hg)	16 ± 3	0.01	24 ± 7	19 ± 6	NS	21 ± 9
Urine (mL/kg/min)	1.8 ± 1.04	0.05	1.12 ± 0.90	1.1 ± 0.67	NS	1.51 ± 0.92
Dopamine (mcg/kg/min)	5.83 ± 2.83	0.01	14.13 ± 3.38	8.60 ± 3.18	0.01	19.4 ± 10.1
Fio_2	0.71 ± 0.14	0.01	0.9 ± 0.1	0.63 ± 0.18	NS	0.77 ± 0.27
Pao_2	169 ± 94	NS	168 ± 134	106 ± 22	0.01	75 ± 33
Ventilator rate	22.3 ± 4.2	NS	25 ± 6	26.5 ± 6.1	NS	26.1 ± 8.8
pH	7.36 ± 0.05	0.01	7.26 ± 0.11	7.41 ± 0.09	NS	7.33 ± 0.18

*NS = not significant.
†NA = not applicable.
Reprinted with permission from Klein MD, Whittlesey GC, Pinsky W, Arciniegas E. Extracorporeal membrane oxygenation (ECMO) for the circulatory support of children after repair of congenital heart disease. J Thorac Cardiovasc Surg 1990;100:498–505.

failed and needed to be replaced during the ECMO run.

Arrythmias occurred on ECMO in three patients. Two cases were controlled with pacing, and one patient survived. One patient developed a nodal rhythm which was temporarily controlled with core cooling while on ECMO, but effective myocardial function did not return and the patient died.

Bacteremia occurred in two patients and was effectively controlled with appropriate antibiotic therapy.

Follow-up Follow-up information is available on all but one survivor. Nine of the patients are entirely normal on evaluation in cardiology clinic, considering their associated problems, such as Down syndrome. The others have various degrees of cardiac disability requiring digoxin and diuretics, which is consis-

TABLE 21.4 Average blood volume administered on ECMO

	mL/kg/h
All cardiac ECMO patients	3.10 ± 4.93
Survivors	1.50 ± 1.13
Nonsurvivors	5.63 ± 7.0
Neck cannulation	3.14 ± 5.36
Chest cannulation	3.01 ± 1.82
Cannulated in operating room from CPB*	7.46 ± 8.29
Cannulated >4 h after CPB	1.50 ± 1.15

*CPB = cardiopulmonary bypass.

tent with their cardiac disease. No long-term problems have been attributable to ECMO. Similar follow-up results have been reported by the St. Louis University group (41).

Other Centers

Other major published series employing cardiac ECMO also report optimistic results. The group from St. Louis University (33) published the first series of cardiac patients, reporting the survival of six of 13 patients supported with ECMO following cardiac surgery. Their patients were somewhat older than ours and were cannulated through the chest (eight cases) or the groin (five cases). The University of Pittsburgh group (34) reported on 10 pediatric patients, with seven survivors. They used transthoracic cannulation of the right atrium and aortic arch in six patients, standard neck cannulation in three, and left axillary artery cannulation in one. The Washington University group at the St. Louis Children's Hospital (32) reported 13 patients, with five survivors. Five patients had transthoracic cannulation of the aortic arch and right atrium; femoral artery and vein cannulation was used in three patients and standard neck cannulation in five.

CONCLUSION

Prevention remains the best method for the treatment of low cardiac output and pulmonary vasoreactive crisis following surgery for congenital heart disease. Currently, the mainstays of prevention are early diagnosis and treatment and intraoperative myocardial protection. There remains, however, a small group of patients who undergo adequate anatomic repair but have early postoperative low cardiac output or severe hypoxemia. The development of neonatal ECMO teams has made it feasible to apply ECMO to this group of patients for temporary circulatory support.

In 1981, the group from Birmingham (30) made a statement that referred to the postoperative care of children following open heart surgery, with respect to fluid and pharmacologic management. We would like to adopt this and apply it to the mechanical support of such children: "... our experience indicates to us that cardiac performance often improves 24 to 72 hours after operation in these small infants.... The augmentation of cardiac output in the early postoperative hours by various interventions allows some patients to survive and do well who would otherwise die of acute heart failure."

REFERENCES

(1) Carrell A, Lindbergh CA. The culture of organs. New York: Hoeber, 1938.

(2) Gibbon JH Jr. Application of a mechanical heart and lung apparatus to cardiac surgery. Minn Med 1954;37:171.

(3) Murray G. Surgery in the making. London: Johnson Publishers, Ltd., 1964.

(4) Dobell ARC, Mitri M, Glava R, et al. Biologic evaluation of blood after prolonged recirculation through film and membrane oxygenators. Ann Surg 1965;161:617.

(5) Lee WH Jr, Krumhaar D, Fonkalsrud EW, et al. Denaturation of plasma proteins as a cause of morbidity and death after intracardiac operations. Surgery 1961;50:29.

(6) Clowes GHA Jr, Hopkins AL, Neville WE. An artificial lung dependent upon diffusion of oxygen and carbon dioxide through plastic membranes. J Thorac Surg 1956;32:630.

(7) Kolobow T, Bowman RL. Construction and evaluation of an alveolar membrane artificial

heart lung. Trans Am Soc Artif Intern Organs 1963;9:238.

(8) Dennis C. Certain methods for artificial support of the circulation during intracardiac surgery. Surg Clin North Am 1956;36:423.

(9) Kantrowicz A, Tjonneland S, Freed PS, et al. Initial clinical experience with intraaortic balloon pumping in cardiogenic shock. JAMA 1968;203:135.

(10) Veasy LG, Blalock RC, Orth JL, Boucek MM. Intra-aortic balloon pumping in infants and children. Circulation 1983;68:1095–1100.

(11) Spence PA, Peniston CM, Mihic N, Jabr AK, Salerno TA. A rational approach to the selection of an assist device for the failing right ventricle. Ann Thorac Surg 1986;41:606–8.

(12) Magovern GJ, Park SB, Maher TD. Use of a centrifugal pump without anticoagulants for postoperative left ventricular assist. World J Surg 1985;9:25–36.

(13) Fisher EIC, Willshaw P, Armetano RL, Delbo MIB, Pichel RH, Favaloro RG. Experimental acute right ventricular failure and right ventricular assist in the dog. J Thorac Cardiovasc Surg 1985;90:580–5.

(14) Toporoff B, Marini CP, Grubbs PE Jr, et al. Pulmonary complication of a roller pump right ventricular assist device. J Surg Res 1988;45:21–7.

(15) Pierce WS, Parr GVS, Myers JL, Pae WE, Bull AP, Waldhausen JA. Ventricular-assist pumping in patients with cardiogenic shock after cardiac operations. N Engl J Med 1981;27:1606–10.

(16) Taenaka Y, Takano H, Nakatani T, et al. Ventricular assist device (VAD) for children: in vitro and in vivo evaluation. Trans Am Soc Artif Intern Organs 1984;30:155–8.

(17) Klein MD, Andrews AF, Wesley JR, et al. Venovenous perfusion in ECMO for newborn respiratory distress: a clinical comparison with venoarterial perfusion. Ann Surg 1985;201:520–6.

(18) Wampler RK, Moise JC, Frazier OH, Olson DB. In vivo evaluation of a peripheral vascular access axial flow blood pump. Trans Am Soc Artif Intern Organs 1988;34:450–4.

(19) Baffes TG, Fridman JL, Bicoff JP, Whitehill JL. Extracorporeal circulation for support of palliative cardiac surgery in infants. Ann Thorac Surg 1970;10:354–63.

(20) Hill JD, de Leval MR, Fallat RJ, et al. Acute respiratory insufficiency: treatment with prolonged extracorporeal oxygenation. J Thorac Cardiovasc Surg 1972;64:511–62.

(21) Soeter JR, Mamiya RT, Sprague AY, McNamara JJ. Prolonged extracorporeal oxygenation for cardiorespiratory failure after tetralogy correction. J Thorac Cardiovasc Surg 1973;66:214–8.

(22) Pyle RB, Helton WC, Johnson FW, et al. Clinical use of the membrane oxygenator. Arch Surg 1975;110:966–70.

(23) Bartlett RH, Gazzaniga AB, Fong SW, Jeffries MR, Roohk V, Haiduc N. Extracorporeal membrane oxygenator support for cardiopulmonary failure: experience in 28 cases. J Thorac Cardiovasc Surg 1977;73:375–86.

(24) Cullen M, Splittgerber F, Sweezer W, Hakimi M, Arciniegas E, Klein MD. Pulmonary hypertension postventricular septal defect repair treated by extracorporeal membrane oxygenation. J Pediatr Surg 1986;21:675–7.

(25) Bartlett RH, Gazzaniga AB, Wetmore NE, Rucker R, Huxtable RF. Extracorporeal membrane oxygenation (ECMO) in the treatment of cardiac and respiratory failure in children. Trans Am Soc Artif Intern Organs 1980;26:578–80.

(26) Pennington DG, Golding L, Hill D, et al. Temporary mechanical support for cardiogenic shock. Trans Am Soc Artif Intern Organs 1986;2:629–32.

(27) Pennington DG, McBride LR, Kanter KR, et al. Bridging to heart transplantation with circulatory assist devices. J Heart Transplant 1989;8:116–23.

(28) Milliken JC, Laks H, George B. Use of a venous assist device after repair of complex lesions of the right heart. J Am Coll Cardiol 1986;8:922–9.

(29) Klein MD, Whittlesey GC, Pinsky W, Arciniegas E. Extracorporeal membrane oxygenation (ECMO) for the circulatory support of children after repair of congenital heart disease. J Thorac Cardiovasc Surg 1990;100:498–505.

(30) Kirklin JK, Blackstone EH, Kirklin JW, McKay R, Pacifico AD, Bargeron LM Jr. Intracardiac surgery in infants under age 3 months: predictors of postoperative in-hospital mortality. Am J Cardiol 1981;48:507–12.

(31) Rizzoli G, Blackstone EH, Kirklin JW, Pacifico AD, Bargeron LM Jr. Incremental risk factors in hospital mortality rate after repair of ventricular septal defect. J Thorac Cardiovasc Surg 1980;80:494–505.

(32) Weinhaus L, Canter C, Noetzel M, McAlister W, Spray TL. Extracorporeal membrane

oxygenation for circulatory support after repair of congenital heart defects. Ann Thorac Surg 1989;48:206–12.

(33) Kanter KR, Pennington DG, Weber TR, Zambie MA, Braun P, Martychenko V. Extracorporeal membrane oxygenation for postoperative cardiac support in children. J Thorac Cardiovasc Surg 1987;93:27–35.

(34) Rojers AJ, Trento A, Siewers RD, et al. Extracorporeal membrane oxygenation for postcardiotomy cardiogenic shock in children. Ann Thorac Surg 1989;47:903–6.

(35) Bavaria JE, Ratcliff MB, Gupta KB, Wenger RK, Bogen DK, Edmunds LH. Changes in left ventricular systolic wall stress during biventricular circulatory assistance. Ann Thorac Surg 1988;45:526–32.

(36) Eugene J, McColgan SJ, Moore-Jeffries EW, Ott RA, Haiduc NJ, Roohk HV. Cardiac assist by extracorporeal membrane oxygenation with in-line left ventricular venting. Trans Am Soc Artif Intern Organs 1984;30:98–101.

(37) Nowlen TT, Salley SO, Whittlesey GC, et al. Regional blood flow distribution during extracorporeal membrane oxygenation (ECMO) in rabbits. J Thorac Cardiovasc Surg 1989;98:1138–40.

(38) Smith HG, Whittlesey GC, Kundu SK, et al. Regional blood flow during extracorporeal membrane oxygenation (ECMO) in lambs. Trans Am Soc Artif Intern Organs 1989;35:657–60.

(39) Kolobow T, Rossi F, Borelli M, Foti G. The use of a percutaneous spring in the pulmonary artery position to decompress the left heart. Trans Am Soc Artif Intern Organs 1988;34:485–90.

(40) Wickline SA, Soeter JR, McNamara JJ. Oxygenation of the cerebral and coronary circulation with right axillary artery perfusion during venoarterial bypass in primates. Ann Thorac Surg 1977;24:560–5.

(41) Ruzevich SA, Kanter KR, Pennington DG, Swartz MT, McBride LR, Termuhlen DF. Long-term follow-up of survivors of postcardiotomy circulatory support. Trans Am Soc Artif Intern Organs 1988;34(2):116.

(42) Pennington DG, Merjavy JP, Codd JE, Swartz MT, Miller LL, Williams GA. Extracorporeal membrane oxygenation for patients with cardiogenic shock. Circulation 1984;70 (Suppl I):I-130–I-137.

(43) Zapol WM, Quist H, Pontoppidan H, et al. Extracorporeal perfusion for acute respiratory failure: recent experience with the spiral coil membrane lung. J Thorac Cardiovasc Surg 1975;69:439.

(44) Zylberberg R, Cook L, Roberts J, Edmonds D, Reese A, Groff D. Total anomalous pulmonary venous return: report of a case diagnosed on ECMO. J Perinatol 1987;7:185–8.

22

ECMO as a Tool for Physiologic Research

Carlos E. Blanco, M.D.

Various extracorporeal systems provide oxygenation or carbon dioxide (CO_2) removal. All these systems remove or add gases independently and are designed to drain blood from the patient or animal and pass it through a gas exchange "membrane" before returning it to the organism. The desired changes in blood gases are achieved by varying the gradients of the different gases across the membrane, varying the blood flow rate, or both. Thus, blood gas parameters may be verified independently of each other, an advantage when performing physiological studies. Various types of extracorporeal circulation (ECC) have been utilized, depending on the effects sought. Some systems use vein-to-artery or vein-to-vein perfusion, both mainly for clinical applications. Artery-to-vein perfusion has been used for research purposes. When umbilical vessels are used, the system is called an "artificial placenta" (1–4). Some investigators use artery-to-vein or vein-to-vein perfusion to load or unload CO_2 (5,6). These systems are known as carbon dioxide membrane lungs (CDML).

Extracorporeal membrane oxygenator (ECMO) systems have proven to be of value in the treatment of pulmonary and/or cardiovascular failure, as extensively discussed in this book.

ECMO systems have been used to study fetal, neonatal, and adult physiology. Of particular interest have been the feasibility studies using ECMO as an artificial placenta.

USE OF EXTRACORPOREAL CIRCULATION AS AN "ARTIFICIAL PLACENTA" OR INCUBATION SYSTEM

The term "artificial placenta" applied to these extracorporeal systems is an unfortunate and confusing one because it assumes that gas exchange is the only placental function. These systems have two purposes: clinical applications for extrauterine support and physiologic studies of the fetoplacental unit.

Feasibility Studies for Clinical Use

Prematurely born infants younger than 28 weeks' gestational age remain a clinical and technical challenge. Despite the decrease in mortality over the last five years, this group continues to present important management problems. Improved perinatal techniques have not reduced the high percentage of chronic morbidity. Since the ideal milieu for the fetus is the uterus, investigators have studied the possibility of creating a system for extrauterine support that reproduces intrauterine conditions.

The favored preparation for this research is the mature fetal lamb: Reasons for this are the size of the animal, the size of its vessels, and our extensive physiologic knowledge regarding this model. These studies attempt to reproduce intrauterine conditions by immersing the fetus in a water bath at 39°C, establishing an arteriovenous shunt (umbilical artery-umbilical vein), perfusing it with blood flow similar to the umbilical flow in utero (150 mL/kg/min), maintaining arterial blood gases and oxygen consumption at fetal levels, and administering glucose as a source of energy.

With these systems, total artificial placentation with a membrane oxygenator was performed in fetal lambs for increasing periods of time from 19 to 24 hours, and ultimately for 55 hours (2,7,8). Recently, Kuwabara et al. (4) reported survival up to 10 days in fetal goats at 112 to 137 days of gestation using an incubation module that is a modified ECMO system with an umbilical artery-to-vein shunt.

Nonetheless, many problems must be solved before the system can be used in clinical practice. The animals in these experiments are very mature and show none of the complications commonly observed in premature infants, such as intraventricular hemorrhage. Fetal sheep of 80 to 90 days' gestation will have to be used to test for these complications (9).

USE OF EXTRACORPOREAL SYSTEMS FOR PHYSIOLOGICAL STUDIES

Studies of Fetal Circulation

Extracorporeal circulation has been used to study the mechanisms involved in the control of circulation prior to birth. Fetal lambs from 115 days' gestation to term (148 to 151 days) were used for these experiments. Extracorporeal support was provided through an artery-to-vein shunt, utilizing the umbilical vessels to conserve physiologic fetal circulatory conditions. After the shunt was completed, the fetuses were delivered, and, in order to maintain constant temperature, they were immersed in a saline bath at 39°C or warmed with radiant heaters. Zapol et al. (10) reported observations on the relationship between arterial Po_2 and ductus arteriosus and pulmonary blood flow in fetal lambs using the artificial placenta system described above. After three to five hours of total extracorporeal support, fetal arterial Po_2 was raised from a range of 13 to 20 mm Hg up to 40 to 60 mm Hg, maintaining fetal pH, Pco_2, and placental flow at unchanged levels. These changes in fetal arterial Po_2 produced constriction of the ductus arteriosus and a marked increase in pulmonary blood flow which reversed when arterial Po_2 was returned to normal fetal levels.

Using a similar system but maintaining fetal temperature with radiant heaters, Siassi et al. (3) reported observations on the responses of baroreceptors and chemoreceptors during cord occlusion at different levels of fetal oxygenation.

Extracorporeal Systems and Control of Respiration

Traditionally, studies on central and peripheral mechanisms involved in the control of breathing after birth have been performed by providing the stimulus through the respiratory system. Responses to known stimuli, like hypercapnia or hypoxia, have been induced by offering the human or experimental animal gas mixtures containing low concentrations of oxygen or high concentrations of CO_2 to breathe. This approach introduces extraneous variables, such as stimulation of airway receptors and stimulation of reflexes, because of changes in pulmonary volumes. This methodology does not permit study of the role of CO_2 production or oscillations in blood gases in the maintenance of breathing. Extracorporeal systems allow variations in blood gases to be produced independently of lung function, therefore providing the opportunity to study these mechanisms.

During hemodialysis, mild hypoxemia is

observed as the result of alveolar hypoventilation (11) caused by removal of CO_2 during the procedure. This observation suggests that extracorporeal systems might be used to study mechanisms involved in the control of breathing. This approach has the advantage of altering only pulmonary CO_2 production (V_{CO_2}) without producing other metabolic, neurologic, or cardiovascular changes that could affect ventilation. Kolobow et al. (5) studied the relationship between CO_2 removal and alveolar ventilation in lambs. They used a subclavian artery-to-jugular-vein shunt. Blood was pumped through a silicone spiral-coiled CDML. CO_2 removal was achieved by changing either gas flow or blood flow to the CDML. Alveolar ventilation could be related directly to the amount of CO_2 removed.

Further studies were performed to assess the importance of peripheral stimuli on the initiation of breathing. Phillipson et al. (6) used CDML techniques with a vein-to-vein shunt (inferior vena cava and both jugular veins to superior vena cava) on adult sheep to examine the dependence of respiratory rhythm generation on the rate of CO_2 production.

Extracorporeal Systems for Studies in Perinatal Physiology

Chronic instrumentation of fetal sheep permits their study under physiologic conditions. For many years, it has been possible to obtain chronic recordings in fetal sheep at different gestational ages. This preparation has permitted observations on the mechanisms involved in the control of fetal breathing. Studying these mechanisms is important to our understanding of the initiation of breathing at birth and its maintenance thereafter.

Breathing differs pre- and postnatally in several respects. After birth, breathing is continuous, and, although it is influenced by many excitatory and inhibitory neural inputs from central and peripheral sources, it persists regardless of the electrocorticogram (ECoG) activity state. In contrast, fetal breathing movements (FBM) are episodic during low-voltage ECoG activity and disappear with the appearance of high-voltage ECoG activity (12,13). Postnatally, breathing is stimulated initially during mild hypoxia, but FBM are inhibited during periods of hypoxia (14).

These differences have long been thought to involve central neuroinhibitory mechanisms. When the fetal brain stem is transected at the level of the colliculi or when lesions are placed in the rostrolateral pons, the incidence of FBM increases; FBM are present during both high- and low-voltage ECoG activity. Moreover, FBM persist or increase during hypoxia (15,16). These observations suggest that the absence of FBM during hypoxia results from the action of inhibitory processes which originate above the pons or which require that an area above the pons be intact for their occurrence. As the inhibition occurs in fetuses in which the peripheral arterial chemoreceptors have been denervated (17), the nature and location of the receptors that sense the change in arterial P_{O_2} are unknown. The extent to which they constitute "central chemoreceptors" has not been defined.

Normocapnic hypoxia (14), hypercapnia (18), and a modest degree of hyperoxia (19) can be achieved in the fetus by altering the gas mixture breathed by the mother. Periods of asphyxia can be produced by altering uterine or umbilical flow. These methods produce maternal or placental changes, making it difficult to alter fetal blood gases independently.

The possibility of having direct access to the fetus and changing its blood gases without altering maternal or placental physiology is very attractive. Using an ECMO system, observations have been made in chronically instrumented fetal sheep in utero (128 to 132 days of gestation) (20). Questions concerning the mechanisms involved in the control of fetal behavior, fetal breathing activity, and the establishment of continuous respirations after birth are all currently under study in our laboratory.

A Model Employing Extracorporeal Circulation to Study the Physiology of Fetal Lambs

We have established a model that allows us to alter physiologic parameters in the fetal lamb independent of each other and of maternal factors by controlling fetal circulation through an ECMO circuit. Texel-bred sheep were operated at 125 to 130 days of gestation under general anesthesia (thiopental 1 g intravenously, maintained with halothane 1%). Wire electrodes (AS 632 Cooner Wire, Chatsworth, California) were sewn into the diaphragm and the neck extensors to record electromyographic activity (EMG), and were implanted bilaterally on the fetal parietal cortex to record the ECoG. Catheters were placed in the right axillary artery and carotid artery (oriented toward the head) to measure blood pressure and heart rate and to sample blood gases. Catheters were placed in the fetal trachea to measure tracheal pressure and in the amniotic cavity to measure amniotic pressure. A #14 cord occluder was placed at the base of the umbilical cord for cord occlusion experiments. For the ECMO system, two silastic catheters were placed at midneck level; one for drainage to the ECMO system (12 Fr gauge) was advanced 10 cm into the right external jugular vein (right atrium level), and one for return of oxygenated blood to the fetus (9.6 Fr gauge) was advanced in the right carotid artery 5 cm toward the heart. Each of these catheters was connected to a 10-mm diameter tube which was capped at one end, permitting connection to the ECMO circuit later. All catheters, tubes, and electrode cables were exteriorized through a small incision in the flank of the ewe. Antibiotics were given to the ewe for five days after surgery.

After operation, the ECMO catheters were flushed twice daily with heparinized saline solution (100 U/mL). On the third day after operation, recordings of ECoG, cervical EMG activity, and fetal breathing from tracheal pressure and diaphragmatic EMG activity were obtained. This provided baseline data on the incidence of fetal breathing activity, its relationship to high-voltage ECoG activity, and the distribution of fetal activity states. Changes in fetal temperature were achieved by raising or decreasing the temperature of the thermostatically controlled box as required for each protocol.

The ECMO system consisted of a 10-mm internal diameter silastic circuit that contained a venous reservoir/bladder, a peristaltic pump, and a membrane lung (SciMed/Kolobow 0.8 m^2, SciMed Life Systems, Inc., Minneapolis, Minnesota). The circuit was enclosed in a thermostatically controlled box to maintain the blood temperature at 39°C (Figures 22.1 and 22.2). The membrane was flushed with 100% CO_2 for 10 minutes, then the priming solution (lactated Ringer's 300 mL) was circulated through the system. The CO_2 was replaced by air, and the priming solution was replaced by fresh adult sheep blood treated with citrate-phosphate-dextrose. Before the circuit was connected, blood was adjusted to the appropriate hematocrit and pH, and the activated coagulation time (ACT) was adjusted to 200 to 300 seconds. Heparin was then infused continuously (50 U/kg/h) to maintain ACT between 200 and 300 seconds.

After the fetus was connected to the bypass circuit, the extracorporeal flow was started at 50 mL/min and was slowly increased to 200 to 250 mL/min as required to obtain the desired fetal blood gases. The membrane lung was supplied with a warmed and humidified gas mixture at a total flow rate of 1.5 L/min. Normocarbia was maintained by adding small amounts of CO_2 to the gas mixture (150 to 200 mL/min). When the experimental design required an alteration to produce fetal hypo- or hypercapnia, the CO_2 flow rate to the membrane was increased or decreased. Blood samples were drawn hourly from the cephalad carotid artery catheter and from venous blood returning to the pump.

This innovative model has been used to ask a number of relevant questions about fetal physiology. Several of these are summarized here.

What is the role of fetal arterial Po_2 in determining fetal behavior and the periodicity of fetal breathing activity? If oxygen-sensitive cells that govern this inhibition are present above the medulla, it could be speculated that fetal Pao$_2$ (20 to 30 mm Hg) might exert a tonic inhibition, limiting breathing activity and wakefulness with the aim of protecting oxygen availability since both activities increase fetal oxygen consumption (21). The presence of breathing activity during episodes of low-voltage ECoG could then be explained as behavioral control overriding biochemical control. Moreover, it could explain the establish-

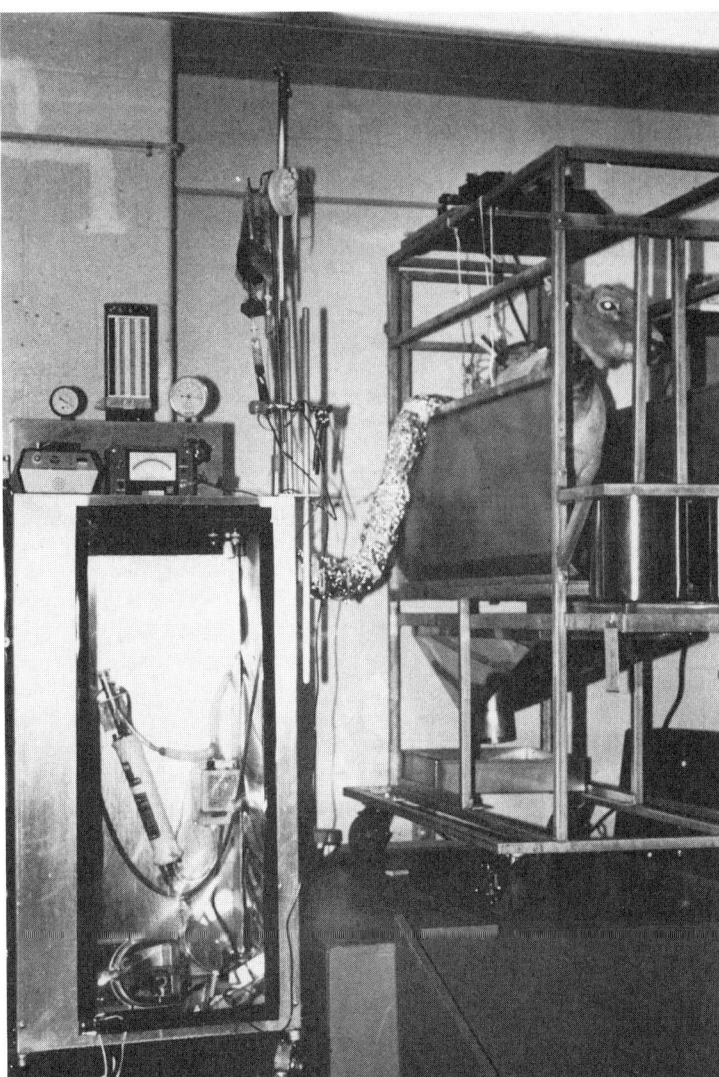

FIGURE 22.1 An experimental setup. The ewe is elevated to facilitate venous drainage. The ECMO system is placed in a thermostatically controlled box.

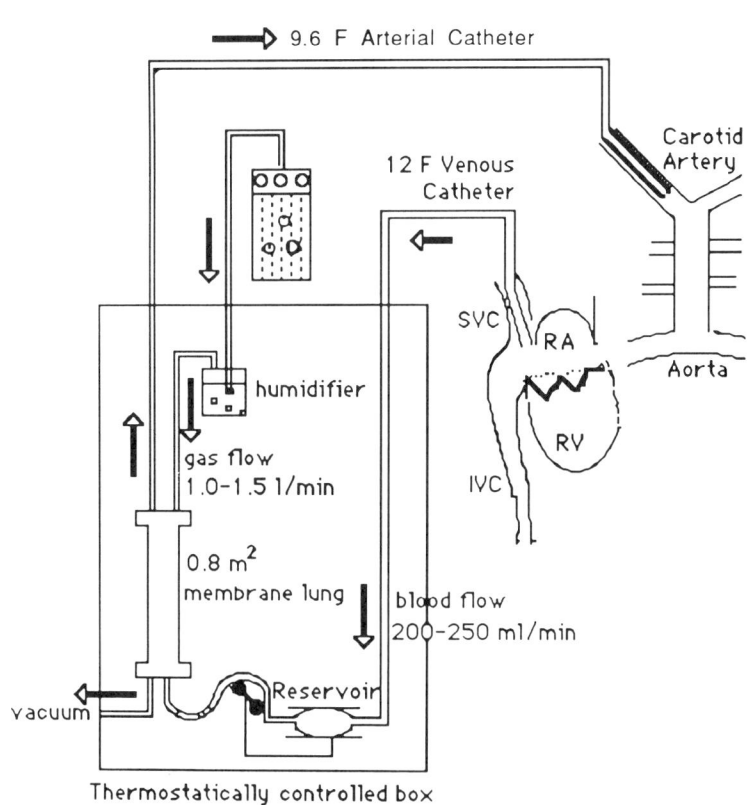

FIGURE 22.2 Drawing of the system used for experiments, showing the position of the catheters and the direction of the blood flow.

ment of continuous breathing after cord clamping at birth.

Table 22.1 shows arterial blood gases, pH, ECoG, and fetal breathing activity during control and ECMO periods. Fetal Pao_2 was the only variable that changed (from 24.7 ± 1.82 mm Hg to 65 ± 4.4 mm Hg). During the experimental period, neither the incidence of high-voltage ECoG activity (48.5% vs. 52.8%) nor the incidence of fetal breathing activity (37%/h vs. 24%/h) changed significantly. In no instance did fetal breathing activity not become continuous. In conclusion, oxygen availability appears not to determine fetal breathing patterns. Other factors, like peripheral afferent input (decreased in utero, increased at and after birth), may play a more important role.

What is the effect of fetal hypocapnia or hypercapnia on fetal breathing movements? It is known from experiments in which maternal hypercapnia was produced that fetal breathing activity is affected by changes in fetal Pco_2 (13). However, this approach, because it is indirect, may introduce unknown variables. ECMO enables one to alter fetal Pco_2 independent of the ewe's blood gases. Fetal Pco_2 can be changed by manipulating the flow of CO_2 to the membrane. Figure 22.3 demonstrates fetal breathing activity in response to direct hypercapnia. These responses may be observed at various levels of fetal Pco_2 or with a combination of hypercapnia and changes in fetal temperature. The latter context is relevant when studying the initiation of breathing at birth.

What are the effects of decreases in fetal core temperature on breathing movements and on fetal activity states? Cold is known to be a

TABLE 22.1 Arterial blood gases, pH, and incidence of high-voltage and fetal breathing movements during control and ECMO periods

Control							ECMO Hyperoxia					
RT*/h	pH	PaO$_2$ (mm Hg)	PaCO$_2$ (mm Hg)	% HV/h	% FB/h		RT/h	pH	PaO$_2$ (mm Hg)	PaCO$_2$ (mm Hg)	% HV/h	% FB/h
27	7.381	21.1	36.0	45.0	28.3		19	7.31	63.8	31.7	64.0	28.3
13	7.404	30.0	38.7	55.2	36.7		15	7.42	61.1	40.5	56.7	15.5
23	7.424	24.5	48.1	51.3	47.8		8	7.41	58.8	47.9	48.9	48.7
14	7.379	30.3	38.8	45.0	40.0		15	7.40	52.3	41.2	56.0	5.6
26	7.293	20.2	51.2	49.5	35.8		19	7.32	58.7	49.9	51.1	21.4
22	7.398	22.2	46.3	43.1	35.5		10	7.38	76.9	46.8	40.2	23.3
							6	7.33	85.0	51.0	—	40.0
Mean	7.38	24.7	43.3	48.5	37.3			7.37	65.2	44.1	52.8	23.8†
Sem	0.02	1.8	2.5	2.0	2.6			0.02	4.4	2.6	3.3	5.9

*RT = recording time; HV = high-voltage movements; FB = fetal breathing movements.
†$P > 0.06$ Wilcoxon.

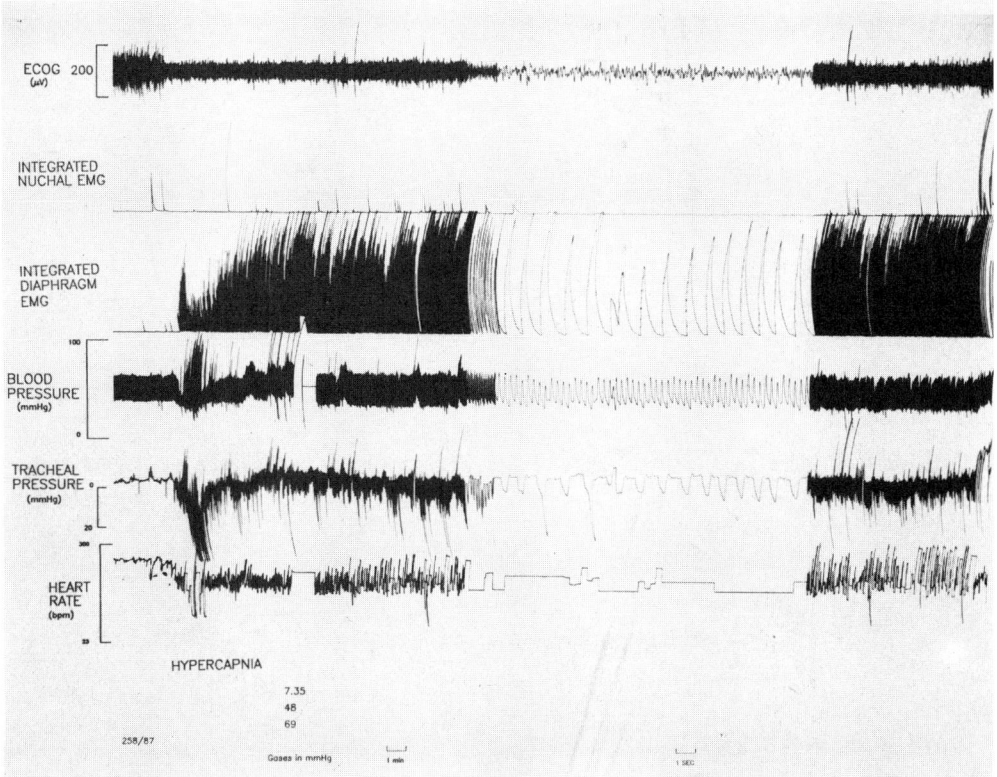

FIGURE 22.3 Recording in utero of a fetal sheep of 130 days' gestational age during hyperoxia three days postsurgery. There is an increase in breathing activity (positive deflections in diaphragm and negative deflections in tracheal pressure) after raising fetal P_{CO_2} from 42 to 48 mm Hg. The first channel shows fetal ECoG activity; the cycling between high- and low-voltage activity can be seen. The second channel shows neck muscle activity. Note that breathing activity is present during low-voltage ECoG activity.

potent respiratory stimulus. In utero, cutaneous cold stimulation produces long periods of fetal breathing activity which may be inhibited by fetal hypoxia. Decreases in core temperature do not have the same effect (22). Interestingly, fetal breathing was stimulated by lowering core temperature (by decreasing the temperature of the blood in the ECMO circuit) and raising fetal P_{CO_2} (Figure 22.4). This respiratory stimulation may result either from the increase in P_{CO_2}, or from the effect of hypothermia in fetal oxygen consumption, or both.

What is the role of umbilical cord clamping in the establishment of continuous breathing at birth? At birth, continuous breathing must be started in order to establish an area of gas exchange. Many stimuli are present at the same time: mild asphyxia, increase in afferent input from peripheral and central receptors, and cord clamping. It has been suggested that the placenta might exercise an inhibitory role on fetal breathing activity such that cord clamping would exclude this inhibitory effect (23,24). Previously, cord clamping experiments have necessarily induced fetal hypercapnia, complicating interpretation of the results. Experiments using ECMO permit observations during cord clamping to be conducted in the presence of normal fetal P_{CO_2}. These studies have failed to demonstrate any regulatory role of the placenta over fetal breathing activity (Figure 22.5) (25).

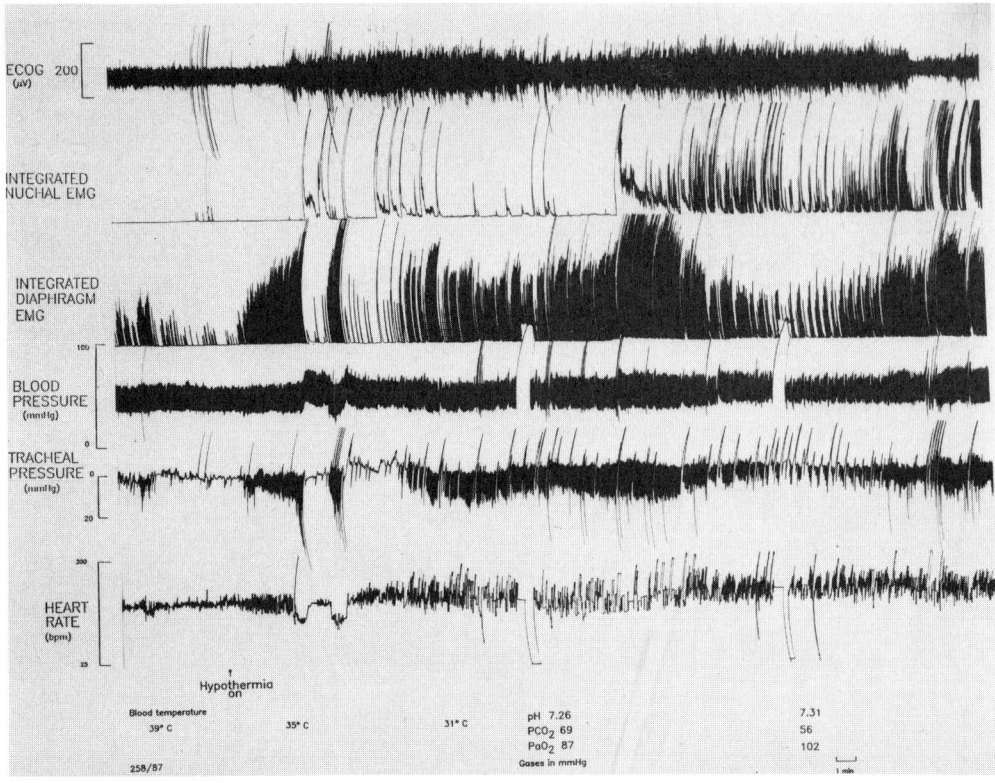

FIGURE 22.4 Recordings in utero from the same fetal lamb shown in Figure 22.3. Fetal breathing activity increases as the temperature falls and P_{CO_2} increases (see diaphragmatic and tracheal pressure deflections). Note that breathing occurs during high-voltage ECoG.

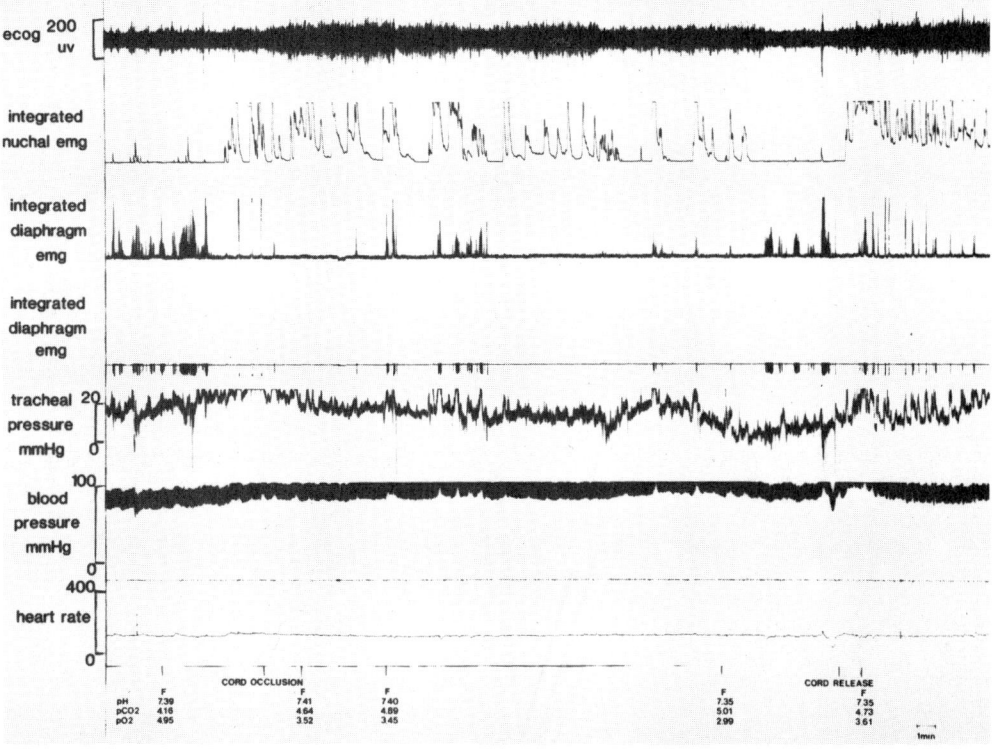

FIGURE 22.5 Fetal lamb of 132 days of gestational age, four days after surgery. This recording shows the same parameters as in the previous figures. In this experiment, the umbilical cord was occluded by insufflating a cord occluder implanted during surgery. ECMO blood flow was 180 mL/kg/min at occlusion. Fetal blood flow was 180 mL/kg/min at occlusion. Fetal blood gases were unchanged, and fetal breathing was not established after occlusion.

ECMO is a powerful tool for research in perinatal physiology since it can establish neonatal conditions in the fetus or fetal conditions in the newborn. These techniques could permit observations on the role of oxygenation at birth, since immature fetal lambs (80 to 90 days' gestation) could be exposed to neonatal Po_2 conditions in utero. This could provide us with a much deeper understanding of the great drama of birth.

REFERENCES

(1) Lawn L, McCance RA. Ventures with an artificial placenta. I. Principles and preliminary results. In: Widdowson EM, ed. Studies in perinatal physiology. Tunbridge Wells, Kent: Pitman Medical Limited, 1980.

(2) Zapol WM, Kolobow T, Pierce JE, Vurek GG, Bowman RL. Artificial placenta: two days of total extrauterine support of the isolated premature lamb fetus. Science 1969;166:617–18.

(3) Siassi B, Wu PYK, Blanco CE, Martin CB. Baroreceptor and chemoreceptor responses to umbilical cord occlusion in fetal lambs. Bio Neonate 1979;35:66–73.

(4) Kuwabara Y, Okai T, Kozuma S, et al. Artificial placenta: long-term extrauterine incubation of isolated goat fetuses. Artif Organs 1989;13:527–31.

(5) Kolobow T, Gattinoni L, Tomlinson TA, Pierce JS. Control of breathing using an extracorporeal membrane lung. Anesthesiology 1977;46:138–41.

(6) Phillipson EA, Duffin J, Cooper JD. Critical dependence of respiratory rhythmicity on metabolic CO_2 load. J Appl Physiol: Respir Environ Exercise Physiol 1981;50:45–54.

(7) Callaghan JC, Maynex EA, Hug HR. Studies in lambs of the development of an artificial placenta. Review of nine long-term survivors of extracorporeal circulation maintained in a fluid medium. Can J Surg 1965;8:208–13.

(8) Alexander DP, Britton HG, Nixon DA. Maintenance of sheep fetuses by an extracorporeal circuit for periods up to 24 hours. Am J Obstet Gynecol 1968;102:969–75.

(9) Reynolds ML, Evans CAN, Reynolds EOR, Saunders NR, Durbin G, Wigglesworth JS. Intracranial hemorrhage in the preterm sheep fetus. Early Hum Dev 1979;3:163–86.

(10) Zapol WM, Kolobow T, Doppman J, Pierce J. Response of ductus blood flow to blood oxygen tension in immersed lamb fetuses perfused through an artificial placenta. J Thorac Cardiovasc Surg 1971;61:891–903.

(11) Sherlock JE, Yoon Y, Ledwith JW, Letteri JM. Respiratory gas exchange during hemodialysis. In: Schreiner GE, ed. Proceedings of the clinical dialysis and transplant forum. Vol 2. Washington, DC: Georgetown University Press, 1972.

(12) Dawes GS, Fox HE, Leduc BH, Liggins GC, Richards RT. Respiratory movements and rapid eye movements sleep in foetal lambs. J Physiol 1971;220:119–43.

(13) Dawes GS, Gardner WN, Johnston BM, Walker DW. Activity of intercostal muscles in relation to breathing movements, electrocortical activity and gestational age in foetal lambs. J Physiol 1980;307:47p–48p.

(14) Boddy K, Dawes GS, Fisher RL, Pinter S, Robinson JS. Foetal respiratory movements, electrocortical and cardiovascular responses to hypoxaemia and hypercapnia in sheep. J Physiol 1974;243:599–618.

(15) Dawes GS, Gardner WN, Johnston BM, Walker DW. Breathing in fetal lambs: the effects of brainstem section. J Physiol 1983;335:535–53.

(16) Gluckman PD, Johnston BM. Lesions in the upper lateral pons abolish the hypoxic depression of breathing in unanaesthetized fetal lambs in utero. J Physiol 1987;382:373–83.

(17) Moore PJ, Parkes MJ, Nijhuis JG, Hanson MA. The incidence of breathing movements of fetal sheep in normoxia and hypoxia after peripheral chemodenervation and brainstem transection. J Dev Physiol 1989;11:147–51.

(18) Chapman RLK, Dawes GS, Rurak DW, Wilds PL. Breathing movements in fetal lambs and the effects of hypercapnia. J Physiol (London) 1980;302:19–29.

(19) Ritchie K. The fetal response to changes in the composition of maternal inspired air in human pregnancy. Semin Perinatol 1980;4:295–9.

(20) Blanco CE, Maertzdorf W, de Jong DS. Responses in the chronically instrumented fetal sheep to changes in blood gases and temperature produced by an extracorporeal membrane oxygenation system (ECMO) (Abstract). Pediatr Res 1988;23:239A.

(21) Rurak DW, Gruber NC. Increased oxygen consumption associated with breathing activity in fetal lambs. J Appl Physiol 1983;54:701–7.

(22) Gluckman PD, Gunn TR, Johnston BM. The effects of cooling on breathing and shivering in unanaesthetized fetal lambs in utero. J Physiol (London) 1983;343:495–506.

(23) Adamson SL, Richardson BS, Homan J. Initiation of pulmonary gas exchange by fetal sheep in utero. J Appl Physiol 1987;62:989–98.

(24) Blanco CE, Martin CB Jr, Hanson MA, McCooke HB. Determinants of the onset of continuous air breathing at birth. Eur J Obstet Gynecol Reprod Biol 1987;26:183–92.

(25) Blanco CE, Maertzdorf W, de Jong D, Pfaff L, Hanson M. Effects of changes in fetal oxygenation on fetal breathing activity. Reading, England: Society for the Study of Fetal Physiology, 16th meeting. July, 1989.

23

The Economics of ECMO Therapy

❖

Billie Lou Short, M.D.
Gail D. Pearson, SC.D., M.D.

Enormous medical strides have been made in newborn intensive care in the past 25 years, with extracorporeal membrane oxygenation (ECMO) representing one of the most exciting and effective technologies developed during this period. Since the first neonatal survivor in 1975, ECMO has undergone a period of investigation and development, leading to its gradual acceptance as a viable therapy. In the last five years, more than 55 new ECMO centers have opened, and additional programs are in various stages of development.

The cost of health care has become a pressing concern for health professionals and the public. The medical profession is criticized for failure to control costs, and the merits of many expensive procedures are now questioned. High-technology intensive care interventions are often singled out as an important factor contributing to escalating costs. It is clear that ECMO falls into this category (1–4). Given the recent rapid growth in the number of ECMO programs and the relatively high cost of providing this therapy, it is imperative to evaluate financial considerations in concert with ECMO's clinical effectiveness. This chapter will address the costs of developing and operating an ECMO program, as well as the cost-effectiveness of ECMO compared to conventional therapy.

ECMO PROGRAM DEVELOPMENT COST

The first step in developing an ECMO program is to determine the regional need for ECMO and project the number of patients to be treated. Although difficult to determine, it has been estimated in two different regions that one infant in either 2,000 or 3,000 live births will require ECMO (5) (data presented at Fourth Annual ECMO Symposium, February 1988, summary of Washington, D.C. regional need). It is recommended that a minimum of 12 patients per year be treated in order to ensure that clinical skills are maintained for this complicated therapy. Not every neonatal intensive care unit, therefore, should provide ECMO services. Careful assessment of the regional need and existing programs is essential in planning new ECMO centers.

Once the decision has been made to undertake development of a new program, a lead time of approximately one year is required for staff training and administrative preparations before the first patient can be treated. A general summary of the major elements involved in starting an ECMO program are listed in Table 23.1. Specific program development costs will vary, depending on differences among hospitals in such factors as salary, availability of equipment, animal expenses, number of beds planned, and the number of technical staff to be trained. In general, the total cost of developing an ECMO program averages $125,000, with a range of $50,000 to $200,000. Equipment and training costs represent the majority of the expense incurred. As will be discussed in the next section, this is in contrast to the operating budget, where the major expense is for personnel.

Most centers start with only one bed the first year, which allows time for the team to develop the technical expertise needed to manage more than one patient safely. One bed necessitates the purchase of two complete sets of equipment, however, to ensure that proper backup equipment is available.

The number of beds to be operated and the estimated number of patients to be treated in the first year dictate the number and type of technical personnel to be trained during the development phase. Most continuous bedside care required by infants on ECMO is provided by ECMO specialists, who are registered nurses, registered respiratory therapists, or certified perfusionists. The average length of ECMO therapy is 130 hours per patient. Therefore, with one patient a month, approximately 16 eight-hour shifts or 11 twelve-hour shifts are required, as indicated in Table 23.2. Additional patients will necessitate additional staff hours. The specific number of specialists required will also be determined by the proportion who are full-time, rather than part-time.

Most centers train 10 to 15 specialists in the first group, which is a reasonable number to allow enough hands-on experience to ensure individual technical competence. The decision to make the staff full-time or part-time, or a combination, should be tailored to the needs and resources of the hospital planning the program. In practice, most programs have at least some full-time staff. In addition, a full-time coordinator is highly recommended for any program, but is essential for programs with more than one bed.

Table 23.3 lists the essential equipment to develop an ECMO program. Equipment costs range from approximately $20,000 to $30,000, depending on the type of pump preferred and number of additional monitoring systems required. For example, pre- and postmembrane

TABLE 23.1 ECMO program development expense categories

Coordinator's salary

Specialists' salaries during training

Consultants' fees: bioengineer and perfusion

Administrative support

ECMO equipment: two sets

Laboratory training:
  Animals and blood products
  Disposables: tubing packs, membrane lungs, IV supplies and medications, ACT* tubes, etc.
  Laboratory space

Office and storage space

Telephone

Printing of training manuals

Travel to ECMO center for training/consultation

*ACT = activated clotting time.

TABLE 23.2 Number of shifts per month per ECMO patient

Patients per month	Total hours per month	Number of 8-h shifts	Number of 12-h shifts
1	130	16	11
2	260	32	22
3	390	48	33

Note: Average ECMO patient is on 130 hours.

TABLE 23.3 ECMO equipment

Pump and base
Venous return monitor
Bladder box
Oxygen/CO_2 flow meters
Oxygen blender
Heating unit
Coagulation timer
Temperature probe
Pressure-monitoring devices
Venous saturation monitor
TY gun
Tubing clamps
CO_2 or carbogen tank regulators
Membrane mounting board

Note: Average total cost = $30,000.

pressure monitoring can be accomplished easily using the patient's bedside monitor, if available. If not, a separate monitoring system is required.

Once the staff is selected and equipment obtained, initial training of the key physician members of the team, as well as the ECMO specialists and coordinators, can begin. Most centers use at least six to eight animal sessions to train key individuals and to work out any equipment design questions. The cost of these animal training sessions will vary, but, in our institution, an average animal run costs approximately $1,000. This includes animals ($120 each), blood products ($50 per unit), membrane lungs ($400 each), tubing packs ($450 each), laboratory time, and consumable supplies, such as intravenous tubing, intravenous fluids, and medications. Laboratory costs can be decreased by buying tubing and making individual tubing packs instead of purchasing commercially available ECMO packs. In addition, it is important to determine the exact cost of laboratory time. Use of a well-equipped physiology laboratory can cost as much as $100 per day in some facilities.

The initial training program for the ECMO specialists to Children's National Medical Center (CNMC) includes 40 hours of didactic material, 16 hours of laboratory training (12 hours in animal training and four hours of water drills), and 40 hours of bedside training paired with a certified ECMO specialist. At CNMC, this training necessitates about $2,200 in salary expense per specialist. To decrease costs and the number of animals needed for training, animal sessions are conducted over a two- to 3-day period, with training during both day and night shifts.

Other expenses that should not be overlooked during program development are costs of office space for the ECMO coordinator, storage space for the clinical equipment, preparation and printing of training manuals, administrative support, and consultation from perfusionists and biomedical engineers.

ECMO PROGRAM OPERATING COSTS

The operating budget is dependent primarily on the number of patients who will be treated in the ECMO center. Most ECMO centers have two operating budgets: the physician budget and the program operations budget. The major items in a typical ECMO operating budget are listed in Table 23.4. The physician budget may be either incorporated into the department budget or a separate cost center. This budget usually covers the cost of physician salaries and administrative support. Institutions also vary in their approach to allocating ECMO operating expenses. This operating budget may be a subset of the intensive care unit or a separate cost center. The latter arrangement is preferred because it simplifies determination of the program's financial status at any given time.

The cost of running an ECMO program reflects its personnel-intensive nature, with salaries and wages usually accounting for more than 80% of total operating expenses. Replacement of equipment also should be considered in developing the budget, because equipment

TABLE 23.4 ECMO operating budget

Coordinator's salary
Specialists' salaries
Consulting salaries
    Bioengineering
    Perfusionists
Office/telephone
Maintenance and replacement of equipment
Retraining
Supplies: medical/surgical and office

requires replacement within five years. Basic training for new team members and continuing training for existing staff are essential. Most centers have one to two training sessions a year to replace specialists, and all centers have mandatory emergency drill training for all staff members once every one to two months.

One difficulty in managing an ECMO program's budget is determining the number of patients that the program will treat annually, because this directly determines staffing needs. As discussed earlier, the importance of regional planning for ECMO cannot be overemphasized.

POTENTIAL INDIRECT COSTS OF ECMO

The effect of providing ECMO on critical resources such as nursing, respiratory therapy, and perfusion is difficult to evaluate. It has been stated, for example, that recruiting ECMO specialists from the already-limited pool of experienced, critical care nurses is akin to robbing Peter to pay Paul. On the other hand, many observers believe that critical care nurses need a professional change and that participating in ECMO may prevent them from leaving the health care system entirely. At CNMC, those who took full-time positions with the ECMO team were planning to change jobs. Although some may have stayed within the nursing hierarchy, others would have left the nursing profession. There are no studies to date examining this issue, so the effect of ECMO on the pool of critical care resources remains unknown, although the CNMC experience suggests that the effect may well be positive.

Another issue that should be considered before opening a program is its effect on the intensive care unit. If the unit is crowded and has inadequate space between beds, two bed spaces may be needed for one ECMO patient because of the equipment. This should be taken into account when designing the equipment and the base on which it is placed. In addition, the cost implications of bed space loss should be considered when developing the budget.

An ECMO center is likely to attract sizable numbers of patients, many of whom will be critically ill for prolonged periods of time, consuming considerable intensive care resources. Whether the resulting increase in bed utilization and in average patient acuity turns out to be financially beneficial to the institution depends in large measure on the payor mix and funding sources of the referred patients.

COST-EFFECTIVENESS OF ECMO

Many new therapies are considerably more costly than those that they replace, making financial considerations, in concert with clinical effectiveness, increasingly important in the assessment of technological innovations.

An analysis completed at CNMC in 1986 compared the cost of ECMO therapy with the cost of a clinically similar population who had not received ECMO (6). This study showed that the average length of stay for the ECMO population was significantly shorter than for the non-ECMO group (21 vs. 37 days). Therefore, even though ECMO increased the daily charges significantly (average increase of $1,800), it did not increase total charges because the length of stay was shortened. When only survivors were considered, a more dramatic effect of ECMO on length of stay and hence cost was seen. The ECMO group had an average length of stay of 25 days, compared to 76 days in the non-ECMO group, resulting in a 43% decrease in total physician and hospital charges in the ECMO population. The most important finding, however, was that infant survival quadrupled. Moreover, the short-term clinical outcome for ECMO survivors is excellent (see Chapter 16). Not only are acute-care costs lower for infants who receive ECMO rather than maximal medical management, but long-term costs are likely to be lower as well. In addition, the improved survival represents a substantial economic benefit to society because of the opportunity for infants who previously would have died to have productive lives.

The results of the CNMC study have been corroborated by two other studies (7,8). In particular, Bonis evaluated the effect of ECMO on costs in the older pediatric population and found that it resulted in a 36% reduction in costs because of a significant reduction in average length of stay (27 days vs. 11 days).

It must be remembered that these studies were in centers that treated more than 20 patients per year. Although much of the expense associated with ECMO therapy is directly proportional to the number of patients treated, there are economies of scale that accrue to larger programs. For smaller centers that must maintain an expensive team for a few patients, the cost-effectiveness of ECMO has not yet been demonstrated. This is another factor that should be considered before developing a new program.

As with any intensive medical intervention, it probably would be less expensive to prevent pulmonary problems in term infants than to provide ECMO therapy. Of the clinical indications for ECMO, however, only one is clearly amenable to preventive efforts: meconium aspiration syndrome (MAS). In the past decade, better resuscitation techniques in the delivery room have substantially decreased the incidence of meconium below the vocal cords, with a concomitant reduction in MAS requiring neonatal intensive care. Other clinical conditions for which ECMO is used, however, cannot be prevented with current understanding and technology. For example, the causes of persistent pulmonary hypertension of the newborn and congenital diaphragmatic hernia are unknown, so preventive efforts cannot be undertaken.

ECMO PROGRAM FOLLOW-UP COST

The specific costs of care for infants following successful completion of ECMO therapy are difficult to determine because most follow-up care is provided by existing neonatal clinics, without the need for substantial additional resources. All ECMO centers must have an active follow-up program for these infants. (See Chapter 16 for a thorough review of the appropriate follow-up studies for infants receiving ECMO.) It is estimated that annual follow-up expenses per infant at CNMC are $600 the first year and $200 per year thereafter. Another issue to consider is third-party payment. Because these infants usually are doing quite well, there has been difficulty in obtaining reimbursement from third-party payors. At CNMC, part of the follow-up specialists' salaries are paid by the clinical program to ensure that follow-up occurs despite inadequate reimbursement. Recommendations on follow-up requirements for infants receiving ECMO are available from the Extracorporeal Life Support Organization (ELSO) and may help to justify any testing questioned by insurance companies.

SUMMARY

ECMO is one of the most exciting new neonatal therapies to emerge in the past decade. Studies have indicated that it is both clinically successful and cost-effective. It should be developed and organized on a regional basis to maximize these advantages. Once the decision is made to start a new program, substantial lead time and a preliminary budget of approximately $125,000 are required for adequate training of personnel and for administrative activities. Once in operation, the program's budget consists chiefly of personnel expenses, including continuing training costs.

REFERENCES

(1) Boyle MH, Torrance GW, Sinclair JC, et al. Economic evaluation of neonatal intensive care of very-low-birth-weight-infants. N Engl J Med 1983;308:1330–7.

(2) Budetti P, McManus P, Barrand N, et al. The costs and effectiveness of neonatal intensive care (background paper no. 2, case study no. 10). Washington, D.C.: Office of Technology Assessment, 1981.

(3) Fineberg HV, Hiatt HH. Evaluation of medical practices: the case for technology assessment. N Engl J Med 1979;301:1086–91.

(4) Sinclair JC, Torrance GW, Boyle MH, et al. Evaluation of neonatal-intensive care programs. N Engl J Med 1981;305:489–94.

(5) Southgate WM, Howell CG, Kanto WP. The need for and impact on neonatal mortality of extracorporeal membrane oxygenation in infants

greater than 2500 gram birth weight. Pediatrics (In press.)

(6) Pearson GD, Short BL. An economic analysis of extracorporeal membrane oxygenation. J Intens Care Med 1986;2:116–20.

(7) Bonis SL, Palermo M, Adolph VR, et al. The economics of pediatric extracorporeal membrane oxygenation. Beckenridge, CO: Sixth Annual ECMO Symposium, 1990.

(8) Bartlett RH, Schumacher R, Roloff DW. Prospective randomized study of cost effectiveness of neonatal ECMO. Ann Arbor, MI: Charter Meeting, Extracorporeal Life Support Organization, 1989.

24

Prospects for the Future

❖

Robert H. Bartlett, M.D.

At the time that this book is being written, extracorporeal life support (ECLS) is being used routinely for term and near-term newborn infants with respiratory failure in North America, Europe, and Japan. Older children are being treated with ECLS for respiratory failure in several centers in the United States and abroad; ECLS is used for adult respiratory failure quite extensively in Europe but rather cautiously in the United States. Venoarterial bypass is used for cardiac support and for respiratory support in most newborn infants. Venovenous bypass is most commonly used for respiratory failure in children and adults. Sci-Med membrane lungs are used routinely, as are servoregulated roller pumps, direct cut-down vascular access, and systemic heparinization to whole blood activated clotting times in the range of 200 s. Only moribund patients are considered for ECLS, with survival rates in experienced centers of 90% for neonates, 50% for children and adults, and 50% for pediatric cardiac support. Several potential improvements in the technology are under evaluation in various laboratories. In this final chapter, we will speculate on the future of ECLS technology during the next 10 to 20 years.

ARTIFICIAL ORGANS

In the future, variations of microporous membrane lungs will replace the solid silicone rubber membrane because of improved efficiency of gas transfer, lower perfusion pressures, workability of materials, and lower cost of manufacture. The only problem that precludes the use of microporous membranes currently is the plasma leakage that occurs when the micropores have become wet, usually related to condensation of water in the gas phase (in a process very similar to what causes a tent to leak in the rain when it is touched with a damp finger). The problem of plasma leakage will be eliminated through a combination of surface coating and minimizing water condensation (1). The process of heparin bonding to microporous materials may be sufficient to eliminate the problems of wettability and plasma leakage without the need for further modification to sweep gas temperature or humidification (2).

As the systemic heparin dose decreases, manufacturers will pay increasing attention to flow design, minimizing stagnant and eddy current zones, while maintaining low resistance to blood flow. With these modifications, only two sizes of membrane lung will be necessary: a neonatal/pediatric size, with a rated flow of approximately 1 L/min, and a child/adult size, with a rated flow of approximately 5 L/min.

The IVOX, a long, thin capillary membrane oxygenator designed for placement inside the vena cava and right atrium, is entering initial clinical trials (3). The gas exchange capacity of this device is inadequate for total support but may be applied in partial CO_2 removal as an extracorporeal membrane lung that fills the conduit tubing or, with modifications, as the first implantable orthotopic artificial lung.

The servoregulated roller pump is certainly the workhorse of extracorporeal circulation, but is inherently potentially dangerous. The centrifugal pump is equally dangerous because high negative pressure and hemolysis can easily occur. The ECLS pumps of the future will be passive filling, mechanically servoregulated, inexpensive, portable, compact, unable to aspirate or pump air, and durable. As outlined in Chapter 4, the Rhone Poulenc/Collin Cardio pump currently used in Paris has most of these characteristics (4). It is not hard to imagine valved ventricle pumps activated pneumatically, hydraulically, or mechanically that would have the same characteristics. Any of these pumps will require accurate on-line flow meters. Pump speed will be adjusted automatically to maintain adequate systemic oxygen delivery under a wide range of conditions, probably based on mixed venous saturation.

In the future, almost all ECLS for respiratory support will be carried out in the venovenous mode using a single catheter with two lumens (5) or tidal flow systems (6). Venoarterial bypass will be used when cardiac support is required. Percutaneous access will become more common, with the use of dilators to introduce peel-away sheaths through which the access catheters will be placed. The most important advance in the next decade will be in the development of nonthrombogenic prosthetic surfaces. These advances are important only when companies are able to routinely and reliably produce devices with specific coatings. Both Medtronic/Carmeda (7) and Bentley Laboratories (8) have developed methods of surface bonding that permit ECLS without systemic anticoagulation in the laboratory. These systems will make it possible to conduct extracorporeal support with the administration of minimal or no systemic heparin. This will totally change the indications, applications, and complications of extracorporeal support. Various aspects of the technique will have to be changed to allow continuous high flow without bridges or Luer locks, maintaining flow around catheters in access vessels, etc. Although permanent surface bonding of heparin may minimize platelet adherence, adhesion, and aggregation, heparin alone will not be the final answer to nonthrombogenic surface. Some combination of heparin, plasminogen activator, and prostacyclin analog, all bound to the prosthetic surface, will come closer to the normal endothelium and may permit longer perfusion with lower flow rates.

CLINICAL PRACTICE OF ECLS

It will be interesting to see how the clinical supervision of ECLS is managed in the future. By the turn of the century, it is likely that dozens of patients will receive ECLS simultaneously in any major medical center, including premature infants, adult ventilator patients, and patients in cardiogenic and hemorrhagic shock. Common sense would dictate that one professional team should manage this system in conjunction with intensive care nursing. This team may be composed of a distinct new paramedical profession of ECLS specialists (as is currently the practice), or the responsibility might ultimately be taken on by subspecialties in perfusion, respiratory therapy, or nursing. The personnel requirements will be similar to current needs in major centers (three or four deep on-call schedules), but a typical work shift will involve priming circuits, performing emergency cannulations or elective decannulations, managing emergencies, and making rounds to provide general supervision and preventive maintenance for 10 or 20 ECLS patients.

ECLS has become routine practice in the last several years because a standardized system and approach have been developed, as have a new group of health care professionals—ECLS clinical specialists. The need for ECLS specialists arose because the current systems require continuous attendance for monitoring and management, coagulation control, and management of emergencies. Specialists may be trained in medicine, nursing, respiratory therapy, or perfusion. Extensive didactic, laboratory, and bedside experience is required because even individuals from these various professions do not have the backgrounds necessary for ECLS management. The ECLS specialist team is essential to make the technique work, but it is also is the most expensive component of extracorporeal life support. During the next decade, the role of the ECLS specialist will change from continuous bedside supervision to simultaneous supervision of several ECLS patients, generally on an on-call basis. Minute-to-minute and hour-to-hour supervision of the ECLS system will be managed by the bedside nurse, much in the way that mechanical ventilators are managed now. Of course, this will not be possible until the safety features outlined above are incorporated into the circuits and intensive care nurses are educated in the details of prolonged extracorporeal circulation.

With improved circuit safety, single-vein access, and minimal anticoagulation, indications for ECLS will change from moribund status to moderate respiratory failure. ECLS will become an adjunct to conventional ventilation and pharmacologic management, rather than something to try when standard ventilation and pharmacology are failing. ECLS will have a significant role for patients who are difficult to wean from mechanical ventilation. Low-flow venovenous (VV) bypass (or intracaval gas exchange) will be used to facilitate extubation and allow ambulation, eating, and other activities that are often precluded by intubation and mechanical ventilation.

ECLS SPIN-OFF

Many of the lessons learned in ECLS have already been applied to bypass for cardiac surgery (servoregulation, mixed venous saturation monitoring, membrane lungs, and standardized descriptors of vascular access catheters). Heparin-bonded, nonthrombogenic circuits will provide a major advance for cardiac operation and other procedures in which extracorporeal circulation with circulatory arrest or control of local blood flow is desirable. The techniques of cardiac operations without systemic heparin must be worked out in the laboratory. How should blood in the lungs and cardiac chambers be anticoagulated? Will thrombosis occur below an aortic cross-clamp? With heparin-bonded circuits, heparin can be discontinued once the heart is closed, eliminating the dilemma of continued oozing while weaning off bypass versus disconnecting from the circuit prematurely to facilitate clotting. Nonthrombogenic surfaces will find major application for other types of blood-contact artificial organs, including dialysis, hemofiltration, and plasmapheresis. The technology of ECLS will be applied to normothermic organ perfusion.

ECLS has already led to better understanding of pulmonary pathophysiology. The identification of pulmonary hypertension in the newborn as the underlying pathophysiology in virtually all cases of full-term respiratory failure is one example. ECMO studies led to the identification of progressive irreversible fibrosis as the final common pathway in acute adult interstitial lung disease (9). Earlier and more extensive use of ECLS will lead to the study of pharmacologic agents to reverse fibrosis and growth factors to enhance lung generation or regeneration. The study of ECLS has brought proper emphasis to the separation of oxygenation from CO_2 removal and the realization that high peak airway pressure during attempted hyperventilation for CO_2 clearance is the major culprit in ventilator-induced lung injury (10). With this knowledge, a return to pressure-limited mechanical ventilators will occur, and ECLS will be used as an adjunct when low-pressure mechanical ventilation has not achieved CO_2 clearance. The study of oxygen kinetics and the role of mixed venous saturation during ECLS have already found their way to the routine management of intensive care patients. In the intensive care unit (ICU), it is currently common practice to manipulate Do_2 to optimize Do_2/Vo_2 ratio.

During ECLS, it is easy to regulate Vo_2 by regulating temperature, and this technique will find its way to routine ICU management.

The two prospective randomized trials of ECLS in newborn respiratory failure (11,12) used adaptive statistical designs (13,14), bringing randomized clinical trial design to the forefront of discussion (15). This was particularly important because of the evaluation of ECLS as a life support technique, so that ethical as well as statistical considerations guided the planning of these studies. Although the conclusions and the methodology in these studies were initially criticized (16), they stood the test of time, and, in the future, the use of adaptive designs will simplify prospective randomized studies in several areas.

Finally, the general success of ECLS in newborn infants has brought the economics and ethics of high-tech intensive care to center stage. One prominent author questioned whether the cost of ECMO was justified to save a newborn life (17). (He reckoned the cost at $25,000; it is actually about $15,000.) The question is certainly valid, although we commonly spend much more than that in the treatment of a single patient with AIDS, pancreatic cancer, newborn asphyxia, prematurity, or other conditions with less favorable outcomes. A recent study demonstrated that length of hospitalization and hospital costs were actually lower in patients receiving ECLS than in patients receiving conventional ventilation (18). Nonetheless, because ECLS is such a highly visible, complex technology, we will be—and should be—asked constantly, "Is it worth it?"

CLINICAL APPLICATIONS

With the improvements in the system outlined above, ECLS will be applied earlier in respiratory and cardiac failure. It will be used routinely for premature infants, older children, and adults with respiratory failure from a variety of causes. ECLS will be used in conjunction with lung transplantation in two ways: to support the lung transplant patient through acute edema or a later rejection crisis and as a bridge to lung transplant for children and adults with acute irreversible disease.

ECLS will gain wider application as temporary mechanical support of the circulation in children with cardiac failure. Intraaortic balloon pumps and left ventricular assist devices will be preferable for adults with cardiac failure, but, because of the nature of cardiac disease and the variety of sizes, children will do better with venoarterial cardiopulmonary bypass supporting both right and left ventricular function. This application will be most beneficial for cardiac patients postoperatively. Although ECLS can be used as a bridge to cardiac transplantation, the likelihood of obtaining a donor heart of appropriate size and blood type within the two- or three-week duration of uncomplicated ECLS is slight. Consequently, ECLS will probably not be used as a bridge to cardiac transplant until the donor supply is greatly increased (perhaps by ECLS as an organ perfusion system).

New applications of ECLS will include emergency room and catheterization laboratory resuscitation in cardiac failure, resuscitation in trauma and hemorrhagic shock, and use as an adjunct to perfusion and temperature control in other critical illness. Emergency bypass systems are already used in many cardiac catheterization laboratories. There are occasional success stories, but sequential complications often lead to emergency cardiac operations with unfavorable outcomes. In the experience of the author, this relates to the use of ECLS technology by physicians and assistants who have no training, background, or experience in perfusion technology. Even in expert hands, the use of venoarterial bypass for cardiac resuscitation is fraught with problems. The use of the technique should be limited to experienced professionals.

The application of ECLS in the management of trauma and resuscitation from hemorrhagic shock will come with the development of a nonthrombogenic system. Exsanguinating hemorrhage, for example, from a ruptured liver or a duodenal ulcer may be managed by simultaneous transfusion and volume replacement associated with quick cannulation for ECLS. Rapid cooling with perfusion will allow total circulatory arrest or continuous cold perfusion at very low flow rates, permitting identification and repair of the bleeding vessels or organs, followed by rewarming on bypass.

This outline of prospects for the future of ECLS seems at best presumptive and at worst preposterous. However, in the 1970s, there had been no successful cases and it was widely held that prolonged extracorporeal support was impossible. By the 1980s, it had been demonstrated that successful ECLS was possible, although it was widely held that acute lung disease was irreversible in any patient sick enough to need it, and the technique was felt to be impractical or unnecessary. In the 1990s, ECLS is considered standard treatment for some groups of patients. Experience has taught us to predict not the limitations but rather the possibilities of extracorporeal life support.

REFERENCES

(1) Mottaghy K, Oedekoven B, Schaich-Lester D, Poppel K. Non-heparin and heparin bonded systems for ECCO$_2$R. An experimental study. In: Gille JP, ed. Neonatal and adult respiratory failure, mechanisms and treatment. Paris: Elsevier, 1989.

(2) Mottaghy K, Oedekoven B, Poppel K, et al. Heparin free long-term extracorporeal circulation using bioactive surfaces. Trans ASAIO 1989;35:635–5.

(3) Mortensen JD. An intravenacaval blood gas exchange device: a preliminary report. Trans ASAIO 1987;33:570–3.

(4) Durandy Y, Chavalier JY, Lecompte Y. Venovenous extracorporeal lung support: initial experience in paediatric patients. In: Gille JP, ed. Neonatal and adult respiratory failure, mechanisms and treatment. Paris: Elsevier, 1989.

(5) Otsu T, Merz SI, Hultquist KA, et al. Laboratory evaluation of a double lumen catheter for venovenous neonatal ECMO. Trans ASAIO 1989;35:647–50.

(6) Kolobow T, Borell M, Spatola R, Tsumo K, Prato P. Single catheter venovenous membrane lung bypass in the treatment of experimental ARDS. Trans ASAIO 1988;34:35–8.

(7) Olsson P, Larm O, Larsson R, et al. Requirements for thrombo resistance of surface-heparinized materials. Ann NY Acad Sci 1983;416:525–37.

(8) Toomasian JM, Hsu L-C, Hirschl RB, Heiss KF, Hultquist KA, Bartlett RH. Evaluation of Duraflo II heparin coating in prolonged extracorporeal membrane oxygenation. Trans ASAIO 1988;34:410–14.

(9) Pratt PC, Vollmer RT, Shelburn JD, et al. Pulmonary morphology in a multihospital collaborative extracorporeal membrane oxygenation project. Am J Pathol 1979;95:191–212.

(10) Kolobow T. On how to injure healthy lungs (and prevent sick lungs from recovering). Trans ASAIO 1988;34:31–4.

(11) Bartlett RH, Roloff DW, Cornell RG, Andrews AF, Dillon PW, Zwischenberger JB. Extracorporeal circulation in neonatal respiratory failure: a prospective randomized study. Pediatrics 1985;4:479–87.

(12) O'Rourke PP, Krone R, Vacanti J, et al. Extracorporeal membrane oxygenation and conventional medical therapy in neonates with persistent pulmonary hypertension of the newborn: a prospective randomized study. Pediatrics. 1989;84:957–63.

(13) Wei LJ, Durham S. The randomized play-the-winner rule in medical trials. J Am Stat Assoc 1978;73:840–3.

(14) Cornell RG, Landenberger BD, Bartlett RH. Randomized play-the-winner clinical trials. Comm Statist: Theory Methods. 1986;1:159–78.

(15) Meinert CL. Extracorporeal membrane oxygenation trials (commentaries). Pediatrics 1990;85:365–6.

(16) Ware JH, Epstein MF. Extracorporeal circulation in respiratory failure (commentaries). Pediatrics 1985;76:849–51.

(17) Philips JB. Treatment of PPHNS. In: Long WA, ed. Fetal and neonatal cardiology. Philadelphia: W.B. Saunders, 1990.

(18) Roloff DW, Schumacher R, Chapman RA, Snedecor S, Bartlett RH. Neonatal ECMO: A prospective randomized study of cost effectiveness. (In preparation, 1990).

APPENDIXES

1

Cannula Specifications

Steven L. Moulton, M.D.

$$F = \frac{\pi(dP)r^4}{8L\eta}$$

In accordance with Poiseuille's law, the flow (F) through a cannula is directly proportional to the pressure drop from one end to the other (dP), multiplied by the fourth power of its radius (r) and divided by its length (L), where η is the viscosity of the fluid. Optimal flow is achieved by using the shortest cannula with the largest diameter.

The cannula should be manufactured from a smooth, flexible, kink-resistant material. Wire reinforcement helps to prevent kinking but thickens the wall, thereby reducing the internal diameter and lowering the flow. Table A1.1 lists several manufacturers of adult and pediatric cannulas, including the types and sizes of cannulas that are currently available for surgical and percutaneous insertion. Table A1.2 lists the characteristics of several neonatal cannulas. The maximum mean flow rates (MMFR) were determined by maximizing each cannula's flow rate without exceeding certain previously determined limits for shear stress, Reynold's number (turbulence), and velocity (1). The M number is a reference number that allows one to compare the flow characteristics of different cannulas. The M number can be thought of as impedance to flow; the higher the value, the greater the resistance to flow (2,3). The k value is the slope of the equation describing the relationship between flow (y) and pressure (x) for venous cannulas; the higher the the k value, the greater the flow capacity (4).

Acknowledgments Cannula measurements were kindly provided by Mary Hegarty, M.D., Robert Kopotic, R.N., and the manufacturers.

TABLE A1.1 Adult and pediatric cannulas

Manufacturer	Address	Material	Type	Sizes (Fr)	Percutaneous cannula Sizes (Fr)
Argyle	Sherwood Medical 1831 Olive St. St. Louis, MO USA 63178 800-428-4400	Polyvinyl chloride	Arterial* Venous	12–36 (even sizes) 16–36 (even sizes)	20 30
Bard	One Park West Tewksbury, MA USA 01876 800-327-4227	Polyvinyl chloride	Arterial Venous	12–26 (even sizes) 16–36 (even sizes)	18, 20 teflon 18, 20 teflon
Biomedicus	9600 W. 76th St. Eden Prairie, MN USA 55344 800-328-4434	Polyurethane, wire wound	Arterial Venous	12, 14, 15, 17, 19, 21 15, 17, 19, 23, 25, 27, 29	15, 17, 19, 21 15, 17, 19, 21
Cook	P.O. Box 489 Bloomington, IN USA 47402 800-457-4500	Ethylene vinyl acetate	Arterial Venous	12, 16, 18, 20 16, 18, 20, 24, 26, 28	16, 20 22, 30

DLP	P.O. Box 0409 620 Watson, SW Grand Rapids, MI USA 49501-0409 800-253-1540	Polyurethane	Arterial Venous	17, 21 21
ELE-CATH	2100 Felver Court Rahway, NJ USA 07065 800-526-4243	Polyvinyl chloride	Arterial Venous	12, 14, 16 16
Polystan	Vitalcor, Inc. 100 E. Chestnut Ave. Westmont, IL USA 60559 800-874-8358	Polyvinyl chloride	Arterial* Venous	12, 14, 16, 18, 21, 24 16–45
Research Medical	1847 W. 2300 South Salt Lake City, UT USA 84119 800-453-8432	Polyvinyl chloride, wire wound	Venous Arterial	16–40 18, 20, 22, 24	20 teflon 20 teflon

*Cut to size.

TABLE A1.2 Neonatal cannulas for extracorporeal life support

Manufacturer	Address	Material	Type	Sizes (Fr)	Side holes	Bevel	Depth marks
Argyle	Sherwood Medical 1831 Olive St. St. Louis, MO USA 63178 800-428-4400	PVC	Arterial*	10	−	−	+
			Venous*	10, 12, 14	+	−	+
Bard	One Park West Tewksbury, MA USA 01876 800-327-4227	PVC	Arterial	8, 10	−	+	+
			Venous	8, 10, 12	+	+	+
Biomedicus	9600 W. 76th St. Eden Prairie, MN USA 55344 800-328-4434	Polyurethane, wire wound	Arterial	8, 10	−	+	+
			Venous	8, 10, 12, 14	+	+	+
Elecath	2100 Felver Court Rahway, NJ USA 07065 800-526-4243	PVC	Arterial	8, 10	−	+	−
			Venous	8, 10, 12, 14	+	+	−
Gesco Intl.	PO 690188 San Antonio, TX USA 78269 800-531-5814	Silastic	Arterial*	9.6	−	+	+
			Venous*	12, 14	+	+	+
Kendall	15 Hampshire St. Mansfield, MA USA 02048 800-346-7197	Polyurethane	Double-lumen venovenous	10, 12, 14	+	+	+
Polystan	Vitalcor, Inc. 100 E. Chestnut Ave. Westmont, IL USA 60559 800-874-8358	PVC	Venous	12, 14	+	+	−
Research Medical	1847 W 2300 South Salt Lake City, UT USA 84119 800-453-8432	PVC, wire wound	Venous	12, 14	+	+	−

*Cut to size
†ID = inside diameter.
‡OD = outside diameter.
§N/A = not applicable.

Radio-Opaque tip	Size (Fr)	ID† (mm)	OD‡ (mm)	Wall thickness (mm)	Maximum mean flow rate (cc/min)	M number	k value (blood)
+	10	2.2	3.4	0.60	575		3.4
+	12	2.7	4.0	0.65		4.15	3.7
	14	3.2	4.6	0.70			
+	8	N/A§					
	10	N/A					1.5
+	12	N/A					2.8
	14	N/A					3.8
−	8	2.0	3.0	0.50			
	10	2.3	3.4	0.55	900		5.7
+	12	2.9	3.9	0.50			4.4
	14	3.1	4.3	0.60			
+	8	1.6	2.8	0.60	475	4.55	
	10	2.5	3.5	0.50	700	4.10	5
+	12	2.7	4.2	0.75		3.80	3.8
	14	3.0	4.8	0.90		3.70	4.4
+	9.6	1.8	3.2	0.70			1.1
+	12	2.7	4.0	0.65			2.8
	14	3.3	4.6	0.65			4.1
+	14	—	4.05	0.20		4.05	
−	12	2.6	4.0	0.70			
	14	3.2	4.7	0.75			
−	12	2.0	4.0	1.00			
	14	2.6	4.6	1.00			

REFERENCES

(1) Van Meurs KP, Mikesell GT, Winslow RS, Short BL, Rivera O. Maximum blood flow rates for arterial cannulae used in neonatal ECMO. Trans ASAIO 1990;36:M679–81.

(2) Montoya JP, Merz SI, Bartlett RH. A standardized system for describing flow/pressure relationships in vascular access devices. Trans ASAIO (in press.)

(3) Sinard JM, Merz SI, Hatcher M, Bartlett RH. Evaluation of extracorporeal perfusion catheters using a standardized measurement technique: the M-number. (Submitted for publication.)

(4) Ehren H, Frenckner B, Palmer K. In-vitro evaluation of neonatal ECMO cannulae with regard to flow characteristics. Perfusion 1990;5:45–51.

2

Venovenous Extracorporeal Membrane Oxygenation in Neonates Using the Double-Lumen Catheter

❖

Robert H. Bartlett, M.D.

The double-lumen venovenous (VV) catheter provides respiratory support for neonates undergoing ECMO via single-site cannulation of the internal jugular vein. The carotid artery is not cannulated and thus is spared ligation. Since November 1988, we have used ECMO for the treatment of respiratory failure in 117 newborns. Venovenous double-lumen-catheter ECMO was performed in 65 of these patients, with the remaining patients undergoing venoarterial (VA) ECMO because of the inability to cannulate the jugular vein or the need for cardiac support. Gestational age of the patients undergoing venovenous ECMO ranged from 35 to 42 weeks, and weight ranged from 2.5 to 4.9 kg. Patient diagnoses included meconium aspiration syndrome (MAS), sepsis, pneumonia, persistent fetal circulation (PFC), respiratory distress syndrome (RDS), and congenital diaphragmatic hernia (CDH).

Four patients required conversion from venovenous to venoarterial ECMO because of insufficient support (hypotension, hypoxemia, cardiac arrest during initiation of bypass). The remaining 61 patients were supported at flow rates of 125 mL/kg/minute, and bypass time averaged 119 hours (range 55 to 318 hours). Forty-eight percent of cases had complications, which included bleeding, hypotension, hypoxemia, circuit component clotting, seizure, intracranial hemorrhage, kinking of the catheter, raceway rupture, and air entrapment in the venous drainage line. All complications were managed without patient morbidity, and all patients were ultimately decannulated from venovenous ECMO; survival for these patients was 100%.

In conclusion, the double-lumen catheter for venovenous ECMO can provide respiratory support for a majority of newborn patients undergoing ECMO bypass, without cannulation of the carotid artery. Data from the multicenter ELSO study of the double-lumen catheter are included in Table A2.8.

TABLE A2.1 Venovenous ECLS using the double-lumen catheter

117 Patients treated with VA and VV ECLS between November 1988 and February 1991.

73 Patients MET VV criteria (62%). Cannulation was successful in 65 patients (89%).

4 Patients (6%) required conversion to venoarterial bypass because of insufficient support.

The remaining 52 patients were treated with venoarterial ECLS (1 patient recannulated for VA bypass).

TABLE A2.2 Patient diagnoses

Diagnoses	VV	VA
Meconium aspiration syndrome (MAS)	33	13
Persistent fetal circulation (PFC)	6	3
Respiratory distress syndrome (RDS)	12	11
Sepsis/pneumonia	7	7
Congenital diaphragmatic hernia (CDH)	6	15
Other (cardiac anomalies, etc.)	1	4
Totals	65	53

TABLE A2.3 Venovenous vs. venoarterial cases (November 1988 to February 1991)

Diagnoses	VV	VA
Number of patients	65	53
Gestational age (weeks)	40 ± 0.2	38 ± 0.7
Weight (kg)	3.4 ± 0.1	3.1 ± 0.1
Time on bypass (hours)	130 ± 9.7	155 ± 14
Complications (%)	35	38
Survival (%)	98	79

TABLE A2.4 Venovenous ECLS cases: complications

Bleeding	9
Air in circuit	5
Seizures	5
Clotting of circuit	4
VV → VA conversion	4
Kinked catheter	3
Incorrect catheter insertion/placement	4
Intracranial hemorrhage	2
Power loss at pump	2
Hemolysis	1

TABLE A2.5 Limitations/contraindications to venovenous bypass in the newborn

Severe right or left-sided cardiac dysfunction (by echocardiogram, persistent hypotension, metabolic acidosis, anuria)

Need for cardiac support (operation intended)

Cardiac arrest or ongoing CPR

TABLE A2.6 Limitations/contraindications to venovenous double-lumen catheter use in the newborn

Weight < 2.5 kg

Small internal jugular vein size

Cardiac dysfunction (by echocardiogram, persistent metabolic acidosis, anuria)

Vein tears during cannulation

Displacement of mediastinum (i.e., tension pneumothorax)

Prominent first rib

TABLE A2.7 Venovenous bypass

Advantages
  Pulmonary circulation is maintained. Pulmonary circulation oxygenation is maintained.
  Particulate emboli travel to lungs.
  No carotid ligation.
  Pulsatile arterial wave form maintained.
  Efficient CO_2 removal.

Disadvantages
  No control of blood pressure.
  Inefficiency (recirculation). Hypoxemia (low Po_2).
  Dual site access (jugulofemoral access) vs. double-lumen catheter, single-site access.

TABLE A2.8 ELSO double-lumen catheter evaluation protocol: preliminary results

12 centers with 59 venovenous double-lumen catheter cases (and 60 venoarterial cases)

13 centers with only venoarterial cases

Of 59 venovenous double lumen catheter runs, 4 required conversion VV → VA

Two deaths in 59 venovenous cases, 7 deaths in 60 venoarterial cases

TABLE A2.9 ELSO double-lumen catheter evaluation protocol: preliminary results

Diagnosis	VV	VA
MAS	29	22
CDH	5	9
PFC/PPHN*	7	8
RDS	4	10
Pneumonia	4	3
Sepsis	4	4
Cardiac	1	0
?	5	4
Totals	59	60

*PPHN = persistent pulmonary hypertension of the neonate.

TABLE A2.10 ELSO double-lumen catheter evaluation protocol: preliminary results

Catheter complications (59 cases):		
Kinking	1	
Repositioning or malplacement	6	
Totals	7	(12% of cases)

TABLE A2.11 ELSO double-lumen catheter evaluation protocol: preliminary results

	VV	VA
Number	55	60
Hours on bypass	111 ± 8	114 ± 9
Survival (%)	53 (96%)	53 (88%)

Index

ACA. *See* Anterior cerebral arteries (ACA)
Access sites for venovenous ECLS, 265f
Acid-base imbalance, during ECMO, 219–20
ACT. *See* Activated clotting time (ACT)
Activated clotting time (ACT)
  modification on bleeding, 213
  monitoring in perfusion, 99
  monitoring to prevent intracranial hemorrhage, 217
  values for pediatric patients, 279
Acute respiratory failure (ARF)
  definition of, 286
  ECMO for adult patients, NIH study, 42
  pediatric, 183
  therapies for, less conventional, 80–82
Adaptive experimental design, 340
  randomized study, 46–47
ADC. *See* Additional Data Collection (ADC) study

Additional Data Collection (ADC) study, 288
Adenosine, effects in the brain, 140
Adenosine monophosphate (AMP), role in platelet aggregation, 108
Adenosine triphosphate (ATP), NMR measurement of, for evaluation of cerebral injury in infants, 149
Adhesion proteins, tripeptide sequence of, 109
Administrative preparation for new programs, 332
Adult respiratory distress syndrome (ARDS), 43, 179, 286–99
  characteristics of, 287
  in children, 275
  criteria for diagnosis, 276t
  surfactant therapy for, 79–80
Adult respiratory failure, NIH study of ECMO in, 34, 37
Adults
  sources and types of cannulas for, 346–47t

vascular access for ECLS, 175–83
Affective regulation, and damage to the right hemisphere, 248
Afterload, changes in ECMO, 131–32
Agaroses, urokinase bound to, 112
Air embolus as mechanical failure, 210–12
Air leak syndrome, ECLS for infants with, 275
Airway pressure release ventilation, 68
Albolabrin, 109
Albumin
  durability of coating on silicone rubber, 114
  passivation of a surface by, 98, 113–15
  priming a circuit with, 100, 172
  as a source of aluminum toxicity, 234
  for transfusion of neonatal patients, 196, 198
ALEC. *See* Artificial lung-expanding compound (ALEC)
Algorithm, management of

malfunctioning ECMO equipment, 211
Alkaline earth elements as heat stabilizers in medical plastics, 118
Alkalosis
 and phosphofructokinase activity, 141
 respiratory, 94
Aluminum
 in ECMO systems, 234, 235
 particles in emboli, 210
American Academy of Pediatrics, Committee on the Fetus and Newborn, 78–79
Amniotic fluid as a surfactant source, 77
AMP. See Adenosine monophosphate (AMP)
Amphophilic materials for modification of polymers, 116
Anatomic dead space, reduction of, 298
Anemic hypoxia, 139–40
Angiography
 for confirmation of PDA, 221
 for evaluation of carotid artery ligation in neonates, 189
Animal training sessions, cost of, 333
Antacids for gastrointestinal bleeding, 215
Anterior cerebral arteries (ACA), flow velocity in, and pneumothorax, 145
Antiadrenergic drugs in ECC, 24
Antibiotics
 coating the extracorporeal circuit with, 182–83
 for pediatric patients, 279
Anticoagulation, 293
 monitoring of, 102
 for pediatric patients, 279
Antithrombin-heparin mechanism, 107f
Anuria as a complication of ECMO, 234
Apneic oxygenation, 264, 291
 in ARDS patients, 293
Apoproteins in synthetic surfactant, 77
Aprotonin (FUT175), 109–10

Arachidonic acid metabolites, 227
 and intracranial hemorrhage in newborns, 228
ARDS. See Adult respiratory distress syndrome (ARDS)
ARF. See Acute respiratory failure (ARF)
Arginine chloromethyl ketone peptides, selective inactivation of thrombin by, 109
Arginine-glycine-aspartic acid (RGD) sequence, 109
Arrhythmias, during cannulation, 133–34
Arterial blood gases, and fetal breathing activity, 326t
Arterial oxygen saturation versus venous oxygen saturation, 91
Arterial oxygen tension, maintenance with nasal prong CPAP, 52
Arterial pulse contour, and level of venoarterial bypass, 97f
Arterial reservoir, open cardiotomy using (1955), 21t
Arteriovenous bypass
 neonatal, 184, 185
Artificial lung-expanding compound (ALEC) in an artificial surfactant, 76–77
Artificial organs, 337–38
 lungs, 31–32
Artificial placenta, 320–21
Artificial surfaces, interactions of blood with, 105–20
ASD. See Atrial secundum defect (ASD)
Asphyxia, sensitivity of cerebral autoregulation to, 139
Aspiration of gastrointestinal contents underlying ARDS, 287t
Aspirin, effect on platelets, 108
Assist cannulation
 left heart, 303f
 right heart, 304f
Atelectasis
 following ECMO, 200, 202

ATP. See Adenosine triphosphate (ATP)
Atrial naturetic factor, levels in infants on ECMO, 234
Atrial secundum defect (ASD), surgery for
 first successful, 10
 using hypothermia, 11
 using perfusion techniques, 11, 11t
Atrioventricular communis, outcomes of surgery, thirty-year follow-up, 16t
Autogenous lung, 13–14
Autoregulation, cerebral, 139
Avecor Cardiovascular Inc., 34, 207, 337 (formerly Sci-Med Life Systems)
Axillary cannulation, 310–11
Azotemia, management in ECMO, 218
Azygos flow concept, 13
 support from a bubble oxygenator, 19

Baby Bird-2 ventilator, 53
BAER. See Basal auditory evoked response (BAER)
Barotrauma, 43
 in ARDS, 288, 295
 causes of, 272
 in conventional mechanical ventilation, 51, 52
 ECMO use to avoid, 48
 and muscle relaxant use, 56–57
 pulmonary, in tidal volume ventilation, 264
Basal auditory evoked response (BAER), 248
 evaluation prior to discharge, 205
Basal cardiac output versus physiologic flow, 13
Bayley index scores
 correlation with neuroimaging studies, 150
 for evaluation of infants after ECMO, 244
 HFOV study, 73
Bear Cub ventilator, 53
Bedside cart, 172
Beery Test of Visual Motor Integration, outcomes for

ECMO survivors, 245, 245f
Bernoulli principle, 127
Beta-thromboglobulin, effect of disintegrins on, 109
Bias, accommodation to, randomized study, 46
Bias gas flow in HFOVs, 71
Biologic oxygenators, heterologous, 17
Birthweight as a criterion for ECMO, 157
Bladder. See Venous reservoir (bladder)
Bladder bridge for pediatric systems, 277–78
Bladder in the ECMO system, 169
Bleeding
 and ARDS management, 293
 as a cause of death in ARDS, 295
 in CDH patients on ECMO, 259
 in ECMO, 313
  with adult patients, 182
  for cardiac support, 315–16
 esophageal, management of, 215
 indicators of, 213, 215
 management of, 214t, 216f
 in neonatal patients, 197, 199
 in pediatric ECMO, 282
 and selection for ECMO, 158
 and weaning from ECMO, 204–5
Blood, interactions with artificial surfaces, 105–20
Blood coagulation tester, 172
Blood drainage and return, methods for, 292t
Blood flow
 risks of changing patterns during ECMO, 227–28
 total support level, 100
Blood flow rate
 calculated versus measured, 167
 and catheter size and shape, 167
 during ECMO, 130, 130t
 and heparin rate, 199
 in a membrane lung, 171

Blood gases
 arterial values, 203–4
 management on venoarterial ECMO, 202–4
 values in survivors versus nonsurvivors of ECMO, 159t
Blood-gas interface, problems with, 302
Blood pressure in ECMO, 129, 129f
Blood pumps, 167
 for ECMO, 3
Blood reservoir to avoid negative pressure, 95
Blood sampling, 227
Blood-surface interactions, 227
Blood transfusion, risks of, 227
Blood volume
 average ECMO administration, 317
 loss with perfusion techniques for cardiac surgery, 13
Bonding, infant-parent, 199
Bournes BP200 ventilator, 53
BPD. See Bronchopulmonary dysplasia (BPD)
Brain, effects of ECMO on, 138–51
Brain death in CDH infants referred for ECMO, 256
Brain flow studies for evaluation of cerebral injury in infants, 149–50
Brain interstitial fluid, alteration of pH by CO_2, 140–41
Brain metabolism, NMR for evaluation of, 149
Brain-stem function
 auditory responses, 232f
 BAERS in ECMO survivors, 146
 effects of jugular or carotid artery ligation, 231
Bramson membrane oxygenator, 34, 34f
Bronchial divisions, and development of congenital diaphragmatic hernia, 254
Bronchopulmonary dysplasia (BPD), 72
 association with CDH, 256

Bubble oxygenator
 DeWall-Lillehei, 19–23, 20f
 versus membrane oxygenators, 23–24
 open cardiotomy using (1955–1966), 21, 21t
Bubble trap
 incorporation in heat exchanger design, 168
 venous reservoir as, 169
Buffering with sodium bicarbonate in an ECMO system, 173
Bulk additives
 low-level toxic effects of, 118
 for polymers to alter blood compatibility, 116–17
Bunnell Life Pulse High Frequency Ventilator, 71

C5a receptor site on neutrophil membrane, 105
Calcium
 replacement level in neonatal ECMO patients, 198
 serum levels in ECMO, 134
Calf lung surfactant extract (CLSE) in an artificial surfactant, 77
Cannula
 polyurethane double-lumen, 185
 problems with, 209, 209t
 repositioning in pediatric ECMO, 283
 specifications, 345
Cannulation
 adult vascular access schemes, 179
 assist, for the left heart, 303f
 brain-stem auditory responses during, 232f
 cervical, for venoarterial bypass, 189f
 cervical, positioning for, 186f
 chest, in ECMO for cardiac support, 309–10, 309f
 of the femoral vein, 180–81, 181f
 fluid shear stresses at sites of, 119–20
 of the jugular vein, 180, 180f

for neonatal ECLS, detailed description, 186–89, 186f
procedure, 101
single-cannula system for venovenous bypass, 266
techniques for pediatric patients, 278–79
techniques in ECMO for cardiac support, 307–11
two-cannula system for venovenous bypass, 265–66, 266f
vagus nerve manipulation during, and feeding problems, 244
venoarterial, 305f
via iliac or cervical vessels, 184, 184f
for venovenous ECMO, 304f
Capillary permeability, during ECLS, 99
Carbon dioxide (CO_2) levels
and changes in the cerebral blood flow, 228
importance to successful ECLS, 179
and lung damage during VA bypass, 264
management for infants on mechanical ventilation, 57
management with change in gas flow rates, 204
measurement of end tidal, 102
metabolic production of, 91–92
for priming an ECMO circuit, 172
removal by a membrane lung, 264
removal in extracorporeal circulation, 37–39, 93–94, 94f, 292f
contraindications for, 291t
and selection of infants for ECMO, 258
Carbon dioxide membrane lungs (CDML), 264, 320
Carbon dioxide reactivity in the brain, 140–43
Carbon dioxide response curve, effect of fentanyl on, 199–200
Cardiac catheterization
of infants on ECMO, 132
intracardiac pressures of infants on ECMO, 133f
Cardiac changes
abnormal, during ECMO, 133t
output in PPHN, 127
in prolonged ECMO, 126–36
Cardiac disease
ECMO for, 302–17
and selection for ECMO, 158
Cardiac function
changes during ECMO, 136
effect of VV circulation on physiology, 99–100
evaluation of, 128–29, 314
in neonatal ECMO, 231–33
in venoarterial bypass, 218–19
Cardiac patients, survival rates, following ECMO, 4t
Cardiac stun, 132, 134, 135–36, 231, 232
Cardiac tamponade, obstruction to venous return caused by, 213
Cardiomyopathy, temporary, ECMO to treat, 306
Cardiopulmonary bypass (CPB), 89
adult, evaluation of brain changes, 147
original use of heart-lung machine for, 10–11
outcomes, early use of screen oxygenator, 12t
partial, with ECMO, 126, 129
summary (1951–1954), 12t
Cardiorespiratory decompensation in ECMO, 219t
Cardiorespiratory homeostasis, 90–91
Cardiotomy, results, University of Minnesota Hospitals, 21t
Cardiovascular depression in CMV, 51
Carotid artery reconstruction, 189–90, 309
Catecholamines, and oxygen consumption, 90
Catecholamine secretion, during ECLS, 99
Catheters
for ECMO, 3–4, 165–67, 166f
positioning
confirmation by x-ray, 189
documentation of, 133–34
problems with, 209
protection by moderate sedation, 199
size, and M numbers, 97t
Cat model middle cerebral artery occlusion, 142
Cavitation of tubing, 168
CBF. See Cerebral blood flow (CBF)
CDH. See Congenital diaphragmatic hernia (CDH)
CDML. See Carbon dioxide membrane lungs (CDML)
Cellulose acetate, albumin films on, 114
Central nervous system (CNS)
damage from jugular vein or carotid ligation, 228–30
damage in ECMO for infants, 43
insult prior to ECMO in neonates, 242–46
limitation of ECMO damage to, 150–51
management of deterioration, 214t
morbidity, ECMO versus CMV, 49t
in PPHN, follow-up, 65
risks during ECMO, 228–31
Central registry data, ventilator settings, 202
Centrifugal pump
for ECC, 25
for ECLS, 95–96
for neonatal ECMO, 167
Cerebral blood flow (CBF)
changes during ECMO, 243
regulation of, 138–40, 242
Cerebral collateral circulation, testing in venoarterial bypass, 181–82

Cerebral edema, management of, 214t
Cerebral infarction in neonates, 242
Cerebral injury, markers in infants, 148–50
Cerebral ischemia, 142–43
Cerebral oxygen consumption (CMRO$_2$)
 cerebral blood flow in, 140
 as a determinant of CBF, 138
Cerebral palsy, following ECMO, 244
Cerebral vascular reactivity in hypothermia, 140
Certified perfusionists, 332
Cervical cannulation, 189f
 positioning for, 186f
Cetyl alcohol in an artificial surfactant, 76
Chemotaxis, at a neutrophil membrane, 105
Chest cannulation, ECMO for cardiac support, 309–10, 309f
Chest trauma, underlying condition in ARDS, 287t
Children, extracorporeal life support in, 274–84
Children's Hospital, Boston, randomized study of neonatal ECMO, 46–47
Children's Hospital of Michigan
 predictor study, ECLS for cardiac disease, 307
 study of ECMO for cardiac support, 314–17
Children's National Medical Center (CNMC), 157, 333
Chloral hydrate for infants, 199
Chronic instrumentation of fetal sheep, 322
Chronic lung disease
 on follow-up of HFOV versus CMV, 73
 following HFOV or ECMO treatment of infants, 75
 neurodevelopmental outcomes, 246
Chronic obstructive lung disease (COPD), ITV with, 298

Cimetidine for gastrointestinal bleeding, 215
Circuit design
 ECLS, 100–101, 101t
 for pediatric ECMO patients, 277–78
Circulation, effects of mechanical ventilation on, 52
Clinical applications, future of ECMO in, 340–41
Clinical experience with surfactant replacement therapy, 77–78
Clinical outcomes
 brain studies following ECMO, 146–47
 double-lumen VV bypass, 271
 high-frequency ventilation, 72–73
 pediatric ECMO, 280–82
 See also Outcomes; Results
Clinical practice
 ECLS, 338–39
 management of congenital diaphragmatic hernia, 254–56
Clots/clotting
 hemolysis associated with, 221–22
 in a perfusion apparatus, 32
 routine evaluation for risk of, 197
 See also Coagulation
Clotting cascade, 198
Clotting time in polyalkylsufone membranes, 117
Coagulation
 control during perfusion, 98–99
 management in ECMO for cardiac support, 313
 studies of, and criteria for neonatal ECMO, 160
Coagulation cascade, 107f
Coagulation factors, transfusion of, and ACT values, 199
Coagulopathy
 and heparin requirements, 199
 and selection for ECMO, 158
Coatings
 antibiotic, for system surfaces, 182–83

 comparison of polymer surface treatments, 114f
 See also Passivation
Cobe Sentry II single-needle dialysis system, 268
Cold, and fetal breathing activity, 325, 327
Collin Cardio nonocclusive roller pump, 268–69
 operation of, 270f
Color flow Doppler echocardiography for evaluation of PPHN, 128
Color ultrasound for cardiac evaluation
 in ECMO, 314
 in infants with CDH, 255
Complement system, 227
 activation of, 105
 activation of, in infants on bypass, 235
Complications
 definition of, 207
 of ECMO for cardiac support, 315–16
 of neonatal ECMO, 5
 of pediatric ECMO, 282–83
 versus survival rate, ELSO data, 236
 of venovenous ECLS, 352
Compressed spectral array EEG for evaluation of CNS changes in ECMO, 230–31, 231f
Compression ischemia, 142
Computed tomography (CT)
 for documentation of brain lesions in ECMO survivors, 241
 for evaluation of cerebral injury in infants, 149
 for evaluation of CNS damage in ECMO patients, 229–30, 229f
 for evaluation of intracranial abnormalities, 146
Congenital diaphragmatic hernia (CDH)
 data from the National ECMO Registry (1987), 44t
 endocardial cushion defects associated with, 259

management with ECMO, 252–59
survival rate, data from the National ECMO Registry, 45
survival rates, following ECMO, 4t
timing of surgery and ECMO support, 258–59
Congenital heart disease as an exclusionary criterion for ECMO, 160
Constant flow ventilation, 68
Consultation, cost of, 333
Continuous flow versus pulsatile flow, 24
Continuous positive airway pressure (CPAP), 52
future of, 272
Contractility (VCSF), during ECMO, 132
Control trials
ECMO versus conventional therapy, 65
See also Evaluations
Conventional mechanical ventilation (CMV)
versus early and late ECMO for neonates, 48
versus ECMO, 42
versus HFJV, 73
versus HFOV, NIH study, 72
See also Mechanical ventilation
Conventional respiratory support, optimization of, 51–65
COPD. See Chronic obstructive lung disease (COPD)
Cord clamping, experiments in, 327
Cortical blindness, following ECMO, 248
Cost-effectiveness of ECMO, 334–35
Countercurrent flow in a membrane lung, 170, 170f
CPAP. See Continuous positive airway pressure (CPAP)
CPB. See Cardiopulmonary bypass (CPB)
Cranial CT scan for neonates prior to discharge, 205
Cranial ultrasound
for documentation of brain lesions in ECMO survivors, 241
to evaluate intracranial hemorrhage in neonates, 196–97
evaluation with, 217
to screen ECMO candidates, 148
Criteria for patient selection
for cannulation procedure in neonatal ECLS, 190–91
for ECLS for children, 275–77
for ECMO with ARDS, 290
for ECMO with CDH, 255–56, 257–58
for neonatal ECMO, 156–59, 159t
and prematurity, 44
for venovenous bypass in neonates, 352
See also Indications
Cross-circulation
in intracardiac operations, 14–16, 14f
open cardiotomy using (1954–1955), 21t
results, 1954–1955, 16
Cryoprecipitate for transfusion of neonatal patients, 196
CT. See Computed tomography (CT); Cranial computed tomography (CT) scan
Cuprophan, albumin films on, 114
Cushing's response, 139
Cycle length, and tidal flow VV bypass performance, 267
Cyclooxygenase inhibitors, 108
Cystic fibrosis, ECLS with, 183
Cytomegalovirus, pneumonias secondary to, 275

Da Nang lung, 286
Debubbling, step of ECMO circuit priming, 172
Decannulation, 103
laboratory tests following, 205
of neonatal patients, 189
of neonatal pediatric patients, 196
See also Reconstruction
Developmental responses
to anoxia, by immature animals, 141
brain maturation and CO_2 responsivity of the brain, 141
in neonatal ECLS patients, 189
DeWall-Lillehei oxygenator, 19–23, 20f
Dextran, thromboembolism reduction following administration of, 119
Dialysis, indications for, 218
Digital intravenous angiography (DIVA), 150
Dimethylpolysiloxane membrane in early heart-lung machines, 31
Dipalmitoyl phosphatidylcholine in an artificial surfactant, 76
Disintegrins for cell adhesion control, 109
DIVA. See Digital intravenous angiography (DIVA)
Dopamine
dosage as a predictor of cardiac output, 307
for PPHN with oliguria, 58
Doppler echocardiography
color flow, for evaluation of PPHN, 128
for confirmation of PDA, 221
estimation of cardiac output using, 127
for evaluation of cerebral blood flow in infants, 150
for evaluation of patient complications, 221
for evaluation of pulmonary arterial pressure, 132
See also Echocardiography
Double-lumen cannula system, 101, 269–71, 292
evaluation protocol, 352
venovenous (VV) catheter, 351
Down syndrome, ECMO postoperatively for cardiac support, 314

Drainage
    of intrathoracic, abdominal or retroperitoneal hemorrhages, 215
    ratio to infusion time, tidal flow VV bypass performance, 267–68
Drugs
    for passivation of surfaces, 106t
    See also Medications
Ductus arteriosus. *See* Patent ductus arteriosus
Duplex Doppler scan for cardiac evaluation in infants with CDH, 255

ECC. *See* Extracorporeal circulation (ECC)
Echistatin, 109
Echocardiography, of cardiac performance during ECMO, 129–33
    See also Doppler echocardiography
ECLS. *See* Extracorporeal life support (ECLS)
ECLS clinical specialists, 339
ECMO. *See* Extracorporeal membrane oxygenation (ECMO)
ECMO specialists, 332
ECMO system, 161f, 164f
    indications for cardiac support, 306–7
    mechanics of, 3–4
    modification to optimize CNS outcome, 150–51
    neonatal, 43
    priming of the circuit, 172–73
Economics of ECMO therapy, 331–41. *See also* Cost
Eddy flow area, tubing-connector interface, 164f
Edema
    management of, 214t
    in neonatal ECMO patients, 198
Education of an ECMO technical specialist, 208
EEG. *See* Electroencephalograms (EEG); Electroencephalograms (EEG), compressed spectral array

Electroencephalograms (EEG) for evaluation of cerebral injury in infants, 149
Electroencephalograms (EEG), compressed spectral array for evaluation of CNS changes in ECMO, 230–31, 231f
Electrolyte imbalance
    differential diagnosis and management of, 219t
    management of, 214t
ELSO. *See* Extracorporeal Life Support Organization (ELSO)
ELSO National Registry
    complications listed in, 213
    double-lumen catheter evaluation protocol, 352t
    pediatric ECMO data, 283
    preliminary results of studies, 352
ELSO Registry, 207, 226, 256
Emergencies, management of, 207–23
Emerson Airway Vibrator, 71
Endocardial cushion defects, association with congenital diaphragmatic hernia, 259
Endotracheal tube placement for infants on mechanical ventilation, 56
End point attachment for immobilized biologicals, 110
Energy metabolism
    brain, 141–42
    during ECLS, 99
Enteral feedings for neonates after ECMO, 205
Epinephrine for PPHN with hypoxia under ventilation, 58
EPs. *See* Evoked potentials (EPs)
Equipment
    costs of, 332–33
    for ECMO, design at centers, 161, 161t
    for an ECMO program, list, 333t
    types of, in ELSO programs, 207–8
Ethical issues
    in evaluating ECMO outcomes for DCH infants, 257
    prospective randomization, 36
    in randomization, 243
    in statistical design, 46
Di-2-Ethylhexyl phthalate (plasticizer) in the blood of ECMO patients, 235
Evaluations
    adaptive experimental design, 46–47, 340
    adult respiratory failure, NIH study of ECMO in, 34, 37
    double-blind randomized trial of surface treatments, 113–14
    ECMO studies, 1–2, 43–44, 65
    of extracorporeal membrane oxygenation, 178–79
    HFJV comparison with CMV, 73
    play-the-winner randomization, 35–36, 46
    prospective randomized study of ECLS, 340
    prospective randomized study of ECMO in ARF, 289
    ranking versus hypothesis-testing paradigms, 46
    See also Prospective studies; Retrospective studies
Evoked potentials (EPs) for evaluation of cerebral injury in infants, 149
Experimental trials. *See* Evaluations
Extracorporeal assist devices, left-sided and right-sided, 303
Extracorporeal bypass, partial (ECco$_2$)R, 299
Extracorporeal circulation (ECC), 320
    history of development of, 9–26
    potentially detrimental effects of, 217
    for study of fetal lamb physiology, 322–29
    support in heart disease, 302–5
Extracorporeal life support (ECLS), 34

in children, 274–84
gas exchange in, 92–94
spin-off from, 339–40
Extracorporeal Life Support Organization (ELSO), 4, 159
guidelines and standards for ECMO centers, 48
recommendations on follow-up, 335
See also ELSO National Registry; ELSO Registry
Extracorporeal membrane oxygenation (ECMO), 1–6
advantages for cardiac support, 305–6
chronic lung disease following, 75
versus CMV, 42, 45
complications of, 5
criteria for, and previous conventional ventilation, 63
criteria for, Babies' Hospital, 64, 64t
discontinuation in intracranial hemorrhage, 217–18
early versus late, study of, 48
effects on normal and injured brain, 145–50
emergencies, summary, 223t
equipment for, 320
and exogenous surfactant, 79
versus HFOV and CMV, 74–75
problems associated with, 105
Extubation of infants on ventilators, 55–56

Factor X, activation by prostaglandins, 108
Family stress on birth of an ill infant, 248
Fatty acids, affinity of albumin for, 113
Feeding problems, persistent, in ECMO infants, 243–44
Femoral artery, cannulation with allowance for distal perfusion, 182, 182f
Femoral cannulation, 180–81f, 311, 311f

morbidity associated with, 265
Fentanyl
for infants, 199
weaning from, 205
Fetal breathing activity, effects of oxygen and carbon dioxide on, 325
Fetal circulation, animal studies of, 321
Fiberoptic catheter for measuring venous saturation, 101
Fibrin formation, routine evaluation for risk of, 197
Fibrinogen
adsorption at surface crevices, 118
binding to surfaces, 113
thrombogenicity of prosthetic, 98
Fibrinolytic agents for passivation, 112–13
Fick principle of oxygen consumption, 90
Flavoridin, 109
Flow-modulated release of TPA, 119–20
Flow patterns
design to minimize disturbances of, 118
future design, 337–38
red cell preparation in a glass tube, 119f
Flow rate
and clot formation, 98
conventional setting, for an infant ventilator, 53
Flow stabilization, and polysaccharide administration, 119
Fluid balance, management of, 214t
in ECMO for cardiac support, 313
Fluidity enhancement, 118–19
Follow-up
comparison of HFOV and ECMO for neonates, 74–76
costs of, 335
of ECMO for cardiac support, 316–17
of infants after ECMO, 244
of infants with CDH, 257
of intracardiac surgery patients, 16–17

of neonatal ECLS patients, 189–90
of neonatal ECMO patients, 205
of pediatric ECMO patients, 283
right hemispheric evoked potentials post-ECMO, 230
of survivors of intracranial hemorrhage, 217
of tetralogy surgery patients, 19, 21
Food and Drug Administration, approval of ventilators, 71
FPP. *See* Fresh frozen plasma (FFP)
Fractional inspired oxygen, conventional setting, infant ventilator, 53
Fresh frozen plasma (FFP) for transfusion of neonatal patients, 196
Furosemide
for neonatal ECMO patients, 198
for patent ductus arteriosus, 134
response to, and kidney damage, 218
FUT175. *See* Aprotonin (FUT175)

Gamma globulins, binding to surfaces, 113
Gas-blood interface, modification of, in microporous membranes, 116–17
Gas delivery system, 169
Gas flow, matching to blood flow rate in a membrane lung, 171
Gas-permeable membranes, 117–18
Gastrointestinal problems
associated with neonatal ECMO, 234–35
management of bleeding, 215
Geneva pulmonary failure scoring system, 291t
Gestational age
as a criterion for ECMO, 157
and ECMO outcome, 49
and incidence of ROP, 248

and likelihood of intracranial hemorrhage, 217
timing of congenital diaphragmatic hernia development, 253
Glucose
　management of balance, 214t
　substitutes for, in the brain, 141
Glycolysis, resulting from alkalosis, 141

Hand bagging, during mechanical failure, 210
Hard shell bubble oxygenator, 24
Head control, inadequate, after ECMO, 244
Head trauma, sensitivity of cerebral autoregulation to, 139
Head ultrasound for evaluation of intracranial abnormalities, 146
Healthdyne 105 ventilator, 53
Hearing loss in infants following PPHN, 247–48
Heart disease, congenital
　association of abnormalities with CDH, 255
　echocardiography for evaluation of, 127–28
　as an exclusionary criterion for ECMO, 160
　See also Cardiac entries
Heart-lung machines, history, 302
Heart rate in ECMO, 129, 129f
Heaters for ECMO circuits, 167–68
Heat exchange by PFCs, 82
Heat exchanger
　for ECMO systems, 3, 168, 168f
　malfunction of, 210
　for pediatric patients, 277, 277t
Heavy metals as stabilizers in medical plastics, 118
Hematocrit
　desired level in neonates on ECMO, 203
　levels for ARDS management, 293
　as a measure of bleeding, 213
Hemodialysis
　arteriovenous (AV) bypass with, 89
　hypoxemia in, 321–22
Hemodilution, 24
Hemodynamic deterioration
　management of, 220, 220f
　in venoarterial bypass, 218
Hemodynamics
　in cardiac stun, 135f
　cerebral, during ECMO, 150
　of the extracorporeal circuit, 94–98
　of perfusion systems, 118–20
　surface passivation by attention to, 106t
　venovenous bypass, 294
Hemofiltration
　arteriovenous (AV) bypass with, 89
　for renal failure during ECMO, 218
Hemoglobin, 102. See also Hematocrit; Packed red blood cells (PRBCs)
Hemolysis, 221–22
　in centrifugal pump systems, 95, 167
　in early heart-lung machines, 31
　in early oxygenators, 42
　management of, 222f
　from negative pressure in perfusion, 95
　and percutaneous femoral vein access, 182
Hemopericardium, following ECMO, 233
Hemopump axial flow pump, 303, 305
Hemorrhage, differential diagnosis and management of, 219t
Hemorrhage
　intracerebral, 218
　posterior fossa, 231, 232f
　pulmonary, 158
　See also Intracranial hemorrhage (ICH)
Hemostasis, 181, 213
　management of, 108
　and platelet count in perfusion, 99

Heparin, 106–8, 120, 293
　daily management in neonatal patients, 198–99
　in ECMO for cardiac support, 313
　infusion rate, and bleeding, 214–15
　and intracranial hemorrhage, 216–17
　introduction of, 302
　for pediatric patients, 279
　to prevent fibrin formation in ECLS, 98–99
　and risk of intracranial hemorrhage, 228
　titration to a defined clotting time, 32
Heparin-bonded hollow fiber oxygenator, polypropylene, 291
Heparin-bonded systems, 297
　Carmeda, 296
　end point attachment to silicone rubber or PVC, 111–12
　surface immobilization in, 110–12
Heparinized perfusion systems, 299
Heparinless perfusion circuits, 272
Heterologous biologic oxygenators, 17
　canine lung (1955), 21t
HFFIs. See High-frequency flow interrupters (HFFIs)
HFJV. See High-frequency jet ventilation (HFJV)
HFOV. See High-frequency oscillatory ventilation (HFOV)
HFPPV. See High-frequency positive-pressure ventilation (HFPPV)
HFV. See High-frequency ventilation (HFV)
HFV Infant Star ventilator, 71
HIE. See Hypoxic/ischemic encephalopathy (HIE)
High-frequency flow interrupters (HFFIs), 70
　Programmable Volumetric Diffusive Ventilator, 71
High-frequency jet ventilation (HFJV), 70–71

comparison with CMV, randomized prospective study, 73
evaluation in comparison to ECMO, 75
High-frequency oscillatory ventilation (HFOV), 70, 71–72
chronic lung disease following, 75
High-frequency positive-pressure ventilation (HFPPV), 54–55, 70
High-frequency ventilation (HFV), 69–76
HIV. See Human immunodeficiency virus (HIV)
Hollow-fiber membrane oxygenators, 24, 24f, 112
polypropylene heparin-bonded, 291
Homeostasis
cardiorespiratory, 90–91
cross-circulation for maintenance of, 17
Human immunodeficiency virus (HIV), resulting from transfusion during bypass, 244
Humidity
in HFOVs, 71
maintenance for infants on mechanical ventilation, 56
Hummingbird BMO 20N ventilator, 72
Hyaline membrane disease
diagnosis and management of, 65
ECLS for infants with, 275
Hybrid VV/VA bypass, 298
Hydralazine
for control of systemic hypertension in ECMO, 218
to treat hypertension associated with ECMO, 133
Hydrocephalus
following ECMO, 232f
HFOV study finding, 73
Hydroxylation, influence on albumin binding, 114–15, 115f
Hyperalimentation of neonates on ECMO, 198
Hyperbilirubinemia, following ECMO, 235

Hypercapnia
and fetal breathing activity, 325
with hypoxia, effects on the brain, 143–44
Hypercapnic acidosis, sensitivity of cerebral autoregulation to, 139
Hyperemia, following ischemia, 142
Hyperglycemia, and ischemia, 142
Hyperoxia, effects on the brain, 140
Hyperventilation
effects on the neonatal brain, 143
hypocapnia from, 141
with induced alkalosis, 51
lung damage from, 297
for potential ECMO candidates, 242
strategy for neonates, 69
Hypervolemia, management of, 214t
Hypocapnia, from hyperventilation, 141
Hypocapnic alkalosis, following hyperventilation, 143
Hypoglycemia in sick newborn infants, 141–42
Hypotension, associated with ECMO, 133
Hypothermia
for heart surgery, 10
open cardiotomy using (1952–1956), 21t
Hypothermic hemodilution, 24
Hypothesis-testing paradigm versus ranking paradigm, 46
Hypotonia on follow-up after ECMO, 244
Hypoventilation versus ventilation at peak airway pressures, 298
Hypovolemia, management of, 214t
Hypoxemia
as a criterion for ECMO in ARDS patients, 290
refractory, negative-pressure ventilation for, 80
Hypoxia
acute, differential diagnosis

and management of, 219t
at birth, 52
effects on the brain, 139–40
with hypercapnia, effects on the brain, 143–44
sensitivity of cerebral autoregulation to, 139
and thrombocytopenia, 218
Hypoxic hypoxia, 139
Hypoxic/ischemic encephalopathy (HIE), 242

IABP. See Intraortic balloon pump (IABP)
IBM. See International Business Machines Corporation (IBM)
ICH. See Intracranial hemorrhage (ICH)
Idling of blood flow prior to weaning, 204
Iloprost (PGI$_2$), 108
Immobilized biological compounds
for biocompatibility of ECMO circuits, 110–20
for passivation, 106t
Immune reactivity to plasmapheresis equipment, 105–6
Implant, immobilized heparin on, 112
IMV. See Intermittent mandatory ventilation (IMV)
Inadvertent PEEP, 70
Indications
for conventional mechanical ventilation (CMV), 52–53, 53t
for ECCO$_2$R, 291t
See also Criteria
Indirect costs of ECMO, 334
Indwelling vena caval oxygenator, 117
Infection
precautions in ECMO, 196
risk of, in ECMO, 235
Infundibular pulmonary stenosis, outcomes of surgery, thirty-year follow-up, 16, 16t
Inorganic phosphate (Pi) for evaluation of cerebral injury in infants, 149

Inspiratory time, conventional setting, infant ventilator, 54
Inspiratory time with an inspiratory plateau, prolonged, 55
Integrins, 109
Intermittent mandatory ventilation (IMV), 52
 conventional setting, infant ventilator, 53–54
 rate of, 55
Intermittent positive pressure ventilation (IPPV), 288
Intermittent pump operation for a tidal flow system, 268
International Business Machines Corporation (IBM), mechanical pump oxygenator, 18
International ELSO Registry complication reported to, 236–38
 See also ELSO Registry
Intracerebral hemorrhage, protocol for reducing with medical management, 218
Intracranial hemorrhage (ICH)
 and criteria for neonatal ECMO, 158, 160
 management of, 214t, 215
 in neonates on ECMO, 196–97
 and neurodevelopmental prognosis, 146
 in pediatric ECMO, 282
 PET with ^{15}O-labeled water for study of, 150
 risk for, 228
 as a risk of ECMO for neonates, 237
 study of survivors, 242
Intracranial lesions, among ECMO-treated infants, 243
Intraortic balloon pump (IABP), 302–3
Intrapulmonary hemorrhage in pediatric ECMO, 282
Intratracheal pulmonary ventilation (ITPV), 298
Intratracheal ventilation (ITV), 298
Intraventricular hemorrhage (IVH)
 in premature infants, 242
 in surfactant replacement therapy, 78
Inverse ratio ventilation, 68–69
IPPV. See Intermittent positive pressure ventilation (IPPV)
Iron lung (negative-pressure ventilation), 80
Ischemia
 after hypocapnia, 141
 myocardial, differential diagnosis and management of, 219t
 renal, prevention in ECC, 24
 reperfusion injury to tissues, 190
Ischemic myocardial disease, use of an intraortic balloon pump with, 302

Jugular vein
 cannulation of, 180, 180f
 ligation of, and damage to the central nervous system, 228–30

Kallikrein, inhibition by aprotonin, 109–10
Kay-Cross apparatus. See Rotating disc film oxygenator (Kay-Cross apparatus)
Kidneys, ultrasound evaluation of, 218. See also Renal entries
Kolobow Sci-Med membrane oxygenator, 34

Labetalol to treat hypertension associated with ECMO, 133
Laboratory tests
 in clinical management of neonatal patients, 195–96
 following decannulation, 205
Lande-Edwards membrane oxygenator, 34
Lateral asymmetry, follow-up evaluation of, 246–47
Learning curve
 data from the National ECMO Registry, 45
 decrease in patient complications, 236
Lee-White clotting time, comparison between polyalkylsulfone and hydroxylated silicone rubber film, 117
Left ventricular blood flow, response to ECMO, 131, 131f
Left ventricular shortening fraction (LVSF)
 changes after ECMO, 218
 response to ECMO, 130f
Left ventricular systolic wall stress in ECMO, 310
Leg length discrepancies, following femoral vein ligation and cannulation in newborns, 185
Length of hospital stay, ECMO versus non-ECMO patients, 334
Levine rat model, 142
Life support. See Extracorporeal life support (ECLS)
Liquid ventilation, 81
Liver
 changes in function during ECLS, 99
 damage in jugular venous-to-umbilical bypass, 266
 endogenous heparinization in, 120
Logistics of neonatal ECMO centers, 48
Low-frequency positive-pressure ventilation
 with extracorporeal CO_2 removal, 264
 for management of ARDS, 290–91
Lung assist as an emerging concept, 271–72
Lung compliance, 233
 as a criterion for weaning, 204
 studies in neonatal patients, 196
 versus time on ECMO, 202f
Lung function. See Rated flow (lung function)
Lungs
 artificial, 31–32
 effect of congenital diaphrag-

matic hernia on, 253–54
end tidal carbon dioxide as a measure of function, 102
iatrogenic injury to, 288
impairment by prolonged overventilation, 63
management of ARDS, 293
overinflation of, and ARDS, 287
secondary injury to, in neonatal ECMO, 43
See also Pulmonary *entries*
Luxury perfusion syndrome, 142
during cardiopulmonary bypass in adults, 147
LVSF. *See* Left ventricular shortening fraction (LVSF)
Lymphocyte count in infants on bypass, 235

Magnetic resonance imaging (MRI) for evaluation of cerebral injury in infants, 149
Maintenance fluids for neonates on ECMO, 197–98
Management of pediatric ECMO patients, 279–80. *See also* Patient management
Management algorithm for replacement of malfunctioning ECMO equipment, 211f
Mandatory minute volume ventilation, 68
MAP. *See* Mean airway pressure (MAP)
MAS. *See* Meconium aspiration syndrome (MAS)
Maturity, and risk of intracranial abnormalities, 146
Maximum mean flow rates (MMFR), 345
Mayo-Gibbon screen oxygenator, 18, 18f
Mean airway pressure (MAP)
effects on the brain, 145
and oxygen tension, 63

Mechanical circuit
ECMO for cardiac support, 311–12, 312f
See also ECMO system
Mechanical complications
in ECMO, 208–13, 208t
for cardiac support, 315–16
neonatal, 5t
pediatric, 282–83
management of, 209t
Mechanical heart, 15f
Mechanical pump oxygenator, 18
Mechanical ventilation, 52–55, 296–97
adverse effects of, 288
duration, and selection for ECMO, 158
with elevated airway pressures, 287t
initial, of infants with CDH, 255
involvement in ARDS and MOSF, 287
management of infants during, 56–65
prior to ECMO, pediatric patients, 280–81
unconventional use of, 68–69
See also Conventional mechanical ventilation
Meconium aspiration syndrome (MAS), 43, 51
case example, 58–61
data from the National ECMO Registry, 44t
ECMO support for, 43
pre-ECMO x-ray, 200f
prevention of, 335
and risk of complications, 218
survival rates, following ECMO, 4t
Mediastinal tamponade, 313
Medications
effects on the brain, 144–45
introducing into the circuit, 196
Megaesophagus, 234–35
Membrane lung, 169–71
binding of fentanyl to, 199–200
carbon dioxide clearance through, 94, 94f
for ECMO, 3

monitoring of, 102–3
as one of two cardiopulmonary units, 202–3
rated flow through, 100
surface area, rated flow, and patient size, 101t
Membrane oxygenators, 176, 302
versus bubble oxygenators, 23–24
specifications for, 170t
Mental handicaps in PPHN survivors, 243
Meta-analysis of surfactant replacement therapy, 77
Metabolic acidosis, effects on the neonatal brain, 144
Metabolic alkalosis, effects on the brain, 144
Metabolic cascades, following ischemia, 142
Metabolic rate, management of, 102
Microembolization
during ECC, 100
and neurologic complications of cardiopulmonary bypass, 147–48
Microporous oxygenators, film coatings for, 116–17
MMFR. *See* Maximum mean flow rates (MMFR)
M number, 96, 96f, 101, 345
Monitoring methods
in ECLS, 101–2
in ECMO for ARDS, 293–94
Morbidity
in ARDS patients on $ECCO_2R$ and LFPPV, 294–95
in ARF/ARDS, 288–89
in early or late ECMO, and CMV, 48–49, 49t
in ECMO support for infants, 43–44
in infants of less than twenty-eight weeks gestational age, 321
of neonatal ECMO, 47
from postoperative bleeding, 235
Mortality rates
in ARDS, 79, 294–95

in ARF/ARDS, 288–89
eighty percent criterion for selecting ECMO patients, 158–59
HFOV study versus conventional ventilation, 72
prediction of, 45–46
during transport to regional centers, 159
See also Survival rates
MOSF. See Multiorgan system failure (MOSF)
Motor handicaps in PPHN survivors, 243
MRI. See Magnetic resonance imaging (MRI)
MUGA. See Multiple gated acquisition (MUGA) nuclear scan
Multiorgan system failure (MOSF), 287, 288
experimental induction of, 297
Multiple gated acquisition (MUGA) nuclear scan
for evaluation of cardiac function, 314
Muscle relaxants for infants on mechanical ventilation, 56–57
Myocardial ischemia, differential diagnosis and management of, 219t
Myocardial stun during venoarterial bypass, 264. See also Cardiac stun

Narcotic withdrawal for infants on fentanyl, 199
Nasal prong CPAP, 52
case example, 60
Nasotracheal intubation for infants on mechanical ventilation, 56
National Heart, Lung and Blood Institute, adult ECMO trial, 34, 182, 289
National Institutes of Health (NIH)
controlled trial of HFV, 71–72
ECMO evaluation project, 1
ECMO study, Additional Data Collection (ADC) portion, 288–89

HIFI Study Group report on neonatal HFV, 72
prospective randomized study, ECMO, 42
randomized multicenter trial of ECMO, 178–79
National Toxicology Program on DEHP, 118
Native lung function, during VV bypass, 93
Natural lungs, oxygen uptake by, 264
Neck cannulation, ECMO for cardiac support, 307–9
Necrotizing enterocolitis in surfactant replacement therapy, 78
Necrotizing tracheobronchitis (NTB), 73
associated with HFV, 71
Negative-pressure ventilation (NPV), 80–81
Neonatal cannulas, source and types, 348t-49t
Neonatal ECMO, 43
clinical studies, 42–49
patient selection criteria, 2t
randomized studies, 46–47
See also Extracorporeal membrane oxygenation (ECMO)
Neonatal ECMO Registry, 2, 4, 159
data from (1987), 44–46
Neonatal patients
clinical management of, 195–205
pre-ECMO considerations for, 156–73
Neonatal Pulmonary Insufficiency Index (NPII), 43
criterion for ECMO randomized study, 46
Neonatal respiratory failure, 34–36
Neonatal therapy for RDS, 69
Neonatal vascular access, 184–90
Neurodevelopmental outcomes
at age one year, 244, 244t, 245, 245t
correlation with laboratory and imaging measurements, 150
follow-up for ECMO patients, 146
of neonatal ECMO, 241–49

predictors of, 246–48
status of neonates after HFV, 73
See also Clinical outcomes; Outcomes
Neuroimaging, 246
for evaluation of cerebral injury in infants, 148
of intracranial abnormalities in ECMO patients, 146
Neurological examination of neonates on cessation of paralysis, 199
Neurologic damage
as a criterion for ECMO, 161
in neonatal ECMO, 5
Neuromuscular blocking agent, during decannulation, 205
Neuropsychological performance
of adults after cardiopulmonary bypass surgery, 147
specific deficits on follow-up, 248
Neutrophil count in infants on bypass, 235
Neutrophil membrane, C5a receptor site on, 105
NIH. See National Institutes of Health (NIH)
Nitroprusside to treat hypertension associated with ECMO, 133
Nomogram for M number, pressure, and flow relationships, 96
Nonthrombogenic prosthetic surfaces, 338
Normal saline for priming and ECMO circuit, 172
Normothermia, cardiopulmonary bypass at, 13
Nosocomial infection, and prophylactic antibiotics for neonatal patients, 196
NPII. See Neonatal Pulmonary Insufficiency Index (NPII)
NPV. See Negative-pressure ventilation (NPV)
NTB. See Necrotizing tracheobronchitis (NTB)

Nursing care versus sedation, 199
Nutritional support
  of ARDS patients on bypass, 294
  for pediatric patients, 279

Ochsner Medical Institutions, 280
OI. *See* Oxygenation index (OI)
Oliguria
  associated with PPHN, 58
  as a complication of ECMO, 234
  during ECMO, 218
Open heart surgery, 9
  original techniques, 10t
Operating costs, ECMO program, 333–34, 333t
Opiates for pediatric patients, 279
Outcomes
  of ECMO for infants with CDH, 256
  of ECMO for neonates, 4–5, 43–44
  of ECMO for premature infants, 44, 44t
  of heterologous biologic oxygenators, 17
  measurements on open heart surgery patients, 308t
  in PPHN, Babies' Hospital, 64t
  of VA bypass in infants, early study, 42–43
Overventilation, case example, 61–62
Oxygen, cerebral consumption of, 140
Oxygenated blood reservoir, 17–18
Oxygenation
  at birth, 52
  canine lungs for, 17
  DeWall-Lillehei bubble oxygenator, 19–23
  management of decrease in, 203
  with a mechanical pump, 18
  membrane, 1–6
  reservoir of blood for simple intracardiac repairs, 17–18
  rotating disc film oxygenator, 23

  See also Membrane lung
Oxygenation index (OI)
  criterion for imminent mortality, 45
  in hyperventilation, 63
Oxygenators
  deterioration of, 282–83
  failure of, 209–10
Oxygen availability
  and fetal breathing activity, 325
  transfer across silicone rubber membranes, 31–32
Oxygen concentrations
  high inspiratory, underlying condition in ARDS, 287t
  in-line monitoring, in neonatal ECMO, 171–72
  measurement of, 90, 90f
Oxygen consumption, 90
  kinetics of, and tissue respiration, 90–92
Oxygen delivery (Do_2)
  during ECLS, 92–93, 93f
  measurement in CDH, 255
  monitoring in CDH patients on ECMO, 259
  relationship to oxygen consumption, 91, 91f
  systemic, 90–91
  in venovenous ECMO, 263
Oxygen tension
  and mean airway pressure (MAP), 63
  in venovenous ECLS, 93
Oxygen toxicity, ECMO use to avoid, 48
Oxygen uptake in PPHN, 265

Packed red blood cells (PRBCs)
  for transfusion of neonatal patients, 196
  use in priming an ECMO circuit, 172–73
Pancuronium, effects on the brain, 144
Papillary muscle necrosis in PPHN, 263
Partial prothrombin time (PTT), effect of heparin on, 199
Passivation
  blood-system interfaces, 106–10, 106t
  of the ECMO circuit, 120

  summary, 120
  See also Coatings
Passive-filling pump for perfusion, 95
Patent ductus arteriosus (PDA), 134–35
  expected, in ECMO, 221
  and heparin requirement, 199
  management of, 214t
  outcomes of surgery, thirty-year follow-up, 16t
  in the perinatal period, 127
  and shunting patterns in ECMO, 134t
Pathology of ATF, 288
Pathophysiology of ARF/ARDS, 287–88
Patient care for neonates after ECMO, 205
Patient management
  of complications, 214t
  in ECMO, 213–23, 213t
  in ECLS, 102–3
  in ECMO for ARDS patients, 290–94
  protocol in surgery prior to ECMO, 215
Patient selection
  for congenital diaphragmatic hernia, 257–58
  criteria for neonatal ECMO, 2t
  in ECMO studies, 46
Pavulon for paralyzing potential ECMO patients, 242
PCr. *See* Phosphocreatine (PCr)
PDA. *See* Patent ductus arteriosus (PDA)
Peak end-expiratory pressure (PEEP), management in neonates on ECMO, 202
Peak inspiratory pressure (PIP), conventional setting, infant ventilator, 54
Pediatric ECMO, indications for, 275t
Pediatric vascular access, 183–84
PEEP. *See* Peak end-expiratory pressure (PEEP); Positive end-expiratory pressure (PEEP)
PEO. *See* Polyethylene oxide (PEO)

Percent bypass, 203
  and carbon dioxide tension evaluation, 204
Percutaneous cannulation, 179
  of the saphenous vein, 265
  Seldinger technique for, 182
  technique and survival rate, 297
Perfluorochemicals (PFCs) for fluid ventilation, 81–82
Perfusion
  long-term, history of, 1
  support technology, 6
Pericardial tamponade, 220, 221, 313
  differential diagnosis and management of, 219f
Perinatal physiology, study of, 322
Permeability of polyalkylsulfones, 117
Persistent fetal circulation (PFC), ECMO support for, 43
Persistent pulmonary hypertension of the newborn (PPHN), 51, 57–65, 126–27
  association with myocardial dysfunction, 263
  case example, 58–61
  CNS damage in survivors of, 242–43
  ECMO support for, 43
  ECMO versus HFV for treatment of, 73–76
  outcomes, Babies' Hospital (1983–1990), 64
  survival rates, following ECMO, 4t
  treatment with negative-pressure ventilation, 80
pH, and fetal breathing activity, 326t
Phentolamine to treat hypertension associated with ECMO, 133
D-Phenylalanyl-L-prolyl-L-arginyl-chloromethyl ketone (PPACK), 109
Phosphatidyl glycerol in an artificial surfactant, 77
Phosphocreatine (PCr), NMR, for evaluation of cerebral injury in infants, 149
Phospholipids in synthetic surfactants, 77

Physician training, 333
Physiologic considerations
  complications during ECMO, 236t
  flow during perfusion, 13
  in management of ECLS, 100–103
  research on, 320–29
  in venovenous ECMO, 262–71
Physiology
  of extracorporeal life support, 89–103
  perinatal, study of, 322
Pi. See Inorganic phosphate (Pi)
Pierce-GE membrane oxygenator, 34
Piperidine for platelet control, 108–9
Plasma discharge, passivation of polymers with, 116
Plasma leakage, 337
  Carmeda system, 296
  in hollow fiber oxygenators, 292
Plasma proteins, denaturation in early heart-lung machines, 302
Plasmin, inhibition by aprotonin, 109–10
Plasticizers, di(2-ethylhexyl)phthalate (DEHP), 118
Platelet count
  following decannulation, 205
  level desired, 218
  maintenance of, 102
  monitoring of, 102
Platelet fibrin mesh, prevention of growth in perfusion, 98
Platelet granule material, 98
Platelets
  adding, 196
  effect of disintegrins on, 109
  effect of heparin on, 108
  effect of prostaglandins on, 108
  maintaining the level of
    in ARDS patients, 293
    in CDH patients on ECMO, 259
    in neonatal patients, 198
  transfusions of
    and ACT values, 199

in ECMO for cardiac support, 313
in thrombocytopenia, 217
Platelet/white cell emboli, 100
Play-the-winner randomization, 35–36, 46
Plutonium 238 pump for an artificial heart, 25–26, 25f
Pneumocystis carinii, and evaluation of children for ECLS, 275
Pneumonia, underlying ARDS, 287t
Pneumothorax patients, survival rates, following ECMO, 4t
Poiseuille's law, 165, 345
Polyalkylsulfone membranes, oxygenator applications, 117
Polycythemia/hyperviscosity, effects on the brain, 140
Polyether polyurethanes for oxygenator membranes, 118
Polyethylene oxide (PEO)
  films as passivating surfaces, 115–16
  spacer arm for immobilization of heparin, 110–11
Polyhydramnios, survival rate after prenatal diagnosis, 257
Polymer surface treatments, 116–18
  for passivation, 113–16
Polyphosphazenes as biomedical polymers, 117
Polypropylene heparin-bonded hollow fiber oxygenator, 112, 291
Polysaccharides, anticoagulant activity of, 119
Polyurethane conduits, binding of albumin to, 113
Polyvinyl chloride (PVC), toxicity of plasticizers used in, 118
Porcine lung extract in an artificial surfactant, 77
Positive displacement roller pump for neonatal ECMO, 167. See also Roller pump

Positive end-expiratory pressure (PEEP), 179
  conventional setting, infant ventilator, 54
  inadvertent, 70
  and pulmonary problem reduction, 233
  rest setting for, 265
Positive inspiratory pressure (PIP), rest setting for, 265
Positive-pressure ventilation, effects on the neonatal brain, 145
Positron emission tomography (PET)
  for evaluation of carotid artery ligation in neonates, 189
  for evaluation of cerebral injury in infants, 149
Postcardiotomy cardiogenic shock, ECMO in treatment for, 306
Posterior fossa hemorrhages, 231, 232f
Posthypocapnia hyperemia, 143
Postmembrane blood gas levels, 204
Postoperative cardiac ECMO, 314–15
Potassium
  requirement of neonates on ECMO, 198
  serum levels in ECMO, 134
Predictive indicators
  for ARDS patients, 296
  for ECMO, 276
  of neurodevelopmental outcomes, 246–48
Predictive models of complications, 237–38
Predictor study, 316t
  of ECMO support for cardiac patients, 307
Pre-ECMO evaluation, 237
  by the ECMO center, 160–61
Preload, changes in ECMO, 131
Premature infants, outcomes of ECMO support for, 44
Prenatal diagnosis, and survival rate, CDH and polyhydramnios, 257

Preoperative cardiac ECMO, outcomes, 314–15
Preschool testing of ECMO survivors, 245
Pressure
  in an ECLS system, 101
  in an extracorporeal circuit, 95
  monitors for ECMO, 3
Pressure-flow characteristics
  of arterial catheters, 165f
  in vascular access catheters, 96f
Pressure support ventilation, 68
Primary pulmonary failure, pediatric patients, 183
Priming process for a membrane lung, 100
Prognosis for ARDS survivors, 289–90
Program development expenses, 332t
Prolonged inspiratory time with an inspiratory plateau, 55
Prophylactic antibiotics following decannulation, 205
Prospective studies
  of failure of mechanical ventilation (ELSO), 276
  mechanical ventilation versus CMV plus bypass support, 1
  for neonatal use of HFV, 72–73
  randomized
    of ECLS in newborn respiratory failure, 340
    of ECMO in ARF, 289
  See also Evaluations
Prospective risks versus retrospectively evaluated risks, 3
Prostacyclin (PGI$_2$), inhibition of platelet aggregation by, 108
Prostaglandin E$_1$
  inhibition of platelet aggregation by, 108
  for PPHN with hypoxia under ventilation, 58
Protein C, 107f
  role in coagulation, 108
Protein denaturation in early heart-lung machines, 31

Protein metabolism, during ECLS, 99
Psychosocial issues
  in ECMO for neonates, 248
  psychological support for pediatric patients, 280
PTT. See Partial prothrombin time (PTT)
Pulmonary arterial pressure
  correction for pump flow rates, 132–33
  versus ECMO flow rate, 134f
  hypertension, 306
  systolic, in infants on ECMO, 132–33, 132f
Pulmonary barotrauma in tidal volume ventilation, 264
Pulmonary blood flow in VA and in VV bypass, 264
Pulmonary compliance. See Lung compliance
Pulmonary edema
  in autogenous lung oxygenation, 13
  from persistent left-to-right shunt in newborns, 221
Pulmonary embolism as impetus for development of ECC, 31
Pulmonary failure
  primary, in pediatric patients, 183
  summary data for patients with ECMO, 280–81t
Pulmonary function
  criteria for ECMO versus CMV, 49t
  and criteria for neonatal ECMO, 160
  impairment from massive transfusion, 313
  loss on VV bypass, 265
  management of neonatal patients on ECMO, 200–202
  problems in, 233–34
Pulmonary function testing (PFT), 72–73
Pulmonary hemorrhage as an exclusionary criterion for ECMO, 158
Pulmonary hypertension
  in ECMO survivors, 256
  in neonatal respiratory failure, 35

Pulmonary hypoplasia, 253
  in infants with CDH, 258
Pulmonary opacification, 233
  following ECMO, 200, 201f, 202
Pulmonary stenosis, 16t
Pulmonary therapy for pediatric patients, 279–80
Pulmonary vascular resistance (PVR)
  lowering with alkalosis, 63
  in PPHN, 127
Pulmonary vasodilation in a newborn, 127
Pulmonary vasomotor tone in congenital diaphragmatic hernia, 254
Pulmonary vasoreactive crisis, 306
Pulsatile flow
  versus continuous flow, 26
  during VV perfusion, 264
Pulse contour in venoarterial bypass, 96
Pulse pressure in venoarterial bypass, 96
Pumps
  for cardiac support in ECMO, 312–13
  comparison of types, for tidal flow venovenous bypass, 268–69
  design for ECC, 24–25
  failure of, 210, 282
  flow rates, correction of pulmonary artery pressure for, 132–33
  management of malfunction, 212–13, 212f
Purkinje cells of the neocortex, vulnerability to ischemic injury, 142
P-VAT. *See* Visual attention task (P-VAT)
PVC. *See* Polyvinyl chloride (PVC)
PVR. *See* Pulmonary vascular resistance (PVR)
Pyramidal cells of the hippocampus, vulnerability to ischemic injury, 142

Raceway tubing
  selection and maintenance of, 163–65
  specifications, 277

Radiograph to confirm congenital diaphragmatic hernia, 255
Radiographic score versus time on ECMO, 202f
Radioisotope studies for evaluation of carotid artery ligation in neonates, 189
Randomized prospective studies
  double-blind, of surface treatments for pacemaker insulators, 113–14
  of extracorporeal membrane oxygenation, 178–79
  of infants with respiratory distress syndrome, 73
  of neonatal ECMO, 46–47
  play-the-winner technique, 35–36
Ranking paradigm versus hypothesis-testing paradigm, 46
Rated flow (lung function), 92, 92f
RDS. *See* Respiratory distress syndrome (RDS)
Recirculation flow
  in double-lumen cannula systems, 269, 271
  in venovenous ECMO, 263
Recombinant DNA technology as a source of protein for surfactants, 78
Reconstruction
  carotid artery, 189–90, 309
  of the femoral artery, 278
  of the femoral vein, 278
Red blood cell count, effect of prolonged ECC on, 99
Regional centers
  need study, 331
  for neonatal ECMO, 48
  utilization processes, 159–61
Registered respiratory therapists, 332
Reherniation, congenital diaphragmatic hernia patient, 196, 197f
Reinfusion pressure, risks associated with increases in, 267
Renal failure
  in ARDS patients, 294

  during ECMO, 221
  management of, 214t
Renal function
  during ECLS, 99
  effect on ACT values, 199
  problems in, 234
  and pulsatile flow, 264
Renal insufficiency
  in pediatric ECMO, 283
  predictors of, 237
Renal ischemia, prevention of, in ECC, 24
Renin
  elevated production in neonatal patients, 198
  levels in infants on bypass, 234
Reperfusion injury, 190
  cardiac stun as, 233
Reptilase test for fibrinogen, 199
Respiration, control of, 321–22
Respiratory acidosis, and mortality rate, 159
Respiratory alkalosis, from carbon dioxide removal from blood, 94
Respiratory distress syndrome (RDS), 51
  data from the National ECMO Registry (1987), 44t
  ECMO support for, 43
  intracranial hemorrhage risk in, 215
  inverse ratio ventilation for, 69
  potential avoidance with HFOV, 72
  and probability of intracranial hemorrhage, 237
  randomized prospective study of infants with, 73
  survival rates, following ECMO, 4t
Respiratory drive, carbon dioxide for maintaining after weaning from ECMO, 205
Respiratory failure
  alternative therapies for, 68–82
  classification scheme (Morel), 290

comparison of HFOV and ECMO, 74
differential diagnosis and management of, 219t
Geneva scoring system for, 291t
neonatal, 34–36
routine evaluation of neonates for ECLS, 275
Respiratory Severity Index (RSI), 276
Respiratory support, venovenous bypass for, 338
Results
ECMO for cardiac support, 314–17
of randomized study of ECMO, 42
See also Outcomes
Retinal vascular changes, following ECMO, 231
Retinopathy of prematurity (ROP), 248
Retrospective studies
of OI as a predictor of mortality, 46
for setting selection criteria, 157
of ventilation in neonates, 276
See also Evaluations
Reversible lung disease, and selection for ECMO, 158
"Re-white-out", following membrane lung change, 233
RGD. See Arginine-glycine-aspartic acid (RGD) sequence
Rhone Poulenc pump, 95
Right-handedness, frequency of, in high-risk populations, 247
Right heart assist cannulation, 304f
Right ventricle, fetal versus older child, 126
Right ventricular failure in older children, 129
Risk-producing procedures in ECMO, 157
Risks
balance with benefits, ECMO for neonates, 2–3
of infection, 235

of intracranial hemorrhage, 198–99, 215–16
in neonatal ECMO, 5, 5t, 226–38
Rockefeller Institute, 302
Roller pump
for neonatal ECMO, 167
for perfusion, 95
servoregulation of, 32
ROP. See Retinopathy of prematurity (ROP)
Rotating disc film oxygenator (Kay-Cross apparatus), 23
Routine care for neonatal ECMO patients, 195
RSI. See Respiratory Severity Index (RSI)
Rygg bubble oxygenator, 23

Safety of ECMO support for infants, 43–44
Saphenous bulb, femoral vein cannulation via, 181, 181f
Sci-Med Life Systems. See Avecor Cardiovascular Inc.
Sechrist IV-100B ventilator, 53
Sedation
effects on the brain, 144
of neonates on ECMO, 199–200
for pediatric patients, 279
Seizures
during ECMO, 237
management of, 214t
Seldinger technique
for drainage catheter placement, 215
for drainage tube placement, 221
for percutaneous cannulation, 182
Self-regulating pump in a tidal flow system, 268–69
SensorMedics 3100 ventilator, 72
Sepsis
data from the National ECMO Registry, 44t
differential diagnosis and management of, 219t
ECLS for children with, 274–75
and oxygen consumption, 90

and probability of seizures during ECMO, 237
and risk of complications, 218
safety and efficacy studies of ECMO in, 43
and selection for ECMO, 158
survival rates, following ECMO, 4t
in venovenous bypass, 294
Serine proteases, inhibition to block coagulation, 109–10
Servoregulators
with a bladder box, 277
in the ECMO system, 168
for prolonged perfusion with a roller pump, 95
See also Autoregulation
Shear-induced release of TPA, 119
Shock, acute respiratory failure associated with, 286
Sigmamotor pump, 20f
Silicone membrane lungs, 170, 291
Silicone membrane oxygenator
carbon dioxide clearance in, 94
for pediatric patients, 277, 277t
Silicone rubber
albumin binding to modified, 114
coating for microporous membranes, 116–17
heparin immobilized to, 110–11
for membrane dialyzers, 31
passivation with an interpenetrating network of PEO, 115–16
Single-cannula systems for venovenous bypass, 266
Single-lumen tidal flow system, 266–69, 269f
SK. See Streptokinase (SK)
SMA. See Surface-modifying additives (SMA)
Social learning disability, and right hemisphere deficits, 248
Sodium bicarbonate to correct metabolic acidosis in neonates, 144

Solvent polishing, 118
SP-A. *See* Surfactant protein A (SP-A)
Spacer arm attachment for immobilized biologicals, 110
Space requirements for an ECMO program, 333
Spastic diplegia in preterm ECMO-treated neonates, 244
Spiral coil membrane lung, 100
Staffing
  for $ECCO_2R$, 294
  per infant requirement for ECMO, 332t
Starling forces, rearrangement of, and pulmonary problems, 233
St. Louis University study, ECMO for cardiac support, 317
"Streaming" oxygen measurement, 209
Streptokinase (SK), immobilized on nylon film, 113
Stroke
  in the newborn, 230
  risk in carotid artery ligation, 278
Stunned myocardium after ECMO, 218. *See also* Cardiac stun
Suctioning for infants on mechanical ventilation, 56
Sulfonated polymers, heparin mimicking, 117–18
Super-Tygon tubing, successful use of, 282
Surface immobilization, 110–20
  of heparin, 111f
Surface-modifying additives (SMA) for polymers, 117f
Surface treatment for passivation, 106t
Surfactant apoprotein levels of infants on ECMO, 202
Surfactant protein A (SP-A) in ECMO patients, 79
  levels, versus time on ECMO, 202f
Surfactant replacement therapy, 76–80
Surfactant-TA. *See* Survanta (Surfactant-TA)

Surfactant therapy for acute respiratory distress syndrome (ARDS), 79–80
Surgery
  ECMO as a bridge to, 306
  for prolonged PDA, 221
Surgical procedures
  and complications of subsequent ECMO, 215
  cutdown technique, advantages and disadvantages of, 180
  for infants with CDH, and ECMO support, 258–59
  See also Cannulation; Reconstruction
Survanta (Surfactant-TA) in an artificial surfactant, 77
Survival rates
  of ARDS patients, long-term, 295t
  and diagnoses, venovenous ECLS, 352–53
  of ECMO patients, 334
  of infants with CDH, 256
  of neonatal ECMO patients, 4t, 207
  of pediatric ECMO patients, 276, 283t
  See also Mortality rates
Synchronized intermittent mandatory ventilation, 68
Synthetic heparin, 117–18
Synthetic surfactants, 76
Systemic alkalosis, treatment for potential ECMO patients, 242
Systemic blood pressure, maintenance of, 102
Systemic hypertension, 234
  during ECMO, 133
Systolic hypertension as a side-effect of ECMO, 218

TAH. *See* Total artificial heart (TAH)
Tension hemothorax, 220–21, 220f
  differential diagnosis and management of, 219t
Tension pneumothorax, 220–21, 220f
  differential diagnosis and management of, 219t

Tetralogy of Fallot
  ECLS for pulmonary failure after repair of, 183
  outcomes of surgery, thirty-year follow-up, 16, 16t
  repair using ECMO, 305
  surgery using azygos flow and bubble oxygenator, 19, 21
Thrombin time (TT), effect of heparin on, 199
Thrombocytopenia
  in ECC, 33
  heparin-induced, 108
  management of, 214t
  as a patient complication of ECMO, 217
  routine management of in neonates on ECMO, 218
Thromboresistant surfaces, 182
Thrombosis
  pressure as an indicator of, 101
  at a prosthetic surface, 98–99
Thromboxane B_2, changes during bypass, 227, 227f
Tidal flow systems, 101
  comparison of, 268–69
Tidal volume (TV)
  determinant of tidal flow VV bypass performance, 267
  in HFV, 69
  Programmable Volumetric Diffusive Ventilator, 71
Tidal volume ventilation, pulmonary barotrauma in, 264
Tissue plasminogen activator (TPA), 107f, 113
  hemodynamic control to induce release of, 119
Tolazoline
  effect on oxygenation, 64
  for PPHN with hypoxia under ventilation, 57–58
Total anomalous pulmonary venous drainage, comparison with PPHN, 127–28
Total aortic blood flow, response to ECMO, 131, 131f
Total artificial heart (TAH), 25–26, 25t

Toxic fume inhalation, underlying condition in ARDS, 287t
Toxicity
  of bulk additives to polymers, 118
  of chemicals leached from foreign surfaces, 227
  from early heart-lung machine functioning, 31
TPA. See Tissue plasminogen activator (TPA)
Tracheal insufflation of oxygen, 68
Training
  cost of manuals for, 333
  of an ECMO technical specialist, 208
  lead time for, 332
Transcutaneous oximetry, 101–2
Transcutaneous oxygen tension, tracings, 61
  for infants with MAS and PPHN, 60f
  for infants on mechanical ventilation, 57
  for infants with PPHN, 59
Transitional circulation of a newborn, 127
Transplantation
  ECC during surgery, 25
  ECMO as a bridge to, 306
Transport of ECMO candidates, 160
"Trial off" prior to weaning, 204
Trials. See Evaluations
Tricuspid insufficiency, during transitional circulation, 127
TT. See Thrombin time (TT)
Tubing
  pack design, 162–63, 162f
  rupture of, 210
  specifications, for pediatric patients, 277, 277t
TV. See Tidal volume (TV)
Two-cannulas system for venovenous perfusion, 265–66, 266f
Two-dimensional echocardiography, 314
Tyloxapol in an artificial surfactant, 76

Ultrasound, evaluation of kidney function, 218
University of Chicago, 280
University of Minnesota, Department of Surgery, 9
University of Pittsburgh, ECMO for cardiac support, 317
Upper airway obstruction in ECMO patients, 233–34
Urine output as a predictor of cardiac output, 307
Urokinase (UK), immobilized on polymers, 112

VA bypass. See Venoarterial bypass (VA bypass)
Valium for infants, 199
Valvular heart disease, open cardiotomy in acquired condition, 25
Variety Club of the Northwest, 9
Vascular access for ECLS, 175–91
Vascular resistance, changes in a neonate, 127
Vasoactive substances
  effects on the brain of drugs, 144–45
  release due to blood-surface interactions, 233
  release on blood-surface interaction, 227
Vasodilators, carbon dioxide, 140
Vasopressin for gastrointestinal bleeding, 215
VCFS. See Velocity of circumferential fiber shortening (VCFS)
VCSF. See Contractility (VCSF)
Velocity of circumferential fiber shortening (VCFS), 128–29, 128f
Vena caval oxygenator, indwelling, 117
Venoarterial bypass (VA bypass), 89, 176, 176f, 181–82, 228
  cannulas for, pediatric, 184t
  for cardiac support, 338
  conversion from VV bypass, 268
  hemodynamic problems, 294
  high-flow, 179f
  hybrid with VV bypass, 298
  neonatal, 184–85
    for ECMO, 42–43
  for pediatric patients, 183–84
  for respiratory support, 338
  single cannula via the internal jugular, 185
  versus venovenous bypass, 98t
    in newborns, 185
  via axillary arteries, 176–77, 177f
  via femoral vessels, 176–77, 177f
Venoarterial cannulation, 305f
  via iliac or cervical vessels, 184, 184f
Venoarterial ECMO
  with a pulmonary artery spring catheter, 310f
  versus venovenous ECMO, 263t
Venous catheter, protection against suction to, 95
Venous oxygen saturation versus arterial oxygen saturation, 91
Venous reconstruction of the femoral vein, 278
Venous reservoir (bladder), 169
Venous return, decreased, management of, 219
Venous return monitor (VRM), 168–69
Venous saturation
  evaluation of values from monitors, 203
  monitoring of, 101–2, 101f
Venovenous bypass (VV bypass), conversion to VA perfusion, 265
Venovenous ECMO, 262–72
  cannulation for, 304f
  for cardiac support in children, 303
  conversion to venoarterial ECMO, 351
  for neonates, 351–53
  in PPHN, 128–29
  for premature infants with respiratory failure, 43
  versus venoarterial ECMO, 263t, 352

Venovenous extracorporeal gas exchange, 38–39
Venovenous-venoarterial bypass, 178, 178f
Venovenous (VV) access, blood flow requirement with, 100
Venovenous (VV) bypass, 89, 180–81
  effect on hemodynamics, 97
  oxygen delivery in, 92–93
Ventilation. *See* Conventional mechanical ventilation (CMV); Mechanical ventilation
Ventilators
  continuing research in strategies for using, 82
  conventional technique, 54t
  settings of, 53–55
    survivors versus nonsurvivors of ECMO, 159t
  types of, 53, 69–70
Ventilatory index, and selection for ECMO, 257
Ventricular septal defect (VSD)
  cross-circulation utilization perfusion, 14–15, 15f
  mortality for, 307
  outcomes of surgery, thirty-year follow-up, 16, 16t
Ventricular stroke volumes, during ECMO, 131f
Viral pneumonia, ECLS for infants with, 275
Virchow's triad, 106
Visual attention task (P-VAT), performance on, and later Bayley scores, 246
Vocal cord paralysis, 234–35
Volume expansion, effects on the neonatal brain, 145
Von Willebrand factor, promotion of platelet adhesion by, 113
VRM. *See* Venous return monitor (VRM)
VSD. *See* Ventricular septal defect (VSD)
VV bypass. *See* Venovenous bypass (VV bypass)

Wall shear rate, effect on anticoagulant potency of bound heparin, 112
Wall stress, and VCFS, 128f
Washington University, ECMO for cardiac support, 317
Weaning
  from ECMO, 204–5
    for cardiac support, 313–14
    failure of, 222f
  from fentanyl, 205
  from an infant ventilator, 55
  from a membrane lung, 103
Wet lung syndrome, 73
White blood cell count
  change on institution of bypass, 235
  during extracorporeal circulation, 99
"White-out" lung, 200, 201f, 202

Xenon 133 clearance for evaluation of cerebral blood flow in infants, 150
Xenotransplantation, 25
X-rays
  meconium aspiration, pre-ECMO, 200f
  verification of catheter placement in neonatal patients, 196

RJ 312 .E95 1993

Extracorporeal life support

NO LONGER THE PROPERTY
OF THE
UNIVERSITY OF R.I. LIBRARY